Breast MRI Interpretation

Text and Online Case Analysis for Screening and Diagnosis

Gillian M. Newstead, MD, FACR
Director of Global Breast Imaging
Former Professor of Radiology
Department of Radiology
University of Chicago
Chicago, Illinois, USA

3479 illustrations

Thieme
New York • Stuttgart • Delhi • Rio de Janeiro

Library of Congress Cataloging-in-Publication Data is available from the publisher.

Important note: Medicine is an ever-changing science undergoing continual development. Research and clinical experience are continually expanding our knowledge, in particular our knowledge of proper treatment and drug therapy. Insofar as this book mentions any dosage or application, readers may rest assured that the authors, editors, and publishers have made every effort to ensure that such references are in accordance with **the state of knowledge at the time of production of the book.**

Nevertheless, this does not involve, imply, or express any guarantee or responsibility on the part of the publishers in respect to any dosage instructions and forms of applications stated in the book. **Every user is requested to examine carefully** the manufacturers' leaflets accompanying each drug and to check, if necessary in consultation with a physician or specialist, whether the dosage schedules mentioned therein or the contraindications stated by the manufacturers differ from the statements made in the present book. Such examination is particularly important with drugs that are either rarely used or have been newly released on the market. Every dosage schedule or every form of application used is entirely at the user's own risk and responsibility. The authors and publishers request every user to report to the publishers any discrepancies or inaccuracies noticed. If errors in this work are found after publication, errata will be posted at www.thieme.com on the product description page.

Some of the product names, patents, and registered designs referred to in this book are in fact registered trademarks or proprietary names even though specific reference to this fact is not always made in the text. Therefore, the appearance of a name without designation as proprietary is not to be construed as a representation by the publisher that it is in the public domain.

Thieme Medical Publishers, Inc.
333 Seventh Avenue, 18th Floor
New York, NY 10001, USA
www.thieme.com
+1 800 782 3488, customerservice@thieme.com

Cover design: Thieme Publishing Group
Typesetting by Thomson Digital, India

Printed in USA by King Printing Company, Inc.   5 4 3 2 1

ISBN 978-1-62623-467-3

Also available as an e-book:
eISBN 978-1-62623-468-0

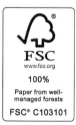

FSC
www.fsc.org
100%
Paper from well-managed forests
FSC® C103101

This book is dedicated to my husband, Bob, for his unwavering help and support; my daughters, Caroline and Jennifer; my son-in-law, Alex; my grandchildren, Kosey, Henry, and Charlotte, who have brought so much joy to my life; and also most importantly, to the patients, who over many years have taught me so much.

Contents

Foreword

In early 1990s, having witnessed the power of MRI to revolutionize assessment of a rapidly expanding list of ailments throughout the body, I became interested in exploring the use of MRI for diagnosing breast cancer. However, my expertise was in MRI, not breast cancer. Fortunately, one of my colleagues, Gillian Newstead, was not only a leading authority on imaging breast cancer, she was also passionate about it, and she had a firm grasp on the benefits and limitations of extant modalities. More importantly, she had a curiosity and an open mind about a potentially transformative role for MRI. Together with Jerry Waisman, a pathologist, we set out to learn and to teach each other about our respective disciplines.

After years of a successful collaboration, I eventually moved on to other areas of endeavor, but Gillian kept plugging away on breast MRI, and she has continued to make important contributions well into the 21st century. Amongst these are her enormous contributions to education. This text is a testament to her innovative and long-standing commitment to education and to advancing the appropriate use of MRI for breast cancer diagnosis.

Jeffrey C. Weinreb, MD, FACR, FISMRM, FSCBT/MR
Professor of Radiology and Biomedical Imaging
Yale School of Medicine
New Haven, Connecticut, USA

Preface

Knowledge of breast magnetic resonance imaging is now an essential requirement for all of us in medicine who screen women for breast cancer and take care of patients with a cancer diagnosis. This is not a new technology. There have been major advances in MRI technique since the mid-1980s when technical breakthroughs first promised a new method for cancer detection. These new advances were made possible primarily by the development of breast surface coils, fast gradient-echo imaging sequences with small flip angles, and use of paramagnetic contrast agents. In subsequent years in Germany, Sylvia Heywang and Wilfried Kaiser pioneered the clinical development and implementation of breast MRI. My involvement with this technique began in 1991 at New York University under the mentorship of Jeffrey Weinreb and since then, rapid expansion of the use of breast MRI throughout most radiology practices has taken place. Further development and application of new and improved hardware and software has led to routine clinical use. This has provided radiologists with excellent spatial and temporal resolution images allowing improved detection and diagnosis. MRI has been shown to be superior to all other imaging methods for detection of both non-invasive and invasive cancer, and will increasingly become the most important imaging method for cancer screening and for the management and follow-up of women with a new cancer diagnosis.

The purpose of this book is to provide practical information for all colleagues involved in the acquisition and interpretation of breast MRI images. I believe that in many ways we have shied away from this technique by making our task too complicated, and we need to simplify routine studies for optimum clinical utility and cost effectiveness. Streamlining of breast protocols based on proven reliable DCE-MRI technology should allow completion of a screening examination in 10 minutes or less and a diagnostic examination in 20 minutes or less with excellent results. In routine practice, concentration on achieving one simple screening series and one standard diagnostic series with optimal technique, rather than chasing the tail of exotic new sequences, is preferable. MR imaging protocols in clinical practice are often long and repetitious, taking 40 minutes or even up to one hour in length in some instances. Learning how to maximize image quality and how to simplify and shorten imaging protocols by stripping down to only the essential series will greatly improve workflow and diagnostic results. The images shown in this book were all acquired at the University of Chicago and almost all at high field strength (3.0T). The images were obtained in the axial plane with identical screening and diagnostic protocols used throughout the book to allow for consistent viewing of all cases and all lesions shown. In the forthcoming chapters, viewing of acquired images for each given case will not only show one single selected image, but additional side-by-side images at different time points and acquisition parameters, in three dimensions. Such a standardized interpretation method using simple workstation tools will help to improve diagnostic performance. In addition to the selected images shown in this book, key cases will be stored in the cloud allowing the reader to access and review the full datasets. Indications for breast MRI will be divided into screening and diagnostic sections with specific protocols for each. Additionally, the image acquisition and image interpretation chapters will focus separately on screening and diagnostic MRI. This distinction will be of increased importance in the next few years as we move into the future with expansion of breast MRI for screening, using shorter, abbreviated MRI acquisitions.

Finally, we are in a period of rapid flux in breast imaging. Technical innovation in the fields of machine learning, biomarkers, and genetic fingerprinting will increasingly guide practice in the next few years. The last section of the book will review advanced acquisition techniques and explore future applications of breast MRI including the possibility of non-contrast imaging, quantitative dynamic imaging, and artificial intelligence using advanced computer analytic methods. Expansion and growth of our specialty from screening and diagnosis to prediction and prognostication will prove to be challenging for all of us, but we must be up to the task—the future is now.

Gillian M. Newstead, MD, FACR

Acknowledgments

No woman is an island. None of us works alone, especially in the diagnosis and treatment of breast cancer. The team approach is probably best epitomized in the management of patients in the breast screening, diagnostic, and therapy domains. I have been privileged to work at the University of Chicago with many gifted physicians and scientists, both researchers and clinicians. I offer special thanks to my colleagues who have prepared their excellent contributions to this book: Hiroyuki Abe, Maryellen L. Giger, Gregory S. Karczmar, Frederico D. Pineda, Milica Medved, Michael Middleton, and Naoko Mori. I have also been helped and supported by many colleagues who deserve particular mention and gratitude: breast radiologists David V. Schacht, Kirti M. Kulkarni, Deepa Sheth, Robert A. Schmidt, and the late Charlene Sennett. Other leading medical colleagues have greatly informed and supported our work in breast imaging: surgeons Nora Jaskowiak and Asha Chhablani; pathologists Jerry Waisman, Hussain Sattar, and Jeffrey Mueller; and medical oncologists Samuel Hellman, Olufunmilayo Olopade, and Gini Fleming.

This book would not have been possible without the support of the many dedicated technologists, nurses, and research staff who have helped patients on a daily basis and contributed mightily toward maintenance of a successful breast imaging practice thus providing all of the high-quality images in this volume.

I would be remiss if I do not recognize certain other colleagues who have collaborated and inspired me along the way: Michael Linver, Ellen Mendelson, Hildegard Toth, Ulrich Bick, Christiane Kuhl, Christopher Comstock, and last, but by no means least, Laszlo Tabar who taught me the fundamentals of breast imaging and breast pathology, which formed the foundation of my work in breast MRI.

I also wish to acknowledge Carole Segal and the Segal Family Foundation for strong support of breast imaging research at the University of Chicago. Carole recognized over 15 years ago the importance of advanced breast imaging with MRI and has supported numerous breast imaging and breast pathology research fellows. She has been instrumental in helping to develop an imaging database, coordinating multiple grant proposals, and has served as an advocate on several of our NIH grants. We owe her enormous gratitude, and I am forever indebted to her.

Special mention is also due to the excellent editorial staff at Thieme for their courtesy, competence, and valuable assistance, with a special thanks to my editors Mary Wilson and Sarah Landis.

Gillian M. Newstead, MD, FACR

Contributors

Hiroyuki Abe, MD, PhD
Professor of Radiology
Department of Radiology
Breast Imaging
University of Chicago
Chicago, Illinois, USA

Maryellen Giger, PhD
A.N. Protzker Professor of Radiology
The Committee on Medical Physics
The College Vice-Chair for Basic Science Research
Department of Radiology
University of Chicago
Chicago, Illinois, USA

Gregory Karczmar, PhD
Professor of Radiology
Committee on Medical Physics and the College
University of Chicago
Chicago, Illinois, USA

Milica Medved, PhD
Associate Professor of Radiology
Department of Radiology
University of Chicago
Chicago, Illinois, USA

Michael S. Middleton, MD, PhD
Project Scientist
Department of Radiology
University of California, San Diego
La Jolla, California, USA

Naoko Mori, MD
Department of Diagnostic Radiology
Tohoku University
Tohokudai
Sendai, Miyagi, Japan

Gillian M. Newstead, MD, FACR
Director of Global Breast Imaging
Former Professor of Radiology
Department of Radiology
University of Chicago
Chicago, Illinois, USA

Frederico D. Pineda, PhD
Department of Radiology
University of Chicago
Chicago, Illinois, USA

1 Breast MRI: Overview

Gillian M. Newstead

Abstract

The first chapter provides a general overview of the clinical applications and diagnostic utility of breast MRI and the need for specific individual technical protocols for both screening and diagnostic indications. The shortcomings of mammographic screening, particularly for those women at high risk or with dense breasts at mammography, have led to increased use of an abbreviated MRI sequence for breast screening. MRI standards, protocols and practice guidelines for screening are reviewed and discussed. MRI is a functional imaging technique and there is growing interest in establishing functional breast imaging methods using dynamic contrast-enhanced MRI (DCE-MRI) with kinetic analyses for classification of tumor biology and correlation with genomic markers. MRI is well suited for this type of analysis, identifying features that may reflect underlying malignant potential, providing an imaging biomarker that could play a key role in the development of precision medical therapy and personalized cancer care.

The diagnostic applications of breast MRI require a standard full protocol and may need additional advanced sequences according to the clinical indication for each individual patient. Indications for diagnostic MRI include assessment of disease extent at the time of initial cancer diagnosis, postoperative evaluation of residual disease following cancer excision, identification of recurrent tumor and monitoring of women undergoing cancer treatment with neoadjuvant chemotherapy. Other applications discussed in this chapter include problem-solving for difficult clinical or imaging findings, nipple discharge, implant assessment and use of MR-Guided biopsy.

Keywords: clinical applications breast MRI, MRI screening techniques, clinical utilization of breast MRI screening, practice guidelines for breast MRI, diagnostic MRI applications, known cancer MRI applications, MRI as a problem-solving tool, MR-Guided therapy, MR imaging biomarker

1.1 Introduction

Breast imaging has played an important role in the rapid development and change in breast cancer management over the past decades, not only by the introduction of new technical tools to aid in cancer detection and improve diagnosis, but also by the use of these tools to provide diagnostic information necessary to guide therapy. Over past years, the role of the radiologist has greatly changed; supervision of breast cancer screening programs using multimodal techniques and increased participation in multidisciplinary conferences have resulted in improved care for women diagnosed with breast cancer. When an abnormality is detected at screening, or when a patient is referred with clinical symptoms, the radiologist performs a diagnostic evaluation, discusses the pertinent findings with the patient and her family, and is usually the first physician to decide if a biopsy is necessary based on imaging findings. The whole gamut of interventional procedures, using stereotactic, ultrasound, or magnetic resonance imaging (MRI) guidance, provide accurate and timely diagnoses of nonpalpable image–detected lesions, with the additional advantage of limited patient morbidity when compared to surgical excision. When a malignant or uncertain finding is diagnosed, the radiologist will communicate the biopsy results with the patient and, in many instances, guide her to treating physicians for further management. New imaging techniques have benefitted patients, not only by allowing detection of an increased number of small cancers, but also by providing important diagnostic information essential for treatment, the goal being to provide optimal treatment for each individual cancer patient.

Mammography has been the tried-and-true breast imaging method for many decades, providing over 80% sensitivity for breast cancer detection in postmenopausal women and even greater sensitivity in the symptomatic population, when combined with breast ultrasound.[1] It would be logical therefore to ask why another imaging modality such as breast MRI is needed. It is well recognized that the sensitivity of mammography is substantially lower in the dense breast, less than 50% even when full-field digital mammography (FFDM) is used, as shown in the Digital Mammographic Imaging Screening Trial (DMIST).[2] Mammography suffers from inherent limitation of image contrast; many suspect lesions are therefore indeterminate and require further imaging evaluation and biopsy. Other important shortcomings of mammographic screening include recognized observer limitations as well as a propensity for detection of lesions with less aggressive histology, which may result in underdiagnosis of biologically aggressive disease. The failure to detect some high-grade breast cancers with mammography is driven largely by the degree of breast tissue density, but also by the very nature of rapidly growing, biologically relevant cancers that exhibit imaging features that are indistinguishable from normal breast tissue. Failure to diagnose these cancers at mammographic screening will result in progression of disease and diagnosis of advanced-stage interval cancers. Breast ultrasound is now commonly used for screening, and although this technique will identify some additional mammographically occult cancers, identification of ductal carcinoma in situ (DCIS) is challenging, and ultrasound suffers from low specificity in the screening setting.[3,4] Breast cancer continues to represent a major cause of cancer death in women; therefore, continued search for improved breast cancer screening methods is needed.

Against this background of mammography and ultrasound imaging, breast MR technology has improved steadily over the last three decades in large part due to research collaboration between radiologists, technologists, physicists, and industry scientists. Continued focus on research and educational efforts aimed toward improving diagnosis and patient care have resulted in increased use of breast MRI as a valued clinical resource for women's health care. The main driver for the increasing adoption of breast MRI in clinical practice is its extremely high sensitivity, approaching 100% for cancer detection. Multiple studies have shown that standard dynamic contrast-enhanced MRI (DCE-MRI) for breast imaging achieves the highest sensitivity of any imaging modality, identifying cancer regardless of radiographic breast density, stage (DCIS or invasive), tumor type, or postsurgical changes.[5,6,7,8] Criticisms of low specificity in the early years of breast MRI might be expected with such a sensitive modality, but with current techniques and protocols, the specificity and positive predictive value (PPV) for malignancy can exceed that of breast ultrasound and mammography. Recognition of the salient MRI features of benign and malignant disease, and the specific morphologic and kinetic characteristics associated with various malignant subtypes, allows radiologists to provide important diagnostic information that can guide therapy. DCE-MRI protocols at both 1.5 and 3.0 Tesla provide excellent spatial resolution and accurate analysis of lesion morphology. Dedicated software providing semiquantitative analysis of lesion kinetics and display of its internal enhancement characteristics can improve diagnostic specificity. Measures of the initial rise and delayed phase of contrast enhancement within lesions are displayed as standard signal-intensity-versus-time-intensity curves (TICs). These computer-aided, semiquantitative, kinetic analysis tools have the advantage of being relatively simple to implement into routine practice and are widely used in the United States.

1.2 Breast MRI as a Biomarker

Traditionally, breast cancer treatment was determined by two major factors: (1) tumor histology, assessed by classifications based on grade and morphology such as ductal, lobular, mucinous tubular etc., and (2) the TNM staging method, based on cancer size, nodal status, and presence or absence of distant metastases. During the last 10 years or so, molecular subtyping of breast cancer has assumed a more important role in treatment planning and cancer classification has moved beyond the basic histologic assessment of prior years, to encompass treatment stratification based on tumor biology and gene expression profiles. There is a growing interest in establishing functional breast imaging methods, using DCE-MRI and its kinetic and morphologic analyses, for classification of tumor biology and correlation with genomic markers. MRI is a functional imaging technique and is well suited for this type of analysis. If MRI is to fulfill this role, the semiquantitative MRI methods used in current practice that document change in signal intensity over time will not be sufficient, and protocols that provide quantitative measurements of concentration of contrast media in tissues will be needed. Quantitative kinetic analysis depends on intrinsic lesion characteristics, acquisition parameters, and concentration, all of which play a role in signal enhancement. This type of analysis is necessary if we want to move beyond the binary choice, "is the lesion in question benign or malignant?" to ask whether a detected tumor has features that may reflect underlying biology and play a key role in precision medicine and personalized cancer care.

There is thus a need for further development of quantitative MRI biomarkers for prediction and prognosis. The goal of an imaging biomarker is to improve risk stratification, provide the right treatment for the right patient at the right time, reduce the variability in interpretation, and avoid trial and error in treatment. Quantitative imaging methods, however, face a key challenge because of the current lack of image standardization. Further development of acquisition standards that are reproducible and measures of signal analysis that are quantitative and

widely available are required. Why are imaging biomarkers important? MRI is able to sample the entire cancer, and quantitative measures display tumor heterogeneity, providing serial noninvasive image data that are complementary to in vitro assay. Clinical trials that monitor drug action during treatment rely on quantitative standardized MRI results. The topic of image standardization and quantitative measures of enhancement will be discussed in detail in Chapter 12.

1.3 Clinical Utilization of Breast MRI in the United States

Overall use of breast MRI has increased over the past decade with 445,434 contrast-enhanced breast MR procedures performed in the United States in 2014. Although the number of breast imaging facilities declined by nearly 7% from 2002 to 2011, facility accreditation has increased. A modest expansion of breast MRI studies is expected in the next few years, driven partly by an increasing number of new breast density notification laws that have resulted in additional supplemental screening procedures for women with dense breasts. These laws have created a growing demand for new technologies that improve diagnostic accuracy.[9]

An observational study reported in 2014 collected MRI and mammography data from 8,931 breast MRI examinations in women aged 18 to 79 years, during a time period of 2005 to 2009.[10] Data were acquired from five national Breast Cancer Surveillance Consortium registries. The overall rate of breast MRI nearly tripled from 2005 to 2009 from 4.2 to 11.5 examinations per 1,000 women, with the most rapid increase from 2005 to 2007 ($p = 0.02$). The list of MR studies by indication for the examination showed that the most common clinical indication was diagnostic evaluation (40.3%), followed by screening (31.7%). Women who underwent screening breast MRI, when compared with women who received mammography alone, were more likely to be younger than 50 years, white non-Hispanic, and nulliparous. Women in the MRI screening group were more likely to have a personal history of breast cancer, a family history of breast cancer, and extremely dense breast tissue (all $p < 0.001$). The proportion of women screened using breast MRI at high lifetime risk for breast cancer (> 20%) increased during the study period from 9% in 2005 to 29% in 2009. The authors concluded that the use of breast MRI for screening in high-risk women is increasing and that there is a need to improve appropriate use, by including more women at high risk who may benefit from screening breast MRI.

Another paper looked at overall rates of breast MRI use, by clinical indication and average annual percent changes, in a retrospective cohort study at a not-for-profit health plan and multispecialty group medical practice in New England.[11] The study enrolled 10,518 women aged 20 years and older in the health plan for at least 1 year. Each woman had at least one breast MRI between January 1, 2000, and December 31, 2011, and breast MRI counts were obtained from claims data. The results showed that breast MRI use increased more than 20-fold from 6.5/1,000 women in 2000 to 130.7/10,000 in 2009, and use then declined and stabilized to 104.8/10,000 by 2011. A published commentary on these two studies by Hwang and Bedrosian noted that in the Wernli study,[10] fewer than 5% of the women at greater than 20% risk were actually screened, indicating that screening with MRI was overused in women who did not meet screening guidelines, while underused in those who could benefit the most.[12]

A study of diagnostic MRI, recently reported among 10,766 older women, compared the frequency and sequencing of breast imaging and biopsy use for the diagnostic and preoperative work-up of women with newly diagnosed breast cancer. SEER-Medicare data from 2004 to 2010 were used and results indicated that 20% of women underwent MRI in the diagnostic/preoperative period, 60% received a mammogram and ultrasound, and 20% a mammogram alone. MRI use increased across study years, tripling from 2005 to 2009 (9–29%). Interestingly, among women receiving preoperative MRI, 26% underwent a subsequent biopsy compared with 51% receiving a subsequent biopsy in the subgroup without MRI.[13]

1.4 Practice Guidelines

The American College of Radiology (ACR) Practice guidelines recommend benefits of breast MRI targeted to select patient populations. These recommendations include screening studies for early cancer detection to improve survival, and diagnostic studies for evaluation of extent of disease, better diagnosis for improved treatment planning, and improved prediction for early assessment of response to therapy. It is apparent from published data that both for screening and diagnostic indications, a large variability in recommendations and utilization for breast MRI studies exists, despite existing clear guidelines regarding the use of MRI for screening and for clinical management of patients with breast cancer. This problem is clearly evident in the variability in use of diagnostic MRI for preoperative work-up of women with a new cancer. These discrepancies in recommendations for MRI exist not only in older women but in young women as well. There is a need to increase standardization of referrals to optimize clinical management and care for all women.[14]

The need for improved screening methods for women at average to intermediate risk has come into focus in recent years, due to the passage of breast density legislation in over half of the U.S. states, requiring that women be informed about the possible benefit of additional screening methods. Historically, the main barriers to MRI use have included limited availability, high costs, long examination times, and limited exposure of the benefits of MRI to the medical community and to patients. In an ideal world, cancer screening should be accurate, inexpensive, and widely available; however, many radiologists use lengthy breast MRI protocols lasting 30 minutes or more and costs are high in the United States. Counseling of high-risk women at the time of a recommendation for MR screening is beneficial, and many cities today have genetic counseling clinics for this purpose. Referring physicians and radiologists may also use a risk assessment model for patient guidance.

ACR guidelines recommend MRI screening for high-risk women at a greater than 20% lifetime risk of breast cancer starting at age 30. MRI is the best method for detection of early node-negative breast cancer, and many clinical trials conducted in the United States and Europe showed significantly improved cancer detection in high-risk women, finding small cancers that

were occult on clinical, mammographic, and ultrasound examinations (▶ Fig. 1.1).[5,7,15,16,17,18,19,20,21,22] In the United States, 28 (56%) states have already passed breast density legislation and the number is growing. State laws now require that women be informed if their breasts prove to be heterogeneously or extremely dense at mammography suggesting that supplemental breast cancer screening could be considered. Given that approximately 50% of women younger than 50 years and 33% of women older than 50 have dense breasts at imaging, the need for improved screening methods is clearly needed.

1.5 Screening MRI

As use of breast MRI has matured, there is now evidence to suggest that the indication for breast MRI will dictate the type of MR protocol to be used. Just as many years ago mammography services were divided into a screening or a diagnostic indication, this same distinction could now be applied to MRI examinations. An abbreviated screening examination could be used for cancer detection in asymptomatic women, and a full standard diagnostic study could be used for other indications such as the evaluation of a clinical problem when conventional imaging is uncertain and assessment of disease extent in patients with newly diagnosed breast cancer. Radiologists could therefore develop and implement dedicated acquisition protocols for screening and diagnosis, and create new patient and imaging workflow.

I think it is fair to say that the basic MRI acquisition protocols for breast imaging have not changed greatly over the last two decades although hardware and software improvements have led to greatly improved image quality over time. Most clinical breast MR practices today do not distinguish between screening and diagnostic indications. In general, a screening study could consist of an abbreviated acquisition protocol performed within a time limit of 3 to 10 minutes, and a basic diagnostic acquisition within 15 to 20 minutes. Screening MRI studies must be efficient and affordable with short imaging time. Designated magnet availability and well-organized patient workflow can deliver short screening studies at a lower financial cost. It is possible that, in the future, dedicated breast MR systems optimized on a scale for population-based screening will be developed and used extensively in breast practices for screening. Dr Kuhl and colleagues have successfully pioneered an early proof-of-concept study involving interpretations of an abbreviated breast MRI protocol (AB-MR) and have shown equivalent sensitivity for cancer detection in women at mild and moderate risk when compared to a full standard breast MRI.[23] Other early studies involving interpretations of an AB-MR protocol have demonstrated equivalent sensitivity for cancer detection when compared to a full standard MRI, with only minimal decrease in specificity.[24,25,26,27,28] Further research on the outcome of screening results using an abbreviated protocol is needed.

1.5.1 Technical Considerations

Standard Protocols

As we look at the key technical components of any breast MRI protocol, abbreviated or standard, it is clear that an excellent T1-weighted (T1w) dynamic series with injection of a gadolinium-based contrast agent is essential for cancer detection.

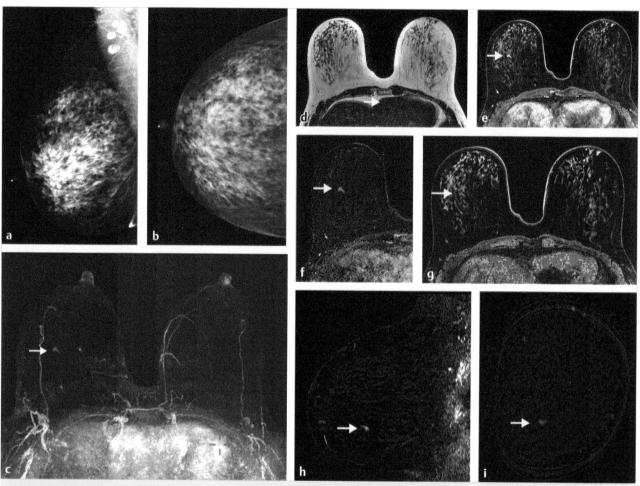

Fig. 1.1 Screening MRI: Asymptomatic woman age 57 years with a personal history of left breast DCIS, treated with BCS in 2004. RT breast screening mammogram MLO and CC views show extremely dense breast tissue, but no suspicious finding. **(a, b)** The MIP image demonstrates a small enhancing focus with irregular morphology **(c)**. Although axial T2-weighted image **(d)** shows no abnormal finding, the corresponding T1-weighted contrast-enhanced images show a focal area of NME, 9 × 8 × 6 mm, visible on the source 140 s postcontrast series **(e)**, subtracted series angiomap **(f)**, persistent enhancement **(g)**, and on the sagittal and reformatted coronal images in subtraction mode **(h, i,** *arrows*). MR-guided biopsy yielded DCIS solid type, high-grade, ER (+) PR (–).

These contrast agents act by reducing the T1 in the microenvironment, increasing the signal in a T1w acquisition, so that regions or lesions with increased blood flow and permeability accumulate contrast media to a greater extent than the surrounding tissue, resulting in higher signal increase. The technical details outlined in the Breast Magnetic Resonance Imaging Accreditation Program sponsored by the ACR require both a T2w sequence and a multiphase T1w series. The dynamic series must include a precontrast T1w series, an early phase (first) postcontrast T1w series to be completed within 4 minutes of contrast injection, and a late phase T1w series with features matching the precontrast T1w series.[29] Measures of the rate of uptake and washout of contrast media within breast lesions have been shown to contain diagnostically useful information and the shape of the TIC is widely used in the classification of enhancing lesions.[30]

Screening Protocols

The ACR Accreditation Program does not provide a specific protocol for screening indications. With this in mind, an AB-MR screening protocol could be constructed by shortening the dynamic component of a diagnostic examination to 2 to 3 minutes, acquiring data in the initial phase of enhancement only. An AB-MR study should fulfill the following requirements: standardized contrast administration based on kilogram weight using a power injector, total scan time of shorter than 10 minutes (including localizer), one pre- and one or two postcontrast gradient echo (GRE) fat-suppressed T1w axial acquisitions, with in-plane resolution of 1 mm or less, slice thickness of 3 mm of less. Addition of an axial T2w sequence with in-plane resolution matching the GRE sequences and 3 mm or less slice thickness is useful for improved specificity. The T1w dynamic sequence in diagnostic protocols would remain the same, and the traditional acquisition of dynamic data for 5 to 7 minutes following contrast injection and acquisition of DCE data in both the initial and delayed phase, as specified in the ACR Accreditation Program, would remain.

In the near term, however, a new focus on adaptation and modification of the basic DCE T1w sequence has yielded promising results. Implementation of a short sequence for screening, using an abbreviated dynamic sequence (AB-MR), and use of ultrafast perfusion imaging in the initial dynamic phase are both relatively new methods, adapted for screening, and have already begun to be implemented in some radiology practices. A new ECOG/ACRIN trial "Comparison of Abbreviated Breast MRI and Digital Breast Tomosynthesis in Breast Cancer Screening in Women with Dense Breasts (EA1141)" opened in October 2016, and patient recruitment is now completed for the initial round. Details of the protocols used for screening and diagnostic indications will be provided in ensuing chapters.

1.6 Diagnostic MRI: Clinical Applications

Diagnostic applications of breast MRI will be discussed below and include assessment of disease extent at time of initial cancer diagnosis, postoperative evaluation of residual disease following cancer resection, identification of recurrent tumor, and monitoring of women undergoing cancer treatment with neoadjuvant chemotherapy. Other applications include problem solving for difficult clinical or imaging findings, nipple discharge, implant assessment, and use of MR-guided biopsy.[14] High-quality images are essential for accurate diagnoses of breast disease. This goal is challenging in MRI because all current breast protocols require DCE-MRI sequences, accurate contrast administration, and optimal standard acquisitions. Sensitivity for cancer detection is already very high, and various new innovative acquisition protocols, such as diffusion-weighted imaging (DWI) and fat suppression methods using short TI inversion recovery (STIR) and high spectral and spatial resolution (HiSS) imaging, raise the future possibility of improved diagnostic specificity and cancer detection, without the use of contrast agents. These advanced imaging techniques will be discussed further in Chapter 11.

1.6.1 Preoperative Breast MRI

Can preoperative breast MRI help reduce reoperation rates by providing careful mapping of disease extent? It has been shown in many studies that the use of multimodality imaging, including mammography, ultrasound, and especially MRI along with the additional use of percutaneous biopsy techniques, can produce a precise map of the extent and localization of breast disease for surgical guidance. Although no large studies have proved a survival advantage with use of preoperative MRI and questions remain as to reduction of re-excision and recurrence rates, the potential benefit of preoperative MRI is valuable. MRI can identify foci of invasive disease with greater sensitivity than other imaging methods allowing precise identification of multicentric and multifocal, invasive and noninvasive disease that would otherwise go undetected. (▶ Fig. 1.2). Identification of additional foci of cancer may lead to a more extensive lumpectomy than originally planned, or even to mastectomy. Surgeons need to know if there is any malignant nipple involvement because if tumor is present, resection of the nipple–areola complex is usually needed. MR can identify DCIS lesions exhibiting linear enhancement extending into the subareolar region close to the nipple, which are occult at mammography (▶ Fig. 1.3).

MRI may also demonstrate axillary and internal mammary lymphadenopathy and chest wall invasion, which can affect surgical and radiotherapy management. Historically, some treating physicians have acted on MRI findings and altered surgical plans without prior histologic confirmation. Optimal patient care in most of these cases requires tissue sampling before definitive treatment, when additional disease identified on MRI is located beyond the location of the known malignancy.

Complete assessment of the tumor burden requires measurement of not only the size of the tumor component(s), but also the full volume of the extent of disease, both invasive and in situ. Multifocal disease may consist of in situ cancer only, multiple invasive cancers with intervening normal tissue, or multiple invasive cancers associated with an in situ component (▶ Fig. 1.4). Accurate tumor measurements are important for surgical and oncologic therapy planning; they are necessary not only at time of initial presentation, but also for monitoring during subsequent chemotherapeutic treatments. Two large studies that carefully examined newly diagnosed breast cancers with serial tumor sectioning at pathology found the majority of tumors to be multifocal (66 and 63%) with tumor foci extending beyond the known index cancer.[31,32] It is evident that tumor multifocality identified at MRI cannot be accurately assessed by a single maximum diameter measurement of the cancer in most cases. Newer computer-generated volume and surface area calculations reflect a more accurate estimate of tumor burden. Radiologists can facilitate removal of all malignant tissue and provide surgical guidance, by using image-guided biopsy methods with clip placement to identify additional disease prior to surgical excision. Translation of imaging data to the surgical environment, however, may be challenging, and although knowledge of the true extent of cancer is an important requisite for successful surgery, the literature is varied as to whether identification of additional ipsilateral or contralateral occult malignancy is beneficial.

1.6.2 Postlumpectomy with Positive Margins

Breast-conserving therapy with partial mastectomy is one of the most commonly performed cancer operations in the United States and estimates indicate that 60 to 75% of breast cancer cases undergo partial mastectomy as the initial treatment.[33] The challenge for breast imagers, surgeons, oncologists, and pathologists is to adopt evidence-based strategies that aim to conserve the breast if possible, minimize reoperations, and maintain good cosmesis. In any given case, the extent of surgery for tumor removal may range from a simple gross excision to a wide lumpectomy or quadrantectomy.

Ideally, all cancer should be removed at the time of initial surgical excision and failure to achieve appropriate pathological margins at initial operation usually necessitates additional surgery.[34,35,36,37] The appropriate treatment for patients with close histologic margins at tumor excision is not yet completely established, and an extensive literature, mostly retrospective, shows wide variation in definitions of surgical technique, specimen processing, and outcome reporting of acceptable margin status. Definitions such as "no tumor within 1, 2, 5, or 10 mm of the margin" are still used in clinical practice; however, in a recent paper, the Society of Surgical Oncology—American Society for Radiation Oncology guideline defines "no tumor on ink"

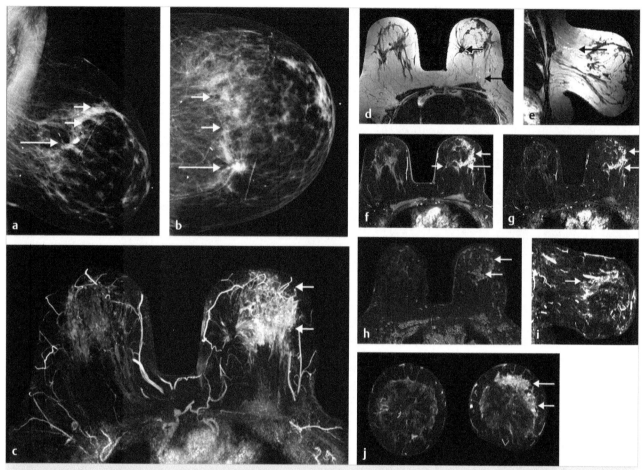

Fig. 1.2 Diagnostic MRI: Age 64 years, referred for "thickening" in the lateral left breast. History of left BCS in 2004 for low-grade DCIS. Left MLO and CC mammographic views (**a, b**) show distortion and calcification at site of prior lumpectomy (*long arrows*), and developing asymmetry in the superior left breast (*short arrows*). MIP image shows diffuse nonmass enhancement in the left breast. (**c**) T2-weighted axial image demonstrates distortion and a small postsurgical seroma in the medial left breast (*short arrows*) and linear fluid extending posteriorly from the mid to the posterior breast, (distended lymphatic vessels), also seen to advantage in the sagittal reconstructed image (**d, e,** *long arrow*). T1-weighted correlative postcontrast 120-second image shows distortion at the prior surgical site (*short arrows*) and diffuse nonmass enhancement in the anterolateral breast, shown to advantage on both the source and the subtracted correlative image (**f, g,** *long arrow*). Angiomap shows mostly persistent enhancement (**h**). The sagittal and coronal reconstructed images (**i, j**) provide three-dimensional visualization of tumor extent. Histology at mastectomy yielded diffuse invasive and noninvasive ductal cancer grade 2. Micropapillary DCIS extended for 9 cm, with scattered foci of ILC and pleomorphic LCIS.

as an adequate margin.[38] Factors contributing to positive surgical margins include the size and location of the primary tumor, and the presence of an extensive intraductal component (EIC) within an invasive ductal carcinoma (IDC).[31,39,40,41] It is generally accepted that the presence of microscopically positive margins necessitates re-excision surgery in order to decrease the risk of local recurrence.[42,43,44,45,46]

Reoperation Rates

There are large variations in reoperation rates following cancer excision among surgeons and institutions, and reoperation rates have been shown to be high in the United States.[47,48] Current estimates of the frequency of surgical re-excisions range from 30 to 60%,[42,43,44,45] and the burdens of reoperation are considerable, with increased patient morbidity and costs. Additional operations may delay the use of recommended adjuvant therapy and cause psychological, physical, and economic stress

for patients, especially when more extensive surgery such as mastectomy is required. Once re-excision surgery is performed, a review of the literature indicates that the frequency of tumor in second surgical excision specimens ranges from 32 to 63%, microscopic residual disease being found in only about 50% of patients overall.[40,41] Residual tumor has been shown to be associated with an increasing risk of recurrent cancer in the ipsilateral breast, for both invasive and noninvasive cancer, with some investigators showing increased local recurrence rates,[49,50] whereas others have indicated no increase in recurrence rates.[51,52,53]

Today, even with declining reoperation rates, too many women still end up back in the operating room after a partial mastectomy. A recent editorial in the *New England Journal of Medicine* stressed that the rate of reoperation can and should be reduced, and the authors further point out that even a reduction of 10% in the re-excision rate nationwide could result in reoperation being avoided for 10,000 to 20,000 women

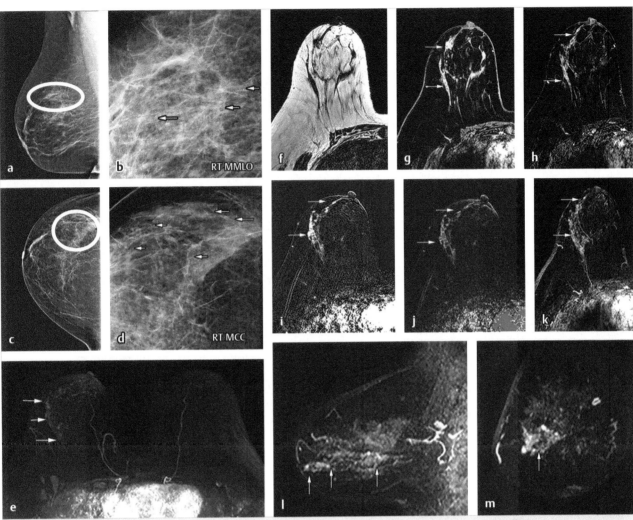

Fig. 1.3 Diagnostic MRI: Asymptomatic 48-year-old woman underwent screening mammography. Grouped pleomorphic calcifications were identified in the superolateral aspect of the right breast in a segmental distribution. **(a–d)** Stereotactic biopsy yielded low and intermediate-grade DCIS. MRI for assessment of disease extent demonstrates extensive segmental nonmass enhancement in the right breast on the MIP image **(e)**, corresponding to the distribution of the mammographic calcifications. T2-weighted image of the right breast shows no significant finding. **(f)** However, T1-weighted postcontrast source and subtracted images at 120 seconds show nonmass enhancement extending anteriorly to the base of the nipple **(g–i)**, with a persistent enhancement pattern seen on the angiomap **(j)**. Creation of thin MIP images and multiplanar reformatting allow visualization of the disease extent in three dimensions **(k–m)**. This type of image reconstruction is very helpful for display of nonmass enhancement. Simple mastectomy yielded cribriform, papillary, and micropapillary DCIS, 7 cm in extent, with calcification, necrosis, and extension into subareolar ducts. Two foci of microinvasion were identified, and sampled axillary lymph nodes were negative for cancer.

annually.[54] The variability in reoperation rates among surgeons and institutions speaks to the important need for professional societies to provide guidelines and further education for surgeons and their trainees.

Diagnosis of Residual Disease

Clinical examination of the breast after tumor resection is usually limited because of focal thickening, pain, and swelling at the surgical site. Patient discomfort, breast edema, postoperative inflammatory changes, and postsurgical hematoma and seroma fluid collections all may limit the value of mammographic and ultrasound studies in the immediate postoperative period.[55,56] Mammography, however, using minimal

compression, may detect residual malignant microcalcifications, which may prove useful in guiding re-resection in certain cases.[57] MRI is the primary imaging modality for this task. Findings suspicious for residual tumor include irregular thickening of the seroma wall and adjacent mass or nonmass enhancement (▶ Fig. 1.5). MRI is very sensitive to the detection of residual disease, despite normal postoperative changes that may limit the positive predictive value and specificity of residual cancer detection in some cases. Limiting factors include contrast enhancement caused by postsurgical inflammatory changes and fat necrosis.[58,59] Although the overlapping features of postsurgical changes and malignant lesions remain as limitations, DCE-MRI has proved to be a useful tool for identification and guidance of residual disease.[60,61]

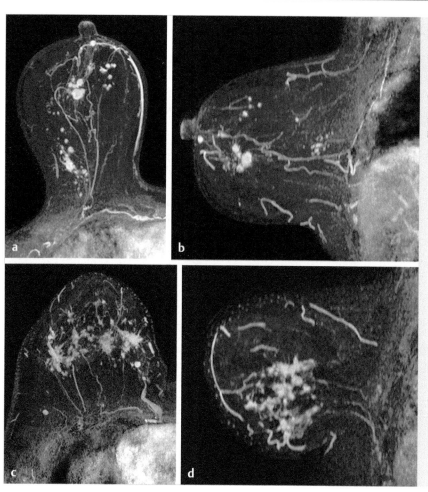

Fig. 1.4 Diagnostic MRI: Use of multiplanar reconstruction and slab or thin MIP technique is very helpful for demonstrating disease extent. Using this technique, two examples of the main patterns of multifocal/multicentric and diffuse disease are shown; multiple invasive cancers presenting as masses of various sizes with intervening normal tissue (**a, b**), and diffuse invasive lobular carcinoma (**c, d**).

1.6.3 Assessment of Neoadjuvant Chemotherapy Treatment

Neoadjuvant chemotherapy treatment (NACT) before surgery for local regional control is the standard recommended treatment for locally advanced breast carcinoma (stage III B and C). NACT is widely used prior to surgery for invasive cancer, the goal being to improve overall survival by eradication of micrometastases with the additional potential benefit of tumor volume reduction during treatment that might allow for more conservative surgery. Large, long-term clinical trials (NSABP 18 and 27)[62] have shown no statistically significant difference in relapse-free and overall survival between adjuvant and neoadjuvant treatment groups, although a trend toward an increased benefit in women younger than 50 years of age was shown in the NACT group. Patients with stage II and IIIA disease may also receive a benefit because of an increased likelihood of successful breast conservation as a result of a decrease in the size of the index lesion following NACT.[63] Favorable long-term outcomes are associated not only with a decrease in the index tumor size as evidenced on imaging during NACT, but also with successful treatment of axillary lymphadenopathy. Change in tumor size has been shown to be a clinically useful measure of tumor response and is predictive of patient survival.

MRI is the most accurate imaging method for monitoring treatment response during therapy and for assessment of the extent of residual disease at the end of therapy, prior to surgical treatment. In vivo monitoring with MRI is noninvasive and allows physicians to test the effects of treatment and to change the treatment in case of nonresponse. MRI studies are generally repeated three times: a pretreatment study serving as a baseline examination for comparison with posttreatment studies, a second study after one or two treatments, and a third study after the final treatment before surgery. Response to treatment is based on accurate pre- and posttreatment documentation of any decrease or increase in overall tumor size and volume, compared to the pretreatment MRI. There is variability in the imaging appearance of tumors as they respond to treatment. Invasive cancers presenting as masses on MRI often exhibit concentric shrinkage, are easier to measure, and accord good histologic and imaging concordance after therapy (▶ Fig. 1.6). Other invasive cancers, presenting initially as multifocal lesions or as nonmass enhancement, may exhibit an overall volume decrease with heterogeneous tumor regression following therapy, but without a significant change in maximum tumor diameter (▶ Fig. 1.7). Assessment of tumor volumes and surface areas using computerized analytical software can provide more accurate comparison measures than traditional linear measure of maximum tumor diameter.[63,64] MRI documentation of treatment response is traditionally recorded as follows. Absence of any enhancement at the site of the prior index lesion(s) is recorded as a complete response (CR). Reduction in the index

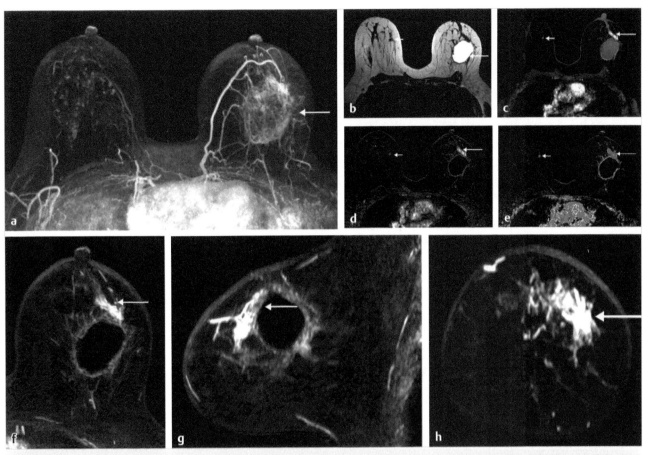

Fig. 1.5 Diagnostic MRI: A 44-year-old woman underwent BCS for newly diagnosed left breast IDC grade 2 with associated high-grade DCIS, lumpectomy histology yielding an inferior surgical margin positive for invasive carcinoma. No preoperative MRI was done. MIP image from the postoperative MRI shows a postoperative seroma cavity in the left breast extending from 12 to 2 o'clock position measuring 49 × 38 mm **(a)**. T2-weighted images show the seroma cavity **(b)**. T1-weighted postcontrast images demonstrate irregular nonmass enhancement with persistent late-phase kinetics adjacent to the anterior, inferomedial, and inferolateral margin of the seroma cavity **(c–e)**, suggesting postsurgical residual cancer (*arrows*). Note the benign focus in the medial right breast **(c–e**, *short arrow*). Thin MIP axial image **(f)**, reformatted in the sagittal and coronal plane **(g, h)**, shows to advantage the location and extent of the residual disease (*arrows*). Re-excision lumpectomy histology yielded residual IDC, grade 3 with associated ductal carcinoma in situ, high nuclear grade, solid and micropapillary types, and two microscopic foci of invasive carcinoma (largest 5 mm). Specimen margins were free of tumor.

cancer size by greater than 30% is recorded as a partial response (PR). Decrease in the size of the index cancer less than 30% is recorded as no response (NR). MR studies performed after the first cycle of chemotherapy often provide the best opportunity for the radiologist to assess early tumor response. In the event that a tumor shows no response or even progression of disease on imaging after the first treatment, modifications to the treatment protocol can be considered, thus sparing the patient from prolonged and ineffective chemotherapy.

1.6.4 Breast Cancer Recurrence

The main goal of breast conservation is local control. The 10-year rates of local recurrence after breast-conserving surgery (BCS) are already quite low, 6% among patients with node-negative disease[65] and 9% among those with node-positive disease.[66] Furthermore, modern adjuvant therapy for breast cancer has improved so much that it has become very challenging to show an improvement in outcomes as evidenced by local recurrence rates. As previously discussed, current surgical practice

mandates that no tumor be present on inked specimen margins at BCS, and re-excision surgery to achieve "no tumor on inked margins" is frequently employed. Furthermore, many patients receive adjunctive systemic chemotherapy and/or long-term antihormonal treatment. Therefore, current advances in treatment of breast cancer are unlikely to reduce recurrence rates much further.

Breast MRI is the preferred method for detection of a recurrent or new malignancy among women who have been treated for breast cancer and is useful when clinical or other imaging studies are suspicious or inconclusive for diagnosis of recurrence. Tumor may be identified either in the native treated breast or in the autologous reconstructed breast following mastectomy. Women with a personal history of breast cancer are at high risk for additional cancer in the ipsilateral or contralateral breast, and increasingly, many of these women undergo MRI screening annually.[67] The breast treated with BCS, radiation therapy, and chemotherapy exhibits a variable decrease in background parenchymal enhancement (BPE) when compared with the contralateral, nontreated breast. This finding may be

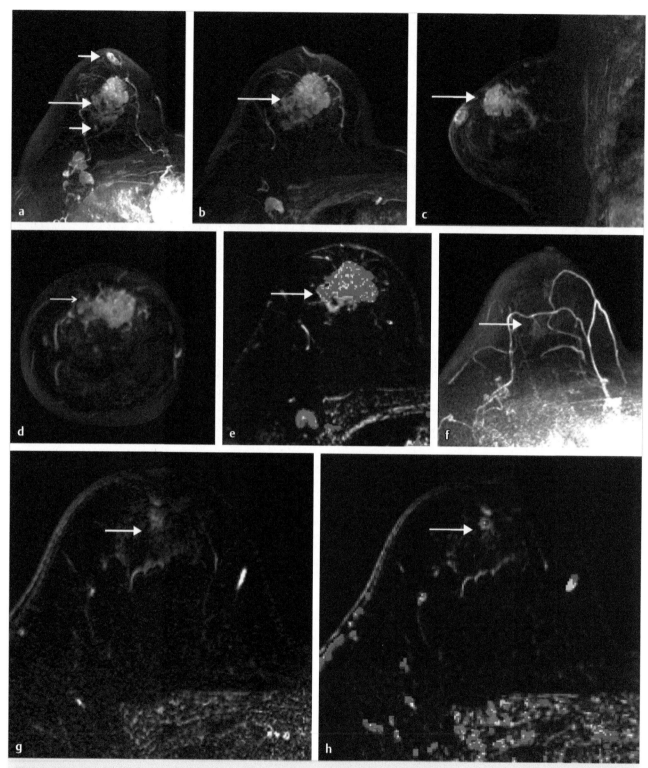

Fig. 1.6 Diagnostic MRI: Age 45 with a right breast palpable mass, biopsy yielding IDC with lobular features grade 2, ER/PR(+), HER-2/neu(−). MR images, before and after neoadjuvant chemotherapy treatment, are shown. The index mass lesion measures 2.6 cm (*long arrow*) with satellite lesions (*short arrow*) and enlarged axillary lymph nodes with skin thickening, skin enhancement, and axillary adenopathy (**a**). Multiplanar reformatting allows accurate pretreatment measurements (**b–d**). Angiomap axial image identifies heterogeneous enhancement with washout kinetics (**e**). Posttreatment, presurgery MRI shows concentric shrinkage of the index mass with minimal residual enhancement on the MIP image (**f**), decrease in size of axillary nodes, and absent skin enhancement (**g, h**). Final histology at mastectomy found minimal residual scattered foci of IDC and four positive axillary nodes (4/33).

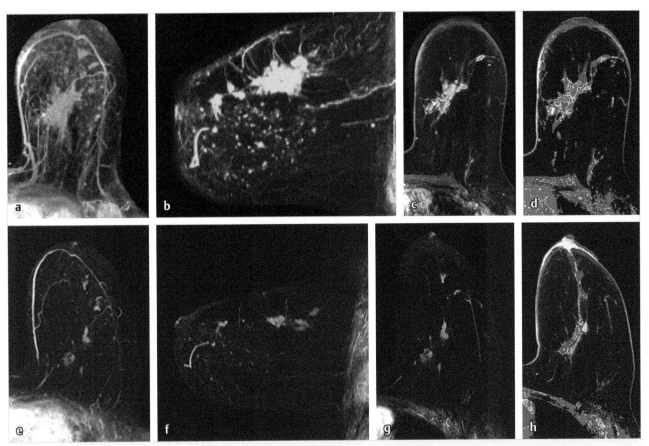

Fig. 1.7 Diagnostic MRI: A 48-year-old woman presented with a left breast palpable mass, biopsy yielding IDC grade 3, ER/PR(−) Her2/neu (FISH)(+), Ki-67: 25%. MRI imaging before neoadjuvant chemotherapy identified on MIP images, an irregular, extensive nonmass enhancement extending from the posterior breast to the nipple, in the axial plane **(a)** and the sagittal plane **(b)**. Axial T1-weighted postcontrast (70 seconds) image demonstrates heterogeneous enhancement with skin thickening and skin enhancement **(c)** and heterogeneous internal enhancement with washout kinetics **(d)**. MRI following completion of chemotherapy and before surgery found decreased tumor volume on the T1-weighted postcontrast MIP images, in the axial plane **(e)** and the sagittal plane **(f)** without any overall change in the maximum diameter measurement. Correlative postcontrast (120 seconds) axial image **(g)** and angiomap **(h)** show decrease in lesion signal intensity due to treatment effect. Histology at mastectomy identified multiple foci of IDC grade 3, the largest focus was 1.1 cm in size, scattered throughout the tumor bed, associated with high-grade DCIS, solid with necrosis. Tumor involved the nipple–areola complex and the axillary lymph nodes were negative for carcinoma.

particularly conspicuous in younger women, and usually persists on subsequent MRI examinations (► Fig. 1.8). Li et al[68] reviewed MRI findings in patients who had undergone BCS with radiation therapy. In their study, they found not only a decrease in BPE in the treated breast, reflecting a decrease in vascularity due to radiation therapy, but also a lesser effect in the untreated breast, suggesting an additional systemic effect from endocrine therapy or chemotherapy.

Normal postoperative MRI findings include postradiation edema, skin and parenchymal enhancement, and rim-enhancing seromata at the surgical site, which may remain visible for many months. Benign focal or postsurgical scar enhancement, with or without architectural distortion, is often present at the lumpectomy site in the immediate postoperative period; however, in some cases such changes may be minimal. Postoperative findings usually peak at 3 months after therapy, decrease by 6 months, and completely resolve within 12 to 18 months. Enhancement may remain at the surgical site for several years in some cases signifying the presence of fat necrosis. Recurrent tumor is generally easily identified in the setting of diminished

BPE, as a new or increasing mass or area of nonmass enhancement, prompting biopsy (► Fig. 1.9). Fat necrosis may present as an irregular enhancing mass, requiring biopsy for definitive diagnosis (► Fig. 1.10). Signal voids are often noted at the surgical site reflecting the presence of surgical clips (► Fig. 1.11).

At the present time, it is uncertain as to whether recognition of occult malignancy by use of preoperative MRI could improve local failure rates and improve patient outcomes. Two retrospective studies, Solin et al ($n = 756$), with 8-year follow-up,[69] and Hwang et al ($n = 472$), with 4.5-year median follow-up,[70] each compared two patient groups following BCS, one group with and one group without preoperative MRI. Long-term follow-up found no significant difference in local failure rates between the two groups. The failure rates were low in both studies, with 3 and 2% recurrence rates in the MRI groups, and 4 and 3% rates in the non-MRI groups. Another study compared the rate of recurrent cancer between two patient cohorts, one with a group of 121 patients undergoing preoperative breast MRI, and a second group of 225 patients undergoing surgical excision without MRI. A significant reduction in local

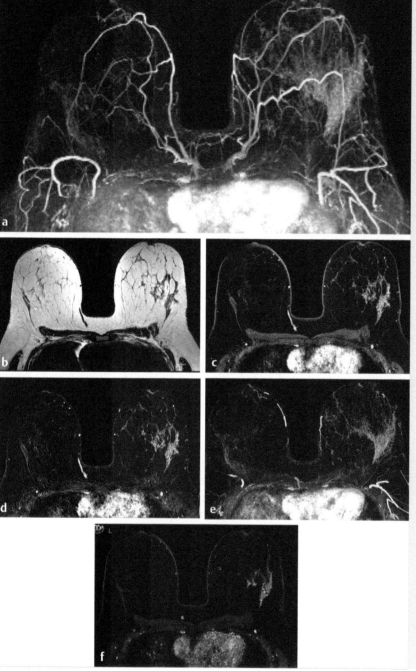

Fig. 1.8 Screening MRI: Asymptomatic woman, age 38, presents for screening MRI. History of right breast BCS, radiation and chemotherapy 2 years ago, for grade 3 IDC/DCIS, ER/PR negative, Her2/neu (FISH) positive. Axial MIP image at 120 seconds postcontrast injection shows increased nonmass enhancement in the left breast compared to the right breast **(a)**. T2-weighted image shows asymmetric parenchyma, left breast greater than right breast, **(b)** and T1-weighted postcontrast nonsubtracted and subtracted images show asymmetric normal parenchyma with enhancing terminal ductal lobular units (TDLU) **(c, d)**, shown also on the thin MIP image **(e)**. BPE in the left breast exhibits persistent enhancement in the delayed phase **(f)**. The findings of diminished enhancement in the treated breast are typical for patients following BCS, radiation and chemotherapy, and any future enhancing findings in the treated breast found on follow-up MRI should be carefully evaluated to exclude a new or recurrent cancer.

recurrences was found in the preoperative MRI group, 1%, compared to 7% in the non-MRI group ($p < 0.001$). The relatively short follow-up period of 3.4 years only is a limitation of this study.[71] It is important to consider that local cancer recurrence rates are already low (5–10% at 10 years), so that use of potential change in recurrence rates as a metric for determining the clinical efficacy of preoperative MRI is not meaningful. A study with a very long-term follow-up period might be able to elicit some measure of improvement in recurrence rates beyond the already low failure rates. Breast MRI should be a prerequisite for every patient under consideration for treatment with a localized radiation therapy protocol. Confirmation of unifocality at MRI is necessary to exclude areas of multifocal or multicentric disease, which could remain untreated if partial radiation treatment is employed.[72,73,74,75]

1.7 MRI as a Problem-Solving Tool

1.7.1 Cancer of Unknown Primary (CUPax) Syndrome

When metastatic cancer is diagnosed, and the primary is unknown and suspected to be of breast origin, MRI is useful if mammography and ultrasound studies are normal. These patients usually present with axillary adenopathy, and no other

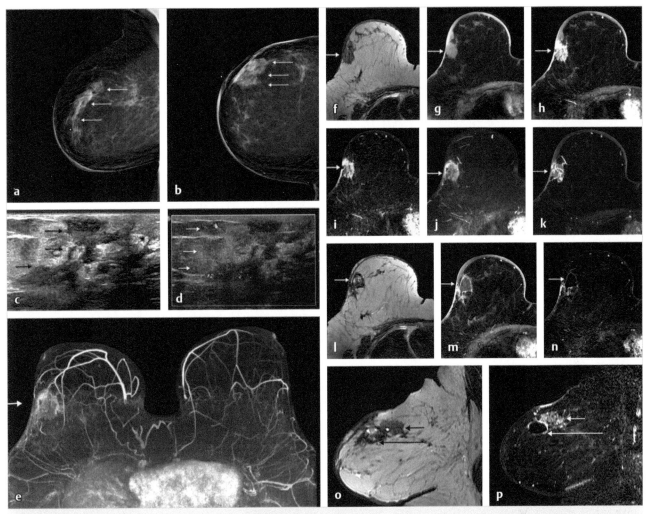

Fig. 1.9 Diagnostic MRI: Age 42 with history of triple negative IDC right breast treated with BCS 5 years ago, now presents with "thickening" in the upper outer right breast. ML and CC mammographic views (**a, b**) show a focal asymmetry, with associated distortion and a marker clip, at the site of prior BCS (*arrows*). Targeted ultrasound at this site demonstrates a predominantly hyperechoic lesion measuring. 2.6 × 1.8 × 2.9 cm with internal irregular hypoechoic/anechoic areas and peripheral increased vascularity located just superior to the surgical scar (**c, d**). Core biopsy of the palpable finding yielded triple negative IDC, presumed to represent recurrent tumor. MRI shows two lesions, immediately adjacent to one another: Lesion 1 is shown as an enhancing malignant mass located superior and posterior to the resection site as seen on MIP image (**e**). T2-weighted image shows a medium-intensity round irregular mass with diffuse postoperative skin thickening (**f**). T1-weighted pre- and postcontrast source and subtraction images (**g–k**) exhibit an irregular mass with heterogeneous washout contrast enhancement and focal skin enhancement representing skin invasion. Lesion 2 is located immediately adjacent to the inferior and anterior aspect of the cancer. The T2-weighted image shows a postoperative seroma/hematoma (**l**). T1-weighted postcontrast images show normal rim enhancement of the seroma wall (**m, n**). Sagittal reformatting of the T2- and T1-weighted postcontrast images (**o, p**) demonstrates to advantage, the relative juxtaposition of the enhancing cancer and the postoperative seroma with fat necrosis.

imaging or physical findings of primary breast carcinoma are present. Clinical trials have shown that MRI can locate a primary breast cancer, regardless of breast density at mammography, in over half of women presenting with metastatic axillary adenopathy and an occult primary[76,77,78,79] (▶ Fig. 1.12). Adenocarcinomas rarely present as isolated axillary metastases from sites other than breast, thus extensive search for disease elsewhere is usually not indicated.[80]

1.7.2 Nipple Discharge

Nipple discharge is usually benign and a relatively common clinical breast complaint, accounting for approximately 7 to 10%

of all breast symptoms.[81,82] It may be caused by benign conditions such as papilloma, periductal inflammation, duct ectasia, hyperplasia, and fibrocystic change. Further investigation is warranted when the discharge is spontaneous, bloody, or serous and emanating from a single duct, because underlying malignancy may be found in up to 25% cases.[83,84] Bloody nipple discharge may be a benign finding when associated with physiologic conditions, such as pregnancy or breast-feeding.[85] Typically, mammography and ultrasound imaging are the initial diagnostic methods used for evaluation of the patient with significant nipple discharge. Ultrasound can often identify a specific intraductal mass near the nipple; however, when mammography and ultrasound are unrevealing, a blind central duct

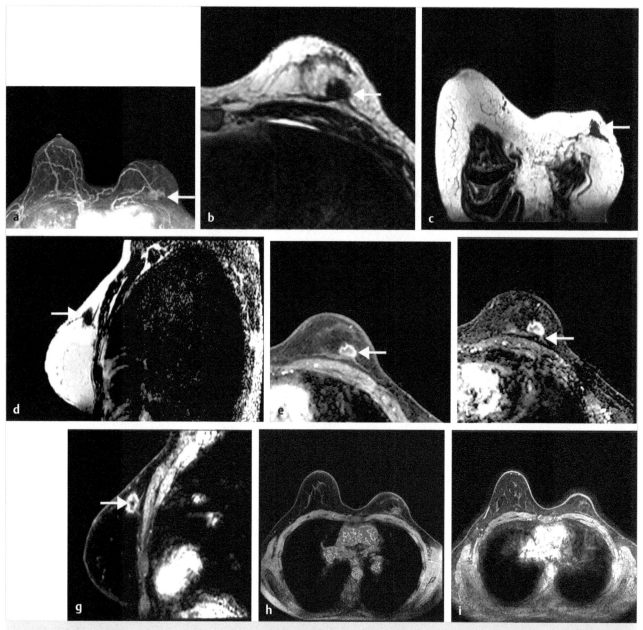

Fig. 1.10 Screening MRI: Age 43. History of left mastectomy 10 years ago when screening MRI detected DCIS with microinvasion. Patient underwent annual screening MRI thereafter. Autologous reconstruction of the left breast was performed 5 years prior to the current study. MIP image shows a new mass enhancement in the lateral posterior left breast **(a)**. T2-weighted image demonstrates an irregular low-signal mass, without internal fat, shown in the axial, sagittal, and coronal plane **(b–d)**. T1-weighted postcontrast, source, and subtracted images in the axial plane **(e, f)**, and the sagittal plane **(g)** show an irregular rim-enhancing mass with persistent kinetics **(h)**. The prior examination obtained 1 year ago shows a normal-appearing seroma with a very thin, smooth enhancing wall **(i)**. Identification of a new enhancing mass prompted MR-directed ultrasound; the lesion was identified and biopsied, histology yielding extensive fat necrosis.

surgical excision is the current procedure of choice for patient treatment. Galactography has long been considered the gold standard for diagnosis of patients with nipple discharge.[86,87] It is a safe and economical method, providing direct visualization of the secreting duct, and identification of intraductal lesions. Technical expertise and experience are needed for successful duct injection by radiologists. Some ducts may be difficult to cannulate especially when the nipple is inverted or when the discharge is intermittent and cannot be elicited on the scheduled appointment day.

From a clinical perspective, most patients with bloody or serous nipple discharge do not have breast cancer; the overwhelming majority have a benign diagnosis. Central duct excision is an invasive procedure with potential for a poor cosmetic result. At surgery, the specific duct with bloody discharge is cannulated to the level of an obstructing lesion, and if blood cannot be elicited, a blind procedure is performed with removal of approximately 4 cm of tissue deep to the nipple.[88] Side effects from this surgical procedure include patient morbidity, disturbance of lactation, cosmetic effects, and increased costs.

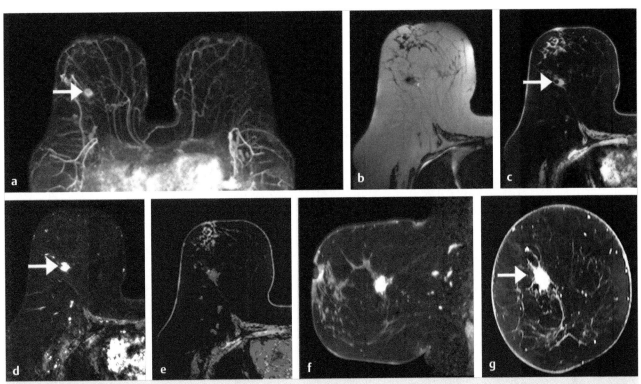

Fig. 1.11 Diagnostic MRI: Age 50. Screening mammography detected a right upper, outer quadrant, mid-depth, partially circumscribed mass, measuring 15 mm, with a correlative irregular mass with indistinct margins, and posterior acoustic enhancement visible at ultrasound and biopsied with clip placement. Histology yielded triple negative IDC grade 2and 3 and MRI was recommended for evaluation of disease extent. A correlative irregular, unifocal, enhancing mass is noted on the MIP image measuring 13 × 14 × 19 mm (**a**). T2-weighted image shows a high signal mass with a round low signal biopsy clip located at the lateral margin of the mass (**b**, *arrow*). T1-weighted precontrast source and postcontrast subtraction images (**c, d**) show a lateral marker clip. The subtraction image (**d**) shows rim enhancement and homogeneous washout kinetics within the cancer on the angiomap (**e**). Sagittal subtracted reformatted image shows rim enhancement without clip visualization (**f**); however, the coronal source image clearly demonstrates the biopsy clip at the lateral aspect of the rim-enhancing cancer (**g**, *arrow*).

An important factor contributing to the failure to identify a causative lesion in women with nipple discharge is often related to the location of the lesion. Peripheral lesions causing nipple discharge may not be visible at conventional imaging but are readily identified at MRI including both benign lesions associated with ductal disease, such as papilloma (▶ Fig. 1.13), and malignant lesions, in situ and invasive. When malignancy is found, the extent of involvement can be documented, and in contrast to a blind surgical excision, an image-guided biopsy or needle localization procedure can be used to guide the surgeon and assist in complete disease removal. A recent study evaluated 103 women with nipple discharge who underwent conventional imaging and MRI. Of these women, 88% (*n* = 91) underwent surgical excision or had clinical and/or radiographic follow-up for at least 2 years after presentation. Among the 11 patients diagnosed with malignancy in this study, 64% (*n* = 7) had a negative mammographic and ultrasound work-up. The sensitivity and specificity of MRI for the detection of malignancy were 100% (11 of 11) and 68% (54 of 80), respectively. The positive predictive value (PPV) and negative predictive value (NPV) were 37 and 100%, respectively.[89] The authors conclude that MRI is a valuable diagnostic tool for the evaluation of pathologic nipple discharge when conventional imaging is negative, and importantly, that a negative MRI in this symptomatic population may obviate the need for duct exploration and excision.

A second recent retrospective report looked at 200 patients with bloody nipple discharge and normal mammographic and ultrasound studies.[90] Among these symptomatic patients, 115 were referred directly to surgery and 85 underwent MRI before surgery. In the non-MRI group, eight (7%) cancers (seven DCIS) and seven high-risk lesions were found, with six of the eight patients requiring re-excision surgery for positive margins. In the 85 patients who underwent MRI, 8 cancers (9.4%) were identified at either core biopsy or surgery, all representing DCIS. One cancer was found by surgical nipple biopsy (false-negative) and three (3.5%) unsuspected contralateral cancers were identified.

Criticism of MRI often includes the financial costs associated with false-positive diagnoses. The Sanders paper,[90] however, found indeterminate/suspicious findings prompting additional core biopsies in just five patients (5.9%); the remaining patients underwent surgery either with or without a preoperative needle localization of an MRI finding, and the authors concluded that the extremely high NPV of MRI would support the view that a negative study could obviate central duct excision in most patients, unless overriding clinical factors prevail. These recent studies support an increasing trend for use of MRI as a primary diagnostic tool for women with clinically significant nipple discharge. The high NPV of breast MRI examinations could allow women to be safely followed without surgical intervention in some cases, if abnormal enhancement is absent and clinical symptoms are not severe.

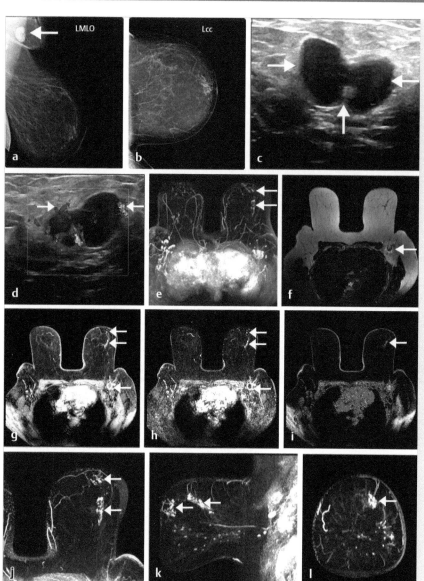

Fig. 1.12 Diagnostic MRI, CUPAx syndrome: Age 70. Palpable large left axillary lymph node noted on clinical examination, biopsy yielding poorly differentiated cancer consistent with a breast cancer primary. Left MLO and CC mammographic views (**a, b**) show fatty breast tissue composition without abnormal mammographic findings except for an enlarged axillary lymph node identified in the MLO view (**a**). Ultrasound of the axilla shows an enlarged lymph node with diffuse cortical thickening (**c**) and nonhilar increased blood flow noted on color Doppler imaging (**d**). MRI was recommended for detection of a breast primary. MIP image at 120 seconds postcontrast injection (**e**) shows linear nonmass enhancement in the lateral anterior left breast extending to the subareolar region. T2-weighted image shows a postbiopsy seroma with surrounding edema in the left axilla (**f**), seen also on T1-weighted pre- and postcontrast source and subtracted images (**g, h**, *long arrows*). Linear nonmass enhancement is seen in the lateral anterior left breast extending to the subareolar region (**g, h**, *short arrows*), with mixed persistent and washout kinetics (**i**). Thin MIP multiplanar reformatted images clearly identify the extent of the nonmass enhancement, in axial, sagittal, and coronal planes (**j–l**). MRI-guided core biopsy of the left breast at 2:00 found invasive ductal carcinoma, grade 2–3/3 with associated ductal carcinoma in situ, intermediate grade, solid type. Immunohistochemical stains for p63 and myosin heavy chain show an absence of myoepithelial cells associated with the invasive carcinoma, ER (+), PR (−), and Her2/neu (+).

1.7.3 Incidental Extramammary Lesions

When radiologists interpret breast MRI, the main focus is to evaluate the breast tissue, chest wall, skin, and axillary lymph nodes. Search patterns should, however, also include a survey of other anatomical structures in the field of view (FOV) such as the upper abdomen, neck, lung, mediastinum, spine, ribs, and sternum. Extramammary findings are frequently seen and may require additional clinical information and/or additional imaging studies to achieve a final diagnosis. Before further work-up is initiated, correlative prior images for comparison should be obtained, if possible, in order to evaluate lesion stability. Two recent papers found the frequency of these findings on breast MRI studies to be 10.7% (140 of 1,305) and 16.8% (391 of 2,334), respectively. Both studies showed that benign liver lesions were the predominate finding; however, important lesions, those that would affect patient management, were found in only eight women (0.6%) and nine women (0.4%), respectively.[91,92]

1.7.4 Challenging Clinical or Imaging Diagnoses

Problem-solving studies in the diagnostic domain require exclusion of a breast cancer diagnosis. According to current practice guidelines, MRI has a very limited role for further diagnostic assessment of any type of mammographic or ultrasound finding. Despite the high sensitivity and NPV of breast MRI, there is no agreement regarding the use of MRI as a problem-solving tool for assessment of equivocal findings on conventional imaging. Current ACR parameters for the performance of contrast-enhanced MRI in the United States recommend that, in rare cases, breast MRI may be indicated when other imaging examinations such as ultrasound and mammography and physical examination are inconclusive for the presence of breast cancer, and biopsy cannot be performed (e.g., possible distortion on only one mammographic view without an ultrasound correlate). Additional recommendations conclude that

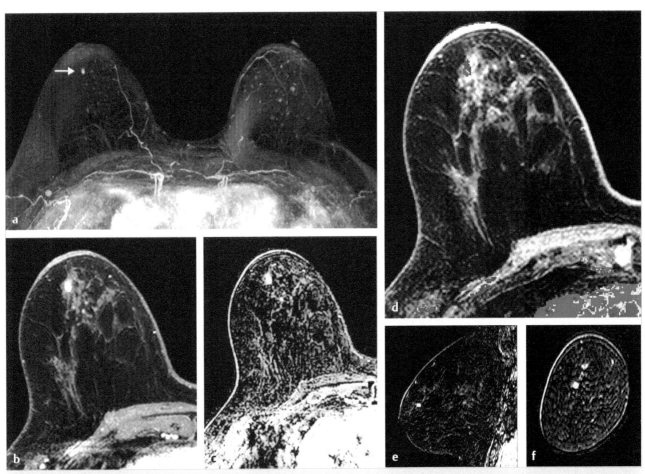

Fig. 1.13 Screening MRI: Age 72 with a *BRCA2* gene mutation, presents for screening MRI (10th examination). MIP image **(a)** shows a single new focus of enhancement at 10:00 in the anterior right breast. Correlative T1-weighted axial source and subtraction images **(b, c)** show a 5-mm homogeneously enhancing mass with circumscribed margins and washout kinetics **(d)**. Sagittal and coronal reformatted images show correlative mass enhancement **(e, f)**. MR-guided biopsy of this small mass proved to be a large duct papilloma without atypia. Papillomata in the large subareolar ducts often present as small, circumscribed masses with washout kinetics. Biopsy of this type of lesion in a high-risk patient is usually recommended, and MRI-guided biopsy is often the preferred method for tissue sampling.

MRI should not replace ultrasound or diagnostic mammography to evaluate clinical focal signs or symptoms in the breast or to evaluate lesions identified on screening mammography.[14] Moreover, because of concerns that MRI will miss some cancers that mammography will detect, guidelines recommend that MRI cannot "overrule" a decision to biopsy based on an abnormal mammogram or clinical examination, nor supplant careful problem-solving mammographic views or ultrasound in the diagnostic setting. European guidelines also indicate that there is no evidence in favor of breast MRI for characterizing equivocal findings at conventional imaging when needle biopsy procedures can be performed.[88] Another report recommended judicious indications for breast MRI in problem-solving situations, because falsely negative results were found in patients with suspicious findings on mammogram and ultrasound in their study.[93]

Recent research has shown that MRI could improve diagnostic accuracy beyond conventional imaging, and could possibly eliminate the need for interventional procedures in some cases. In a prospective study of 340 asymptomatic women, comprehensive, conventional, imaging work-up resulted in 353 BIRADS 4 assessments and then patients underwent MRI. When BIRADS 4 or 5 category assessments were confirmed at MRI, biopsy was done. However, if MRI rated the finding as BIRADS 1, 2, or 3, then biopsy was performed only if the initial finding presented as microcalcification at mammography, otherwise a systematic follow-up imaging protocol was conducted for the remaining cases every 6 months for 2 years. The results of this study showed that MRI helped to avoid an "unnecessary" biopsy in 92% of women (264 of 287), was able to diagnose unsuspected invasive breast cancers in 3 women (unrelated to the initial conventional imaging assessment), and failed to diagnose low-grade DCIS in 3 women (a false-negative rate of 4% [3/66]).[94]

A second study investigated 111 consecutive patients with inconclusive conventional breast imaging diagnoses categorized as BIRADS 0, who underwent subsequent MRI. MRI results yielded 15 true-positive, 85 true-negative, 11 false-positive, and zero false-negative breast MRI findings. Sensitivity of MRI was 100% (15/15), specificity 88.5% (85/96), PPV 57.7% (15/26), and NPV 100% (85/85). Breast density and reasons for referral had no significant influence on the diagnostic performance of breast MRI ($p > 0.05$).[95] This study showed that MRI was able to exclude malignancy reliably, and thus improve diagnostic accuracy when mammographic and ultrasound imaging studies were inconclusive. Further research is needed; however, it is likely that MRI will increasingly be used in the future to increase diagnostic accuracy and improve patient selection for interventional procedures.

1.8 MRI-Guided Biopsy

MRI is an essential guidance method for access to lesions that are occult on mammography or ultrasound and demonstrable only with MRI. Interventional procedures, such as vacuum-assisted biopsy, are minimally invasive and preferable to open surgical biopsy for diagnosis. The advantages of percutaneous biopsy procedures include reduced morbidity, superior cosmesis, less tissue scarring, and improved accuracy comparable to that of open surgical biopsy. MRI-guided breast intervention is suitable for most MRI-depicted suspicious abnormalities; however, in clinical practice, search for an ultrasound correlate is usually done before selection of an MR-guided biopsy. An MRI-directed ultrasound study, also known as "second-look ultrasound," has the advantage of an ultrasound-guided biopsy in terms of cost, time, and patient comfort, if a correlative lesion is found. However, certain lesion types are less well identified on ultrasound than on MRI; these include foci or small masses less than 5 mm, and small nonmass lesions less than 10 to 15 mm in size. When ultrasound investigation is thought unlikely to lead to identification of an imaging correlate, then it is usually appropriate to proceed directly to MR-guided biopsy. When nonmass enhancement suggesting a DCIS diagnosis is found, retrospective review of prior mammograms to search for a calcification correlate may allow a stereotactic biopsy under radiographic guidance.

Successful use of MRI-guided breast interventional procedures relies on high-quality imaging, and experience in MRI-guided techniques. Accurate lesion localization and sampling and histopathologic correlation for concordance are necessary for accurate diagnosis.[96] As with any image-guided biopsy, radiology/pathology concordance must be established and should be documented by the physician performing the biopsy in the procedure report. Collaboration between the radiologist and the pathologist is especially important when evaluating the extent of disease for a patient with a newly diagnosed cancer. MRI often identifies additional tumor that may not be identified initially by the pathologist, and a "second-look pathology" evaluation may be needed. A decision to repeat MRI-guided percutaneous sampling, as an alternative to surgical biopsy, may be required in cases when initial biopsy results are unsuccessful resulting in nondiagnostic findings, or when the pathology results are discordant with the imaging findings.

Preoperative wire localization using MRI guidance can also be used to guide excision of malignant lesions seen only on MRI, or when discordant or nondiagnostic findings are found on MRI-guided vacuum core biopsy. MRI-guided needle localization can also be useful when lesions are not technically amenable to MRI-guided core biopsy, because of difficulty in positioning the patient, or far posterior location of the lesion. In these cases, bracketing of a lesion with more than one wire under MR guidance may ensure accurate guidance and complete surgical removal.

1.9 MRI to Evaluate Implants

MRI is the best method for evaluating implant integrity and diagnosis of rupture. It is not generally recommended for routine "screening" of silicone implants and is not recommended for evaluation of saline implants because clinical and mammographic findings can provide the diagnosis of rupture. MRI is also not recommended before mammography or if rupture is already diagnosed by mammography and/or ultrasound. The clinical scenario and impact of MRI should be taken into account before MRI studies are recommended.

1.10 Summary

Breast imaging radiologists now assume much of the responsibility of primary care for patient breast health. Central to this care is the discussion of individual breast density at mammography, choice of screening methods, and assessment of individual cancer risk. Furthermore, supervision and conduction of cancer screening, diagnostic imaging, patient counseling, image-guided biopsy, and pathology consultation all fall under the purview of the breast radiologist. MRI is now an integral part of all aspects of breast imaging and will additionally contribute image-related prognostic and predictive biomarkers using advanced computer analytic methods, thus aiding our treating physicians in the therapy-planning process. This potentially important new MRI-based contribution to clinical management for women with breast cancer should further strengthen the utility of breast MRI in years to come.

References

[1] Britton P, Warwick J, Wallis MG, et al. Measuring the accuracy of diagnostic imaging in symptomatic breast patients: team and individual performance. Br J Radiol. 2012; 85(1012):415–422

[2] Pisano ED, Gatsonis C, Hendrick E, et al. Digital Mammographic Imaging Screening Trial (DMIST) Investigators Group. Diagnostic performance of digital versus film mammography for breast-cancer screening. N Engl J Med. 2005; 353(17):1773–1783

[3] Berg WA, Zhang Z, Lehrer D, et al. ACRIN 6666 Investigators. Detection of breast cancer with addition of annual screening ultrasound or a single screening MRI to mammography in women with elevated breast cancer risk. JAMA. 2012; 307(13):1394–1404

[4] Berg WA, Bandos AI, Mendelson EB, Lehrer D, Jong RA, Pisano ED. Ultrasound as the primary screening test for breast cancer: analysis from ACRIN 6666. J Natl Cancer Inst. 2015; 108(4):1–8

[5] Kriege M, Brekelmans CT, Boetes C, et al. Magnetic Resonance Imaging Screening Study Group. Efficacy of MRI and mammography for breast-cancer screening in women with a familial or genetic predisposition. N Engl J Med. 2004; 351(5):427–437

[6] Lehman CD, Isaacs C, Schnall MD, et al. Cancer yield of mammography, MR, and US in high-risk women: prospective multi-institution breast cancer screening study. Radiology. 2007; 244(2):381–388

[7] Warner E, Plewes DB, Hill KA, et al. Surveillance of BRCA1 and BRCA2 mutation carriers with magnetic resonance imaging, ultrasound, mammography, and clinical breast examination. JAMA. 2004; 292(11):1317–1325

[8] Saslow D, Boetes C, Burke W, et al. American Cancer Society Breast Cancer Advisory Group. American Cancer Society guidelines for breast screening with MRI as an adjunct to mammography. CA Cancer J Clin. 2007; 57(2):75–89

[9] Imaging Technology News. Breast Density. February 19, 2019

[10] Wernli KJ, DeMartini WB, Ichikawa L, et al. Breast Cancer Surveillance Consortium. Patterns of breast magnetic resonance imaging use in community practice. JAMA Intern Med. 2014; 174(1):125–132

[11] Stout NK, Nekhlyudov L, Li L, et al. Rapid increase in breast magnetic resonance imaging use: trends from 2000 to 2011. JAMA Intern Med. 2014; 174 (1):114–121

[12] Hwang ES, Bedrosian I. Patterns of breast magnetic resonance imaging use: an opportunity for data-driven resource allocation. JAMA Intern Med. 2014; 174(1):122–124

[13] Onega T, Weiss JE, Buist DS, et al. Breast MRI in the diagnostic and preoperative workup among Medicare beneficiaries with breast cancer. Med Care. 2016; 54(7):719–724

[14] ACR Practice Parameter for the Performance of Contrast- enhanced Magnetic Resonance Imaging (MRI) of the Breast. Revised 2018 (Resolution 34). https://www.acr.org/-/media/ACR/Files/Practice-Parameters/mr-contrast-breast.pdf.

[15] Morris EA, Liberman L, Ballon DJ, et al. MRI of occult breast carcinoma in a high-risk population. AJR Am J Roentgenol. 2003; 181(3):619–626

[16] Leach MO, Boggis CR, Dixon AK, et al. MARIBS study group. Screening with magnetic resonance imaging and mammography of a UK population at high familial risk of breast cancer: a prospective multicentre cohort study (MARIBS). Lancet. 2005; 365(9473):1769–1778

[17] Lehman CD, Blume JD, Weatherall P, et al. International Breast MRI Consortium Working Group. Screening women at high risk for breast cancer with mammography and magnetic resonance imaging. Cancer. 2005; 103(9): 1898–1905

[18] Lehman CD, Gatsonis C, Kuhl CK, et al. ACRIN Trial 6667 Investigators Group. MRI evaluation of the contralateral breast in women with recently diagnosed breast cancer. N Engl J Med. 2007; 356(13):1295–1303

[19] Warner E, Messersmith H, Causer P, Eisen A, Shumak R, Plewes D. Systematic review: using magnetic resonance imaging to screen women at high risk for breast cancer. Ann Intern Med. 2008; 148(9):671–679

[20] Weinstein SP, Localio AR, Conant EF, Rosen M, Thomas KM, Schnall MD. Multimodality screening of high-risk women: a prospective cohort study. J Clin Oncol. 2009; 27(36):6124–6128

[21] Kuhl C, Weigel S, Schrading S, et al. Prospective multicenter cohort study to refine management recommendations for women at elevated familial risk of breast cancer: the EVA trial. J Clin Oncol. 2010; 28(9):1450–1457

[22] Sardanelli F, Podo F, Santoro F, et al. High Breast Cancer Risk Italian 1 (HIB CRIT-1) Study. Multicenter surveillance of women at high genetic breast cancer risk using mammography, ultrasonography, and contrast-enhanced magnetic resonance imaging (the high breast cancer risk Italian 1 study): final results. Invest Radiol. 2011; 46(2):94–105

[23] Kuhl CK, Shrading S, Strobel K, et al. Abbreviated breast MRI: first postcontrast subtracted images and MIP—a novel approach to breast cancer screening with MRI. J Clin Oncol. 2014; 32(22):2304–2310

[24] Machida Y, Shimauchi A, Kanemaki Y, et al. Feasibility and potential limitations of abbreviated breast MRI: an observer study using an enriched cohort. Breast Cancer. 2017; 24(3):411–419 2016

[25] Heacock L, Melsaether AN, Heller SL, et al. Evaluation of a known breast cancer using an abbreviated breast MRI protocol: correlation of imaging characteristics and pathology with lesion detection and conspicuity. Eur J Radiol. 2016; 85(4):815–823

[26] Moschetta M, Telegrafo M, Rella L, Stabile Ianora AA, Angelelli G. Abbreviated combined mr protocol: a new faster strategy for characterizing breast lesions. Clin Breast Cancer. 2016; 16(3):207–211

[27] Harvey SC, Di Carlo PA, Lee B, Obadina E, Sippo D, Mullen L. An abbreviated protocol for high-risk screening breast MRI saves time and resources. J Am Coll Radiol. 2016; 13(4):374–380

[28] Mango VL, Morris EA, David Dershaw D, et al. Abbreviated protocol for breast MRI: are multiple sequences needed for cancer detection? Eur J Radiol. 2015; 84(1):65–70

[29] American College of Radiology Breast Magnetic Resonance Imaging Program. https://www.acraccreditation.org/modalities/breast-mri

[30] Kuhl CK, Mielcareck P, Klaschik S, et al. Dynamic breast MR imaging: are signal intensity time course data useful for differential diagnosis of enhancing lesions? Radiology. 1999; 211(1):101–110

[31] Holland R, Veling SH, Mravunac M, Hendriks JH. Histologic multifocality of Tis, T1–2 breast carcinomas. Implications for clinical trials of breast-conserving surgery. Cancer. 1985; 56(5):979–990

[32] Tot T. The metastatic capacity of multifocal breast carcinomas: extensive tumors versus tumors of limited extent. Hum Pathol. 2009; 40(2):199–205

[33] Katipamula R, Degnim AC, Hoskin T, et al. Trends in mastectomy rates at the Mayo Clinic Rochester: effect of surgical year and preoperative magnetic resonance imaging. J Clin Oncol. 2009; 27(25):4082–4088

[34] Fisher B, Anderson S, National Surgical Adjuvant Breast and Bowel Project. Conservative surgery for the management of invasive and noninvasive carcinoma of the breast: NSABP trials. World J Surg. 1994; 18(1):63–69

[35] Veronesi U, Banfi A, Del Vecchio M, et al. Comparison of Halsted mastectomy with quadrantectomy, axillary dissection, and radiotherapy in early breast cancer: long-term results. Eur J Cancer Clin Oncol. 1986; 22(9):1085–1089

[36] Fisher B, Anderson S, Bryant J, et al. Twenty-year follow-up of a randomized trial comparing total mastectomy, lumpectomy, and lumpectomy plus irradiation for the treatment of invasive breast cancer. N Engl J Med. 2002; 347 (16):1233–1241

[37] Veronesi U, Cascinelli N, Mariani L, et al. Twenty-year follow-up of a randomized study comparing breast-conserving surgery with radical mastectomy for early breast cancer. N Engl J Med. 2002; 347(16):1227–1232

[38] Moran MS, Schnitt SJ, Giuliano AE, et al. Society of Surgical Oncology, American Society for Radiation Oncology. Society of Surgical Oncology-American Society for Radiation Oncology consensus guideline on margins for breast-conserving surgery with whole-breast irradiation in stages I and II invasive breast cancer. J Clin Oncol. 2014; 32(14):1507–1515

[39] Solin LJ, Fourquet A, Vicini FA, et al. Mammographically detected ductal carcinoma in situ of the breast treated with breast-conserving surgery and definitive breast irradiation: long-term outcome and prognostic significance of patient age and margin status. Int J Radiat Oncol Biol Phys. 2001; 50(4):991–1002

[40] Schnitt SJ, Connolly JL, Khettry U, et al. Pathologic findings on re-excision of the primary site in breast cancer patients considered for treatment by primary radiation therapy. Cancer. 1987; 59(4):675–681

[41] Beron PJ, Horwitz EM, Martinez AA, et al. Pathologic and mammographic findings predicting the adequacy of tumor excision before breast-conserving therapy. AJR Am J Roentgenol. 1996; 167(6):1409–1414

[42] Kotwall C, Ranson M, Stiles A, Hamann MS. Relationship between initial margin status for invasive breast cancer and residual carcinoma after re-excision. Am J Surg. 2007; 73(4):337–343

[43] Morrow M, Jagsi R, Alderman AK, et al. Surgeon recommendations and receipt of mastectomy for treatment of breast cancer. JAMA. 2009; 302(14): 1551–1556

[44] Waljee JF, Hu ES, Newman LA, Alderman AK. Predictors of re-excision among women undergoing breast-conserving surgery for cancer. Ann Surg Oncol. 2008; 15(5):1297–1303

[45] Cellini C, Hollenbeck ST, Christos P, et al. Factors associated with residual breast cancer after re-excision for close or positive margins. Ann Surg Oncol. 2004; 11(10):915–920

[46] Lovrics PJ, Cornacchi SD, Farrokhyar F, et al. Technical factors, surgeon case volume and positive margin rates after breast conservation surgery for early-stage breast cancer. Can J Surg. 2010; 53(5):305–312

[47] McCahill LE, Single RM, Aiello Bowles EJ, et al. Variability in reexcision following breast conservation surgery. JAMA. 2012; 307(5):467–475

[48] Isaacs AJ, Gemignani ML, Pusic A, Sedrakyan A. Association of breast conservation surgery for cancer with 90-day reoperation rates in New York state. JAMA Surg. 2016; 151(7):648–655

[49] Freedman G, Fowble B, Hanlon A, et al. Patients with early stage invasive cancer with close or positive margins treated with conservative surgery and radiation have an increased risk of breast recurrence that is delayed by adjuvant systemic therapy. Int J Radiat Oncol Biol Phys. 1999; 44(5): 1005–1015

[50] Smitt MC, Nowels KW, Zdeblick MJ, et al. The importance of the lumpectomy surgical margin status in long-term results of breast conservation. Cancer. 1995; 76(2):259–267

[51] Cowen D, Houvenaeghel G, Bardou V, et al. Local and distant failures after limited surgery with positive margins and radiotherapy for node-negative breast cancer. Int J Radiat Oncol Biol Phys. 2000; 47(2):305–312

[52] Gage I, Schnitt SJ, Nixon AJ, et al. Pathologic margin involvement and the risk of recurrence in patients treated with breast-conserving therapy. Cancer. 1996; 78(9):1921–1928

[53] Peterson ME, Schultz DJ, Reynolds C, Solin LJ. Outcomes in breast cancer patients relative to margin status after treatment with breast-conserving surgery and radiation therapy: the University of Pennsylvania experience. Int J Radiat Oncol Biol Phys. 1999; 43(5):1029–1035

[54] Cody HS , III, Van Zee KJ. Reexcision—the other breast cancer epidemic. N Engl J Med. 2015; 373(6):568–569

[55] Peters ME, Fagerholm MI, Scanlan KA, Voegeli DR, Kelcz F. Mammographic evaluation of the postsurgical and irradiated breast. Radiographics. 1988; 8 (5):873–899

[56] Dershaw DD, Shank B, Reisinger S. Mammographic findings after breast cancer treatment with local excision and definitive irradiation. Radiology. 1987; 164(2):455–461

[57] Waddell BE, Stomper PC, DeFazio JL, Hurd TC, Edge SB. Postexcision mammography is indicated after resection of ductal carcinoma-in-situ of the breast. Ann Surg Oncol. 2000; 7(9):665–668

[58] Soderstrom CE, Harms SE, Farrell RS , Jr, Pruneda JM, Flamig DP. Detection with MR imaging of residual tumor in the breast soon after surgery. AJR Am J Roentgenol. 1997; 168(2):485–488

[59] Lee JM, Orel SG, Czerniecki BJ, Solin LJ, Schnall MD. MRI before reexcision surgery in patients with breast cancer. AJR Am J Roentgenol. 2004; 182(2):473–480

[60] Chae EY, Cha JH, Kim HH, et al. Evaluation of residual disease using breast MRI after excisional biopsy for breast cancer. AJR Am J Roentgenol. 2013; 200 (5):1167–1173

[61] Frei KA, Kinkel K, Bonel HM, Lu Y, Esserman LJ, Hylton NM. MR imaging of the breast in patients with positive margins after lumpectomy: influence of the time interval between lumpectomy and MR imaging. AJR Am J Roentgenol. 2000; 175(6):1577–1584

[62] Rastogi P, Anderson SJ, Bear HD, et al. Preoperative chemotherapy: updates of National Surgical Adjuvant Breast and Bowel Project Protocols B-18 and B-27. J Clin Oncol. 2008; 26(5):778–785

[63] Kaufmann M, von Minckwitz G, Bear HD, et al. Recommendations from an international expert panel on the use of neoadjuvant (primary) systemic treatment of operable breast cancer: new perspectives 2006. Ann Oncol. 2007; 18(12):1927–1934

[64] Eisenhauer EA, Therasse P, Bogaerts J, et al. New response evaluation criteria in solid tumours: revised RECIST guideline (version 1.1). Eur J Cancer. 2009; 45(2):228–247

[65] Wapnir IL, Anderson SJ, Mamounas EP, et al. Prognosis after ipsilateral breast tumor recurrence and locoregional recurrences in five National Surgical Adjuvant Breast and Bowel Project node-positive adjuvant breast cancer trials. J Clin Oncol. 2006; 24(13):2028–2037

[66] Anderson SJ, Wapnir I, Dignam JJ, et al. Prognosis after ipsilateral breast tumor recurrence and locoregional recurrences in patients treated by breast-conserving therapy in five National Surgical Adjuvant Breast and Bowel Project protocols of node-negative breast cancer. J Clin Oncol. 2009; 27(15): 2466–2473

[67] Brennan S, Liberman L, Dershaw DD, Morris E. Breast MRI screening of women with a personal history of breast cancer. AJR Am J Roentgenol. 2010; 195(2):510–516

[68] Li J, Dershaw DD, Lee CH, Joo S, Morris EA. Breast MRI after conservation therapy: usual findings in routine follow-up examinations. AJR Am J Roentgenol. 2010; 195(3):799–807

[69] Solin LJ, Orel SG, Hwang WT, Harris EE, Schnall MD. Relationship of breast magnetic resonance imaging to outcome after breast-conservation treatment with radiation for women with early-stage invasive breast carcinoma or ductal carcinoma in situ. J Clin Oncol. 2008; 26(3):386–391

[70] Hwang N, Schiller DE, Crystal P, Maki E, McCready DR. Magnetic resonance imaging in the planning of initial lumpectomy for invasive breast carcinoma: its effect on ipsilateral breast tumor recurrence after breast-conservation therapy. Ann Surg Oncol. 2009; 16(11):3000–3009

[71] Fischer U, Zachariae O, Baum F, von Heyden D, Funke M, Liersch T. The influence of preoperative MRI of the breasts on recurrence rate in patients with breast cancer. Eur Radiol. 2004; 14(10):1725–1731

[72] Al-Hallaq HA, Mell LK, Bradley JA, et al. Magnetic resonance imaging identifies multifocal and multicentric disease in breast cancer patients who are eligible for partial breast irradiation. Cancer. 2008; 113(9):2408–2414

[73] Tendulkar RD, Chellman-Jeffers M, Rybicki LA, et al. Preoperative breast magnetic resonance imaging in early breast cancer: implications for partial breast irradiation. Cancer. 2009; 115(8):1621–1630

[74] Kühr M, Wolfgarten M, Stölzle M, et al. Potential impact of preoperative magnetic resonance imaging of the breast on patient selection for accelerated partial breast irradiation. Int J Radiat Oncol Biol Phys. 2011; 81(4):e541–e546

[75] Kowalchik KV, Vallow LA, McDonough M, et al. Classification system for identifying women at risk for altered partial breast irradiation recommendations

[76] Buchanan CL, Morris EA, Dorn PL, Borgen PI, Van Zee KJ. Utility of breast magnetic resonance imaging in patients with occult primary breast cancer. Ann Surg Oncol. 2005; 12(12):1045–1053

[77] Obdeijn IM, Brouwers-Kuyper EM, Tilanus-Linthorst MM, Wiggers T, Oudkerk M. MR imaging-guided sonography followed by fine-needle aspiration cytology in occult carcinoma of the breast. AJR Am J Roentgenol. 2000; 174(4): 1079–1084

[78] Olson JA , Jr, Morris EA, Van Zee KJ, Linehan DC, Borgen PI. Magnetic resonance imaging facilitates breast conservation for occult breast cancer. Ann Surg Oncol. 2000; 7(6):411–415

[79] Orel SG, Weinstein SP, Schnall MD, et al. Breast MR imaging in patients with axillary node metastases and unknown primary malignancy. Radiology. 1999; 212(2):543–549

[80] Pentheroudakis G, Lazaridis G, Pavlidis N. Axillary nodal metastases from carcinoma of unknown primary (CUPAx): a systematic review of published evidence. Breast Cancer Res Treat. 2010; 119(1):1–11

[81] Santen RJ, Mansel R. Benign breast disorders. N Engl J Med. 2005; 353(3): 275–285

[82] Sauter ER, Schlatter L, Lininger J, Hewett JE. The association of bloody nipple discharge with breast pathology. Surgery. 2004; 136(4):780–785

[83] Kilgore AR, Fleming R, Ramos MM. The incidence of cancer with nipple discharge and the risk of cancer in the presence of papillary disease of the breast. Surg Gynecol Obstet. 1953; 96(6):649–660

[84] Piccoli CW, Feig SA, Vala MA. Breast imaging case of the day. Benign intraductal papilloma with focal atypical papillomatous hyperplasia. Radiographics. 1998; 18(3):783–786

[85] Dinkel HP, Trusen A, Gassel AM, et al. Predictive value of galactographic patterns for benign and malignant neoplasms of the breast in patients with nipple discharge. Br J Radiol. 2000; 73(871):706–714

[86] Tabár L, Dean PB, Péntek Z. Galactography: the diagnostic procedure of choice for nipple discharge. Radiology. 1983; 149(1):31–38

[87] Van Zee KJ, Ortega Pérez G, Minnard E, Cohen MA. Preoperative galactography increases the diagnostic yield of major duct excision for nipple discharge. Cancer. 1998; 82(10):1874–1880

[88] Sardanelli F, Boetes C, Borisch B, et al. Magnetic resonance imaging of the breast: recommendations from the EUSOMA working group. Eur J Cancer. 2010; 46(8):1296–1316

[89] Bahl M, Baker JA, Greenup RA, Ghate SV. Evaluation of pathologic nipple discharge: what is the added diagnostic value of MRI? Ann Surg Oncol. 2015; 22 Suppl 3:S435–S441

[90] Sanders LM, Daigle M. The rightful role of MRI after negative conventional imaging in the management of bloody nipple discharge. Breast J. 2016; 22(2): 209–212

[91] Phadke S, Thomas A, Yang L, Moore C, Xia C, Schroeder MC. Frequency and clinical significance of extramammary findings on breast magnetic resonance imaging. Clin Breast Cancer. 2016; 16(5):424–429

[92] Niell BL, Bennett D, Sharma A, Gazelle GS. Extramammary findings on breast MR examinations: frequency, clinical relevance, and patient outcomes. Radiology. 2015; 276(1):56–64

[93] Yau EJ, Gutierrez RL, DeMartini WB, Eby PR, Peacock S, Lehman CD. The utility of breast MRI as a problem-solving tool. Breast J. 2011; 17(3): 273–280

[94] Strobel K, Schrading S, Hansen NL, Barabasch A, Kuhl CK. Assessment of BI-RADS category 4 lesions detected with screening mammography and screening US: utility of MR imaging. Radiology. 2015; 274(2): 343–351

[95] Spick C, Szolar DHM, Preidler KW, Tillich M, Reittner P, Baltzer PA. Breast MRI used as a problem-solving tool reliably excludes malignancy. Eur J Radiol. 2015; 84(1):61–64

[96] ACR Practice parameter for the performance of magnetic resonance imaging-guided breast interventional procedures. Revised 2016 (resolution 35) https://www.acr.org/-/media/ACR/Files/Practice-Parameters/MR-Guided-Breast.pdf

2 Screening MRI: Who Should Be Screened?

Gillian M. Newstead

Abstract

Mammography screening trials have shown the decreased mortality benefit of early diagnosis. Nonetheless there is certainly room for improvement with new screening methods. This chapter will discuss the relative efficacy of breast screening using mammography (including digital tomosynthesis), handheld and automated-ultrasound and MRI. Results from the breast screening trials using single or a combination of these various modalities are reviewed. In recent years, studies of high-risk women have shown that, when compared with mammography and ultrasound, dynamic contrast-enhanced magnetic resonance imaging (DCE-MRI) is the most sensitive method for detecting breast abnormalities and is an excellent screening tool. Data concerning recent trials using MRI for women at moderate risk (15–20%), women with a prior history of breast cancer and women with mammographically dense breasts, have shown excellent results with increased cancer detection rates when compared with other modalities.

Further discussed in this chapter is the importance of not only consideration of the number of cancers detected by various methods, but also consideration of the *biology* of screen-detected cancers, specifically those with adverse pathologic profiles. It is increasingly evident that identification of small aggressive cancers at screening will have the greatest likelihood of achieving improved breast cancer mortality reduction, and in this respect, MRI has a distinct advantage.

Keywords: mammographic screening, digital breast tomosynthesis (DBT) screening, breast density assessment, hand-held ultrasound screening (HHUS), automated breast ultrasound screening (ABUS), MRI screening trials of high-risk women, screening of women at moderate-risk (15-20%), screening of women with a personal history of breast cancer, screening of women with dense breasts at mammography, women with diagnosis of a high-risk lesion, women at average-risk (< 25%)

2.1 Background

Breast cancer is the most common type of malignancy found among women in both developed and developing countries and remains the second leading cause of cancer death in women. According to estimates from the International Agency for Research on Cancer (IARC) there will be about 1.2 million new breast cancer cases worldwide in 2018, accounting for almost 1 in 4 cancer cases among women, and about 626 thousand breast cancer deaths.[1] Approximately one in eight women (about 12%) in the United Sates will develop invasive breast cancer over the course of her lifetime. In 2017, the American Cancer Society (ACS) estimates that 252,710 new cases of invasive cancer and 63,410 cases of in situ disease will be diagnosed in women in the United States.[3,4] The lifetime risk of breast cancer in men is about 1 in 1,000, with the ACS estimating that 2,470 new cases of invasive breast cancer in men will be diagnosed in 2017. Despite a decrease in breast cancer death rates

since 1989, about 40,610 women in the United States are still expected to die from this disease in 2017. The decrease in death rates is likely the result of earlier cancer detection through screening, increased awareness, and improved treatment. As of March 2017, there are more than 3.1 million women living with a personal history of breast cancer in the United States, including women currently undergoing treatment and those who have completed treatment.[3]

There is known to be a close association between the stage of breast cancer at diagnosis and cancer survival, even when discounting the confounding impact of various histologic tumor types and treatment regimens. Women with small cancers, less than 15 mm in size, are highly curable with 10-year survival rates greater than 90%. Women with regional disease confined to the breast and axillary nodes can expect a 10-year survival of about 80%; however, survival rates for women with metastatic disease are greatly reduced. Earlier detection of breast cancer through mammography screening results in a significant decrease in the number of advanced breast cancers, better disease-specific survival, relapse-free survival, and overall survival. Indeed, early detection allows a higher frequency of breast-conserving surgery (BCS) and fewer patients requiring severe forms of adjuvant therapy.

2.2 Mammographic Screening

Mammography has been the primary large-scale screening method for breast cancer detection in the general female population over the past five decades. The goal and expectation that early detection of breast cancer will decrease breast cancer death has been validated in multiple randomized clinical trials.[5,6,7,8] Mammography screening as shown in the Swedish trials resulted in a decrease in breast cancer mortality by about 30%, detecting small node-negative cancers before their clinical presentation, with the additional benefit of improving patient treatment options allowing less aggressive therapy.[5] A 30% breast cancer mortality decrease has been achieved not only in randomized controlled mammography trials but also in observational and service studies as well, with meta-analyses confirming that a decrease in breast cancer mortality begins about 5 to 7 years after the institution of screening.[6,9] It is important to note, however, that of the mammography screening trials, none were specifically directed toward screening of women at a high risk for breast cancer.

Despite these important gains in reducing breast cancer death, mammography has limitations, notably decreased sensitivity in women with dense breast tissue. Mammographic technique creates radiographic images of the breast that produce two-dimensional X-ray projection images that do not penetrate dense breast tissue effectively. Cancers may thus be obscured by dense overlapping tissue. The sensitivity of mammography in young high-risk women with dense breasts is low, as shown in the ACRIN-DMIST trial. Almost 50,000 women were recruited into this investigation, which was designed to compare the clinical performance of film-screen mammography with that of digital mammography.[10] The overall sensitivity of screening mammography for women with dense breasts, ACR category (c) heterogeneously dense and (d) extremely dense, ranged between 36 and 38%.

Multiple retrospective and prospective screening studies have demonstrated the limitations of mammography in high-risk patients, especially in those with a BRCA mutation. Compared to the sporadic breast cancers identified in women of average risk, cancers detected in high-risk women, those with a genetic predisposition, are usually more difficult to detect at mammography. These cancers exhibit unique imaging features and pathologic profiles; often presenting as masses at a younger age (premenopausal), with rapid growth and a tendency to present a more benign appearance by exhibiting "pushing" rather than spiculated or irregular margins. These aggressive lesions are generally noncalcified, high grade, receptor negative, and frequently favor a posterior location in the breast where detection is more difficult.[11] The majority of these cancers are larger than 1 cm in size at diagnosis, with a 20 to 56% incidence of metastatic axillary node involvement.[12,13]

2.2.1 Breast Density

Breast density has been shown to be an independent risk factor for breast cancer. A meta-analysis in 2006 showed that women with dense breasts were at a four- to fivefold increased risk compared with other women.[14] Evidence concerning the limitations of mammography has prompted the majority of U.S. states to pass national breast density legislation. These laws generally require that women be informed if they are known to have heterogeneously dense or extremely dense breasts on mammography and that consideration of adjunctive imaging screening methods should be considered.[15] These laws impact a very large number of women because it is estimated that more than 50% of women fall into the dense breast category. Although mammography is an effective screening test for many women, the shortcomings of mammography, particularly for those women at high risk and with dense breasts, have led to an interest in pursuing adjunctive supplementary screening methods. The requirement for any alternative or supplemental screening method must be validated by studies, which document their ability to detect small node-negative cancers. Current candidate methods for adjunctive breast cancer screening include digital breast tomosynthesis (DBT), ultrasound (US), and magnetic resonance imaging (MRI).

Digital Breast Tomosynthesis Screening

DBT is a Food and Drug Administration (FDA)-approved mammographic technique and is a recent improvement, now increasingly a replacement to conventional 2-dimensional (2D) digital mammography. DBT employs quasi-cross sectional x-ray images of the breast allowing the depiction of masses that might otherwise be obscured by dense fibroglandular tissue. Several large clinical studies have shown an added cancer yield of about 1.25 per 1,000 women, an average 30% increase in breast cancer detection, when DBT is compared to screening with standard full-field digital mammography (FFDM). A study reported in 2019 from the Oslo Tomosynthesis Screening Trial found that addition of DBT to digital mammography resulted in significant gains in sensitivity and specificity. Additionally, synthetic mammography in combination with DBT had similar sensitivity and specificity to digital mammography in combination with DBT.[3] DBT also has the added important advantage of reducing recall rates and improving the positive predictive value (PPV) of recall and biopsy recommendations.[16,17,18] Central to the outcome of a screening program is the consideration not only the number of cancers detected, but also the biologic profile of those detected. Although more research is needed, the studies show that DBT has a propensity to identify cancers that are associated with well-differentiated lower-grade disease, when compared with small higher grade cancers that are found with screening MRI.

Ultrasound Screening

Studies have consistently shown that whole breast ultrasound (WBUS) will detect an additional 2 to 4 cancers per 1,000 women screened beyond those detected at mammography.[19,20,21] Supplemental WBUS in addition to mammography is now the most commonly used method for adjunctive screening of women with dense breasts. Multiple prospective ultrasound screening studies have found an increased cancer detection rate of about 4 per 1,000 women compared with mammographic screening in the same group of individuals, with a concomitant reduction in the interval cancer rate.

Handheld Ultrasound Screening

The additive value of handheld ultrasound screening (HHUS) in women with heterogeneously dense or extremely dense breast tissue and at least one other high or intermediate risk factor was evaluated in the ACRIN-sponsored 6,666 trials.[19] Berg and colleagues investigated 2,662 women who underwent three rounds of annual mammography and HHUS screenings between April 2004 and February 2006. Cancer yield overall was 111, 33 (30%) detected on mammography only, 32 (29%) by ultrasound only, and 26 (23%) by both mammography and ultrasound; 11 (12%) were not detected by either screening method. Supplemental screening ultrasound identified 3.7 cancers/1,000 screenings. Of the cancers found only at ultrasound, 94% were invasive with a median size of 10 mm and 96% were node negative. The reported interval cancer rate was low at 8%. However, rates of biopsy for findings seen only on ultrasound were high (5%) on incidence screens, with a low malignancy rate (7.4%). It is important to note that after three negative consecutive mammographic and ultrasound screening rounds, a subset of 612 women underwent a single MRI screening examination. Cancer yield among these women was 14.7/1,000, a significant increase when compared to the 4.2/1,000 detection rate in the same cohort of women who received mammographic and ultrasound screening in the prevalent round. Of the MRI-detected cancers, 89% were invasive, median size was 8.5 mm, and 100% (of those staged) were node negative.

Automated Breast Ultrasound Screening

A large multicenter study comparing mammography screening with automated breast ultrasound screening (ABUS) was conducted between 2009 and 2011 and included a total of 15,318 women with heterogeneously or extremely dense breasts; 112 cancers were identified, 82 on mammography and 30 on ultrasound. The additional cancer yield with ultrasound was 1.9/1,000 women screened; 62.2% of the mammography-detected cancers were invasive compared with 93.3% of the cancers identified at ABUS. Ultrasound increased the recall rate from 15 to 28.5% (285/1000), mammography yielding 1 cancer for every 28.1 recalls, and ultrasound yielding 1 cancer for every 68.7 recalls. An additional 552 biopsies were performed to identify 30 "US-only" cancers.[20]

Limitations of Screening with Ultrasound

Although current screening practice for women with dense breasts now consists of annual mammography supplemented by WBUS, there are several limiting factors. These are principally due to the high biopsy rates and unwieldy short-term follow-up rates of screening with WBUS and increased radiologist interpretation time.[19,20] Other limiting factors include the time to conduct the examination; on average, a bilateral ultrasound screening study in the 6666 ACRIN took just under 20 minutes to complete. The low PPV of WBUS-generated biopsies and the high rates of short-term interval follow-up recommendations result in increased downstream costs.[21] Sprague et al estimated the cost per QALY gained by screening women with mammography and supplemental ultrasound to be $320,000, a significant burden on health care costs.[22]

Because of the limitations of WBUS outlined above, alternative supplemental screening tests have been investigated to screen women with dense breasts, notably abbreviated breast MRI (AB-MR). A short MRI scan time, reduced to less than 10 minutes, has been shown to be equivalent in time and cost to the standard combination of mammography and WBUS. Early studies involving interpretations of an abbreviated MRI protocol (AB-MR) have shown equivalent sensitivity for cancer detection when compared to a full standard MRI, with only minimal decrease in specificity.[23,24] The growing evidence for an abbreviated MR protocol suggests a strong benefit for the expanded use of breast MRI for screening of a larger section of the female population. The abbreviated MRI technique will be discussed further in Chapter 3.

2.3 MRI Screening for High-Risk Women

In recent years, studies have shown that, compared with mammography and ultrasound, dynamic contrast-enhanced magnetic resonance imaging (DCE-MRI) is the most sensitive method for detecting breast abnormalities and is an excellent screening tool. MRI uses magnetic fields to produce cross-sectional images of soft-tissue structures. The contrast between normal breast tissue consisting of adipose and fibroglandular structures, and breast lesions, depends on the mobility and magnetic environment of the hydrogen atoms in the water and fat of these tissues. Gadolinium-based contrast agents (GBCA) are injected intravenously during MRI to improve detection of cancers and other lesions.[25,26,27] The advantages of MRI include its high sensitivity for detection of invasive breast cancers and most in situ cancers and unlike mammography, the sensitivity of MRI is not limited by breast density, postsurgical or postradiation changes or the presence of breast implants.

The superior sensitivity of breast MRI compared to other breast imaging methods has been shown in women with a familial increased risk for breast cancer. This evidence has resulted in recommendations from the ACS, the National Comprehensive

Cancer Network (NCCN), and joint recommendations from the Society of Breast Imaging (SBI) and the American College of Radiology (ACR) that MRI be used as an adjunct to mammography screening to improve breast cancer detection in high-risk women.[28,29,30,31,32] Supplemental screening with breast MRI is recommended for those women who are carriers of *BRCA1*, *BRCA2*, mutation, for their first-degree relatives with a BRCA mutation (tested or untested), for those with a lifetime risk of 20 to 25% or greater, and for those with a clinical history of chest irradiation between ages 10 and 30 years.[31,33] Annual screening with MRI and mammography is also recommended for women with less common, specific genetic mutations such as Li–Fraumeni syndrome, Cowden's and Bannayan–Riley–Ruvalcaba syndromes (*TP53* gene mutations) or their first-degree relatives.

2.3.1 Women with a Genetic Predisposition for Breast Cancer

Clinical features indicating that a woman may be at high risk for breast cancer caused by a high-penetrance gene include close relatives with a history of breast or ovarian cancer (two or more) occurring before age 50. Harmful mutations of the BRCA tumor suppressor genes result in a greater lifetime risk of malignancy particularly for breast and ovarian cancers, and are estimated to account for 5 to 10% of all newly diagnosed breast cancers.[34] The BRCA gene mutation can be inherited from either parent and passed on to both daughters and sons in an autosomal dominant pattern of transmission. Each first-degree relative of a BRCA mutation carrier has a 50% chance of also being a carrier of the mutated gene. Women with no known risk factors have an average lifetime breast cancer risk of 12.3%, whereas women with a BRCA mutation have a 55 to 65% (*BRCA1*) and a 45% (*BRCA2*) risk of developing breast cancer by age 70. An increased risk of up to 63% for development of a second ipsilateral cancer or a contralateral breast cancer is found in women with a *BRCA1*-associated breast cancer, the highest risk conferred in women with a primary cancer diagnosed before age 40.[35,36,37,38] A woman's risk nearly doubles if a first-degree relative (mother, sister, and daughter) is known to have a personal history of breast cancer. Genetic counseling should be recommended for women who are found to be at increased risk of carrying a BRCA gene mutation.

Fewer than 15% of women diagnosed with breast cancer have a history of breast cancer in a family member. Breast cancer is more common in African-American women than white women, when diagnosed under age 45, and have an increased likelihood of dying from breast cancer. Asian, Hispanic, and Native American women have a lower risk of developing and dying from breast cancer. Women with known genetic mutations are associated with a high lifetime risk of breast cancer estimated at 50 to 80%. Supplemental MRI screening of BRCA mutation carriers should begin at an early age and is essential for early and accurate cancer diagnosis. Management options for women with a BRCA mutation include enhanced screening with MRI, prophylactic mastectomy, and/or oophorectomy, and chemoprevention. Treatment with tamoxifen has been shown to reduce the risk of receptor-positive tumors for women who are known *BRCA1* or *BRCA2* mutation carriers.

The BRCA1 Gene

The *BRCA1* gene located on chromosome 17 is thought to be responsible for the hereditary breast and ovarian cancer syndrome (HBOC). *BRCA1*-associated breast cancers account for 50% of familial breast cancers and 5 to 8% of all breast cancers. The associated cancer risk is known to decrease with increasing age. These cancers are usually high grade and invasive, differing from sporadic cancers in that they are often aneuploid and of the basal type triple negative molecular subtype,[39,40] and exhibit 19% prevalence for the medullary subtype of invasive ductal carcinoma (IDC), a subtype rarely diagnosed in women with sporadic cancers (< 1%). *BRCA1*-associated breast cancers constitute 15% of medullary cancers in the general female population.

The BRCA2 Gene

The *BRCA2* gene located on chromosome 13 accounts for approximately 35% of familial breast cancers. *BRCA2* carriers have been known to confer a high risk for other cancers including prostate, colon, bladder, pancreatic, fallopian tube, and male breast. *BRCA2*-associated cancers are estrogen receptor positive (> 75%) and triple negative (16%).[41] They have been found to be of a higher histologic grade than tumors identified in age-matched control studies compared to sporadic cancers[42] and their rates of associated ductal carcinoma in situ (DCIS) are similar to rates found in sporadic breast cancers.[43,44] No increase in frequency of the medullary IDC subtype is found in these lesions. Mutations in other less common genes, such as the *TP53* and *PTEN* genes, are also known to confer a high risk for breast cancer, and women with these gene mutations should benefit from supplemental MRI screening as well.

An important metric for judging the success of breast cancer screening is not only the sensitivity of cancer detection and cancer size at diagnosis, but also the interval cancer rate. For average-risk women, the interval cancer rate at mammography screening is generally between 30 and 50%, the rate is about 20% in breast ultrasound screening and 0 to 6% rate for MRI screening of high-risk women. The low interval cancer rate at MRI screening is especially important, given that these cancers tend to be rapidly growing and aggressive. Rapid tumor growth, especially in young BRCA mutation carriers, accounts for the high interval cancer rate found at mammography screening, double that of nonmutation carriers.[13,45]

Women with a Lifetime Risk of 20 to 25% or Greater

How do we identify women with a risk of 20 to 25% or greater? The majority of high-risk women selected to undergo supplemental screening with MRI do not have an identified genetic mutation, but rather a strong family history of breast cancer. Estimation of breast cancer risk is usually calculated by applying models that primarily evaluate family history. The prediction model of breast cancer is a mathematical equation designed to quantify the risk that an individual woman would develop breast cancer within a defined period. Risk-prediction models that are commonly used in clinical practice include the Gail, Claus, and Tyrer–Cuzick BOADICEA and BRCRAPRO

models.[46,47,48,49,50] Among these prediction models, various factors are incorporated to quantify breast cancer risk and they differ from one model to another. For example, the Gail model factors in only a first-degree relative,[46] whereas the Tyrer–Cuzick model includes both family history and a history of a high-risk lesion diagnosis (lobular carcinoma in situ [LCIS] and atypical ductal hyperplasia [ADH]), not included in other risk-prediction models.[48] There are limitations to the consistency and accuracy of breast cancer risk-prediction models as shown in a recent meta-analysis that included 18 prediction models and 7 validating studies. The authors found only poor-to-fair discriminatory accuracy in internal and external validation and recognized an important need for development of a new reliable risk-prediction model.[51]

Nonetheless, although the current risk models are indeed imperfect, they remain the standard means of assessing breast cancer risk for the majority of the female population; indeed, most of the women who participated in the large prospective screening studies that evaluated breast MRI sensitivity and specificity were evaluated by these models. The 2000 and 2005 National Health Interview Survey and the National Cancer Institute Breast Cancer Risk Assessment Tool (Gail model 2) estimate that 880,063 (1.09%) of U.S. women aged 30 to 84 years have a lifetime absolute breast cancer risk of 20% or more, and are thus eligible for MRI screening.[52]

MRI Screening Trials of High-Risk Women

An early MRI screening study published by Kuhl et al in 2000 evaluated a cohort of 192 women with known or suspected carriers of a breast cancer gene mutation and found that of the 9 cancers diagnosed, 6 were visible only on MRI and were occult at mammography and ultrasound.[53] One of the largest MRI screening trials published by Kriege and colleagues in 2004 divided the patient cohort of 1,909 women into mutation carriers (50–85% lifetime risk), and women at high risk of developing breast cancer due to family history (20–29% lifetime risk) and the moderate risk group (15–20% risk). The overall rate of detection for all breast cancers both invasive and in situ was 9.5 per 1,000 woman-years at risk, with the highest rate, 26.5 per 1,000, in women with a known genetic mutation. The overall sensitivity of MRI was 79.5% compared to 17.9% for clinical breast examination and 33% for mammography.[28]

Multiple prospective high-risk screening studies followed these early reports, all aimed to compare the diagnostic accuracy of MRI with screening mammography with or without ultrasound (▶ Table 2.1). The risk factors for women recruited to these later studies varied widely, including women with a known, or likely, genetic mutation, women with a strong family or personal history of breast cancer, and women with a prior diagnosis of a high-risk lesion (LCIS or ADH).[29,30,54,55,56] Despite the differences in the entry risk criteria, reports yielded concordant results, finding that MRI screening was consistently more accurate than screening with mammography and ultrasound. The sensitivity of breast MRI in all studies was approximately 90% range (71–100%), significantly higher than that of mammography range (13–59%). When data from 11 studies were combined in a meta-analysis, it was found that there was an overall sensitivity of 77% for MRI alone, 94% for a combination of MRI and mammography, and 39% for mammography

Table 2.1 High-risk screening: comparative sensitivities

Author (year)	Cancer yield	MG	US	MR	Interval cancers	Cancer yield MR only
Sardanelli (2011)[89]	52/501 10%	50%	52%	91%	3	16/501 3.2%
Rijnsburger (2010)[90]	97/2,157 4%	41%	–	71%	13	44/2,157 2%
Hagen (2007)[91]	25/491 5%	50%	–	86%	5	8/491 1.6%
Lehman (2007)[92]	6/171 3.5%	33%	–	100%	N/A	4/171 2.3%
Kuhl (2005)[29]	43/529 8%	33%	40%	91%	1	19/529 3.6%
Leach (2005)[30]	35/649 5%	40%	–	77%	2	19/649 2.9%
Kreige (2004)[28]	51/1,909[a] 3%	40%	–	71%	4	22/1,909 1.2%
Warner (2004)[93]	22/266 9%	36%	33%	77%	1	7/236 3%

[a]24. 1 of 51 cancers detected was non-Hodgkin's lymphoma.

alone.[57] The relatively low sensitivity (71–77%) observed for MRI in the early screening trials can be explained in part by false-negative MRI diagnoses of DCIS. This problem is likely due to older technology with limited spatial resolution and lack of knowledge concerning the interpretive criteria necessary for recognition of the subtle nonmass findings seen in DCIS. A criticism of MRI in the early years of high-risk screening trials concerned the lower specificity of MRI than mammography. In recent years, the specificity of MRI has improved as radiologist experience has increased, and the current PPV3 of biopsy rates and short interval follow-up rates for MRI are comparable to those of mammography.

The EVA trial, published in 2010, studied intermediate- to high-risk women, investigating the respective contributions of screening with mammography, ultrasound and MRI, to the individual diagnosis of breast cancer.[58] The sensitivity of mammography alone was about 33%, similar to the findings in the ACRIN-DMIST trial[10] for digital mammography screening of women with BIRADS category (C) and (D) breast tissue density. The addition of ultrasound to mammography screening yielded an overall sensitivity of 48%, whereas MRI alone yielded a sensitivity of 93%. Three low-grade DCIS cancers in this trial were undetected at MRI. Nonetheless, the authors concluded that MRI could be used as a stand-alone imaging method because the missed cancers in this trial were low-grade lesions, considered "insignificant," thus preventing *overdiagnosis* of lesions that, if followed, would not harm the patient. The high sensitivity of MRI for biologically significant disease in this study could be viewed as a method of avoiding the problem of *underdiagnosis*, by identifying and treating small node-negative aggressive lesions that would harm the patient if left undetected.

Riedl et al conducted a prospective, nonrandomized comparison study in 2015, reporting on 559 women with 1,365 complete imaging rounds (2.45 rounds per woman) who underwent annual high-risk screening with mammography, ultrasound, and MRI.[59] Women entered into the study were high risk, either *BRCA1* or 2 mutation carriers (28%) (n = 156) or

those found to have a greater than 20% lifetime risk based on family history. MRI sensitivity (90%) was significantly higher than the sensitivity of mammography (37.5%), ultrasound (37.5%), and mammography combined with ultrasound (50%), (p < 0.001 for all methods). MRI identified all 14 cases of DCIS, mammography and ultrasound each detected 5 cases (35.7%), and a combination of mammography and ultrasound methods detected 7 cases (50%). No cancers were detected by ultrasound alone. The authors concluded that MRI allows early detection of breast cancer in high-risk patients regardless of patient's age, breast density, or risk status, and also proffered the opinion that when MRI screening is utilized, the added value of mammography is limited and there is no added value of ultrasound.

Today, the recommended screening protocol for women at high lifetime risk for breast cancer is a combination of annual mammography beginning at age 30 and MRI screening beginning at age 25. The two annual examinations can be scheduled at 6-month intervals.[60] Adding ultrasound to this protocol has not shown to increase cancer detection rates.[58] With increasing breast MRI expertise and technologic advances, routine use of screening mammography in high-risk women undergoing screening breast MR imaging is under question. A clinical service study by Lo and colleagues in Canada, published in 2017, sought to evaluate the added value of cancer detection of mammography when high-risk women undergo screening with MRI.[61] The cancer detection rate for MRI was 21.8 cancers per 1,000 examinations (95% confidence interval [CI]: 15.78, 29.19) and that for mammography was 7.2 cancers per 1,000 examinations (95% CI: 3.92, 11.97; p = 0.001). MRI detected smaller cancers than those detected on mammography. Sensitivity and specificity of MRI were 96 and 78% respectively, and those of mammography were 31% and 89%, respectively (p = 0.001). PPV for imaging recalls was 9.3% for MRI and 6.5% for mammography. The authors found no mammography screening benefit, that is, mammography depicted no MRI-missed cancers and concluded that the routine use of screening mammography in women undergoing screening breast MRI warrants reconsideration.

2.4 Women with a History of Chest Irradiation

Breast cancer is the leading cause of death in long-term survivors of mediastinal and chest irradiation, many of whom were treated for Hodgkin's lymphoma at a young age. The risk of subsequent development of breast cancer is greatest in those women who were treated between the ages of 10 and 30 years, because radiation sensitivity is highest in this age group.[62,63] Breast cancer risk has been shown to be highest among women treated during the time period from the early 1960s to the mid-1970s when higher radiation doses were used compared to subsequent years.[64] Studies have shown that the incidence of breast cancer in women with a history of irradiation is similar to that of women with a BRCA mutation, breast cancer occurring in about 13 to 20% of women by the age of 40 to 45. The ACS, ACR, and the Children's Oncology Group recommend annual screening MRI as an adjunct to mammography in women with a history of chest irradiation.[31] The screening protocol for women who have been treated with moderate- to high-dose mediastinal and/or chest irradiation includes annual screening with mammography and MRI beginning at 8 years following completion of treatment but not before age 25.[65,66] The cumulative radiation risk depends on the dose and volume of the radiation field and the time interval since therapy was completed.[62]

Two retrospective studies reported on the utility of supplemental breast MRI screening in women with a history of mediastinal/chest irradiation. Sung and colleagues performed a review of 247 screening examinations in 91 women and reported a 4.4% incremental cancer detection rate increase with MRI when compared to mammography. Ten cancers were identified in the study period. Among these, four cancers were seen on MRI alone (early-stage T1 invasive cancers) and three with mammography alone (DCIS and DCIS with microinvasion). The authors concluded that MRI is a useful adjunct to mammography screening in women with this history.[67] Other investigators reviewed the medical records of 98 patients with a prior history of chest radiation therapy; all had undergone both screening mammography and MRI between January 2004 and July 2010.[68] Analysis of 558 screening examinations (296 mammograms and 262 MRI) yielded an incremental cancer detection rate of 4.1% (95%, CI 1.6–10%). Of the 13 cancers detected, 12 (92%) were found on MRI and 9 (69%) by mammography. The median latency from completion of radiation to detection of the breast cancer was 18 years (range, 8–37 years). The authors concluded that both MRI and mammography should be used to screen women in this high-risk group.

Despite the recommendation that women with a history of chest irradiation benefit from screening with mammography and MRI, many women in this category are not adequately screened. Lack of compliance with MRI screening recommendations is evident in a study of women participating in the Childhood Cancer Survivor Study (CCSS), a North American cohort of long-term survivors diagnosed from 1970 to 1986.[66] In this group of women, 63.5% of those aged 25 through 39 years, and 23.5% of those aged 40 through 50 years, failed to be screened with mammography during the prior 2 years. Screening MRI was not included in the study design.

2.5 Women at Moderate Risk (15–20%)

Women who fall into this category include women with a personal history of invasive or in situ breast cancer, women with a prior biopsy or excision yielding a high-risk lesion such as ADH or lobular neoplasia, and women with heterogeneously dense or extremely dense breasts on mammography. Recent literature supports the use of screening MRI in addition to mammography in patients with a moderate risk of developing breast cancer. The 2018 ACR Practice Parameters for Breast MRI state that screening MRI may be considered as a supplement to mammography to screen women at intermediate (moderately elevated) risk of breast cancer (15%-20%). Annual screening MRI is also recommended for women with a personal history of breast cancer, those with dense tissue at mammography, or those women diagnosed with breast cancer under the age of 50.[32] Current guidelines also recommend that individual facilities in conjunction with referring clinicians may be in the best position to decide whether to screen these patients.[69] The NCCN and SBI/ACR guidelines also state that screening MRI should be considered in these moderate-risk patients.

2.5.1 Women with a Personal History of Breast Cancer

Women with a personal history of breast cancer are generally classified as moderate risk; the current recommendations by ASCO, the ACS, and the NCCN for surveillance of women with a personal history of breast cancer are clinical examination and mammography.[31,33,70,71] These women are at a higher risk of developing a breast cancer recurrence or a second breast cancer, depending on their age at cancer diagnosis and the presence of other risk factors. A retrospective review of breast MRI examinations in 144 women with a personal history of breast cancer, without a family history, evaluated the stage at diagnosis of recurrent lesions. Cancer was detected in 12% of women ($n = 18$) and of these, 10/18 cancers were solely identified on MRI. Of the 10 "MRI-only" cancers, 4/10 were noninvasive and 7/10 were minimal cancer lesions, defined as DCIS or node-negative invasive cancer less than 1 cm in size. The PPV of MRI screening was 39%.[72] Another study conducted between January 2008 and March 2012 in Korea followed 607 consecutive women (median age, 48 years; age range, 20–72 years) who had undergone BCS. Preoperative MRI was performed in 92% of the study cohort. All women had negative mammography and US findings and underwent posttreatment surveillance MRI. Of the cancers detected at MRI screening, 11 additional cancers were found, (18.1 cancers per 1,000 women), 8 invasive, 3 DCIS (median invasive size, 0.8 cm, range, 0.4–1.4 cm), all node negative. Results specified a PPV for recall of 9.4%, PPV for biopsy of 43.5%, sensitivity 91.7%, and specificity 82.2%.[73] Other beneficial supporting evidence for MRI screening in this group is found in a study that showed recurrent tumor to be more likely to be mammographically occult if the primary tumor before treatment was not visible at mammography.[74] A recent report on breast MRI screening in women ($n = 1,521$), by Lehman and colleagues,[75] found equally high cancer detection rates in women with a personal history (PH) but no known genetic or family history (GFH) of breast cancer, compared to the detection rates of patients of breast cancer in the GFH group. The overall MRI sensitivity was 79.4% for all cancers and 88.5% for invasive cancers. False-positive examinations were lower in the PH versus the GFH group (12.3 vs. 21.6%, $p < 0.001$), specificity was higher (94 vs. 86%, $p < 0.001$). Sensitivity and cancer detection rate were not statistically different ($p > 0.99$). More than half of the cancers detected were invasive, the latency period being 5 years after treatment. The authors concluded that the diagnostic performance of screening MRI is superior in women with a personal history of breast cancer compared with women with a genetic or family history of breast cancer.

The MRI screening results conducted on women with a personal history of breast cancer as shown above provide convincing evidence that MRI benefits these patients by detecting breast cancers while they are still small, node negative, and undetectable by other imaging methods (▶ Fig. 2.1).

2.5.2 Women with Diagnosis of a High-Risk Lesion

Breast biopsies performed for diagnosis of mammographic or ultrasound-detected abnormalities yield a diagnosis of ADH, LCIS, atypical lobular hyperplasia (ALH), or other high-risk lesions, in about 10% of biopsies.[76] Studies have shown that the lifetime risk of breast cancer in women with prior diagnosis of a high-risk lesion is about 30% when followed for 25 years.[77,78,79] Supplemental MRI surveillance is often recommended for these women in clinical practice.[80,81]

LCIS is usually an incidental histologic diagnosis without an imaging correlate, found in image-guided percutaneous biopsy specimens or surgical excisions. A diagnosis of LCIS is associated with a 7 to 12 increased relative risk of breast cancer[82,83] and is regarded to be a risk indicator for subsequent breast cancer in either breast, and a nonobligate precursor for development of invasive lobular carcinoma.[83,84] A few retrospective MRI studies have investigated patients with a history of LCIS. One review of 445 examinations in 198 patients reported that MRI detected malignancy in 3.8% (5/133) of patients with LCIS, with a median size of 0.8 cm. The authors concluded that breast MRI helped identify breast cancer in LCIS patients, at a rate similar to that shown in high-risk populations for whom screening breast MRI is consistently recommended.[85] Another retrospective review of 670 screening studies in 220 women with a history of LCIS found 17 cancers at screening MRI; 12 were identified only by MRI, the majority were small cancers (9 invasive; 3 DCIS). The results yielded a 4.5% incremental cancer detection rate at MRI.[80]

Scant data exist on the efficacy of screening MRI in patients with a history of ADH, yet many centers across the United States do provide MR screening for women with history of an ADH diagnosis.[86]

2.6 Women at Average Risk (<25%)

Current guidelines do not recommend breast cancer screening with MRI for women with a lifetime risk of less than 15%. A report by Kuhl et al, in 2017, however, investigated the efficacy of supplemental breast MRI screening of women at average lifetime risk (<15%).[87] This prospective observational study was conducted at two academic breast centers in women aged 40 to 70 years with a calculated lifetime breast cancer risk of 6 to 12% according to the Gail model. Women with normal conventional imaging findings (screening mammography with or without screening ultrasonography) were invited to undergo supplemental MRI screening; 2,120 women were recruited and underwent 3,861 screening MRI studies; 60 additional breast cancers

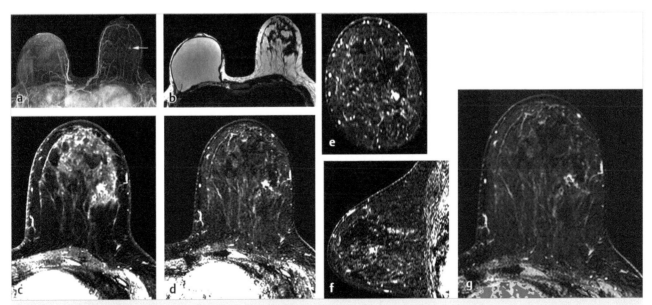

Fig. 2.1 Screen-detected cancer in a woman with a personal history of breast cancer. Patient age 37, without a family history of breast cancer, was treated for right breast DCIS 2 years ago, undergoing mastectomy and reconstruction with a silicone implant. MIP image (**a**, *arrow*) shows a 4-mm irregular enhancing mass in the left breast, without a correlate on the T2w series. A right breast silicone implant is noted (**b**). Postcontrast T1w image (**c**) and subtracted image (**d**) show margin irregularity with persistent kinetics noted on angiomap (**e**). Reformatted sagittal and coronal images are shown. Histology: DCIS intermediate/high grade at MRI-guided biopsy (**f, g**).

were depicted at MRI (DCIS, $n = 20$; invasive carcinoma, $n = 40$) for an overall supplemental MRI cancer detection rate of 15.5 per 1,000 cases (95% CI: 11.9, 20). Forty-eight additional cancers were detected with MRI at initial screening (supplemental cancer detection rate, 22.6 per 1,000 cases). During the 1,741 subsequent screening rounds, 12 of 13 incident cancers were found with MRI alone (supplemental cancer detection rate, 6.9 per 1,000 cases). Cancers diagnosed with MRI were small (median, 8 mm), node negative in 93.4% of cases, and were high grade in 41.7% of cases at prevalence screening and 46% of cases at incidence screening. No interval cancers were observed. MR imaging screening offered high specificity (97.1%) and high PPV (35.7%). Supplemental MRI screening in average-risk women was shown to improve early diagnosis of breast cancer with an additional cancer yield of 15.5 per 1,000 cases, a substantially higher rate than reported for supplemental, US, or digital breast tomosynthesis screening of similar cohorts. Both the biologic profile of the cancers diagnosed with MRI and the absence of interval cancers in this study, suggest that the cancers detected with MRI were prognostically relevant and would have progressed to clinical disease if left undetected.

2.7 Survival Benefit from Screening MRI

The hypothesis that early detection of breast cancer could decrease mortality from breast cancer was investigated in the Swedish trials of mammography screening. These trials showed a decrease in breast cancer mortality of about 30%. It is likely, therefore, that other screening methods, which are able to detect small node-negative breast cancers, should also be able to reduce mortality from breast cancer. Although it has been clearly shown that MRI is the most sensitive modality for breast cancer detection, no randomized clinical trial of MRI screening has been conducted to date; consequently, tumor size, interval cancer rate, and nodal status are used as surrogate markers of mortality. Warner and colleagues reported in 2011 on a prospective clinical trial that investigated the rate of advanced-stage breast cancer in women ($n = 1,275$), with and without MRI screening.[88] Women with a genetic mutation (*BRCA1* and *BRCA2*) were screened with mammography, and a subset of these women, ($n = 4450$) were additionally screened with MRI. All women were followed for a mean of 3.2 years. The cumulative incidence of DCIS, or stage1 breast cancer at 6 years, was 13.8% in the MRI-screened group and 7.2% in the comparison group ($p = 0.01$). The cumulative incidence of stages 2 to 4 grade cancers was 1.9% in the MRI-screened cohort and 6.6% in the comparison group ($p = 0.02$). The authors concluded that annual surveillance with MRI is associated with a significant reduction in the incidence of advanced-stage breast cancer in *BRCA1* and *BRCA2* carriers, and future studies designed to estimate the reduction of breast cancer–specific mortality is warranted.

2.8 Summary

Despite many years of screening, breast cancer still remains the second leading cause of cancer death in women, accounting for many "life years" lost. Mammography screening trials have shown the mortality benefit of early diagnosis; nonetheless, there is certainly room for improvement with new screening methods, such as tomosynthesis, ultrasound, and MRI.

In recent years, criticism of breast screening has focused on the concept of *over*diagnosis, the detection of nonprogressive, self-limiting breast cancers that would likely not result in life-threatening disease. Radiographic breast imaging (mammography and tomosynthesis) exhibits a propensity for detection of less aggressive cancer types such as calcifications and architectural distortions that are related to tumor necrosis or hypoxia, and are generally associated with a lower grade and a good prognosis. Rapidly growing aggressive noncalcified cancers, round or oval in shape, are often difficult to detect at mammography when the breast tissue is dense. MRI depends on contrast enhancement with angiogenesis for cancer detection, thus tending to identify high-grade lesions with a high proliferative index (Ki-67) and rapid growth. Screening trials of MRI that compared the added value of mammography concordantly found that the cancers not diagnosed at MRI were usually low-grade tumors, often DCIS, and of limited prognostic importance.

Finally, as we look beyond identification of the number of cancers found by different screening methods, we should also consider the biology of screen-detected cancers, specifically those with adverse pathologic profiles. It is increasingly evident that identification of small aggressive cancers at screening will have the greatest likelihood of achieving improved breast cancer mortality reduction, and in this respect, MRI has a distinct advantage.

References

[1] Global Cancer Facts & Figures 4th Edition: "Global cancer statistics 2018: GLOBOCAN estimates of incidence and mortality worldwide for 36 cancers in 185 countries, American Cancer Society journal, CA: A Cancer Journal for Clinicians.

[2] Skaane P, Bandos AI, Niklason LT, et al. Digital mammography versus digital mammography plus tomosynthesis in breast cancer screening: The Oslo tomosynthesis screening trial. Radiology. 2019; Feb 19182394, epub ahead of print

[3] Siegel RL, Miller KD, Jemal A. Cancer statistics, 2016. CA Cancer J Clin. 2016; 66(1):7–30

[4] American Cancer Society. Breast Cancer Facts & Figures 2017-2018. Atlanta: American Cancer Society, Inc. 2017.

[5] Tabár L, Vitak B, Chen TH, et al. Swedish two-county trial: impact of mammographic screening on breast cancer mortality during 3 decades. Radiology. 2011; 260(3):658–663

[6] Tabár L, Fagerberg CJ, Gad A, et al. Reduction in mortality from breast cancer after mass screening with mammography. Randomised trial from the Breast Cancer Screening Working Group of the Swedish National Board of Health and Welfare. Lancet. 1985; 1(8433):829–832

[7] Institute of Medicine. Saving Women's Lives: Integration and Innovation: A Framework for Progress in Early Detection and Diagnosis of Breast Cancer. Washington, DC: National Academies Press; 2005

[8] Smith RA, Duffy SW, Gabe R, Tabar L, Yen AM, Chen TH. The randomized trials of breast cancer screening: what have we learned? Radiol Clin North Am. 2004; 42(5):793–806, v

[9] Nickson C, Mason KE, English DR, Kavanagh AM. Mammographic screening and breast cancer mortality: a case-control study and meta-analysis. Cancer Epidemiol Biomarkers Prev. 2012; 21(9):1479–1488

[10] Pisano ED, Hendrick RE, Yaffe MJ, et al. DMIST Investigators Group. Diagnostic accuracy of digital versus film mammography: exploratory analysis of selected population subgroups in DMIST. Radiology. 2008; 246(2):376–383

[11] Tilanus-Linthorst M, Verhoog L, Obdeijn IM, et al. A BRCA1/2 mutation, high breast density and prominent pushing margins of a tumor independently contribute to a frequent false-negative mammography. Int J Cancer. 2002; 102(1):91–95

[12] Scheuer L, Kauff N, Robson M, et al. Outcome of preventive surgery and screening for breast and ovarian cancer in BRCA mutation carriers. J Clin Oncol. 2002; 20(5):1260–1268

[13] Komenaka IK, Ditkoff BA, Joseph KA, et al. The development of interval breast malignancies in patients with BRCA mutations. Cancer. 2004; 100(10):2079–2083

[14] McCormack VA, dos Santos Silva I. Breast density and parenchymal patterns as markers of breast cancer risk: a meta-analysis. Cancer Epidemiol Biomarkers Prev. 2006; 15(6):1159–1169

[15] Price ER, Hargreaves J, Lipson JA, et al. The California breast density information group: a collaborative response to the issues of breast density, breast cancer risk, and breast density notification legislation. Radiology. 2013; 269 (3):887–892

[16] Skaane P, Bandos AI, Eben EB, et al. Two-view digital breast tomosynthesis screening with synthetically reconstructed projection images: comparison with digital breast tomosynthesis with full-field digital mammographic images. Radiology. 2014; 271(3):655–663

[17] Friedewald SM, Rafferty EA, Rose SL, et al. Breast cancer screening using tomosynthesis in combination with digital mammography. JAMA. 2014; 311 (24):2499–2507

[18] Gilbert FJ, Tucker L, Young KC. Digital breast tomosynthesis (DBT): a review of the evidence for use as a screening tool. Clin Radiol. 2016; 71(2):141–150

[19] Berg WA, Zhang Z, Lehrer D, et al. ACRIN 6666 Investigators. Detection of breast cancer with addition of annual screening ultrasound or a single screening MRI to mammography in women with elevated breast cancer risk. JAMA. 2012; 307(13):1394–1404

[20] Brem RF, Tabár L, Duffy SW, et al. Assessing improvement in detection of breast cancer with three-dimensional automated breast US in women with dense breast tissue: the SomoInsight Study. Radiology. 2015; 274(3):663–673

[21] Hooley RJ, Greenberg KL, Stackhouse RM, Geisel JL, Butler RS, Philpotts LE. Screening US in patients with mammographically dense breasts: initial experience with Connecticut Public Act 09–41. Radiology. 2012; 265(1):59–69

[22] Sprague BL, Stout NK, Schechter C, et al. Benefits, harms, and cost-effectiveness of supplemental ultrasonography screening for women with dense breasts. Ann Intern Med. 2015; 162(3):157–166

[23] Kuhl CK, Schrading S, Strobel K, Schild HH, Hilgers RD, Bieling HB. Abbreviated breast magnetic resonance imaging (MRI): first postcontrast subtracted images and maximum-intensity projection-a novel approach to breast cancer screening with MRI. J Clin Oncol. 2014; 32(22):2304–2310.

[24] Lee CH, Dershaw DD, Kopans D, et al. Breast cancer screening with imaging: recommendations from the Society of Breast Imaging and the ACR on the use of mammography, breast MRI, breast ultrasound, and other technologies for the detection of clinically occult breast cancer. J Am Coll Radiol. 2010; 7(1):18–27

[25] Boetes C, Barentsz JO, Mus RD, et al. MR characterization of suspicious breast lesions with a gadolinium-enhanced TurboFLASH subtraction technique. Radiology. 1994; 193(3):777–781

[26] Orel SG, Schnall MD. MR imaging of the breast for the detection, diagnosis, and staging of breast cancer. Radiology. 2001; 220(1):13–30

[27] Liu PF, Debatin JF, Caduff RF, Kacl G, Garzoli E, Krestin GP. Improved diagnostic accuracy in dynamic contrast enhanced MRI of the breast by combined quantitative and qualitative analysis. Br J Radiol. 1998; 71(845):501–509

[28] Kriege M, Brekelmans CT, Boetes C, et al. Magnetic Resonance Imaging Screening Study Group. Efficacy of MRI and mammography for breast-cancer screening in women with a familial or genetic predisposition. N Engl J Med. 2004; 351(5):427–437

[29] Kuhl CK, Schrading S, Leutner CC, et al. Mammography, breast ultrasound, and magnetic resonance imaging for surveillance of women at high familial risk for breast cancer. J Clin Oncol. 2005; 23(33):8469–8476

[30] Leach MO, Boggis CR, Dixon AK, et al. MARIBS study group. Screening with magnetic resonance imaging and mammography of a UK population at high familial risk of breast cancer: a prospective multicentre cohort study (MARIBS). Lancet. 2005; 365(9473):1769–1778

[31] Saslow D, Boetes C, Burke W, et al. American Cancer Society Breast Cancer Advisory Group. American Cancer Society guidelines for breast screening with MRI as an adjunct to mammography. CA Cancer J Clin. 2007; 57(2):75–89

[32] American College of Radiology Practice Parameter for the Performance of Contrast enhanced Magnetic Resonance Imaging (MRI) of the Breast. Revised 2018 (Resolution 34). https://www.acr.org/-/media/ACR/Files/Practice-Parameters/mr-contrast-breast.

[33] Bevers TB, Anderson BO, Bonaccio E, et al. National Comprehensive Cancer Network. NCCN clinical practice guidelines in oncology: breast cancer screening and diagnosis. J Natl Compr Canc Netw. 2009; 7(10):1060–1096

[34] Foulkes WD. Inherited susceptibility to common cancers. N Engl J Med. 2008; 359(20):2143–2153

[35] Graeser MK, Engel C, Rhiem K, et al. Contralateral breast cancer risk in BRCA1 and BRCA2 mutation carriers. J Clin Oncol. 2009; 27(35):5887–5892

[36] Siegel RL, Miller KD, Jemal A. Cancer statistics, 2016. CA Cancer J Clin. 2016; 66(1):7–30

[37] Chen S, Parmigiani G. Meta-analysis of BRCA1 and BRCA2 penetrance. J Clin Oncol. 2007; 25(11):1329–1333

[38] Antoniou A, Pharoah PD, Narod S, et al. Average risks of breast and ovarian cancer associated with BRCA1 or BRCA2 mutations detected in case Series unselected for family history: a combined analysis of 22 studies. Am J Hum Genet. 2003; 72(5):1117–1130

[39] Rakha EA, Reis-Filho JS, Ellis IO. Basal-like breast cancer: a critical review. J Clin Oncol. 2008; 26(15):2568–2581

[40] Chappuis PO, Nethercot V, Foulkes WD. Clinico-pathological characteristics of BRCA1- and BRCA2-related breast cancer. Semin Surg Oncol. 2000; 18(4):287–295

[41] Mavaddat N, Barrowdale D, Andrulis IL, et al. HEBON, EMBRACE, GEMO Study Collaborators, kConFab Investigators, SWE-BRCA Collaborators, Consortium of Investigators of Modifiers of BRCA1/2. Pathology of breast and ovarian cancers among BRCA1 and BRCA2 mutation carriers: results from the Consortium of Investigators of Modifiers of BRCA1/2 (CIMBA). Cancer Epidemiol Biomarkers Prev. 2012; 21(1):134–147

[42] Bane AL, Beck JC, Bleiweiss I, et al. BRCA2 mutation-associated breast cancers exhibit a distinguishing phenotype based on morphology and molecular profiles from tissue microarrays. Am J Surg Pathol. 2007; 31(1):121–128

[43] Rapin V, Contesso G, Mouriesse H, et al. Medullary breast carcinoma. A reevaluation of 95 cases of breast cancer with inflammatory stroma. Cancer. 1988; 61(12):2503–2510

[44] Eisinger F, Jacquemier J, Charpin C, et al. Mutations at BRCA1: the medullary breast carcinoma revisited. Cancer Res. 1998; 58(8):1588–1592

[45] Tilanus-Linthorst MM, Obdeijn IM, Hop WC, et al. BRCA1 mutation and young age predict fast breast cancer growth in the Dutch, United Kingdom, and Canadian magnetic resonance imaging screening trials. Clin Cancer Res. 2007; 13(24):7357–7362

[46] Gail MH, Brinton LA, Byar DP, et al. Projecting individualized probabilities of developing breast cancer for white females who are being examined annually. J Natl Cancer Inst. 1989; 81(24):1879–1886

[47] Claus EB, Risch N, Thompson WD. Autosomal dominant inheritance of early-onset breast cancer. Implications for risk prediction. Cancer. 1994; 73(3):643–651

[48] Tyrer J, Duffy SW, Cuzick J. A breast cancer prediction model incorporating familial and personal risk factors. Stat Med. 2004; 23(7):1111–1130

[49] Berry DA, Iversen ES , Jr, Gudbjartsson DF, et al. BRCAPRO validation, sensitivity of genetic testing of BRCA1/BRCA2, and prevalence of other breast cancer susceptibility genes. J Clin Oncol. 2002; 20(11):2701–2712

[50] Antoniou AC, Cunningham AP, Peto J, et al. The BOADICEA model of genetic susceptibility to breast and ovarian cancers: updates and extensions. Br J Cancer. 2008; 98(8):1457–1466

[51] Anothaisintawee T, Teerawattananon Y, Wiratkapun C, Kasamesup V, Thakkinstian A. Risk prediction models of breast cancer: a systematic review of model performances. Breast Cancer Res Treat. 2012; 133(1):1–10

[52] Graubard BI, Freedman AN, Gail MH. Five-year and lifetime risk of breast cancer among U.S. subpopulations: implications for magnetic resonance imaging screening. Cancer Epidemiol Biomarkers Prev. 2010; 19(10):2430–2436

[53] Kuhl CK, Schmutzler RK, Leutner CC, et al. Breast MR imaging screening in 192 women proved or suspected to be carriers of a breast cancer susceptibility gene: preliminary results. Radiology. 2000; 215(1):267–279

[54] Warner E, Plewes DB, Hill KA, et al. Surveillance of BRCA1 and BRCA2 mutation carriers with magnetic resonance imaging, ultrasound, mammography, and clinical breast examination. JAMA. 2004; 292(11):1317–1325

[55] Lehman CD, Isaacs C, Schnall MD, et al. Cancer yield of mammography, MR, and US in high-risk women: prospective multi-institution breast cancer screening study. Radiology. 2007; 244(2):381–388

[56] Sardanelli F, Podo F, D'Agnolo G, et al. High Breast Cancer Risk Italian Trial. Multicenter comparative multimodality surveillance of women at genetic-familial high risk for breast cancer (HIBCRIT study): interim results. Radiology. 2007; 242(3):698–715

[57] Warner E, Messersmith H, Causer P, Eisen A, Shumak R, Plewes D. Systematic review: using magnetic resonance imaging to screen women at high risk for breast cancer. Ann Intern Med. 2008; 148(9):671–679

[58] Kuhl C, Weigel S, Schrading S, et al. Prospective multicenter cohort study to refine management recommendations for women at elevated familial risk of breast cancer: the EVA trial. J Clin Oncol. 2010; 28(9):1450–1457

[59] Riedl CC, Luft N, Bernhart C, et al. Triple-modality screening trial for familial breast cancer underlines the importance of magnetic resonance imaging and questions the role of mammography and ultrasound regardless of patient mutation status, age, and breast density. J Clin Oncol. 2015; 33(10):1128–1135

[60] Lowry KP, Lee JM, Kong CY, et al. Annual screening strategies in BRCA1 and BRCA2 gene mutation carriers: a comparative effectiveness analysis. Cancer. 2012; 118(8):2021–2030

[61] Lo G, Scaranelo AM, Aboras H, et al. Evaluation of the utility of screening mammography for high-risk women undergoing screening breast MR imaging. Radiology. 2017; 285(1):36–43

[62] Travis LB, Hill D, Dores GM, et al. Cumulative absolute breast cancer risk for young women treated for Hodgkin lymphoma. J Natl Cancer Inst. 2005; 97 (19):1428–1437

[63] Bhatia S, Yasui Y, Robison LL, et al. Late Effects Study Group. High risk of subsequent neoplasms continues with extended follow-up of childhood Hodgkin's disease: report from the Late Effects Study Group. J Clin Oncol. 2003; 21 (23):4386–4394

[64] Wahner-Roedler DL, Nelson DF, Croghan IT, et al. Risk of breast cancer and breast cancer characteristics in women treated with supradiaphragmatic radiation for Hodgkin lymphoma: Mayo Clinic experience. Mayo Clin Proc. 2003; 78(6):708–715

[65] Henderson TO, Amsterdam A, Bhatia S, et al. Systematic review: surveillance for breast cancer in women treated with chest radiation for childhood, adolescent, or young adult cancer. Ann Intern Med. 2010; 152(7):444–455, W144--W1-54

[66] Oeffinger KC, Ford JS, Moskowitz CS, et al. Breast cancer surveillance practices among women previously treated with chest radiation for a childhood cancer. JAMA. 2009; 301(4):404–414

[67] Sung JS, Lee CH, Morris EA, Oeffinger KC, Dershaw DD. Screening breast MR imaging in women with a history of chest irradiation. Radiology. 2011; 259 (1):65–71

[68] Freitas V, Scaranelo A, Menezes R, Kulkarni S, Hodgson D, Crystal P. Added cancer yield of breast magnetic resonance imaging screening in women with a prior history of chest radiation therapy. Cancer. 2013; 119(3):495–503

[69] American College of Radiology ACR Appropriateness Criteria® Date of origin: 2012 Last review date: 2016. Available at: https://acsearch.acr.org/docs/ 70910/Narrative/. Accessed May 20, 2017

[70] Khatcheressian JL, Hurley P, Bantug E, et al. American Society of Clinical Oncology. Breast cancer follow-up and management after primary treatment: American Society of Clinical Oncology clinical practice guideline update. J Clin Oncol. 2013; 31(7):961–965

[71] American Cancer Society; Breast Cancer Prevention and Early Detection. Available at: http://www.cancer.org/acs/groups/cid/documents/webcontent/ 003165-pdf. Accessed November 8, 2016

[72] Brennan S, Liberman L, Dershaw DD, Morris E. Breast MRI screening of women with a personal history of breast cancer. AJR Am J Roentgenol. 2010; 195(2):510–516

[73] Gweon HM, Cho N, Han W, et al. Breast MR imaging screening in women with a history of breast conservation therapy. Radiology. 2014; 272(2): 366–373

[74] Yang TJ, Yang Q, Haffty BG, Moran MS. Prognosis for mammographically occult, early-stage breast cancer patients treated with breast-conservation therapy. Int J Radiat Oncol Biol Phys. 2010; 76(1):79–84

[75] Lehman CD, Lee JM, DeMartini WB, et al. Screening MRI in women with a personal history of breast cancer. J Natl Cancer Inst. 2016; 108(3):djv349

[76] Simpson JF. Update on atypical epithelial hyperplasia and ductal carcinoma in situ. Pathology. 2009; 41(1):36–39

[77] Hartmann LC, Degnim AC, Santen RJ, Dupont WD, Ghosh K. Atypical hyperplasia of the breast—risk assessment and management options. N Engl J Med. 2015; 372(1):78–89

[78] Hartmann LC, Radisky DC, Frost MH, et al. Understanding the premalignant potential of atypical hyperplasia through its natural history: a longitudinal cohort study. Cancer Prev Res (Phila). 2014; 7(2):211–217

[79] Page DL, Schuyler PA, Dupont WD, Jensen RA, Plummer WD , Jr, Simpson JF. Atypical lobular hyperplasia as a unilateral predictor of breast cancer risk: a retrospective cohort study. Lancet. 2003; 361(9352):125–129

[80] Sung JS, Malak SF, Bajaj P, Alis R, Dershaw DD, Morris EA. Screening breast MR imaging in women with a history of lobular carcinoma in situ. Radiology. 2011; 261(2):414–420

[81] Londero V, Zuiani C, Linda A, Girometti R, Bazzocchi M, Sardanelli F. High-risk breast lesions at imaging-guided needle biopsy: usefulness of MRI for treatment decision. AJR Am J Roentgenol. 2012; 199(2):W240:-W2:50

[82] Simpson PT, Gale T, Fulford LG, Reis-Filho JS, Lakhani SR. The diagnosis and management of pre-invasive breast disease: pathology of atypical lobular hyperplasia and lobular carcinoma in situ. Breast Cancer Res. 2003; 5(5):258–262

[83] Arpino G, Laucirica R, Elledge RM. Premalignant and in situ breast disease: biology and clinical implications. Ann Intern Med. 2005; 143(6):446–457

[84] Rosen PP, Kosloff C, Lieberman PH, Adair F, Braun DW , Jr. Lobular carcinoma in situ of the breast. Detailed analysis of 99 patients with average follow-up of 24 years. Am J Surg Pathol. 1978; 2(3):225–251

[85] Friedlander LC, Roth SO, Gavenonis SC. Results of MR imaging screening for breast cancer in high-risk patients with lobular carcinoma in situ. Radiology. 2011; 261(2):421–427

[86] Bassett LW, Dhaliwal SG, Eradat J, et al. National trends and practices in breast MRI. AJR Am J Roentgenol. 2008; 191(2):332–339

[87] Kuhl CK, Strobel K, Bieling H, Leutner C, Schild HH, Schrading S. Supplemental breast MR imaging screening of women with average risk of breast cancer. Radiology. 2017; 283(2):361–370

[88] Warner E, Hill K, Causer P, et al. Prospective study of breast cancer incidence in women with a BRCA1 or BRCA2 mutation under surveillance with and without magnetic resonance imaging. J Clin Oncol. 2011; 29(13):1664–1669

[89] Sardanelli F, Podo F, Santoro F, et al. High Breast Cancer Risk Italian 1 (HIB-CRIT-1) Study. Multicenter surveillance of women at high genetic breast cancer risk using mammography, ultrasonography, and contrast-enhanced magnetic resonance imaging (the high breast cancer risk Italian 1 study): final results. Invest Radiol. 2011; 46(2):94105

[90] Rijnsburger AJ, Obdeijn IM, Kaas R, Tilanus-Linthorst MM, et al. BRCA1-associated breast cancers present differently from BRCA2-associated and familial cases: long-term follow-up of the Dutch MRISC Screening Study. J Clin Oncol. 2010 Dec 20;28(36):5265–5273

[91] Hagen AI, Kvistad KA, Maehle L, et al. Sensitivity of MRI versus conventional screening in the diagnosis of BRCA-associated breast cancer in a national prospective series. Breast. 2007 Aug;16(4):367–374. Epub 2007 Feb 21

[92] Lehman CD, Isaacs C, Schnall MD. Cancer yield of mammography, MR, and US in high-risk women: prospective multi institution breast cancer screening study. Radiology. 2007 Aug;244(2):381–388

[93] Warner E, Plewes DB, Hill KA, et al. Surveillance of BRCA1 and BRCA2 mutation carriers with magnetic resonance imaging, ultrasound, mammography, and clinical breast examination. JAMA. 2004 Sep 15;292(11):1317–1325

3 Screening MRI: DCE-MRI Methods

Federico D. Pineda, Gregory S. Karczmar, and Naoko Mori

Abstract

Dynamic contrast-enhanced MRI (DCE-MRI) is the most effective method for detection of breast cancer. MRI contrast agents are injected intravenously, and significantly decrease the longitudinal relaxation time (T1) of water. This increases signal intensity in heavily T1-weighted images. Large and rapid signal increases (enhancement) are detected in cancers relative to surrounding normal tissue, due to the increased blood supply and capillary permeability of cancers. Experienced radiologists can use DCE-MRI to efficiently and reliably identify lesions that are very likely to be cancers. In this chapter we review mechanisms of contrast enhancement and the distribution of contrast agents in the micro-environment of the breast. Then we discuss the MRI methods used to follow the uptake and washout of contrast agents and the physiologic parameters obtained from DCE-MRI. We discuss new approaches to sampling and reconstruction that can accelerate image acquisition and improve image quality. Very rapid imaging during the first 60 seconds after contrast injection, referred to as ultrafast DCE-MRI, increases sensitivity to cancers, facilitates quantitative, standardized image analysis, and allows measurement of new physiologic and morphologic parameters. Various methods of acquiring and reconstructing ultrafast (UF) DCE-MRI data will be discussed. These methods include ultrafast imaging with conventional Fourier sampling, sliding window or view sharing methods, and compressed sensing. While most commonly used MRI methods detect contrast agents using heavily T1-weighted images, contrast agents also produce large local magnetic field gradients that can be detected by susceptibility weighted MRI. We will discuss potential advantages of dynamic susceptibility weighted scans.

Keywords: Dynamic contrast enhanced MRI, T1-weighted images, blood flow, capillary permeability, image reconstruction, ultrafast DCE-MRI, view sharing reconstruction, sliding window reconstruction, compressed sensing, dynamic susceptibility weighted MRI

3.1 Introduction

Routine interpretation of dynamic contrast-enhanced magnetic resonance imaging (DCE-MRI) studies is based on signal intensity and how it changes with time after the injection of contrast media. Intrinsic lesion characteristics, acquisition parameters and concentration all play a role in signal enhancement. While the discrete categorization of lesion kinetics has been shown to be diagnostically useful, investigators have found that the descriptors of curve shape vary significantly between different scanners and acquisition parameters in malignant lesions. In this chapter, we will review the basic physiologic parameters for DCE-MRI and present new strategies based on significant improvements in MR hardware and new methods for image sampling and reconstruction. Various methods of acquiring ultrafast (UF) DCE-MRI will be discussed.

3.2 Rationale for Clinical Use of DCE-MRI

DCE-MRI is based on measurement of changes in the water proton signal following intravenous (IV) injection of MRI contrast agents. In routine clinical practice, the contrast agents are not detected directly, but rather through their effects on water proton relaxation. Most clinical applications rely on decreases in the longitudinal relaxation time (T1) of water molecules produced by low-molecular-weight chelates of gadolinium (III). Gadolinium (III) is strongly paramagnetic with seven unpaired electrons, and thus provides strong MRI contrast.[1,2,3] DCE-MRI data are generally acquired with gradient echo sequences with short repetition time (TR) and relatively large pulse angle, so that water proton magnetization is highly saturated.[4,5] As contrast agent passes through the arterial blood supply, arrives in each image voxel and leaks out of capillaries into the extracellular, extravascular space, the T1 of the water protons is shortened due to interactions with the large and fluctuating local magnetic field produced by the gadolinium.[2,3] This produces very easily detectable enhancement of the water signal, often as much as 300% of baseline intensity in routine clinical practice. The rate of enhancement following IV injection is used as a surrogate measure of perfusion as well as other physiologic and anatomic parameters such as contrast media distribution volume. Breast cancers are characterized by increased blood flow and increased capillary permeability associated with neoangiogenesis, resulting in more rapid enhancement and increased peak enhancement.[6] Thus, degree and rate of enhancement are primary markers for cancer on DCE-MRI.

The sensitivity of DCE-MRI of the breast has been uniformly high across many studies and meta-analyses. A recent analysis by Medeiros et al of 69 different studies found a pooled sensitivity of 90% (95% confidence interval [CI] 88–92%).[7] Individual studies have reported sensitivity ranging from 71 to 100%. Specificity of DCE-MRI, however, has a wide range of reported values, with individual studies finding specificity between 37% and 89%.[7] Medeiros et al reported a pooled specificity of 73% (95% CI 67–79%). However, this number is based on studies of high-risk women. The United States Preventative Task Force [8] cited the lack of studies of intermediate-risk women with MRI and the higher number of false-positives compared to mammography, as well as MRI's higher cost, as a basis for their decision that there is insufficient evidence to recommend MRI as a screening modality for all women.[9,10]

Recent studies have demonstrated the potential for advances in screening with DCE-MRI. Most of the studies cited above were performed at magnetic field strengths of 1.5 Tesla (T). While the majority of breast MRI examinations are currently performed at 1.5 T,[11] there has been a recent increase in the use of higher field strengths, specifically 3 T. Elsamaloty et al reported increased sensitivity and specificity of DCE-MRI performed at 3 T, finding values of 100 and 93.9%, respectively.[12] The authors noted that specificity increased from 92.8 to 94.5%

over the duration of the study. This is an indication that growing experience in the field may lead to an overall increase of specificity. In the first study of its kind, Kuhl et al recently reported on the results of an abbreviated MRI protocol for the screening of women at mildly to moderately increased risk.[8] The goal of this study was to determine the feasibility of replacing mammography with MRI screening. The abbreviated protocol consisted of one precontrast and one postcontrast acquisition. This protocol can be completed in less than 10 minutes, and thus the true cost of the scan is modest. This protocol was used to screen 443 women with sensitivity of 100% and specificity of 94.3%. These values demonstrate the potential of this technique for breast cancer screening of an intermediate-risk population and/or women with dense breasts.

3.3 How Contrast Media Distributes in the Breast

3.3.1 Perfusion, Capillary Permeability, Extracellular Distribution

Contrast media reaches various areas within the breast between 5 and 15 seconds after IV injection, approximately 6 to 30 seconds after reaching the heart. Cancers often enhance before normal breast tissue due to greater arterial blood supply and higher capillary permeability.[13] Clinically used contrast agents—usually gadolinium chelates—are believed to remain primarily in the extracellular space, although recent studies demonstrated some uptake by cells.[14] The commonly used two-compartment method models[15,16] delivery of contrast media to tissue using a plasma compartment in the blood and an extracellular, extravascular compartment. Both compartments are assumed to be well mixed on the MRI time scale, so that the amount of contrast media in each compartment can be represented by a single concentration. The two-compartment model is discussed in more detail in Chapter 12.

In fact, this simple model may not be consistent with normal mammary gland anatomy and the distribution of low molecular weight contrast agents. In normal mammary glands, capillary networks traverse the stroma and reach the edge of epithelia surrounding the mammary ductal lumens. Contrast media

molecules are released initially in the stroma, and then leak into the extracellular space in the epithelia. There is evidence to suggest that, after diffusing through stroma and into epithelium, contrast media eventually leaks into ductal lumens.[17,18] This is demonstrated by the fact that the contrast media is found in breast milk.[19] X-ray fluorescent studies of the distribution of gadolinium in mouse models of breast/mammary cancer provide important information regarding the contrast media distribution of contrast media in the mammary gland over time. To obtain X-ray fluorescent microscopic (XFM) images of gadolinium concentration in the mammary gland microenvironment as a function of time, mice were sacrificed at various times after contrast media injection and mammary gland tissue samples were frozen and prepared for XFM.[18,20] XFM results show a very heterogeneous distribution of contrast agent molecules (based on gadolinium concentration) in the stroma and epithelia surrounding ductal lumens (▶ Fig. 3.1). This supports the work of Yankeelov et al[21] suggesting that diffusion of contrast agent in the extravascular space may significantly affect the results of pharmacokinetic analysis. In addition, XFM shows leakage of contrast media in ductal lumens, with increasing concentrations in ducts with in situ cancer. This suggests that ductal permeability may be a marker for early preinvasive cancer.

In general, the concentrations of contrast media in the stroma, epithelia, and lumen of mouse mammary glands measured by XFM are very different, and the relative concentrations of contrast media in these compartments change as a function of time postinjection. If this is the case in the human breast, then a simple two-compartment model does not accurately describe the uptake and washout of contrast media in the breast.

A number of more complicated models for contrast media dynamics have been proposed and tested.[13,16,22] Addition of more compartments can improve fits to data, but the correspondence between the compartments in these models and the structural elements of mammary glands is not well understood. In addition, complicated models with multiple adjustable parameters can only be used effectively when signal-to-noise ratio (SNR) is very high, and this is rarely the case in routine clinical imaging.

The unidirectional flow model is an alternative to the use of multiple compartments.[23,24,25,26,27] This method applies to data acquired during the very early phase of contrast media uptake

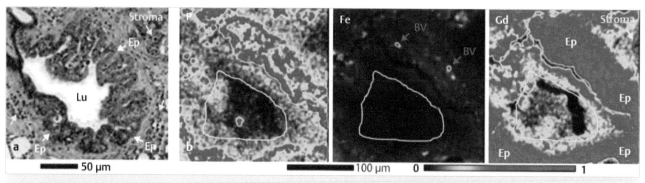

Fig. 3.1 Ex vivo H&E and XFM images of an excised mammary gland from a SV40 mouse with early in situ cancer. The mouse was sacrificed at 2 minutes after gadodiamide injection. (a) An H&E image of a mouse mammary gland; Epithelium ("Ep"), lumen ("Lu") and surrounding stroma (yellow arrows) are labeled. (b) XFM images of P, Fe, and Gd distributions (with 0.3 μm in-plane resolution) in mouse mammary stroma, epithelium and lumen containing an in-situ cancer. Yellow lines indicate the ductal lumen. The orange-red areas (high concentrations) in the Gd map are in the epithelial layer ("Ep") but there is also significant Gd in the lumen and stroma, blood vessels (BV) are indicated by red arrows in the Fe image.

and approximates that the flow of contrast media is exclusively from the capillaries into tissue, with minimal backflow. This is a simple method that does not require a detailed understanding of contrast media distribution in the extravascular space but can only be used when very high temporal resolution imaging is performed to detect the early contrast media kinetics (more details are provided later in this chapter).

3.4 Data Acquisition Methods

3.4.1 Contrast Agent Injection

Contrast media is injected I.V. using an automated syringe at speeds of 2 to 3 mL/s. The concentration of contrast media in the injection solution is typically 500 mM in gadolinium. Therefore, a dose of 0.1 mM/kg is injected in approximately 15 mL of contrast media solution (about 7.5 mM for a 75 kg person), followed by a 20 mL saline flush. The entire dose is injected over 10 to 15 seconds. The contrast media bolus is broadened as it passes through the heart, lungs and vasculature, so that the width of the bolus when it reaches the tissue of interest is typically increased by an additional 5 to 10 seconds by the time it reaches the breast. Therefore, the width at half-height of the contrast media bolus when it reaches the breast is 20 to 30 seconds.[28,29] However, Gadavist (gadobutrol), the only contrast agent approved specifically for breast imaging to date,[30] contains 1 M gadolinium, and therefore injection volume is about 7.5 mL, and injections require 7 to 8 seconds. This is expected to produce a somewhat sharper arterial input function (AIF) in the breast. For conventional clinical DCE-MRI, with temporal resolution of 60 to 90 seconds per image, the width of the arterial input function has no influence on diagnostic accuracy. However, when ultrafast DCE-MRI is used to detect the early kinetics of contrast media injection, shorter injections with more concentrated contrast agent solutions may be helpful.[31,32,33,34,35]

3.4.2 Standard Acquisition Protocols: 60 to 120 Second Scans

Standard DCE-MRI acquisition protocols consist of a series of T1-weighted (short repetition and echo times) spoiled gradient echo acquisitions before and after the administration of GBCA (see contrast injection section above), with or without fat suppression. The American College of Radiology recommends imaging with an in-plane resolution of at least 1 mm × 1 mm with a slice thickness of no more than 3 mm, with scans run bilaterally (i.e., both left and right breast present in the same series), and data acquired at intervals of 120 seconds or less. Typically, DCE-MRI protocols have temporal resolutions ranging from 60 to 120 seconds, and with imaging for 5 minutes or longer after the injection of contrast media. ▶ Table 3.1 compares parameters for conventional clinical DCE-MRI with the ultrafast protocol currently used clinically at the University of Chicago.

A number of different methods have been developed to separate the water signal from the very large fat signal and allow detailed evaluation of the water-containing tissues where almost all cancers are found. Spectrally selective fat saturation (e.g. CHESS[36,37,38]) takes advantage of the frequency difference between fat and water resonance to minimize the fat magnetization. To further improve fat suppression, spectrally selective

inversion recovery methods take advantage of the frequency and T1 differences between fat and water to acquire signal when the fat signal is nulled.[36,39,40] Dixon-type sequences are used to provide images with low spectral resolution, and a number of different algorithms are used to calculate relatively pure fat and water images from these data.[41,42,43] Data acquired with higher spectral resolution, as in high spectral and spatial resolution imaging (HiSS[44,45]), provide improved fat and water separation at the cost of increased run times. Both spectrally selective excitation methods and spectroscopic methods are sensitive to the T2* effects of contrast agents that result in decreased signal intensity during the first pass of the contrast media bolus. All these methods entail a tradeoff between fat suppression efficiency, sensitivity to T2* effects of contrast media, power deposition, SNR, and run time. The optimal fat suppression method will vary depending on the characteristics of the MRI scanner, especially field strength. An understanding of the different fat-suppression options allows radiologists to adopt the most appropriate technique for their clinical practice.

3.4.3 High Temporal-Resolution ("Ultrafast") DCE-MRI

Standard clinical contrast enhanced scans are performed with high spatial resolution to facilitate morphological evaluation of lesions and detect small cancers.[46,47,48] The high spatial resolution required, combined with the large fields-of-view necessary to acquire bilateral images, leads to low temporal resolution. As a result, important kinetic information is obscured.

Acquiring DCE-MRI with high temporal resolution is important, as it allows accurate classification of contrast media dynamics in suspicious lesions, and thus aids discrimination between malignant and benign lesions. In addition, high temporal resolution allows accurate measurement of the AIF for each patient, a critical step in quantitative pharmacokinetic analysis.[29,49,50,51,52,53,54] However, the early events in contrast

Table 3.1 Acquisition parameters for fast and high spatial resolution sequences

Parameter	Fast	High spatial resolution
TR/TE (ms)	3.2/1.6	4.8/2.4
Acquisition voxel size (mm³)	1.5 × 1.5 × 3.0	0.8 × 0.8 × 1.6
SENSE acceleration factor (RL)	4	2.5
SENSE acceleration factor (FH)	2	2
Halfscan (partial Fourier) factor	0.75 (ky); 0.85 (kz)	0.85 (ky); 1 (kz)
Temporal resolution range (s)	3.5–9.9	60–79.5
Number of slices	100–120	187–225
Flip angle	10°	10°
Field-of-view (mm)	300–370	300–370
Fat suppression method	SPAIR (TR: 155 ms; inversion delay: 80 ms)	SPAIR (TR: 155 ms; inversion delay: 80 ms)

Abbreviations: TE, echo time; TR, repetition time.

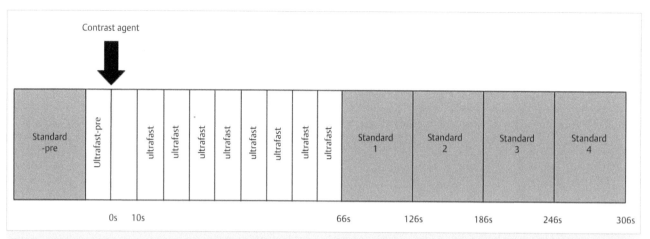

Fig. 3.2 Scanning protocol for 3 T (7-second ultrafast scanning).

media uptake in normal breast and breast lesions have not been well characterized. Thus, it is difficult to know what temporal resolution is optimal for breast MRI. Ultrafast imaging can be included in both a screening and a diagnostic protocol. One standard acquisition after the ultrafast sequence is sufficient for an abbreviated protocol, whereas the standard 4 or 5 sequences can be added to ultrafast for a diagnostic examination. A diagram of an example protocol including ultrafast imaging can be seen in ▶ Fig. 3.2. Recently several groups have reported promising results with ultrafast protocols,[31,32,33,35,54,55] and some groups have substituted the first post-contrast DCE-MRI phase in standard protocols with a series of ultrafast images, some of these results and approaches are summarized in the following sections.

Conventional Fourier Sampling Ultrafast Methods

Jansen et al,[35] Pinker et al,[54] and Planey et al[56] used the conventional Fourier sampling methods to image contrast media uptake in the breast at high temporal resolution. Improvements in temporal resolution in these studies came at the expense of either greatly reduced coverage, or lower spatial resolution than standard clinical scans (e.g., Pinker et al reduced spatial resolution from 1 mm to 1.7 mm isotropic voxels).[54] Nevertheless, these studies showed advantages in conspicuity of pre-invasive lesions, and estimation of pharmacokinetic parameters compared to standard, low temporal resolution, clinical scans.

Studies at the University of Chicago characterized the kinetics of early enhancement in arteries, veins, malignant lesions, benign lesions, and normal-appearing parenchyma; and evaluated the performance of parameters descriptive of early kinetics in differentiating malignant versus benign lesions. Potential advantages in lesion detectability were also investigated. The protocol used the conventional Fourier sampling to allow robust quantitative analysis and a novel filtering and analysis method to identify rapidly enhancing lesions. The acquisition protocol used in these studies can be easily implemented in a clinical setting, regardless of vendor or scanner type. Images were acquired at lower spatial resolution and relatively high SENSE (parallel imaging) acceleration factors during

the first minute postcontrast injection, to produce full bilateral, fat-suppressed breast images with temporal resolution ranging between 6.2 and 9.9 seconds (higher temporal resolutions are possible with this protocol, particularly at 3 T). Following an initial 60 seconds of fast imaging, subsequent images were acquired using a standard clinical protocol with high spatial resolution, intermediate SENSE factors, and low temporal resolution. ▶ Table 3.1 compares acquisition parameters for the conventional DCE-MRI and the ultrafast imaging.

The ultrafast images during the first minute after contrast media injection provide detailed information regarding the early kinetics in the breast, while later high spatial resolution acquisitions allow assessment of the morphology of small lesions. The results provide new information regarding contrast media uptake kinetics during the first minute after injection and demonstrate the potential diagnostic utility of high temporal resolution imaging.

In an initial pilot study,[31,32] ultrafast DCE-MRI was performed on 23 patients with biopsy proven lesions or lesions detected on prior imaging, including a mix of ductal carcinoma in situ (DCIS), invasive cancers, and benign lesions. The study was performed on a Philips Achieva 3T-TX scanner using a 16-channel bilateral breast coil. The DCE series consisted of one standard clinical acquisition, ultrafast acquisitions for 50 to 80 seconds after injection, followed by four standard clinical acquisitions (with the protocols described in ▶ Table 3.1). Contrast media (0.1 mM/kg gadobenate dimeglumine; MultiHance, Bracco, NJ) was injected IV at 2 mL/s.

Arterial enhancement was easily visualized in maximum intensity projections (MIPs), identifying the time at which the contrast media reaches the breast. Thus, lesion enhancement was measured relative to the time of arrival of the contrast bolus in the mammary arteries, rather than the time of injection. This removed variability due to systemic physiology, for example, cardiac output. A digital filter was developed to identify significantly enhancing voxels, and to reduce spurious enhancement due to noise or artifacts. Only pixels with significant and stable enhancement were used for kinetic analysis.

Regions of interest (ROIs) were drawn around the lesions on ultrafast and standard clinical images (at each time point), under radiologists' guidance, and average signal enhancement was measured at each time point. Background parenchymal enhancement (BPE) was measured for all cases by manually segmenting the parenchyma in a slice in the central part of the breast without any lesions present and measuring the average signal intensity at each time-point. The signal intensity in the blood vessels feeding the lesions was also measured for each time point. Percent signal enhancement (PSE) versus time data were fit to a truncated (uptake only) empirical mathematical model (EMM) for malignant lesions, benign lesions, and parenchyma,[57,58] for only the high temporal resolution time-points[57,58,59]

$$PSE(t) = A(1 - \exp(-\alpha t)), \qquad (3.1)$$

where A is the upper limit of percent enhancement, and α is the uptake rate (sec^{-1}). From the EMM parameters, three secondary parameters were calculated: (1) initial area under the contrast enhancement versus time curve (iAUC),[60] (2) time to 90% of maximum enhancement (T90), and (3) initial slope (defined as the product of the uptake rate and the upper limit of enhancement). T90 was used as a surrogate for time-to-peak enhancement.

Lesion conspicuity was quantified by calculating the ratio of signal increase in the lesion to the signal increase of normal parenchyma at each time-point:

$$r(t) = \frac{(S(t) - S_0)_{lesion}}{(S(t) - S_0)_{parenchyma}}. \qquad (3.2)$$

MIPs from ultrafast DCE-MRI (▶ Fig. 3.3 a-d) standard subtractions, (▶ Fig. 3.3g,h) enhancement gradient, show signal increase in the vessels, including very early enhancement in tortuous vessels directly feeding tumors followed by signal increase in the tumors. The enhancement gradient images (each image subtracted from the immediately succeeding image) show a slowing signal increase in the arteries, and in ▶ Fig. 3.3g a blood vessel posterior and lateral to the lesions is seen enhancing immediately after enhancement of the lesion; this is likely a vein draining the tumor. For most cases (19 out of 20), significant arterial enhancement (> 20%) was measured in the second or third ultrafast postcontrast image, in the internal mammary artery. For three cases, the vessel feeding the lesion began to enhance at the same time as the internal mammary artery. In all other cases, the vessel feeding the lesion enhanced later than the internal mammary artery.

The average percentage of significantly enhancing voxels in the whole field-of-view (FOV) started at 0.4% of the FOV at the first time-point post injection (when in most cases only the heart was enhanced) and monotonically rose to 5.7 ± 1.9% at the fourth time point, and 7.3 ± 2.5% of the entire FOV by the

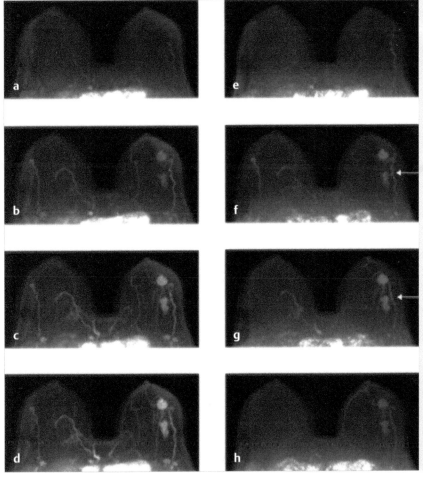

Fig. 3.3 Maximum-intensity projections (MIPs) of ultrafast subtractions (**a–d**) and enhancement gradient images (**e, g, h**). Two invasive ductal carcinomas are visible on the right in each image. Images were acquired with 9 second temporal resolution. *Arrows* point to vessels feeding and draining a lesion (**f**) in the arterial and venous phases.

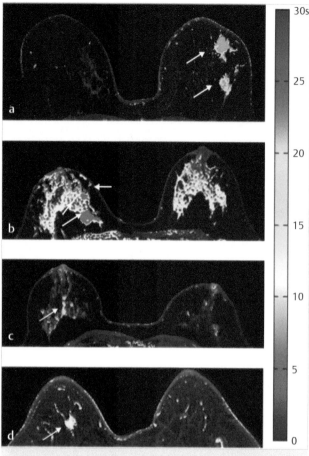

Fig. 3.4 Examples of time-to-enhancement (TTE) maps, lesions marked with arrows: (**a, b**) IDC; (**c**) complex sclerosing lesion; and (**d**) fibroadenoma.

last ultrafast acquisition. This means that enhancement at early times after contrast injection is very sparse.

Time-to-enhancement (TTE) maps were created as a way of visualizing the time at which lesions began enhancing and the heterogeneity of the TTE within lesions. Examples of these maps can be seen in (▶ Fig. 3.4), for both malignant and benign lesions. The results shown are typical of the lesions imaged; the average TTE was much shorter ($p < 0.01$) for malignant lesions (18.4 ± 12.9 seconds) than for benign lesions (43.5 ± 36.1 seconds). Intralesion heterogeneity in TTE can also be appreciated in these maps. In benign ROIs, the average intralesion coefficient of variation in TTE was 0.58 ± 0.37, and in malignant lesions was 0.38 ± 0.51. Thus, heterogeneous enhancement patterns at early times after injection may be an additional marker for cancers that is only available from ultrafast DCE-MRI.

Average signal enhancement from the ROIs, as a function of time relative to the time of injection, is plotted in (▶ Fig. 3.5) for malignancies ($n = 18$), benign findings ($n = 15$), and BPE ($n = 20$). On average malignancies enhanced strongly throughout the first minute relative to benign lesions and parenchyma. The average EMM fits to the data from malignant lesions, benign lesions, and parenchyma are also plotted as solid lines, using the average value of arterial time-of-arrival, 11.6 ± 5.8 seconds relative to the injection time, for illustration purposes. Significant differences (post-Bonferroni corrections) were found

between benign and malignant lesions for EMM parameters related to the rate of early enhancement.

Lesion conspicuity (across all lesions) was highest during the early ultrafast acquisitions, particularly at the fourth ultrafast acquisition postinjection, where its average was 11:1. The difference between ultrafast and conventional acquisitions was most pronounced in cases with marked BPE. For all these cases, the maximum conspicuity of the lesions occurs too early to be detectable in the standard clinical protocol. Subtraction images for three-time points sampled with ultrafast imaging and the first time-point of the standard clinical protocol, from two of the cases (a fibroadenoma and a satellite invasive ductal carcinoma [IDC]) can be seen in (▶ Fig. 3.6).

These preliminary results show that ultrafast imaging accurately measures the early kinetics of enhancement in lesions, blood vessels, and parenchyma. Ultrafast imaging allowed analysis of the TTE data with respect to the time of initial arterial enhancement. In addition the speed of propagation of the arterial bolus can be measured - and used to estimate arterial blood flow. This is not possible in conventional DCE-MRI with temporal resolution more than 1 minute. As a result, ultrafast imaging allows evaluation of the local vasculature characteristics while reducing the influence of global variables such as cardiac output. The results suggest that ultrafast imaging may detect early enhancement of lesions that occurs before parenchymal enhancement, thus making lesions more conspicuous; this is especially useful in cases with marked parenchymal enhancement (i.e., younger women).[61,62,63] This is consistent with earlier results obtained by scanning a limited number of slices (include suspicious lesions and their surroundings) with 7-second temporal resolution and demonstrating that this approach detects significant differences between the early enhancement of DCIS and normal parenchyma, thus improving conspicuity of small diffuse cancers. The differences in average values of some of the kinetic parameters between benign and malignant lesions were very large, suggesting a large dynamic range for ultrafast parameters.

Although the current protocol used clinically at the University of Chicago allows detection of approximate "initial time of enhancement" in arteries and veins, the temporal resolution is not adequate to resolve the detailed shape of the contrast media bolus. Higher temporal resolution would allow accurate measurement of the AIF and precise arrival time of the bolus. These parameters can be combined with standard measures of contrast media uptake to increase diagnostic accuracy.

This study was performed on a 3 T scanner, while the majority of clinical scans in the United States are performed at 1.5 T.[11] A similar protocol has been implemented on a 1.5 T scanner with somewhat lower temporal resolution (at least 9 seconds) and good image quality. The protocol described here is used as the clinical protocol at the University of Chicago (at both 1.5 T and 3 T).

Mori et al implemented a similar ultrafast protocol at 1.5 T with a temporal resolution of 10 seconds (▶ Table 3.2). Image quality and enhancement kinetics of lesions were evaluated in a study of 33 patients imaged with this protocol, with 33 lesions present (15 benign and 18 malignant). SNR was calculated for each case using the method described by Yu et al.[64] The SNR of the ultrafast DCE MRI was found to be lower than that of the standard DCE-MRI acquisition, however the difference was not

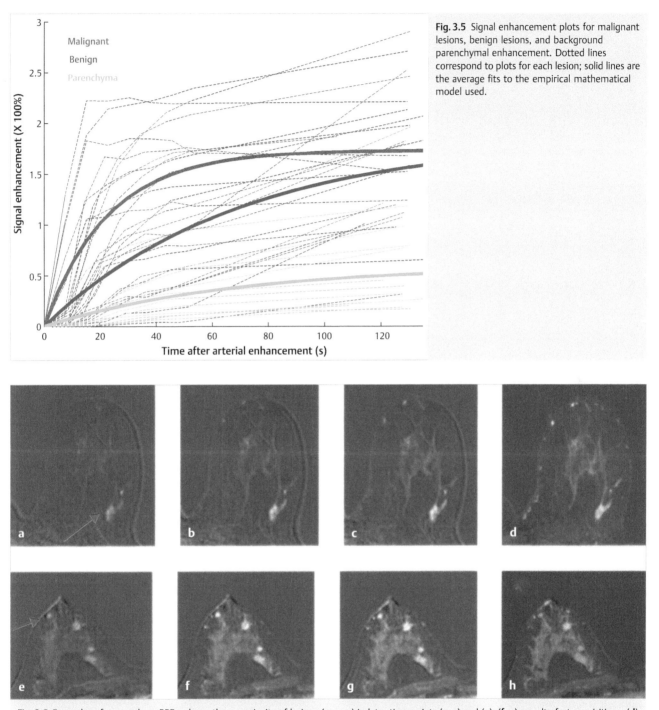

Fig. 3.5 Signal enhancement plots for malignant lesions, benign lesions, and background parenchymal enhancement. Dotted lines correspond to plots for each lesion; solid lines are the average fits to the empirical mathematical model used.

Fig. 3.6 Examples of cases where BPE reduces the conspicuity of lesions (*arrows*) in later time points (**a–c**) and (**e**); (**f, g**) are ultrafast acquisitions; (**d**) and (**h**) high spatial resolution images acquired approximately 2 minutes post-injection. Lesions were (**a, b**) and (**d**) a fibroadenoma that is visible as an oval circumscribed mass in the early images, and (**e–h**) a satellite invasive ductal carcinoma clearly defined in (**f**) and (**g**) but is less conspicuous in (**h**).

statistically significant (▶ Fig. 3.7a). Lesion contrast-to-noise ratio was calculated by comparing the signals in the fibroglandular tissue and the lesions of interest (as described by Song et al).[65] The CNR in the phase when enhancement in the aorta was first detected, and in the time point immediately following it were lower than in the rest of the ultrafast phases and in the initial standard DCE phase (▶ Fig. 3.7b). Lesion conspicuity with respect to BPE was also calculated; lesion conspicuity (or contrast ratio) was higher in the ultrafast images than in the early standard images. However, these differences were not significant (▶ Fig. 3.7c). The difference in the lesion conspicuity between ultrafast and conventional images was most pronounced in cases with marked BPE.

In another study by Mori et al,[66] this one performed on a 3T scanner (▶ Table 3.3), the performance of using early lesion enhancement for classification of lesions was assessed.

Table 3.2 Acquisition parameters for ultrafast and standard scans: 1.5 T system

Parameter	Ultrafast	Standard
TR/TE (ms)	4.7/2.3	5.5/2.7
Voxel size (mm³)	1.5 × 1.5 × 3.5	0.8 × 0.8 × 2
SENSE acceleration factor (RL)	4	3
SENSE acceleration factor (FH)	2	2
Half-scan factor	0.75 (ky); 0.85 (kz)	0.85 (ky); 1 (kz)
Temporal resolution	10	60
Number of slices	110	200
Flip angle	12	
Field-of-view (mm)	360	
Fat-suppression method	SPAIR (TR: 245 ms; inversion delay: 110 ms)	

Abbreviations: TE, echo time; TR, repetition time.

Table 3.3 Acquisition parameters for ultrafast and standard scans: 3 T system

Parameter	Ultrafast	Standard
TR/TE (ms)	2.8/1.5	5.2/2.6
Voxel size (mm³)	1.1 × 1.7 × 4	0.7 × 1.2 × 1.8
SENSE acceleration factor (RL)	3.2	1.6
SENSE acceleration factor (FH)	2.2	1
Half-scan factor	0.7 (ky); 0.7 (kz)	0.75 (ky); 0.8 (kz)
Temporal resolution (s)	3	60
Number of slices	80	170
Flip angle	10	
Field-of-view (mm)	350	
Fat-suppression method	SPAIR (TR: 153 ms; inversion delay: 57 ms)	

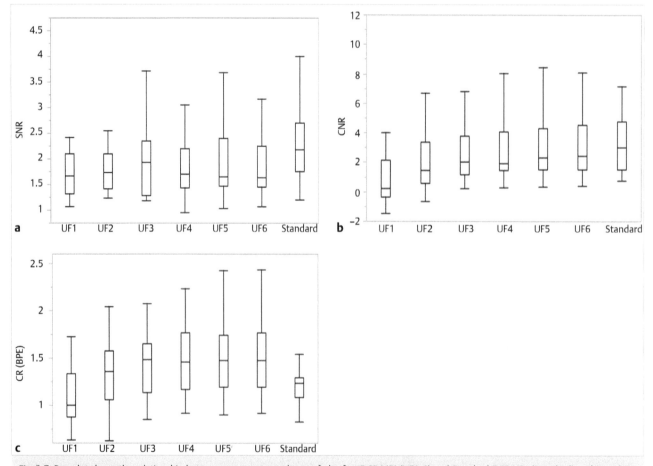

Fig. 3.7 Box-plot shows the relationship between post-contrast phases of ultrafast DCE-MRI (UF1-6) and Standard DCE-MRI (Standard) and Signal-to-noise ratio (SNR) **(a)**, Contrast noise ratio (CNR) **(b)** and Contrast Ratio (CR) to background parenchyma (BPE) (CR (BPE)) **(c)**. In **(a)** there was no significant difference between SNR of ultrafast DCE-MRI (UF1-6) and standard DCE-MRI (Standard). In **(b)** CNR of UF1 and UF2 was lower than that of UF 3, UF4, UF5, UF6 and standard DCE-MRI (Standard). **(c)** shows that CR (BPE) of UF2, UF3, UF4, UF5 and UF6 was higher than that of standard DCE-MRI (Standard).

Thirty-seven patients with 15 benign and 22 malignant lesions were included in this analysis. Axial maximum projection images using this 3 second ultrafast protocol at 3 T are shown in ▶ Fig. 3.8. Relative enhancement rate was calculated in a voxel-by-voxel basis in each lesion ROI. The percent lesion enhancement in the different ultrafast phases was compared between benign and malignant lesions by analyzing the histograms of relative enhancement for the entire ROI. The values from the 50th percentile of the histograms up to the maximally enhancing voxels were calculated for each lesion. Statistically significant differences were found between the relative enhancement of benign and malignant lesions, especially in the first 2 time points following aortic enhancement. For example, the 90th percentile values of enhancement in the first time-point following aortic enhancement were 111 ± 67%, and 26 ±

29% for malignant and benign lesions, respectively. For the following ultrafast phase, these values were 160 ± 61% and 57 ± 53%, again for malignant and benign lesions, respectively. These two phases were recommended by the authors as the most effective in which to detect the differential leakage of contrast agent between benign and malignant lesions.

Pinker et al reported that a combined high temporal and high spatial resolution protocol (similar to the ones described above) allowed accurate detection and assessment of breast lesions, with a sensitivity of 100% and specificity of 72.2%.[54] In this study, ultrafast DCE images were acquired from 34 patients with a temporal resolution of roughly 13 seconds, and contrast media kinetics were sampled for 3.5 minutes after the injection of contrast.

In addition to potentially increased sensitivity, ultrafast imaging may also improve specificity by ruling out cancer in cases

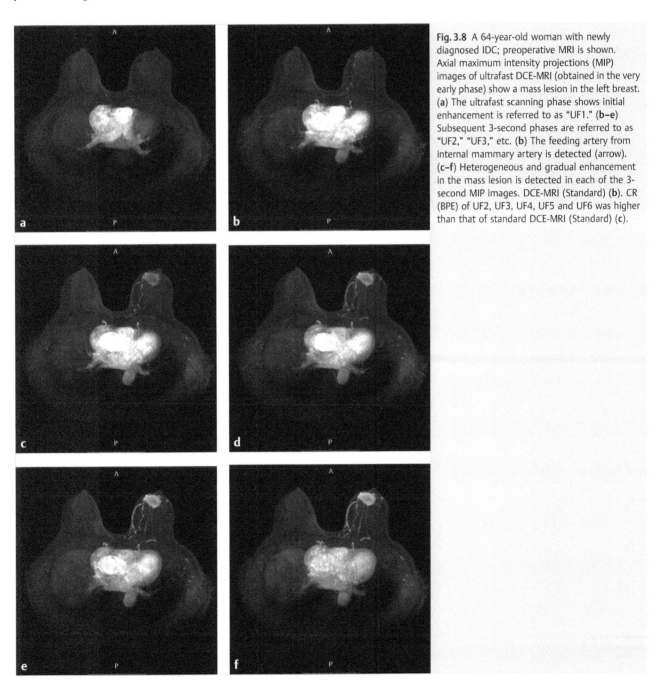

Fig. 3.8 A 64-year-old woman with newly diagnosed IDC; preoperative MRI is shown. Axial maximum intensity projections (MIP) images of ultrafast DCE-MRI (obtained in the very early phase) show a mass lesion in the left breast. (a) The ultrafast scanning phase shows initial enhancement is referred to as "UF1." (b–e) Subsequent 3-second phases are referred to as "UF2," "UF3," etc. (b) The feeding artery from internal mammary artery is detected (arrow). (c–f) Heterogeneous and gradual enhancement in the mass lesion is detected in each of the 3-second MIP images. DCE-MRI (Standard) (b). CR (BPE) of UF2, UF3, UF4, UF5 and UF6 was higher than that of standard DCE-MRI (Standard) (c).

where there is no significant lesion enhancement at early times after arrival of the contrast bolus in the breast.

Sliding Window and View-Sharing Methods

A number of nonstandard acquisition methods have been used to increase the temporal resolution of DCE-MRI. Many investigators have focused on view-sharing or sliding window reconstruction techniques (e.g. DISCO, TWIST, TRICKS, 4D-TRAK),[67,68,69,70] that acquire the center of k-space more frequently than the periphery and combine k-space data from a few acquisitions to obtain higher-resolution images. A diagram of one of these acquisition methods can be seen in (▶ Fig. 3.9), where different regions of k-space are acquired at different temporal resolutions, and then combined to form a fully sampled image.

Mus et al[71] used the TWIST (time-resolved angiography with stochastic trajectory[72]) technique to achieve a temporal resolution of 4.3 seconds for bilateral imaging during the initial part of the DCE series. They found that all the lesions were visible on both the ultrafast and standard images, and that the maximum slope of the kinetic curve performed well in classifying lesions, with an area under the ROC curve of 0.83. Platel et al used the TWIST protocol and found that adding morphological information to the kinetic parameters increased the classification accuracy and performed better than analysis of low temporal resolution data alone. They evaluated the "time to reach maximum slope" as a marker for cancer and found that this performed well (alone) in discriminating benign and malignant lesions (Az = 0.73). Mus et al.[71] evaluated DCE data acquired with TWIST (4.3 seconds temporal resolution) from 157 women and found that "time to enhancement" performed better than kinetic curve type analysis in discriminating benign and malignant lesions. These results confirm that the time and rate at which lesions begin to enhance may have significant clinical importance.

DISCO (differential subsampling with Cartesian ordering) has also been used to accelerate DCE-MRI. This sequence samples elliptical k-space regions; different regions of k-space are sampled at different rates, and images are reconstructed by combining signal from the different k-space regions. Saranathan et al[73,74] used this approach to acquire data with temporal resolution of 9 seconds per volume, while maintaining 1.1 mm in-plane resolution and 1.2 mm slice thickness. The results showed improvement in the image quality (as scored by a radiologist) when compared to a conventional fully sampled acquisition with the same temporal resolution but lower spatial resolution.

While these approaches generate excellent images and capture the initial rate of signal enhancement in lesions, they sample outer portions of k-space at relatively low temporal resolution, and this makes it difficult to interpret kinetics of enhancement, especially for small features with high spatial frequency components. Thus, the acquired images may not reflect the true changes in signal intensity and may, in turn, complicate quantitative analysis of lesion kinetics.

Compressed Sensing

Compressed sensing approaches have also been proposed as an alternative for accelerating DCE-MRI without significant sacrifices in spatial resolution.[75,76,77,78] Compressed sensing exploits the sparsity of the acquired data (or more specifically, that the images are sparse in some appropriate transformation) to reconstruct images from undersampled data. These methods yield useful images when data are randomly sampled so that there are no coherent artifacts from undersampling. For breast DCE-MRI, compressed sensing applications focus on the fact that the enhancement in the breast following contrast media injection is relatively sparse, and therefore images can be decomposed into a baseline component and a sparse time-varying component. Wang et al[77] proposed a reference image based compressed sensing (RICS) technique for acquisition of ultrafast breast DCE-MRI. In this method, fully sampled data (acquired before the administration of contrast media and after the entire DCE series) are used to form a reference image. Randomly undersampled data are then acquired post-contrast. The time-varying components of the images are reconstructed following subtraction of the (sparsified) reference images from the post-contrast data. Finally, the DCE series is constructed by adding the reconstructed time-varying component to the baseline reference images. The RICS method was shown to produce contrast media uptake curves that were highly correlated with the curves measured from fully sampled data, and up to a 10-fold acceleration factor was achieved without significantly degrading spatial resolution.

Otazo et al[79,80] suggested the use of a low-rank plus sparse (L + S) matrix decomposition method for the acceleration of DCE-MRI of the breast. In this method, the background

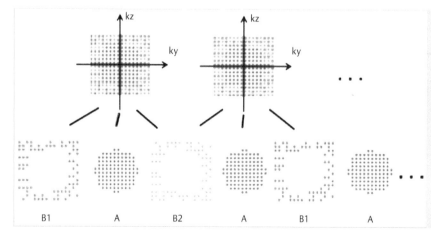

Fig. 3.9 Diagram of a TWIST acquisition scheme for high temporal resolution imaging, where k-space is divided into three regions, a central portion "A" and two peripheral regions "B1 and B2." The effective frame rate of the reconstructed images is given by the time in between "A" acquisitions. Each reconstructed image is made up of an "A" region along with the "B1 and B2" regions that were acquired closest to the given central region. "B1 and B2" are updated less often than "A."

component of the images is captured in the low-rank component, and the time-varying signal in the sparse component. This method was used to acquire bilateral images with 2.6 seconds of temporal resolution and in-plane resolution of roughly 1.1 mm isotropic, and 4 mm slice thickness. Otazo et al showed that the L + S method led to images better suited for the visualization of fine structures in the breast, when compared to standard compressed sensing.

While compressed sensing methods yield high-quality images with high acceleration factors, there remain some drawbacks to these methods. They are susceptible to artifacts that are often incompletely suppressed by compressed sensing reconstruction, especially aliasing artifacts and blurring that is similar to noise.[81,82] Several of these methods require image reconstruction offline, which may hinder clinical workflow. These techniques are currently not widely available or may require specialized software patches. Compressed sensing remains an active area of research, and some of these challenges may be moot in the coming years, especially as vendors incorporate these methods into standard acquisition software. However, careful analysis of compressed sensing techniques is necessary to understand the effect of these methods on the reconstructed images. Smith et al[75] analyzed the effect of compressed sensing on quantitative parameters extracted from DCE-MRI data, and found that at acceleration factors of 4 × the mean error in the pharmacokinetic parameter K^{trans} of tumors was 12% when compared to the full sampled data as the "gold standard." These results highlight the importance of validation studies for new methods for the acceleration of DCE-MRI, especially if quantitative analysis is to be performed on the images.

The results from the studies of ultrafast DCE-MRI discussed in this section suggest that the timing and speed of early signal enhancement are valuable markers for malignancy. The ultrafast images provide new information on early contrast uptake dynamics that could be valuable in classifying breast lesions, while the high spatial resolution images acquired at longer times after contrast media injection provide the level of detail necessary to evaluate morphology of small lesions. Larger clinical trials are necessary to assess the sensitivity and specificity of the various parameters measured from these ultrafast acquisitions. Recently Kuhl et al demonstrated the value of an abbreviated DCE-MRI protocol for breast cancer screening.[8] Addition of ultrafast DCE imaging to the abbreviated protocol could aid in the detection and classification of lesions, without significantly increasing scan time. MIPs of subtraction and enhancement gradient images as well as TTE maps could provide an efficient method for the evaluation of early kinetics by radiologists.

3.4.4 Dynamic Susceptibility

Most clinical protocols detect changes in longitudinal relaxation time (T1) as contrast agent molecules flow into a suspicious lesion. However, MRI contrast agents also produce local magnetic field gradients, due to their high magnetic susceptibility. This is especially true of gadolinium-based contrast agents. As a result, contrast agent molecules decrease T2*. Changes in T2* are largest when most of the contrast agent molecules are in blood vessels, during the first pass of the contrast media bolus, so that there is a large and rapidly changing difference in local magnetic field between the intravascular and extravascular

space. These changes can be detected with T2*-weighted gradient echo sequences,[83,84] including gradient echo sequences with two or more echoes. Changes in T2* can be used to track the contrast media bolus as it enters lesions, and clearly show lesion vasculature. This method was originally used to evaluate cerebral blood flow and brain abnormalities,[84,85,86] but has also been used by a number of research groups to detect and evaluate breast cancer. Kuhl et al reported that T2* changes are very modest in healthy breast parenchyma, while there are large T2* changes in malignant tumors, presumably reflecting dense vasculature.[87] The relationship of T2* changes to contrast media concentration depends on the geometry of blood vessels, including orientation with respect to the main magnetic field. As a result, quantitative analysis of dynamic susceptibility data is challenging. However, dynamic susceptibility and conventional T1-weighted imaging can be combined using multiple gradient echo methods to allow quantitative analysis based on changes in T1 and increased sensitivity to tumor vasculature from changes in T2*.[83]

3.5 Summary

Strategies for DCE-MR imaging are changing rapidly due to significant improvements in MR hardware, particularly parallel imaging, enhanced gradient performance, and improvements in preamplifiers and digitizers, as well as new methods for image sampling and reconstruction. This new technology is significantly increasing the sensitivity and specificity of breast MRI and has potential to significantly reduce morbidity and mortality due to breast cancer. However, the wide variety of new methods pose a challenge for the development of standardized, quantitative metrics that can be used widely in clinical practice to diagnose breast cancer, regardless of the type of scanner and the methods used for data acquisition and analysis. This problem can be addressed in part with quantitative methods for data analysis, and these are discussed in detail in Chapter 12.

References

[1] Weinmann HJ, Brasch RC, Press WR, Wesbey GE. Characteristics of gadolinium-DTPA complex: a potential NMR contrast agent. AJR Am J Roentgenol. 1984; 142(3):619–624

[2] Koenig SH. Molecular basis of magnetic relaxation of water protons of tissue. Acad Radiol. 1996; 3(7):597–606

[3] Koenig SH, Brown RD , III. Relaxometry of magnetic resonance imaging contrast agents. Magn Reson Annu. 1987:263–286

[4] Marino MA, Helbich T, Baltzer P, Pinker-Domenig K. Multiparametric MRI of the breast: a review. J Magn Reson Imaging. 2018; 47(2):301–315

[5] Pinker K, Helbich TH, Morris EA. The potential of multiparametric MRI of the breast. Br J Radiol. 2017; 90(1069):20160715

[6] Buckley DL, Drew PJ, Mussurakis S, Monson JR, Horsman A. Microvessel density of invasive breast cancer assessed by dynamic Gd-DTPA enhanced MRI. J Magn Reson Imaging. 1997; 7(3):461–464

[7] Medeiros LR, Duarte CS, Rosa DD, et al. Accuracy of magnetic resonance in suspicious breast lesions: a systematic quantitative review and meta-analysis. Breast Cancer Res Treat. 2011; 126(2):273–285

[8] Kuhl CK, Schrading S, Strobel K, Schild HH, Hilgers RD, Bieling HB. Abbreviated breast magnetic resonance imaging (MRI): first postcontrast subtracted images and maximum-intensity projection-a novel approach to breast cancer screening with MRI. J Clin Oncol. 2014; 32(22):2304–2310

[9] Force USPST, US Preventive Services Task Force. Screening for breast cancer: U.S. Preventive Services Task Force recommendation statement. Ann Intern Med. 2009; 151(10):716–726, W-236

[10] Nelson HD, Tyne K, Naik A, Bougatsos C, Chan BK, Humphrey L, U.S. Preventive Services Task Force. Screening for breast cancer: an update for the U.S. Preventive Services Task Force. Ann Intern Med. 2009; 151(10):727–737, W237–42

[11] Bassett LW, Dhaliwal SG, Eradat J, et al. National trends and practices in breast MRI. AJR Am J Roentgenol. 2008; 191(2):332–339

[12] Elsamaloty H, Elzawawi MS, Mohammad S, Herial N. Increasing accuracy of detection of breast cancer with 3-T MRI. AJR Am J Roentgenol. 2009; 192(4):1142–1148

[13] Brix G, Kiessling F, Lucht R, et al. Microcirculation and microvasculature in breast tumors: pharmacokinetic analysis of dynamic MR image series. Magn Reson Med. 2004; 52(2):420–429

[14] Rogosnitzky M, Branch S. Gadolinium-based contrast agent toxicity: a review of known and proposed mechanisms. Biometals. 2016; 29(3):365–376

[15] Tofts PS. Modeling tracer kinetics in dynamic Gd-DTPA MR imaging. J Magn Reson Imaging. 1997; 7(1):91–101

[16] Sourbron S. Compartmental modelling for magnetic resonance renography. Z Med Phys. 2010; 20(2):101–114

[17] Mustafi D, Ward J, Dougherty U, et al. X-ray fluorescence microscopy demonstrates preferential accumulation of a vanadium-based magnetic resonance imaging contrast agent in murine colonic tumors. Mol Imaging. 2015; 14:14

[18] Jansen SA, Paunesku T, Fan X, et al. Ductal carcinoma in situ: X-ray fluorescence microscopy and dynamic contrast-enhanced MR imaging reveals gadolinium uptake within neoplastic mammary ducts in a murine model. Radiology. 2009; 253(2):399–406

[19] Rofsky NM, Weinreb JC, Litt AW. Quantitative analysis of gadopentetate dimeglumine excreted in breast milk. J Magn Reson Imaging. 1993; 3(1):131–132

[20] Mustafi D, Gleber SC, Ward J, et al. IV Administered Gadodiamide Enters the Lumen of the Prostatic Glands: X-Ray Fluorescence Microscopy Examination of a Mouse Model. AJR Am J Roentgenol. 2015; 205(3):W313–9

[21] Yankeelov TE, Rooney WD, Li X, Springer CS , Jr. Variation of the relaxographic "shutter-speed" for transcytolemmal water exchange affects the CR bolus-tracking curve shape. Magn Reson Med. 2003; 50(6):1151–1169

[22] Brix G, Salehi Ravesh M, Zwick S, Griebel J, Delorme S. On impulse response functions computed from dynamic contrast-enhanced image data by algebraic deconvolution and compartmental modeling. Phys Med. 2012; 28(2):119–128

[23] Patlak CS, Blasberg RG, Fenstermacher JD. Graphical evaluation of blood-to-brain transfer constants from multiple-time uptake data. J Cereb Blood Flow Metab. 1983; 3(1):1–7

[24] Donaldson SB, West CM, Davidson SE, et al. A comparison of tracer kinetic models for T1-weighted dynamic contrast-enhanced MRI: application in carcinoma of the cervix. Magn Reson Med. 2010; 63(3):691–700

[25] Sourbron SP, Buckley DL. On the scope and interpretation of the Tofts models for DCE-MRI. Magn Reson Med. 2011; 66(3):735–745

[26] Sourbron SP, Buckley DL. Tracer kinetic modelling in MRI: estimating perfusion and capillary permeability. Phys Med Biol. 2012; 57(2):R1–R33

[27] Sourbron SP, Buckley DL. Classic models for dynamic contrast-enhanced MRI. NMR Biomed. 2013; 26(8):1004–1027

[28] Parker GJ, Roberts C, Macdonald A, et al. Experimentally-derived functional form for a population-averaged high-temporal-resolution arterial input function for dynamic contrast-enhanced MRI. Magn Reson Med. 2006; 56(5):993–1000

[29] Wang S, Fan X, Medved M, et al. Arterial input functions (AIFs) measured directly from arteries with low and standard doses of contrast agent, and AIFs derived from reference tissues. Magn Reson Imaging. 2016; 34(2):197–203

[30] Sardanelli F, Newstead GM, Putz B, et al. Gadobutrol-Enhanced Magnetic Resonance Imaging of the Breast in the Preoperative Setting: Results of 2 Prospective International Multicenter Phase III Studies. Invest Radiol. 2016; 51(7):454–461

[31] Abe H, Mori N, Tsuchiya K, et al. Kinetic Analysis of Benign and Malignant Breast Lesions With Ultrafast Dynamic Contrast-Enhanced MRI: Comparison With Standard Kinetic Assessment. AJR Am J Roentgenol. 2016; 207(5):1159–1166

[32] Pineda FD, Medved M, Wang S, et al. Ultrafast Bilateral DCE-MRI of the Breast with Conventional Fourier Sampling: Preliminary Evaluation of Semi-quantitative Analysis. Acad Radiol. 2016; 23(9):1137–1144

[33] Vreemann S, Rodriguez-Ruiz A, Nickel D, et al. Compressed Sensing for Breast MRI: Resolving the Trade-Off Between Spatial and Temporal Resolution. Invest Radiol. 2017; 52(10):574–582

[34] Mann RM, Mus RD, van Zelst J, Geppert C, Karssemeijer N, Platel B. A novel approach to contrast-enhanced breast magnetic resonance imaging for

screening: high-resolution ultrafast dynamic imaging. Invest Radiol. 2014; 49(9):579–585

[35] Jansen SA, Fan X, Medved M, et al. Characterizing early contrast uptake of ductal carcinoma in situ with high temporal resolution dynamic contrast-enhanced MRI of the breast: a pilot study. Phys Med Biol. 2010; 55(19):N473–N485

[36] Miyazaki M, Wheaton A, Kitane S. Enhanced fat suppression technique for breast imaging. J Magn Reson Imaging. 2013; 38(4):981–986

[37] Koh DM, Blackledge M, Burns S, et al. Combination of chemical suppression techniques for dual suppression of fat and silicone at diffusion-weighted MR imaging in women with breast implants. Eur Radiol. 2012; 22(12):2648–2653

[38] Frahm J, Haase A, Hänicke W, Matthaei D, Bomsdorf H, Helzel T. Chemical shift selective MR imaging using a whole-body magnet. Radiology. 1985; 156(2):441–444

[39] Merchant TE, Thelissen GR, Kievit HC, Oosterwaal LJ, Bakker CJ, de Graaf PW. Breast disease evaluation with fat-suppressed magnetic resonance imaging. Magn Reson Imaging. 1992; 10(3):335–340

[40] Tanaka S, Yoshiyama M, Imanishi Y, et al. Measuring visceral fat with water-selective suppression methods (SPIR, SPAIR) in patients with metabolic syndrome. Magn Reson Med Sci. 2007; 6(3):171–175

[41] Dixon WT. Simple proton spectroscopic imaging. Radiology. 1984; 153(1):189–194

[42] Wengert GJ, Pinker-Domenig K, Helbich TH, et al. Influence of fat-water separation and spatial resolution on automated volumetric MRI measurements of fibroglandular breast tissue. NMR Biomed. 2016; 29(6):702–708

[43] Glover GH. Multipoint Dixon technique for water and fat proton and susceptibility imaging. J Magn Reson Imaging. 1991; 1(5):521–530

[44] Fan X, Abe H, Medved M, et al. Fat suppression with spectrally selective inversion vs. high spectral and spatial resolution MRI of breast lesions: qualitative and quantitative comparisons. J Magn Reson Imaging. 2006; 24(6):1311–1315

[45] Medved M, Li H, Abe H, et al. Fast bilateral breast coverage with high spectral and spatial resolution (HiSS) MRI at 3 T. J Magn Reson Imaging. 2017; 46(5):1341–1348

[46] Kuhl CK, Schild HH, Morakkabati N. Dynamic bilateral contrast-enhanced MR imaging of the breast: trade-off between spatial and temporal resolution. Radiology. 2005; 236(3):789–800

[47] Newstead GM, Weinreb JC. Critical pathways for the future: MR imaging and digital mammography. Radiographics. 1995; 15(4):951–962

[48] Newstead GM. MR imaging of ductal carcinoma in situ. Magn Reson Imaging Clin N Am. 2010; 18(2):225–240, viii

[49] Fan X, Karczmar GS. A new approach to analysis of the impulse response function (IRF) in dynamic contrast-enhanced MRI (DCEMRI): a simulation study. Magn Reson Med. 2009; 62(1):229–239

[50] Heisen M, Fan X, Buurman J, van Riel NA, Karczmar GS, ter Haar Romeny BM. The use of a reference tissue arterial input function with low-temporal-resolution DCE-MRI data. Phys Med Biol. 2010; 55(16):4871–4883

[51] Yang C, Karczmar GS, Medved M, Oto A, Zamora M, Stadler WM. Reproducibility assessment of a multiple reference tissue method for quantitative dynamic contrast enhanced-MRI analysis. Magn Reson Med. 2009; 61(4):851–859

[52] Yang C, Karczmar GS, Medved M, Stadler WM. Estimating the arterial input function using two reference tissues in dynamic contrast-enhanced MRI studies: fundamental concepts and simulations. Magn Reson Med. 2004; 52(5):1110–1117

[53] Yang C, Karczmar GS, Medved M, Stadler WM. Multiple reference tissue method for contrast agent arterial input function estimation. Magn Reson Med. 2007; 58(6):1266–1275

[54] Pinker K, Grabner G, Bogner W, et al. A combined high temporal and high spatial resolution 3 Tesla MR imaging protocol for the assessment of breast lesions: initial results. Invest Radiol. 2009; 44(9):553–558

[55] Pineda F, Medved M, Fan X, Karczmar G. Unfolding of aliased dynamic acquisitions for the acceleration of breast dynamic contrast enhanced MRI (DCE-MRI). Paper presented at: American Association of Physicists in Medicine; Washington, DC; 2016

[56] Planey CR, Welch EB, Xu L, et al. Temporal sampling requirements for reference region modeling of DCE-MRI data in human breast cancer. J Magn Reson Imaging. 2009; 30(1):121–134

[57] Fan X, Medved M, River JN, et al. New model for analysis of dynamic contrast-enhanced MRI data distinguishes metastatic from nonmetastatic transplanted rodent prostate tumors. Magn Reson Med. 2004; 51(3):487–494

[58] Fan X, Medved M, Karczmar GS, et al. Diagnosis of suspicious breast lesions using an empirical mathematical model for dynamic contrast-enhanced MRI. Magn Reson Imaging. 2007; 25(5):593–603

[59] Jansen SA, Fan X, Karczmar GS, Abe H, Schmidt RA, Newstead GM. Differentiation between benign and malignant breast lesions detected by bilateral dynamic contrast-enhanced MRI: a sensitivity and specificity study. Magn Reson Med. 2008; 59(4):747–754

[60] Evelhoch JL. Key factors in the acquisition of contrast kinetic data for oncology. J Magn Reson Imaging. 1999; 10(3):254–259

[61] DeMartini WB, Liu F, Peacock S, Eby PR, Gutierrez RL, Lehman CD. Background parenchymal enhancement on breast MRI: impact on diagnostic performance. AJR Am J Roentgenol. 2012; 198(4):W373–W380

[62] Delille JP, Slanetz PJ, Yeh ED, Kopans DB, Garrido L. Physiologic changes in breast magnetic resonance imaging during the menstrual cycle: perfusion imaging, signal enhancement, and influence of the T1 relaxation time of breast tissue. Breast J. 2005; 11(4):236–241

[63] Amarosa AR, McKellop J, Klautau Leite AP, et al. Evaluation of the kinetic properties of background parenchymal enhancement throughout the phases of the menstrual cycle. Radiology. 2013; 268(2):356–365

[64] Yu J, Agarwal H, Stuber M, Schär M. Practical signal-to-noise ratio quantification for sensitivity encoding: application to coronary MR angiography. J Magn Reson Imaging. 2011; 33(6):1330–1340

[65] Song X, Pogue BW, Jiang S, et al. Automated region detection based on the contrast-to-noise ratio in near-infrared tomography. Appl Opt. 2004; 43(5):1053–1062

[66] Mori N, Pineda FD, Tsuchiya K, et al. Fast temporal resolution dynamic contrast-enhanced MRI: histogram analysis versus visual analysis for differentiating benign and malignant breast lesions. AJR Am J Roentgenol. 2018; 211 (4):933–939

[67] Petkova M, Gauvrit JY, Trystram D, et al. Three-dimensional dynamic time-resolved contrast-enhanced MRA using parallel imaging and a variable rate k-space sampling strategy in intracranial arteriovenous malformations. J Magn Reson Imaging. 2009; 29(1):7–12

[68] Willinek WA, Hadizadeh DR, von Falkenhausen M, et al. 4D time-resolved MR angiography with keyhole (4D-TRAK): more than 60 times accelerated MRA using a combination of CENTRA, keyhole, and SENSE at 3.0 T. J Magn Reson Imaging. 2008; 27(6):1455–1460

[69] Ramsay E, Causer P, Hill K, Plewes D. Adaptive bilateral breast MRI using projection reconstruction time-resolved imaging of contrast kinetics. J Magn Reson Imaging. 2006; 24(3):617–624

[70] Han S, Paulsen JL, Zhu G, et al. Temporal/spatial resolution improvement of in vivo DCE-MRI with compressed sensing-optimized FLASH. Magn Reson Imaging. 2012; 30(6):741–752

[71] Mus RD, Borelli C, Bult P, et al. Time to enhancement derived from ultrafast breast MRI as a novel parameter to discriminate benign from malignant breast lesions. Eur J Radiol. 2017; 89:90–96

[72] Hennig J, Scheffler K, Laubenberger J, Strecker R. Time-resolved projection angiography after bolus injection of contrast agent. Magn Reson Med. 1997; 37(3):341–345

[73] Saranathan M, Rettmann DW, Hargreaves BA, Clarke SE, Vasanawala SS. DIfferential Subsampling with Cartesian Ordering (DISCO): a high spatio-temporal resolution Dixon imaging sequence for multiphasic contrast enhanced abdominal imaging. J Magn Reson Imaging. 2012; 35(6):1484–1492

[74] Saranathan M, Rettmann DW, Hargreaves BA, Lipson JA, Daniel BL. Variable spatiotemporal resolution three-dimensional Dixon sequence for rapid dynamic contrast-enhanced breast MRI. J Magn Reson Imaging. 2014; 40(6):1392–1399

[75] Smith DS, Welch EB, Li X, et al. Quantitative effects of using compressed sensing in dynamic contrast enhanced MRI. Phys Med Biol. 2011; 56(15):4933–4946

[76] Chan RW, Ramsay EA, Cheung EY, Plewes DB. The influence of radial under-sampling schemes on compressed sensing reconstruction in breast MRI. Magn Reson Med. 2012; 67(2):363–377

[77] Wang H, Miao Y, Zhou K, et al. Feasibility of high temporal resolution breast DCE-MRI using compressed sensing theory. Med Phys. 2010; 37(9):4971–4981

[78] Chen L, Schabel MC, DiBella EV. Reconstruction of dynamic contrast enhanced magnetic resonance imaging of the breast with temporal constraints. Magn Reson Imaging. 2010; 28(5):637–645

[79] Kim SG, Feng L, Grimm R, et al. Influence of temporal regularization and radial undersampling factor on compressed sensing reconstruction in dynamic contrast enhanced MRI of the breast. J Magn Reson Imaging. 2016; 43(1):261–269

[80] Otazo R, Candès E, Sodickson DK. Low-rank plus sparse matrix decomposition for accelerated dynamic MRI with separation of background and dynamic components. Magn Reson Med. 2015; 73(3):1125–1136

[81] Yang Y, Liu F, Jin Z, Crozier S. Aliasing Artefact Suppression in Compressed Sensing MRI for Random Phase-Encode Undersampling. IEEE Trans Biomed Eng. 2015; 62(9):2215–2223

[82] Lustig M, Donoho D, Pauly JM. Sparse MRI: The application of compressed sensing for rapid MR imaging. Magn Reson Med. 2007; 58(6):1182–1195

[83] Kuperman VY, Karczmar GS, Blomley MJ, Lewis MZ, Lubich LM, Lipton MJ. Differentiating between T1 and T2* changes caused by gadopentetate dimeglumine in the kidney by using a double-echo dynamic MR imaging sequence. J Magn Reson Imaging. 1996; 6(5):764–768

[84] Belliveau JW, Rosen BR, Kantor HL, et al. Functional cerebral imaging by susceptibility-contrast NMR. Magn Reson Med. 1990; 14(3):538–546

[85] Cha S, Pierce S, Knopp EA, et al. Dynamic contrast-enhanced T2*-weighted MR imaging of tumefactive demyelinating lesions. AJNR Am J Neuroradiol. 2001; 22(6):1109–1116

[86] Manka C, Träber F, Gieseke J, Schild HH, Kuhl CK. Three-dimensional dynamic susceptibility-weighted perfusion MR imaging at 3.0 T: feasibility and contrast agent dose. Radiology. 2005; 234(3):869–877

[87] Kuhl CK, Bieling H, Gieseke J, et al. Breast neoplasms: T2* susceptibility-contrast, first-pass perfusion MR imaging. Radiology. 1997; 202(1):87–95

4 Screening MRI: Clinical Implementation

Gillian M. Newstead

Abstract

Implementation of an abbreviated (AB-MR) technique as a method for breast screening for women at moderate (15–20%) risk and/or mammographically dense breasts is an innovative and challenging endeavor. In this chapter, a practical review of acquisition protocols, technical requirements, recruitment and clinical workflow for AB-MR will be discussed. In order to provide optimal screening, breast imaging facilities need to reconsider and modify their MRI workflow to allow for efficient throughput of women to be screened, while also maintaining technical and interpretive excellence. Approximately 50% of women will fall into the dense breast category [BI-RADS categories C & D], where the sensitivity of mammography is diminished and overlapping dense tissue may increase the false-positive call-back rate. Screening with AB-MR has been shown to be a more sensitive screening method for these patients.

If AB-MR breast screening is successfully implemented, providing lower costs and efficient workflow, women would greatly benefit by the detection of a significantly larger number of high-grade cancers than by other imaging methods while also reducing interval cancers and node positivity. The underlying principles of screening MR interpretation are similar, whether an abbreviated protocol or a full protocol is utilized. Descriptions using the BI-RADS lexicon categories of background parenchymal enhancement (BPE) and selected MRI-detected lesions are shown. Ten case examples of BPE and 21 case examples of MR screen-detected benign and malignant lesions are shown.

Keywords: abbreviated MRI technique (AB-MR), equipment for AB-MR, pre-procedure scheduling and preparation, AB-MR imaging procedure, precautions and contraindications, recruitment for AB-MR screening, costs of AB-MR screening, screening MR interpretation, reporting of screening MR results, breast imaging audit

4.1 Introduction

Breast magnetic resonance imaging (MRI) has become the mainstay method for screening of high-risk women due to its high sensitivity for breast cancer compared to mammography and ultrasound. Although higher field strength magnets, increasing numbers of channels in breast coils, and advanced analytic methods have improved breast MRI greatly over the years, the principal technical acquisition methods used for breast screening have remained basically unchanged. The standard MRI protocol has consistently included a precontrast T2-weighted (T2w) acquisition followed by a dynamic contrast-enhanced MRI (DCE-MRI) sequence, encompassing a series of T1w acquisitions before and for approximately 5 to 7 minutes after the intravenous administration of a gadolinium-based contrast medium (GBCM).[1] Physician referrals for either a screening or a diagnostic indication will generally result in women receiving the same MRI acquisition protocol today. In almost all of the early high-risk screening trials (using a full diagnostic

MRI technique), the sensitivity of MRI was higher than mammography, and the specificity was lower. As the technology has matured, the specificity of MRI screening has increased due to improved technical and radiological expertise. The current 6-month follow-up recommendation rates and positive predictive value (PPV3) of biopsy rates at MRI screening are now comparable to those of mammography.

The advent of breast density legislation has changed the landscape for screening women with dense breasts, and new methods are now sought for supplemental screening.[2] Despite its high sensitivity, MRI use has generally been restricted to the screening of high-risk women only for a number of reasons that primarily include time and costs. The length of time required to complete a standard MRI examination is often 30 minutes or more, the cost of the examination is much higher than mammography, and most clinical radiological practices are not geared toward efficient MRI screening. Large prospective screening studies of high-risk women employed annual mammography and annual MRI, yearly simultaneous screening allowing easy cross-referencing for interpretation and audit purposes.

4.2 Abbreviated MRI Technique

Abbreviated breast MRI (AB-MR) was developed to provide a low-cost, efficient, screening method, streamlined workflow, and short interpretation times being essential requirements for any image-based screening study. An abbreviated protocol usually includes only one or two postcontrast dynamic timepoints with the expectation that cancer enhancement will be most conspicuous at the first postcontrast timepoint, with the added benefit that background parenchymal enhancement will be less evident. The concept of abbreviated MRI was pioneered by Dr. Kuhl who published the results of a prospective clinical study on the use of abbreviated breast MRI in 2014.[3] In this study, use of the maximum-intensity projection (MIP) image to provide a quick overview to check for presence or absence of significant enhancement, significantly reducing radiologist reading times. Individual subtracted images were subsequently reviewed as necessary for further categorization of abnormal enhancement. Although a complete dynamic series was acquired, all rapidly enhancing lesions were identified on the first postcontrast subtracted images. For hundred and forty-three women at mildly to moderately increased risk underwent 606 MRI screening rounds. Of the 11 cancers identified in this study, four (36%) were in the intraductal stage, 7 (64%) invasive, with a median size of 8 mm, and all malignancies were node negative. All participants in the study had received a normal mammogram at time of recruitment and the supplementary cancer yield of MRI was 18.3 per 1000 women. Radiologist's reading time was below 3 seconds for interpretation of a MIP image (is there significant enhancement or not?) and below 30 seconds for interpretation of the complete study when significant enhancement was identified on the MIP image. These short reading times are competitive with batch reading times of screening mammograms, and, for example, are substantially shorter than the time needed for review of tomosynthesis studies. Although the AB-MR protocol is likely not sufficient for a complete diagnostic examination, in the screening setting, this study showed a high detection rate without a corresponding high false-positive rate, an indication of an excellent high-quality screening test. These results have prompted other researchers to consider further development of shorter MRI protocols for screening.

Subsequent studies using AB-MR technique have further supported the concept of shortened acquisitions for screening. Various protocols acquiring a precontrast series, one or possibly two postcontrast series and in some cases a T2w series were employed, results showing that comparison performance between a shortened breast MRI protocol and a standard protocol were similar.[3,4,5,6] In the United States, AB-MR protocols have already been incorporated into some breast practices and modified according to the techniques commonly used in North America. Protocols for AB-MR screening are usually defined as an MRI study with a scan time of less than 10 minutes compared to a longer 20- to 40-minute full diagnostic breast MRI. Generally, a T2w scan followed by one T1w pre- and one postcontrast examination completes the protocol. It is important to note that standard kinetic assessment is not possible with AB-MR technique because delayed dynamic acquisitions(s) are not obtained. An ECOG/ACRIN trial, "EA1141: Comparison of Abbreviated Breast MRI and Digital Breast Tomosynthesis in Breast Cancer Screening in Women with Dense Breasts," is now underway in the United States and Germany and will provide additional data on the efficacy of the AB-MR approach to screening.[7] The abbreviated technique has the potential to achieve not only sensitivities comparable to a full diagnostic protocol but also short imaging times and decreased costs. Introduction of this promising new application of breast MRI will be challenging, evoking memories of the early days of mammography screening when radiologists revamped their practices to improve efficiency and throughput.[8] Ultrafast (UF) (accelerated) MRI enables shorter acquisition times (3-7 seconds) and can be included into an AB-MR protocol. A variety of different UF techniques have been reported and discussed extensively in the previous chapter. Although most of the reported clinical studies are feasibility investigations, one study conducted a multicenter reader investigation of ultrafast screening MRI vs. a full diagnostic protocol.[9] No significant difference in the sensitivity of a full diagnostic protocol vs. an ultrafast protocol (0.86 vs. 0.84, $P = 0.50$) was found and specificity was significantly higher for the ultrafast protocol (0.76 full diagnostic vs. 0.82 ultrafast, $P = 0.002$), A significant decrease in reader time was also noted.

4.3 Recruitment for AB-MR Screening

The target population for adjunctive AB-MR annual screening will be asymptomatic women at mild-to-moderate increased risk (15–20%) and/or with dense breast tissue at mammography, beginning at age 40. It is possible that as the technology progresses, MRI screening of high-risk women with AB-MR may be effective as well; however more data are needed to support this hypothesis. As previously noted, approximately 50% of women will fall into the dense breast category (BIRADS categories C and D), where the sensitivity of mammography is diminished, and overlapping dense tissue may increase the false-positive callback rate. Several risk assessment models can be used to estimate lifetime breast cancer risk as discussed in Chapter 2. Radiologists have implemented their own risk assessment program in some practices, and in large breast centers, a dedicated genetic counselor may be on staff assisting the imaging team. In recent years, more than half of the states in the United States have passed mandatory breast density notification legislation, and several more have introduced a bill.[2] These laws generally recommend that women should consider adjunctive imaging screening methods if they are known to have dense breast tissue at mammography. By Mammography Quality Standards Act national statute,[10] letters in lay language are sent to every woman with dense breast tissue explaining that this finding is common, not abnormal, and that dense breast tissue can make it harder to find cancer on a mammogram and may increase her breast cancer risk. These lay reports inform women and recommend that the benefits of adjunctive screening methods should be discussed with their personal physician.[6]

Education of the medical community is needed to provide information on the benefits of improved cancer detection directed toward women in both the high- and moderate-risk categories. Seminars and conferences emphasizing the benefits and efficiencies of AB-MR and the distinction between a screening and a diagnostic MRI examination could be held at community hospitals, physician practices, and local and national breast health organizations. Relevant publications could be circulated to physicians, genetic counselors, and allied health professionals involved in breast care. In local radiologic practices, informational brochures and printed literature could be distributed among referring physicians and placed in the breast imaging waiting room. Identification of those women within an existing mammography screening practice, who have been shown by a previous full field digital mammography (FFDM) examination to have dense breast tissue, could be directly informed about the value of additional AB-MR screening at the time of their routine mammography appointment.

4.3.1 Equipment

Magnet Strength

The majority of breast DCE-MRI studies are still performed at magnetic field strengths of 1.5 Tesla (T); however, recently there has been an increase in the use of higher field strength magnets, 3 T, and dedicated breast coils with an increasing number of channels.[7] A study by Elsamaloty et al reported increased sensitivity and specificity of DCE-MRI when performed at 3 T, finding values of 100 and 93.9%, respectively.[8] Another study by Rahbar et al reported on breast MRI at 3 T and showed a higher correlation with the final pathologic size of ductal carcinoma in situ (DCIS) lesions, when compared to 1.5 T. The authors concluded that higher field strength might prove to be more accurate for assessment of disease extent in the preoperative setting.[9] Although excellent screening MRI technique is possible at both field strengths, these recent studies suggest that growing experience in scanning at higher field strength could lead to an even greater overall increase of both sensitivity and specificity at MRI.

Contrast Injection Devices

Power injectors are preferable for contrast injection because they provide consistent timing of the injection of a gadolinium-based contrast agent (GBCA), ensuring that the injection rate is the same for every patient, every time. Injection doses are calculated according to body weight, and a standard dose of 0.1 mmol/kg should be administered as a bolus, with an injection rate of 2 mL/s followed by a saline flush of at least 10 mL.[10] Power injectors can be triggered from outside the magnet room, facilitating image timing and minimizing patient motion. Standardized injections are especially important for women undergoing annual screening, because direct comparison of kinetic data from one examination to the next is necessary, and elimination of variation due to differences in the injection rate allows valid comparisons.

4.4 Preprocedure Scheduling and Preparation

Streamlined workflow is critical for well-organized screening, and an efficient breast MRI screening program requires well-trained scheduling and reception staff. FFDM and AB-MR studies can be scheduled contemporaneously, so that both imaging procedures are completed within a 1-hour time frame. It is important to note that current ACS guidelines for breast MRI screening of high-risk women do not address the timing of MRI in conjunction with FFDM. Screening protocols therefore include women who prefer to undergo both procedures together on an annual basis and those who prefer to alternate between AB-MR and FFDM every 6 months.

Preparation beforehand is essential in order to achieve effective streamlined workflow on the day of the AB-MR examination. Women should be prescreened, usually by telephone, for claustrophobia, allergic predisposition or history of prior reaction to contrast agents, presence of implantable devices, and history of renal disease. Some practices deliver a packet of information to the woman by mail or by e-mail before the appointment date, covering topics such as the length of time of the procedure, the need for contrast injection, the possibility of follow-up imaging, or biopsy. Other practices may rely on their website for providing this information. Consent for the MRI procedure and administrative details regarding payment and insurance preauthorization should be arranged by phone in advance of the appointment day. Some women may have further questions about breast MRI screening before consenting for the procedure for the first time; a discussion in the radiology department with either a qualified technologist or radiologist before the examination appointment is confirmed can be helpful.

Scheduling of premenopausal women for screening MRI requires special attention. Although premenopausal women undergoing a diagnostic MRI study are not always scheduled according to their menstrual cycle, preferential scheduling is useful for screening. Although it is often recommended that screening breast MRIs should be performed during the 7 to 10 days of the menstrual cycle in order to minimize the degree of background parenchymal enhancement (BPE), some recent studies have suggested that the degree of BPE does not impact MRI sensitivity or specificity. Investigations have shown that BPE typically increases during the fourth week of the menstrual cycle, thus, if at all possible, imaging should be avoided in the premenstrual phase of the cycle. Decreased BPE is found in postmenopausal women and those treated with radiation therapy and antiestrogen therapy (tamoxifen and aromatase inhibitors). The goal is to image when the background enhancement of normal fibroglandular breast tissue is lower, abnormal findings are more conspicuous, and false-positive findings are less frequent.[11,12,13] Scheduling of screening appointments for premenopausal women requires flexibility, and appointments may need to be adjusted on an individual basis. Women using oral contraceptives should observe the menstrual cycle imaging recommendations. Certain women may experience irregular menses, particularly in the perimenopausal years, thus encountering difficulty in selecting the appropriate timing for their examination. In these instances, blood sampling for estimation of serum progesterone levels is helpful for determination of the optimal time for breast MRI. This method may also prove to be particularly useful when earlier examinations have been deemed nondiagnostic because of marked BPE.[14] It is interesting to note that a recent report indicates that hormone replacement therapy has negligible effect on the BPE of postmenopausal women who undergo MRI.[15]

When a woman is referred for MR examination and it is questionable as to whether she will fit into the magnet bore and the breast coil, the issue can be resolved by inviting her to view the magnet and breast coil and attempting to position her in the device. If positioning and placement prove unsuccessful, then alternate screening or diagnostic methods should be employed. All such questions and concerns should be managed, if at all possible, prior to the day of the screening appointment. Attempts must be made to obtain all prior breast image examinations in advance,[16] and these studies should be uploaded onto the picture archiving and communication system (PACS) before the patient arrives for her screening examination.

4.5 Imaging Procedure

Women presenting for screening MRI will often experience increased anxiety, fearing the possibility of a finding that might be malignant. A separate check-in line will minimize the anxiety of waiting with other patients and expedite workflow. Women should receive clear instructions and a complete explanation of the MR procedure by a radiology technologist or nurse once she enters the MRI suite. She will be asked to fill out a detailed questionnaire to confirm that she has no contraindications to the MR examination or to the contrast injection and will be asked to sign a specific informed consent. She will then be directed to the dressing area where she will change into a patient gown, having removed her brassiere, jewelry, and any clothing zippers or other metallic objects.

In the preparation room of the MRI suite, a technologist or nurse will provide venous access and inform the woman that she might experience a warm or tingling sensation in her arm, possibly extending throughout her body, both during and following the injection. She will also be instructed to avoid any movement during scanning, emphasizing the importance of remaining still and avoiding the need for repeat examination.

Once the woman is positioned prone on the MRI table, the technologist will position her so that her breasts are symmetrically placed into the wells of the coil with nipple, palpable masses, and scar markers applied, if requested by the radiologist. Folds or overlapping of breast tissue at the edges of the coil should be avoided, and slight breast compression may be used to reduce motion artifacts. The scanning procedure is intermittently noisy, and the woman should be informed that she can be given earplugs or earphones with a choice of music, if she wishes to minimize the noise during image acquisition. It is important that a method of verbal communication between the woman and the technologist or radiologist is established before scanning takes place. An alarm system device should be provided to her, so that she is aware that when she activates the alarm, the procedure will be stopped, and she will immediately receive assistance.

Following completion of imaging, the intravenous line is removed, the puncture site is compressed, and the woman will then be asked to sit on the table for a moment to avoid any dizziness, and then exit from the magnet room. Once she is dressed in her own clothes, she may be asked to remain in the department for about 15 minutes to check for any possible delayed reaction to the GBCA before leaving the facility.

4.5.1 Precautions and Contraindications

Claustrophobia

Claustrophobia may be experienced by some women when they are asked to enter, and remain immobile, inside the narrow bore of the magnet, for a period of about 10 minutes.[17] Claustrophobia is usually mild and generally less severe when she is able to enter the scanner with her feet first rather than her head first. Moveable trolleys with built-in breast coils are designed to enter the magnet feet first and are especially useful in this regard (▶ Fig. 4.1). These trolleys also allow streamlined workflow when two are available on site; one can be used in the scanning room during image acquisition, and a second

trolley can be used to position the patient in the coil ready for scanning. Women are usually able to tolerate the study without difficulty, and verbal reassurance from the technologist may help her to remain immobile in between acquisition sequences. Women who are extremely anxious may benefit from a viewing of the scanning room and magnet before the examination is scheduled. Sedation may be needed for women with a history of severe claustrophobia, and this is usually arranged by consultation with her referring physician. When sedation is provided, arrangements must be made for another individual to accompany the woman home after the procedure.

Allergic Predisposition

GBCAs are extremely well tolerated by the vast majority of patients who undergo DCE-MRI. Acute adverse reactions are rare, and reports indicate a lower frequency than is reported following administration of iodinated contrast media. Women with a history of multiple allergies, bronchial asthma, or previous allergic reactions to GBCAs have a higher risk for allergic reactions. These women should discuss their allergic history with their referring physicians. Precautionary methods can be taken in these cases, including preprocedure administration of antihistaminic and corticosteroid drugs. In women with serious allergic symptoms, a balance between the potential advantages of MRI and the potential risks of serious allergic reaction should be considered. It is important to note, however, that here is no cross-reactivity between GBCAs and iodinated contrast media.

Foreign Bodies

Absolute contraindications to MRI include the presence of ferromagnetic intracranial aneurysm clips and MR-incompatible implanted electronic devices, such as pacemakers, implantable cardioverter defibrillators, and neurostimulators. Women with intravascular stents or metal screws or plates for osteosynthesis can safely undergo breast MRI 6 weeks following surgical implantation. Questions regarding a history of prior eye injury

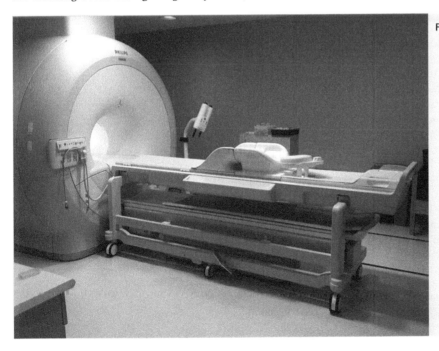

Fig. 4.1 Coil trolley.

from a metal object (metal slivers, metal shavings) are routine before any MRI examination is undertaken, and orbital radiographs may be necessary to document the presence or absence of metal foreign bodies in some cases. Enquires should also be made concerning body tattoos or permanent makeup, including tattooed eyeliner. If the tattoos are extensive or very dark, they may contain iron pigments, and the woman may experience radiofrequency (RF) heating of the tattooed tissue causing local burns. Burning may occur if the tissue in question is located within the volume in which the body coil is being used for RF transmission. Cold compresses or ice packs placed over the tattooed areas, locally applied throughout the MRI examination, may alleviate the heat effect. Additional information may be found in the ACR guidance document on MR safe practices.[18]

Renal Function

Renal function test, obtaining a creatinine level and estimating the glomerular filtration rate (GFR), is recommended within 30 days of the scheduled examination for women over the age of 60. Testing should also be obtained for younger women with a history of bladder or kidney disease, diabetes mellitus, or cardiovascular disease.[19,20] AB-MR screening should be avoided in women with severely impaired renal function because injection of a GBCA may lead to a rare condition known as nephrogenic systemic fibrosis.[21] DCE-MRI is generally contraindicated in pregnant women and AB-MR should be avoided during pregnancy and lactation.[22]

Costs

Although MRI may eventually become a routine method for breast cancer surveillance, the high cost of the examination is currently a major impediment to wider application of its use. Studies of the cost-effectiveness of annual screening with both MRI and mammography have only incorporated to date; those women deemed to be at the highest risk of developing breast cancer. The costs associated with screening MRI, as with other screening methods, include not only those associated with the procedure itself, but also include the downstream costs generated by repeat MRI examinations, targeted ultrasound studies, and image-guided biopsies of screen-detected breast lesions.

Plevritis and colleagues reported in 2006 that the addition of breast MRI to a screening regimen was cost-effective in both *BRCA1* and *BRCA2* mutation carriers.[23] They showed that although the cost–benefits were greatest in patients aged 40 to 49 years for both mutation types, the cost–benefits per quality-adjusted life year (QALY) for women aged 35 to 54 were greater in women with *BRCA1* ($55,420) than for *BRCA2* carriers ($130,695), and if women with dense breasts were considered, the costs decreased for *BRCA1* ($41,183) and for *BRCA2* carriers ($98,454).

Another report in 2014 by Ahern and colleagues studied various options for integrating mammography and MRI schedules into a screening protocol for women with a strong family history of breast cancer and a lifetime risk of greater than 25% or higher. Using current costs of MRI examinations and an incremental cost-effectiveness ratio of $100,000 per QALY, they found that the most cost-effective strategy was an alternating schedule of MRI and mammography examinations plus a clinical breast examination every year from age 30 to 74. For those

women with a 50% lifetime risk, the recommended strategy was to follow the same screening protocol but to alternate these examinations every 6 months, provided there was a 70% reduction in MRI costs. At 75% risk, the recommended strategy became biennial MRI combined with mammography plus clinical breast examination every 6 months.[24]

Health care reimbursement for breast MRI screening is variable among developed countries across the world. When considering costs of screening women at intermediate or average risk, it is certainly essential that the imaging time must be shorter and workflow efficient in order to decrease costs. Future cost-benefit analyses of AB-MR breast screening need to take into account the proven low-interval cancer rate and early detection rate of biologically aggressive cancers, which allow lower downstream costs when compared to treatment of larger tumors. Analyses must consider also that although ultrasound procedure costs are lower, the method is less sensitive and is associated with substantial costs associated with recalls and biopsies.

4.6 Screening Interpretation

Interpretation of screening MRI examinations is one of the most demanding in all of breast imaging and excellent technique, and interpretive experience is of the utmost importance. The high prevalence of benign enhancing lesions observed in young women at high risk is challenging for the radiologist and the "atypical" appearance of many BRCA-associated breast cancers may be mistaken for benign lesions. There is a deep learning curve for interpretation of these studies, and double reading can be helpful for an observer new to screening interpretation. Joint reading of screening studies may benefit a new reader until confidence is established.

The primary difference in interpreting an AB-MR study compared to a full MR diagnostic study is that only one, or at the most two, postcontrast series is obtained. If ultrafast (UF) technique is used during the first postcontrast minute time point, then a second standard acquisition may be used in the second time point, allowing two postcontrast acquisitions but keeping to the 10-minute time limit. The delayed phase of enhancement is not acquired in an abbreviated study, thus standard kinetic analysis cannot be used as an interpretation tool. Small cancers are visible on AB-MR in the initial enhancement phase; however, there are no set criteria yet for defining the actual threshold percentage increase in enhancement. Invasive cancers usually exhibit early enhancement of 50% or more, and additional measures of the enhancement slope and quantitative measures derived from UF techniques are under development.

Although investigations have shown that there is considerable overlap in the kinetic patterns of benign and malignant lesions on standard diagnostic examinations, invasive cancers classically demonstrate early and intense enhancement in the initial phase.[25,26,27] Benign masses exhibiting rapid enhancement include lymph nodes, papillomata, and fibroadenomata in premenopausal women. Interpretation should therefore be based primarily on the morphology and internal composition of suspect lesions. Invasive cancers that present as masses are generally small in size (<1 cm) when visible only on MRI, whereas noninvasive cancers presenting as nonmass enhancement (NME) may be small or large and still remain occult on mammography (MG) and ultrasound (US). Careful morphological analysis is critical for maintaining high sensitivity and specificity with AB-MR.

4.6.1 Assessment of Fibroglandular Tissue

The second edition of the MRI Breast Imaging Reporting and Data System (BIRADS) Atlas requires that a description of the amount of breast fibroglandular tissue (FGT) is included in every MR report.[16] The amount of FGT is considered to be the amount of normal breast parenchyma, as it relates to the amount of normal fatty tissue within the breast and is similar to the mammographic assessment of breast density. FGT is best assessed on a non–fat-saturated T1w or T2w image, or alternatively, the fat-saturated T1w images in the dynamic sequence may be used. The amount of FGT is classified into four categories: (1) almost entirely fat, (2) scattered FGT, (3) heterogeneous FGT, and (4) extreme FGT, based on the ratio of fat and parenchyma (▶ Fig. 4.2).

4.6.2 Background Parenchymal Enhancement

The accuracy of MR interpretation may be affected by the variable enhancement of normal breast tissue, which usually enhances slowly initially, generates a persistent kinetic curve, and is referred to as BPE. The hormonal response of breast tissue in premenopausal women varies during the menstrual cycle. Marked BPE can limit the sensitivity of the examination because enhancing abnormalities maybe less conspicuous and present a diagnostic challenge. For this reason, it is recommended that premenopausal women should be scanned ideally during the second week of the menstrual cycle and week 4 should be avoided if at all possible. The BI-RADS Atlas recommends that each breast MRI report includes a description of the level of BPE. BPE is considered to be the amount and degree of enhancement of the normal breast parenchyma according to approximate quartiles, and is classified as (1) minimal (<25% of glandular tissue demonstrating enhancement), (2) mild (25–50% enhancement), (3) moderate (50–75% enhancement), or (4) marked (>75% enhancement), and symmetric or asymmetric enhancement (▶ Fig. 4.3).

It is important to note that the degree of BPE does not correlate with the amount of FGT. Glandular tissue consists of hormonally influenced terminal ductal lobular units (TDLUs), which enhance on MRI and can be distinguished from surrounding nonenhancing parenchymal fibrosis. A very dense breast exhibiting extreme FGT may exhibit minimal BPE, whereas a fatty breast composed of scattered FGT may show moderate or marked BPE.[28] Early reports studying the relationship between cancer risk and BPE suggest that BPE is a risk marker, the odds of breast cancer risk increasing with increasing levels of BPE.[29]

BPE usually exhibits bilateral scattered foci of enhancement (▶ Fig. 4.4) often with symmetric preferential enhancement located at the periphery of the breast parenchyma seen at the fibroglandular/fat junction (▶ Fig. 4.5). The arterial blood supply to the breast is primarily from the periphery of the breast tissue from perforating branches of the internal thoracic artery (internal mammary) and branches of the lateral thoracic artery and

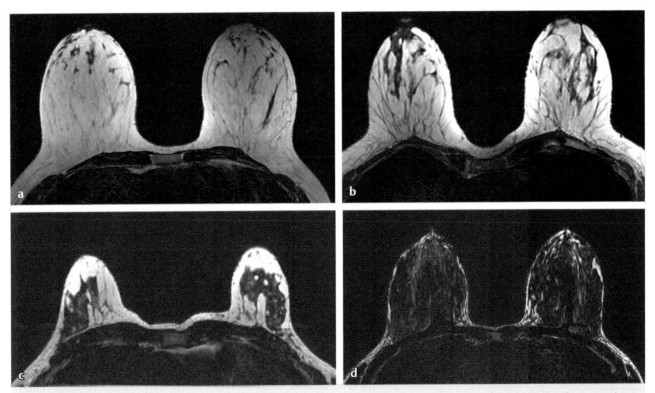

Fig. 4.2 Amount of FGT assessed on fat-saturated T1w imaging or non–fat-saturated T1w, or T2w imaging. **(a)** Almost entirely fat. **(b)** Scattered FGT. **(c)** Heterogeneous FGT. **(d)** Extreme FGT.

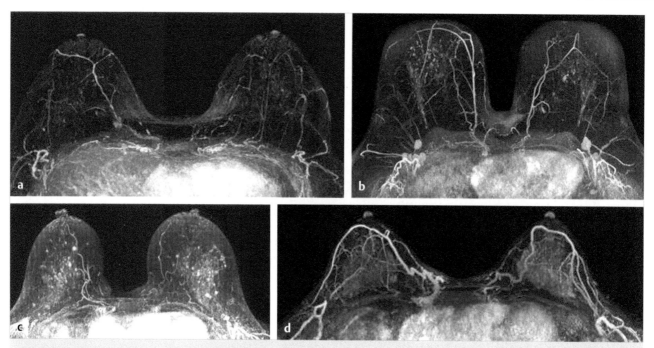

Fig. 4.3 Background parenchymal enhancement (BPE). High-risk screening: BPE can be described as minimal, mild, moderate, or marked. BPE refers to the normal enhancement of the patient's fibroglandular tissue, and assessment occurs on the first postcontrast image. **(a)** Minimal. **(b)** Mild. **(c)** Moderate. **(d)** Marked.

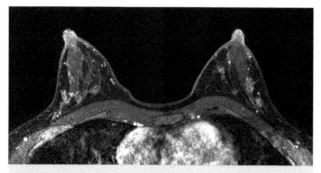

Fig. 4.4 Scattered foci of enhancement. High-risk screening: Axial source postcontrast image reveals bilateral scattered foci of BPE.

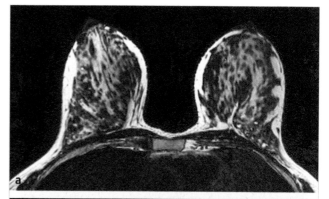

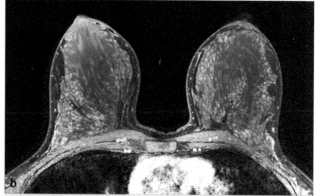

Fig. 4.5 BPE: Peripheral enhancement. High-risk screening: Extreme FGT is seen on T2w non–fat-suppressed precontrast image **(a)** and peripheral enhancement is noted at the fibroglandular/fat junction on T1w postcontrast source image **(b)**.

lateral cutaneous branches of the intercostal arteries. This pattern of vascular inflow accounts for the preferential visualization of BPE at the periphery of the breast tissue cone with later central and retroareolar enhancement. BPE usually demonstrates slow early initial enhancement and progressive delayed enhancement kinetics.[30] BPE may exhibit asymmetric, regional, or focal enhancement, and unilateral asymmetric focal BPE may prompt biopsy in some cases (▶ Fig. 4.6). Patients treated with BCS often exhibit diminished enhancement in the posttreated breast due to radiation change and fibrosis (▶ Fig. 4.7; ▶ Fig. 4.8). A report has also shown similar findings in women treated with aromatase inhibitors.[31] Bilateral similar areas of enhancement, regardless of their distribution, are more characteristic of benign enhancement than of malignancy (▶ Fig. 4.9). BPE increases in postmenopausal women undergoing hormone replacement therapy.[32,33] Marked increase in BPE has been

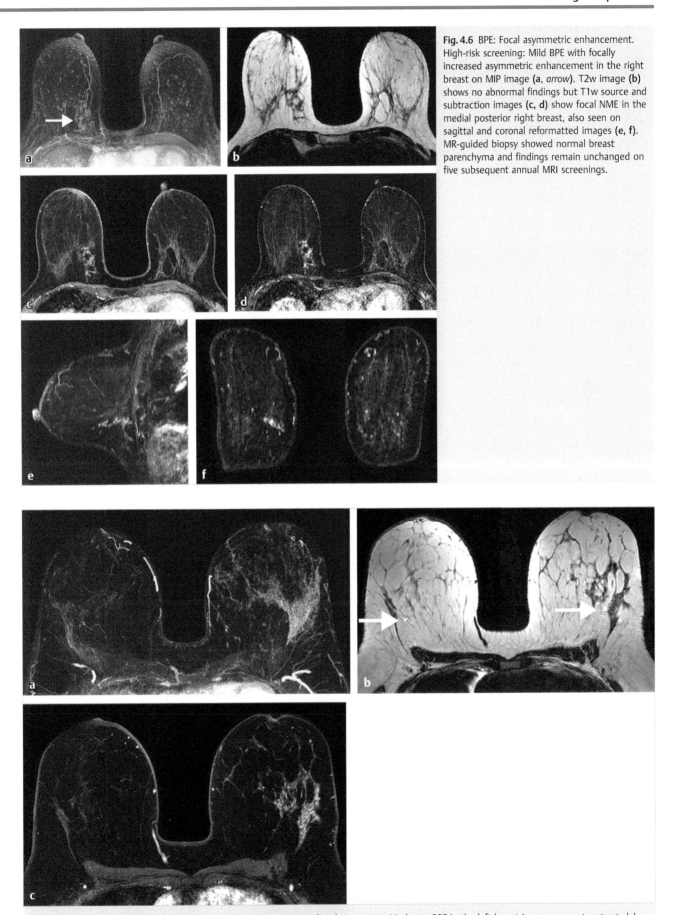

Fig. 4.6 BPE: Focal asymmetric enhancement. High-risk screening: Mild BPE with focally increased asymmetric enhancement in the right breast on MIP image (**a**, *arrow*). T2w image (**b**) shows no abnormal findings but T1w source and subtraction images (**c, d**) show focal NME in the medial posterior right breast, also seen on sagittal and coronal reformatted images (**e, f**). MR-guided biopsy showed normal breast parenchyma and findings remain unchanged on five subsequent annual MRI screenings.

Fig. 4.7 BPE: Asymmetric enhancement post–cancer treatment. High-risk screening: Moderate BPE in the left breast is seen on postcontrast slab image (**a**) with diminished enhancement seen in the right breast due to prior surgery and radiation therapy. T2w image shows asymmetric parenchyma and small, scattered bilateral cysts (**b**, *arrows*). Postcontrast source image (**c**) exhibits tiny punctate areas of parenchymal enhancement within the normal fibroglandular tissue.

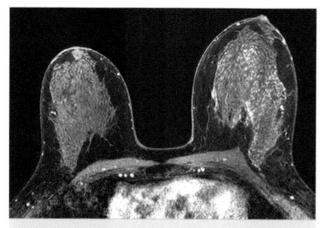

Fig. 4.8 BPE: Asymmetric enhancement post–cancer treatment. High-risk screening: Postcontrast T1w source image shows moderate BPE in the left breast, with diminished enhancement and volume loss noted in the right breast due to BCS and radiation therapy.

shown in lactating women; however, the findings usually resolve completely in the postlactation phase (▶ Fig. 4.10). Viewing of the source and subtraction MIP images generated from the pre- and first postcontrast series is a good way of providing an overview of enhancement for both breasts and for assessment of the level of BPE.

4.7 Cancer Detection

Once the amount of FGT and the level of BPE have been established, the next step in interpretation is to identify any abnormal enhancement that is distinct from the enhancement pattern of BPE. Search for abnormal morphology in addition to increased enhancement is critical for diagnosis, and it is important to recognize that very small lesions may not be visible on MIP images but only seen on individual postcontrast acquisition series. MIP images are created by using a processing method that projects the pixel with the highest signal onto a projection

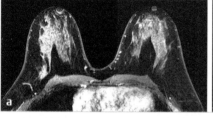
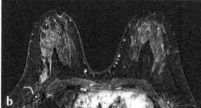

Fig. 4.9 BPE: Similar bilateral patterns of BPE. High-risk screening: Normal study showing moderate BPE with varying distribution, as seen on T1w source and subtracted postcontrast images (a, b).

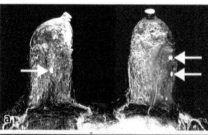
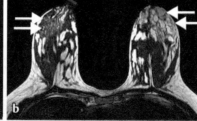

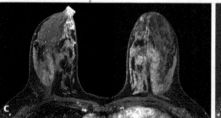
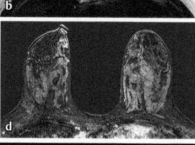

Fig. 4.10 BPE: 2 weeks and 12 months postlactation. High-risk screening, seventh module: MRI study performed at 2 weeks postcessation of breast-feeding shows marked BPE on MIP image (a) and bilateral stable circumscribed benign lesions (arrows). T2w image demonstrates bilateral high signal within enlarged subareolar ducts representing fluid (b, arrows). Source and subtraction T1w postcontrast images exhibit marked BPE (c, d). MIP image (e) obtained 12 months after lactation shows minimal BPE and no evidence of duct dilation is seen on the T2w precontrast image (f). Postcontrast T1w source and subtraction images (g, h) reveal complete resolution of the previously marked BPE with minimal BPE now seen bilaterally.

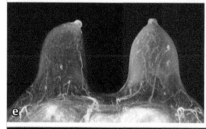
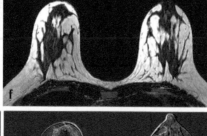

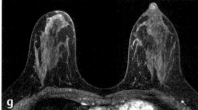
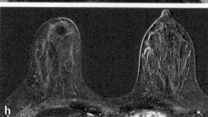

plane, using data from the precontrast and the postcontrast dynamic series (usually the first). Source and subtraction MIP images demonstrate lesion enhancement reflecting increased vascularity.

Enhancing lesions can be characterized as focus, mass, and nonmass enhancement. Most invasive cancers that are visible only on MRI are small and usually present as a focus or a small mass. Noninvasive cancers visible only on MRI may be small or large, because noncalcified DCIS may be occult on mammographic images. Lesion characterization is based on assessment of lesion morphology, the internal signal characteristics on the precontrast T1w and T2w images and the enhancement pattern on the source and subtraction post-contrast series. One of the most difficult aspects of AB-MR interpretation is the task of distinguishing the various presentations of BPE from abnormal NME that represents pathology. In order to maintain high specificity, care must be given to minimize MR biopsy of normal enhancing parenchyma. Availability of a prior MRI examination for comparison is greatly beneficial in this regard.

4.7.1 Focus

A focus is defined as a "spot" of enhancement less than 5 mm in size that is too small to characterize further in terms of its margins or internal enhancement pattern, due to insufficient spatial resolution or volume averaging. These lesions are often too small to be characterized morphologically and often fail to exhibit a corresponding finding on precontrast T2w or T1w

series. A focus may be benign or malignant and must be differentiated from the tiny "spots" of enhancement representing BPE. The distribution pattern of foci may prove helpful for diagnosis; multiple foci widely separated by intervening normal unenhancing breast parenchyma represent a common pattern of BPE, whereas a grouping of foci concentrated in one area in a linear distribution should be considered to represent clumped or linear NME and should be biopsied. Multiple scattered, similar-appearing foci require no additional analysis and MRI should be interpreted as normal.

As previously noted, a focus cannot be further characterized by its margins or internal enhancement pattern; therefore, a single focus may be deemed suspicious if it represents a solitary "spot" of enhancement or if its degree of enhancement is greater than that of the surrounding foci of BPE. Assessment of enhancement kinetics to characterize a focus is not standard in all practices. An investigation in 2014 reported on a retrospective review of 111 consecutive patients who underwent short-term follow-up of 136 enhancing foci.[34] Overall, the malignancy rate of an enhancing focus in this study was 2.9% (4/136), kinetic analysis yielding four malignant foci, two exhibiting progressive kinetics and two exhibiting washout kinetics. In the setting of moderate or marked BPE, a dominant single focus or focal area that exhibits suspicious kinetic features should be of greater concern than a focal area with numerous similar findings. A single focus of enhancement identified in a breast with minimal BPE usually represents a definitive lesion, benign or malignant (▶ Fig. 4.11). Early studies routinely disregarded foci

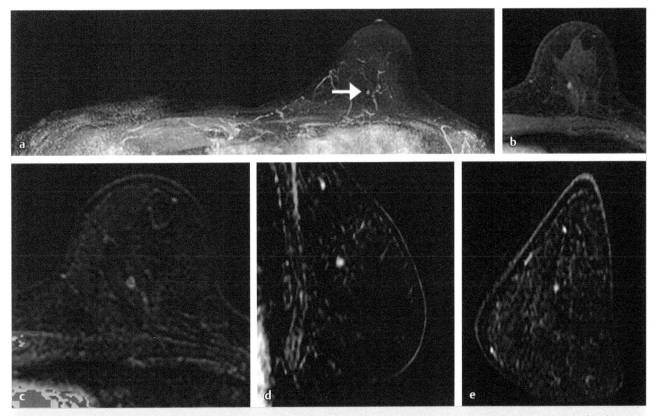

Fig. 4.11 Focus: A single focus in a breast with minimal BPE. High-risk screening, post right mastectomy for prior IDC: A 3-mm persistently enhancing focus is visible at 11 o'clock position in the left breast on MIP image (a) (1.5 Tesla) and postcontrast source and CAD images (b, c), also seen on sagittal and coronal reformatted images (d, e). MR-guided biopsy yielded high-grade DCIS, solid with cancerization of lobules.

as being either benign or probably benign, likely due to the inability at that time to characterize morphology.[35] An investigation by Eby et al in 2009 reported that foci comprised 46% of BIRADS three lesions ($n = 168$) and that only one focus was found to be malignant on follow-up.[36] In recent years, however, imaging with higher field strength magnets (3 T) allows improved visualization of morphology associated with lesions smaller than 5 mm, and such lesions should be classified as small masses, rather than "spots" of enhancement. Although more supporting data are needed, the improved spatial resolution at higher field strength should lead to improved specificity at MRI screening.

4.7.2 Small Masses

A small enhancing mass (< 5 mm in size) and distinct from BPE should be analyzed primarily according to its morphology. Although subtraction T1w postcontrast images are useful for detection, morphologic analysis is best assessed on the postcontrast T1w source images. Raza and colleagues reviewed the outcome of 68 MR-detected small breast masses (≤ 5 mm) biopsied with MR guidance between March 2004 and February 2009.[37] Among these biopsied small masses, 14 (20.6%) were malignant, and of these, 7 (50%) were found in the ipsilateral breast of patients with a newly diagnosed cancer. When the masses were subdivided into lesions 5 mm, 32 (28.1%). The authors concluded that the decision to biopsy small masses should be based on carefully assessed MR features, in the context of examination indication, not solely on mass size.

Mass features that suggest benignity include an oval or round shape, a circumscribed margin, a high signal on T2w series, presence of a fatty hilum, and persistent kinetics. High T2 signal is defined as signal higher than that of the normal glandular tissue and equivalent to the signal of cyst fluid (▶ Fig. 4.12). Appropriate window and leveling is necessary in order to appreciate the internal features of a lesion seen on both T2w and T1w postcontrast series.

Intramammary lymph nodes (IMLN) reliably exhibit washout kinetics, and demonstration of benign morphology is needed for accurate interpretation. A fatty hilum is a salient feature of

an IMLN, and additional features typically found include high signal on T2w series, smooth margins, and washout kinetics on T1w postcontrast series (▶ Fig. 4.13; ▶ Fig. 4.14). The acquisition plane may not identify a fatty hilum, which may only be seen on by reformatting the imaging plane. Features that suggest a probably benign mass on a baseline AB-MR study include a circumscribed margin, homogeneous enhancement, but no high T2 correlate.

Features that suggest malignancy include a mass with an irregular shape, absent bright signal on T2w series, margins that are not circumscribed, and kinetics that exhibit washout (▶ Fig. 4.15). Masses exhibiting rim enhancement need careful evaluation, the differential diagnosis being either an inflammatory cyst (a benign lesion) or a malignancy. Analysis of the T2w series is useful in these cases, because inflammatory cysts may exhibit high signal on either the T1w or T2w precontrast images, matching the dark lesion center on the T1w postcontrast images. Correlation of high spatial resolution T2w images that exactly match the resolution of the T1w series is helpful for diagnosis (▶ Fig. 4.16). Biopsy should be recommended for a circumscribed rim-enhancing mass that is not an inflammatory cyst (▶ Fig. 4.17).

A mass is usually benign if it is stable when compared to a prior study. Biopsy should be considered for any small mass with an irregular shape and margin and for any mass that is new or increased in size when compared to the previous examination (▶ Fig. 4.18). Pseudoangiomatous stromal hyperplasia (PASH) is an uncommon mesenchymal lesion seen at histology as a benign proliferation of fibrous stroma, containing slit-like pseudovascular spaces lined by myofibroblasts. Nodular PASH may appear as a small irregular lesion, visible on MRI as a rapidly enhancing mass (▶ Fig. 4.19). Examples of small masses identified at high-risk MR screening only, subsequently biopsied under MR guidance, are shown in ▶ Fig. 4.20 and ▶ Fig. 4.21. The threshold for MR biopsy should be lowered when a small additional mass is seen in the same breast as an index cancer at the time of initial diagnosis, and this is also true when a new enhancing lesion is found in either breast at follow-up MR screening (▶ Fig. 4.22; ▶ Fig. 4.23), particularly if the finding is found in the previously irradiated breast (▶ Fig. 4.24).

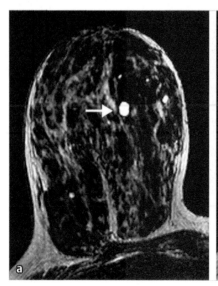
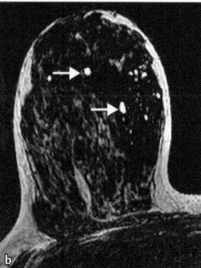

Fig. 4.12 Cysts high-risk screening: Cyst fluid exhibits a signal higher than that of the normal glandular tissue. T2 w non–fat-suppressed images **(a, b)** show extreme FGT and bilateral round and oval high-signal lesions (*arrows*), representing cysts of various sizes. Note that the internal cyst fluid signal is significantly higher than the surrounding fat signal.

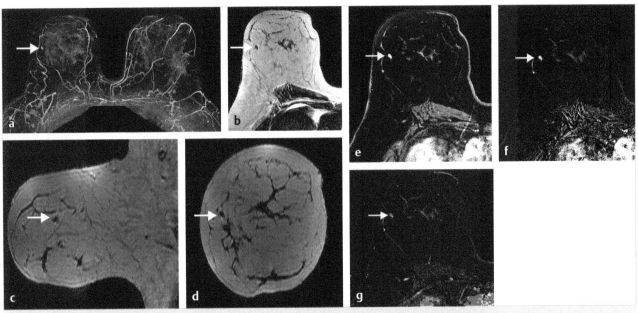

Fig. 4.13 Normal intramammary lymph node (IMLN) high-risk screening: Normal lymph nodes are frequently seen on MR as round or oval masses with circumscribed margins and washout kinetics. MIP image (**a**, *arrow*) shows a rapidly enhancing small mass with an inferolateral notch suggesting a central hilum. T2w non–fat suppressed MPR images (**b–d**, *arrows*) show a correlative isointense mass also seen on postcontrast source and subtracted images (**e, f**, *arrows*). IMLNs have a robust blood supply with a direct feeding artery into the nodal hilum, accounting for washout kinetics seen on CAD image (**g**, *arrow*).

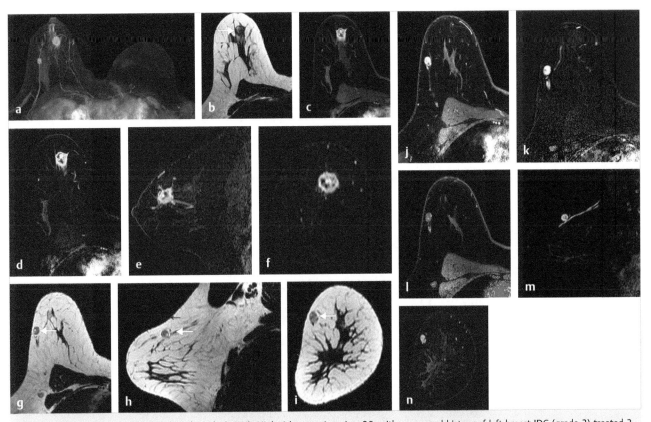

Fig. 4.14 Metastatic intramammary lymph node (IMLN). High-risk screening: Age 36, with a personal history of left breast IDC (grade 3) treated 3 years ago with BCS. MIP image (**a**) reveals a new right anterior mass with rim enhancement and a lateral oval mass with circumscribed margins and a reconstructed left breast. T2w image (**b**) shows an anterior, round high-signal mass (*arrow*), with rim enhancement and a central enhancing nidus seen on postcontrast T1w source and subtraction images (**c, d**) and reformatted sagittal and coronal images (**e, f**). A prominent oval mass with high internal signal representing an enlarged IMLN is seen on T2w axial (**g**, *arrow*) and reformatted images (**h, I**, *arrows*) and postcontrast T1w axial source, subtracted and angiomap images (**j–l**). Reformatted sagittal and coronal images are shown (**m, n**). Histology of the anterior index lesion yielded a triple negative IDC, oncotype DX score = 58. Six axillary sentinel nodes were negative for malignancy (0/6). Ultrasound-guided biopsy of the IMLN yielded metastatic IDC.

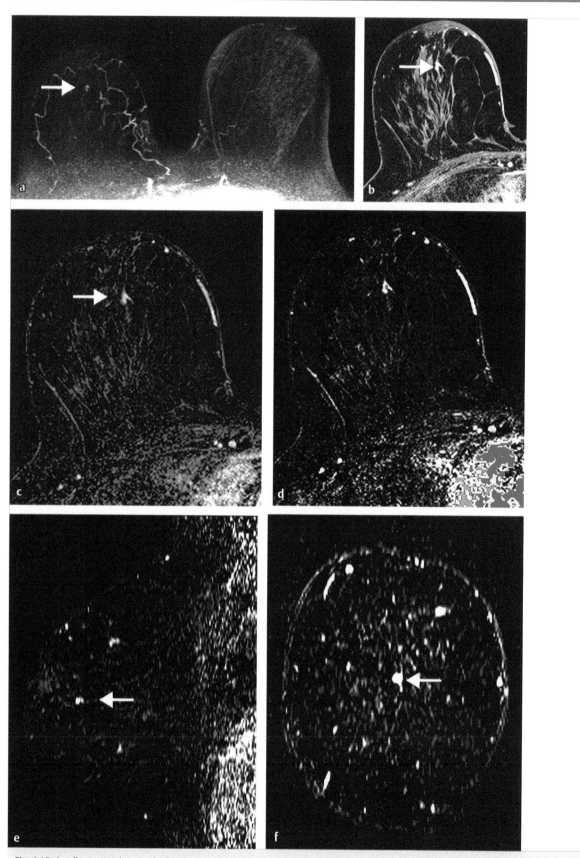

Fig. 4.15 Small mass: Malignant; high-risk screening: Age 73, with a personal history of right breast IDC (grade 3, HER2 positive) 8 years ago, treated with BCS. MIP image (**a**) shows a small irregular enhancing mass in the anterior central right breast (*arrow*). Source postcontrast T1w image (**b**) reveals skin thickening from prior treatment and a new 5-mm irregular mass in the anterior right breast (*arrow*) also seen on subtraction image (**c**, *arrow*). Angiomap (**d**) reveals washout enhancement within the mass and sagittal and coronal reformatted images (**e, f**, *arrows*) are shown. Histology at MR-guided biopsy yielded IBC-mixed ductal and lobular phenotype, intermediate grade, ER/PR (−), HER2/neu (+).

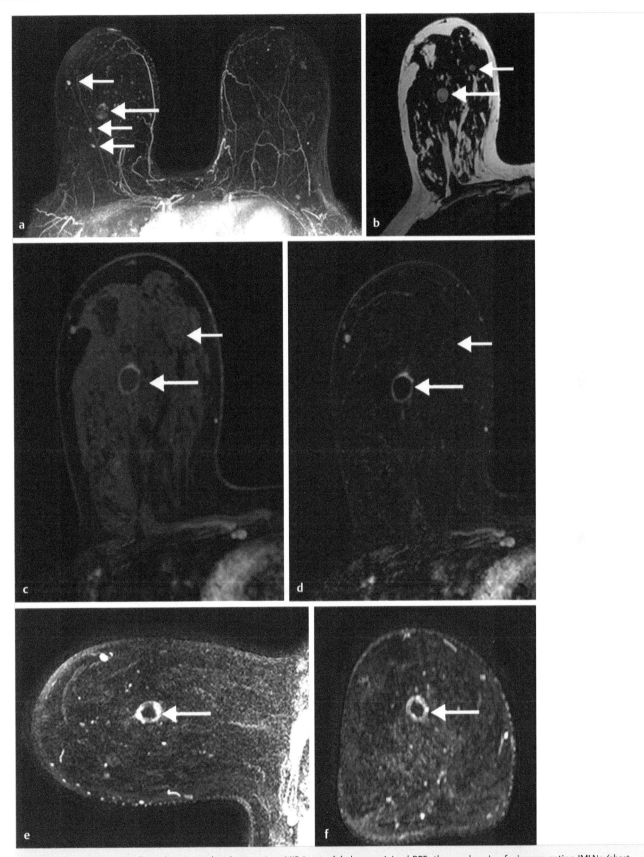

Fig. 4.16 Rim-enhancing inflamed cysts. High-risk screening: MIP image **(a)** shows minimal BPE, three enhancing foci representing IMLNs *(short arrows)* and a new central rim-enhancing round mass *(long arrow)*. T2w non–fat-suppressed image **(b)** shows a round high-signal mass correlating with the MIP finding *(long arrow)* and a second smaller, medial, high-signal mass *(short arrow)*. T1w postcontrast source and subtraction images reveal a thin enhancing rim surrounding a dark lesion center correlating with the high spatial resolution masses seen on the T2w series **(c, d,** *long and short arrows)*. These benign findings are typically seen in inflammatory cysts. Sagittal and coronal images of the larger cyst are shown **(e, f)**.

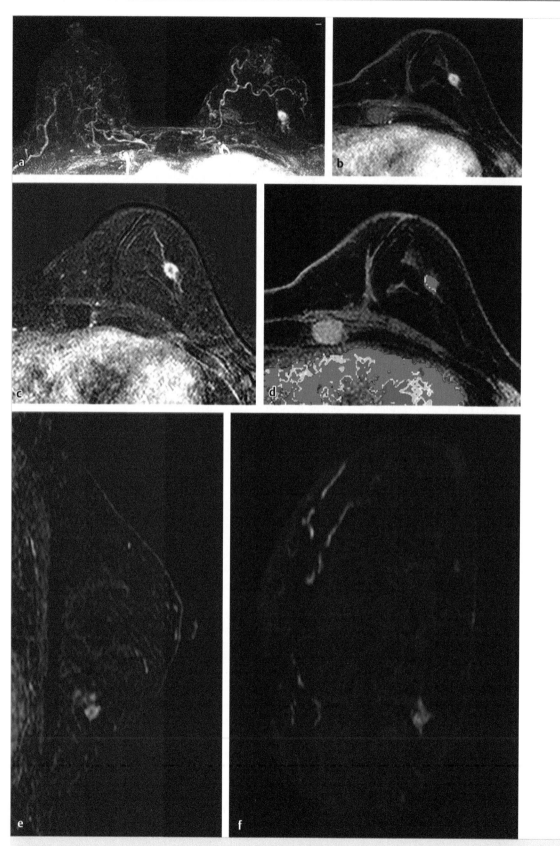

Fig. 4.17 Small mass: Rim-enhancing cancer. High-risk screening, age 62: MIP image **(a)** shows a new, left oval enhancing mass, T1w postcontrast source and subtraction images **(b, c)** revealing a unifocal, 6-mm rim-enhancing mass in the inferolateral left breast in the setting of minimal BPE. Angiomap image **(d)** reveals homogeneous washout kinetics, and reformatted sagittal and coronal images of the small mass are shown **(e, f)**. Histology at MR-guided biopsy yielded IDC grade 2 of 3, lesion size 10 × 13 × 9 mm, with associated internal DCIS, intermediate grade, clinging and cribriform, ER/PR (–), HER2/neu (+), Ki67: 30%. Two axillary sentinel nodes were negative for malignancy (0/2).

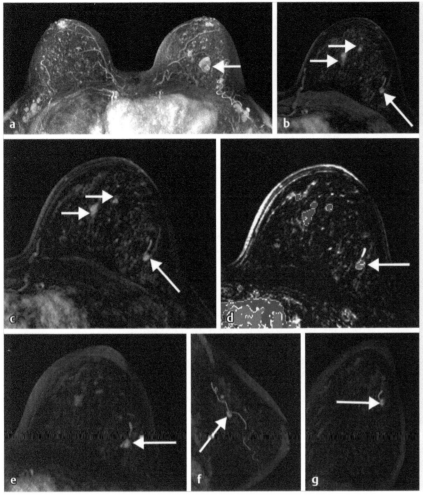

Fig. 4.18 Small mass: Fibroadenoma. High-risk screening: Age 40, fourth module, with a known fibroadenoma (20 × 16 × 14 mm) is demonstrated at 6 o'clock position in the left breast as seen on MIP image (**a**, *arrow*). Postcontrast T1w source and subtraction images (**b, c**) demonstrate two stable enhancing anterior benign lesions (*short arrows*) and a new small 7 mm, round, enhancing mass is identified in the left breast at the 2 o'clock position, posterior depth (*long arrows*). Angiomap (**d**) reveals washout kinetics within the mass and slab axial, sagittal, and coronal images (**e–g**, *arrows*) are shown. MR-guided biopsy yielded fibroadenoma.

4.7.3 Nonmass Enhancement

Nonmass enhancement refers to an area of enhancement that appears distinct from normal surrounding breast parenchyma on postcontrast images. Diagnosis of NME is often challenging, because these lesions do not exhibit mass effect, the enhancing area most often has no correlate on precontrast T2w or T1w images, and the lesion does not demonstrate a clear interface or definitive margins. NME findings are often benign at biopsy with histology yielding adenosis, focal or diffuse fibrocystic change, or high-risk lesions such as atypical lobular hyperplasia (ALH), lobular carcinoma in situ (LCIS), or atypical ductal hyperplasia (ADH). DCIS commonly presents as NME, often without visible associated mammographic calcification. Certain invasive cancers, including invasive lobular carcinoma (ILC), invasive ductal carcinoma (IDC) (more frequently the HER-2/neu positive subtype), and diffuse aggressive invasive cancers, exhibit NME as the presenting finding. Distribution of NME is the key for differentiation of invasive cancer from DCIS. Invasive cancers generally do not exhibit a segmental or linear distribution even though the kinetic behavior of ILC and DCIS lesions may be similar, with progressive enhancement often seen in both cases. IDC lesions usually exhibit rapid uptake and washout. Confounding the difficulty of diagnosis is the lack of robust enhancement, slow uptake, and progressive kinetics frequently making the differential diagnosis between benign lesions and NME more challenging. Nonetheless, very small regions of NME can be diagnosed at MR, and early identification of linear enhancement is often the presenting finding.

The BI-RADS Atlas descriptors characterize NME in terms of their distribution (focal, linear, segmental, regional, multiple regions, or diffuse) and internal enhancement pattern (homogeneous, heterogeneous, clumped, or clustered ring).[16] Multiple studies have correlated BI-RADS descriptors for NME and the likelihood of malignancy, and the results have been variable. A report by Baltzer and colleagues in 2010 concluded that NME was a frequent cause of false-positive biopsies and that BIRADS descriptors were insufficient for differentiating between benign and malignant lesions.[38] In general, I think it is fair to say that linear, focal, and segmental distribution, and clumped and clustered ring internal enhancement, are the most reliable descriptors of DCIS, and a combination of these features can be used

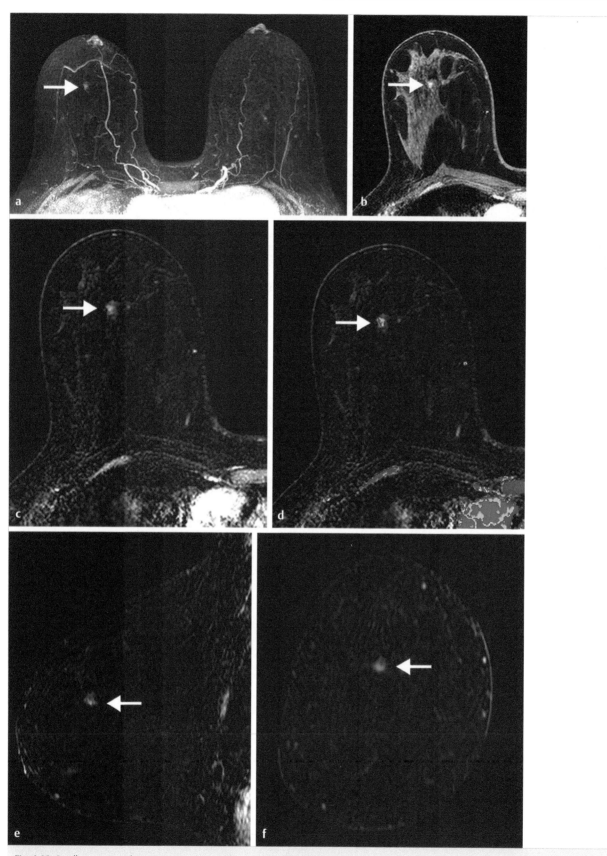

Fig. 4.19 Small mass: pseudoangiomatous stromal hyperplasia (PASH). High-risk screening age 39: MIP image **(a)** shows minimal BPE, and a 3-mm enhancing small mass in the central right breast *(arrow)* with a correlate seen on T1w postcontrast source and subtraction images **(b, c,** *arrows)*. Angiomap shows plateau kinetics **(d,** *arrow)*. Sagittal and coronal reformatted images are shown **(e, f,** *arrows)*. MR-guided biopsy yielded PASH.

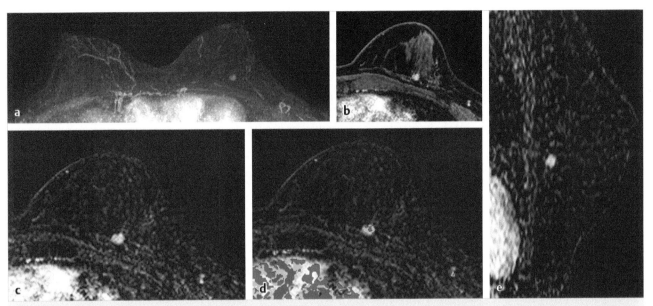

Fig. 4.20 Small mass: Malignant. High-risk screening: MIP image (**a**) shows mild BPE, and a 6-mm enhancing small irregular mass in the posterior left breast with a correlate seen on T1w postcontrast source and subtraction images (**b, c**). Angiomap exhibits washout kinetics (**d**), and a sagittal reformatted image is shown (**e**). MR-guided biopsy yielded histology at IDC grade 2 with lobular features, lesion size 6 mm, ER/PR (+), HER2/neu (−), Ki67: 10 to 15%. Four sentinel nodes were negative for malignancy (0/4).

for a final diagnostic assessment. Lesion types of NME, identified only on screening MRI and subsequently biopsied under MR guidance yielding DCIS, are shown as follows: linear enhancement (► Fig. 4.25; ► Fig. 4.26; ► Fig. 4.27), focal enhancement (► Fig. 4.28; ► Fig. 4.29; ► Fig. 4.30), and segmental enhancement (► Fig. 4.31).

A report in 2013 reviewed MR features of false-negative cases detected on an incident (second or subsequent) round of MR screening.[35] Sixteen cancers were identified, and among these, nine cancers (five foci, two small masses, and two NME) were retrospectively identifiable on the prior MRI examination. All incident cancers showed an increase in size when compared to the prior study (median 80% increase), four showing rapid uptake of contrast on the prior examination and five showing a change in kinetic pattern from slow to rapid uptake. Among the five malignant foci, one was isolated and two of four were located in a background of BPE but could be distinguished by their higher signal intensity. The authors concluded that any lesion that shows an increase in size, rapid uptake kinetics, or a change in kinetic pattern should be viewed with suspicion, and a biopsy should be considered.[44] A retrospective study published in 2017 reported on 163 cancers identified on MRI and found that benign characteristics were present in most of the very small cancers (≤ 5 mm), but that when invasive breast cancers approached 10 mm in size, their characteristics on MRI became increasingly typical of malignancy.[39]

4.8 Reporting

FFDM and MRI screening reports should follow the BI-RADS lexicon developed by the American College of Radiology.[40] In addition to lesion characterization, the report must include the specific MR technique utilized, in summary form, and the type and amount of GBCM administered. The MRI report should include the volume of FGT, the amount of BPE, and when appropriate, the day or the week of the menstrual cycle on which study was obtained. Ideally, studies will be interpreted using double-reading technique for both modalities; however, this is often not possible in routine clinical practice in the United States. When findings are abnormal, the patient should be managed following standard routine clinical practice, after review of all of the findings in both screening studies.

4.8.1 Breast Imaging Audit

Increasing utilization of breast MRI highlights the need for audit and benchmark performance parameters for quality assurance purposes. A breast MRI audit should be conducted as part of routine radiologic practice. The ACR practice parameter for the performance of contrast-enhanced breast MRI recommends that each facility should establish and maintain a medical outcome audit program to follow up positive assessments and to correlate pathology results with the interpreting physician's findings.[10] The recommendations and results of biopsies based on FFDM and MRI screening findings should be recorded to determine the cancer yield, PPV, recall rate, interval cancer rate, and frequency of recommendations for short-term follow-up. Although breast MRI has high sensitivity and can detect smaller tumors than mammography, it has some limitations. Missed cancers may not be detected either because they are very small, or because they do not exhibit sufficient contrast enhancement. Increased recall rates for both additional imaging and biopsy in early studies of high-risk screening populations tend to be higher with MRI ranging from 8 to 17% for imaging and 3 to 15% for biopsy.[41,42,43] As with any new screening technique, radiologic performance can improve with time, factors contributing to accuracy include the technical quality of the acquisition and the experience of the reader. A report on a clinical

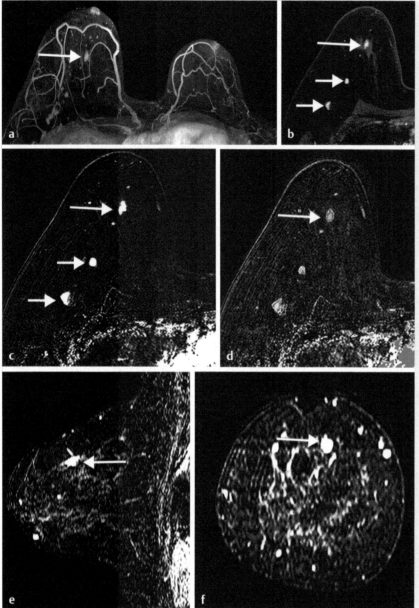

Fig. 4.21 Small mass: Malignant. High-risk screening: MIP image **(a)** exhibits minimal BPE with a 4-mm enhancing irregular mass seen in the anterior right breast at 12 0'clock position (a, *long arrow*). A correlate mass is visible on T1w postcontrast source and subtraction images **(b, c,** *long arrows*) and two enhancing IMLNs are also noted (*short arrows*). Angiomap **(d)** reveals persistent kinetics in the irregular mass (*long arrow*) and two IMLNs exhibit washout kinetics. The irregular mass is also shown on sagittal reformatted image **(e)** and coronal image **(f,** *arrow*). MR-guided biopsy yielded IDC grade 3 with associated high-grade DCIS, solid type with necrosis, ER/PR (−), HER2/neu (−), Ki67: 20%. Six left sentinel nodes were negative for malignancy (0/6).

practice audit of screening examinations from 2010 to 2013 by Strigel et al found that the cancer detection rate, median invasive cancer size, PPV2, and PPV3 all fell within the ACR BI-RADS MRI benchmarks supporting their broader appropriateness for routine practice.[44]

Summary statistics and comparisons generated for each radiologist and for each facility should be reviewed annually by the lead interpreting physician as part of a routine breast MRI screening and diagnostic audit. A report by Lee et al[45] looked at breast MRI BI-RADS assessments and abnormal interpretation rates (AIR) by clinical indication, among a large sample of U.S. community practices. Data were analyzed from 41 facilities across five Breast Cancer Surveillance Consortium imaging registries, between 2005 and 2010, including 11,654 breast MRI examinations in women aged 18 to 79 years. The authors found that the AIR for breast MRI examinations varied by indication

(screening or diagnostic), consistent with the significantly different BI-RADS outcomes for diagnostic and screening mammography.[46,47,48]

Another study by Niell et al evaluated breast MRI performance measures stratified by screening and diagnostic indications in a large study from a single academic institution.[49] A total of 2,444 MR examinations were subdivided into 1,313 screening and 1,131 diagnostic examinations. The cancer detection rates were 14 per 1,000 in the screening setting and 47 per 1,000 in the diagnostic setting ($p < 0.00001$). The AIR was 12% (152 of 1,313) for screening and 17% (194 of 1,131) for diagnostic indications ($p = 0.00008$). The PPVs of MRI were lower for screening (PPV1 [abnormal findings] 12%, PPV2 [biopsy recommended] 24%, PPV3 [biopsy performed] 27%) compared with diagnostic indications, PPV1 28%, PPV2 36%, and PPV3 38%. Performance measures, including PPV, abnormal interpretation

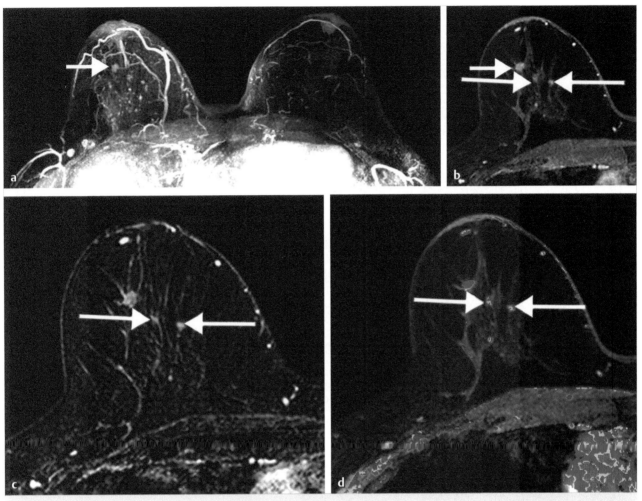

Fig. 4.22 Small masses (3): Malignant. High-risk screening: Age 59, personal history of invasive cancer in the left breast treated with BCS 10 years ago. MIP image **(a)** exhibits mild BPE in the right breast (*arrow*) with diminished BPE in the left breast due to prior cancer treatment. T1w postcontrast source and subtraction images reveal an irregular mass in the anterior right breast **(b, c**, *arrow*) with persistent kinetics noted on angiomap **(d)**. Two additional enhancing masses are located media and posterior to the main mass (*long arrows*). MR-guided biopsy yielded IDC grade 1 and 2 with associated low-grade, cribriform, DCIS. ER/PR (+), HER2/neu (−). Four sentinel nodes were negative for malignancy (0/4).

rate, and cancer detection rate, varied significantly for screening and diagnostic breast MRI examinations (▶ Table 4.1).

Results of these studies clearly show significantly different MRI performance measures for screening and diagnostic indications, thus supporting the practice of stratified rather than aggregate analyses of benchmark measures for breast MRI. The audit should also obtain summary statistics and comparisons generated for each physician and for each facility, and the lead interpreting physician should review the results on an annual basis. The BI-RADS Atlas contains guidance on monitoring outcomes and outlines methods for conducting an audit.[40]

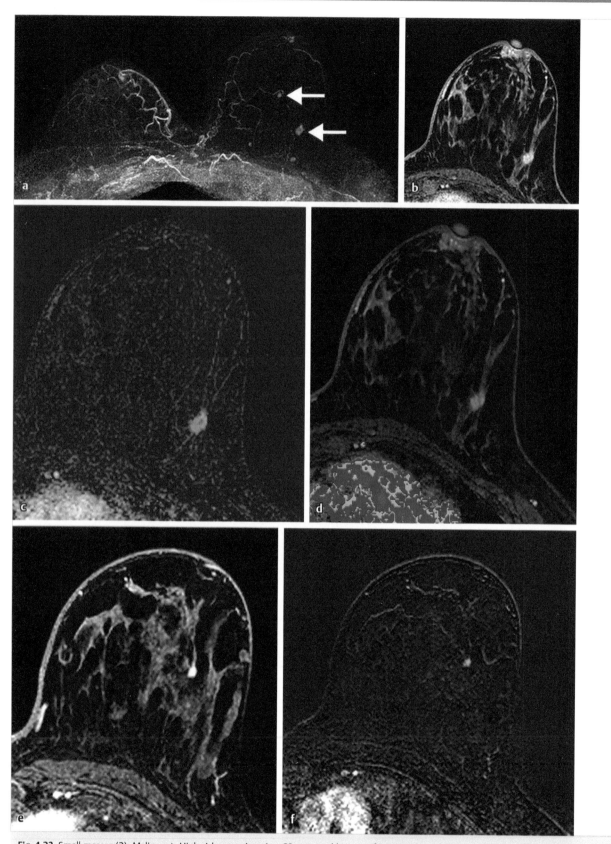

Fig. 4.23 Small masses (2): Malignant. High-risk screening: Age 69, personal history of DCIS in the right breast treated with BCS 12 months ago. MIP image (a) shows right breast volume loss due to prior DCIS treatment and two left breast–enhancing masses; an 8-mm posterior mass at 3 o'clock position and a 3 mm more anterior mass at 12:30 (*arrows*). T1w postcontrast source, subtraction, and angiomap images (**b–d**) show the posterior mass to exhibit irregular shape and margins and no enhancement above threshold kinetics. The more anterior mass exhibits a slightly irregular shape (**e, f**). MR-guided biopsy of both lesions yielded IDC grade 1 and 2 with associated low-grade, cribriform, DCIS. ER/PR (+), HER2/neu (−). Four sentinel nodes were negative for malignancy (0/4).

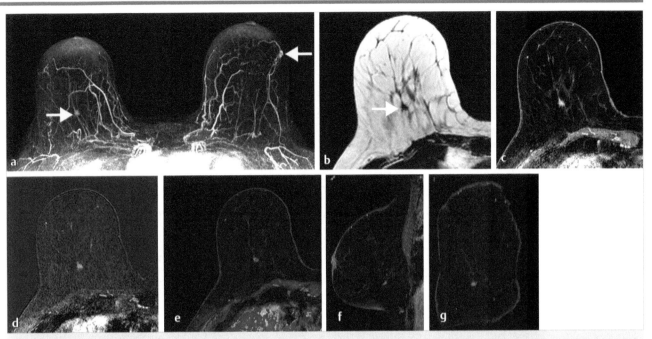

Fig. 4.24 Small mass: Malignant. High-risk screening: tenth module, age 66, personal history of triple negative IDC grade 3 in the right breast treated with BCS 8 years ago. MIP image **(a)** exhibits decreased volume due to prior surgery and a new 6-mm irregular mass in the central right breast, posterior location at 6 o'clock position (*arrow*), in addition to a 6-mm oval, circumscribed mass with a fatty hilum in the upper outer left breast representing an IMLN (*arrow*). A low-signal mass with spiculated margins is seen on T2w image (**b**, *arrow*) and shows irregular shape and persistent kinetics on T1w postcontrast source and subtraction images (**c–e**). Reformatted images **(f, g)** are shown. MR-guided biopsy IDC grade 3, ER/PR (−), HER2/neu (−), Ki67: 15%. Four sentinel nodes negative for malignancy (0/4).

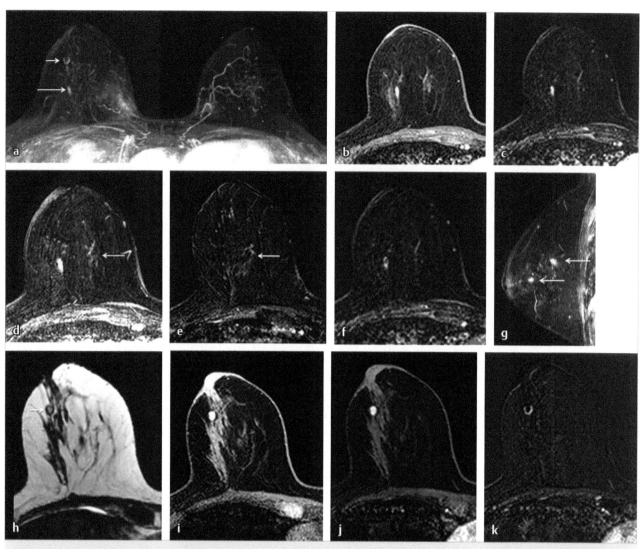

Fig. 4.25 Nonmass enhancement: linear. High-risk screening seventh module: MIP image **(a)** exhibits mild BPE and a 7-mm linear NME in the posterolateral right breast (*long arrow*) and a rim-enhancing small mass in the anterolateral right breast (*short arrow*). T1w axial postcontrast source and subtraction images **(b, c)** reveal linear NME, axial subtraction thin MIP images **(d,** *arrow*), and a more inferior subtraction image **(e)** shows additional medial NME (*arrow*). Angiomap **(f)** shows washout kinetics within the main linear NME, sagittal reformatted image **(g)** demonstrating the segmental extent of NME (*arrows*). MR-guided biopsy yielded DCIS, low and intermediate grade, solid subtype, ER/PR (+), extending for 6 cm in the central right breast. Incidental note is made of a benign rim-enhancing inflamed cyst, present on multiple prior MR screening examinations in the anterolateral right breast: T2w **(h,** *arrow*), precontrast T1w **(i)**, postcontrast T1w **(j)**, and subtraction image **(k)**.

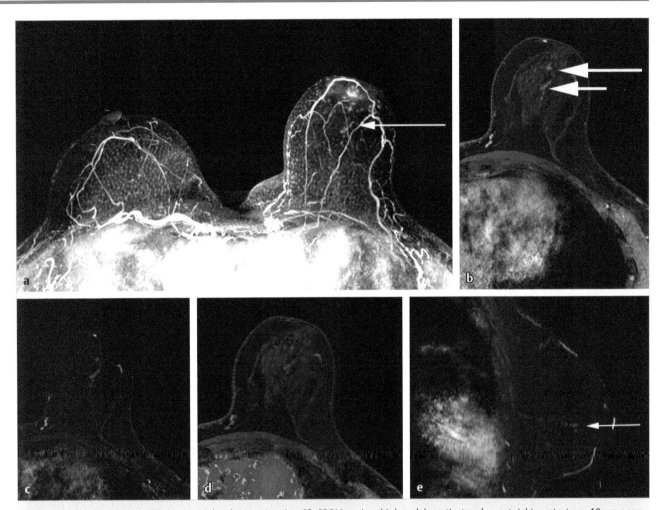

Fig. 4.26 Nonmass enhancement: Linear. High-risk screening: Age 62, *BRCA1* carrier, third module, patient underwent right mastectomy 10 years ago for IDC grade 2 with autologous reconstruction. MIP image **(a)** reveals subtle linear enhancement in the anterior left breast (*arrow*). T1w postcontrast axial source image **(b)** reveals linear NME (*short arrow*) and an anterior focus (*long arrow*) also seen on subtraction image **(c)**, angiomap shows no enhancement above the kinetic threshold **(d)**. The total area of enhancement extends about 7 cm. A sagittal reformatted image is shown **(e,** *arrow*). MR-guided biopsy yielded DCIS, solid subtype, intermediate and high nuclear grade, largest focus 1 cm with disease extending over an area of 8 cm. Five sentinel nodes negative for malignancy (0/5). This case illustrates the importance of morphology. Linear NME requires biopsy despite the absence of robust enhancement.

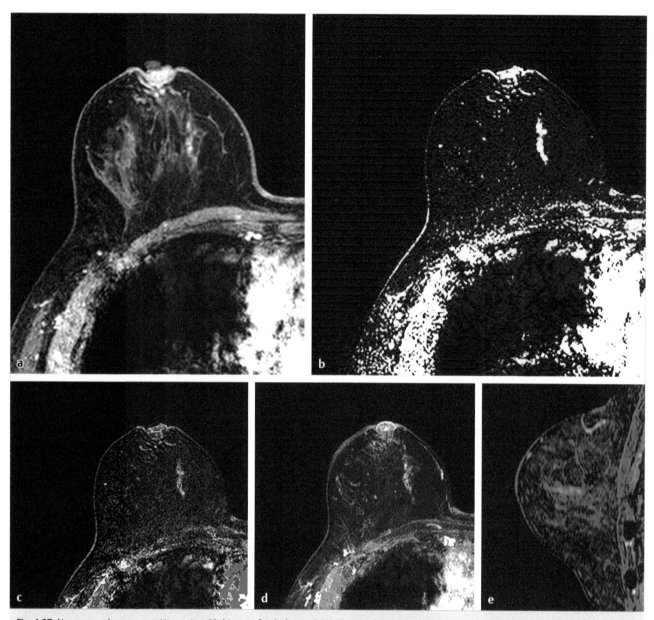

Fig. 4.27 Nonmass enhancement: Linear. Age 62, history of right breast DCIS: T1w axial postcontrast source and subtraction images **(a, b)** reveal 3-cm linear NME in the medial central right breast. Angiomap **(c)** shows persistent kinetics within the main linear NME, and axial slab image shows the extent of NME to advantage **(d)**, a sagittal reformatted image **(e)** is shown. MR-directed mammography identified calcifications at the site of NME, and stereotaxic biopsy yielded DCIS intermediate grade, solid and cribriform types, with associated central necrosis and calcifications, cancerization of lobules and stromal calcifications also identified, ER/PR (+).

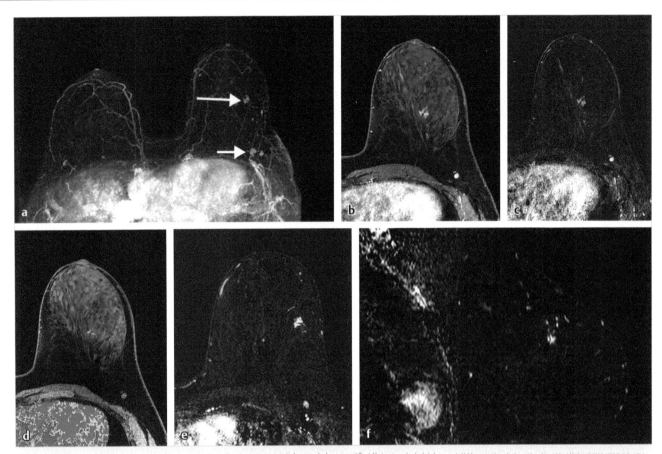

Fig. 4.28 Nonmass enhancement: Focal. High-risk screening, 12th module age 43: History of right breast IDC grade 3, treated with BCS. MIP image **(a)** shows volume loss and decreased BPE, result of prior cancer treatment, also a focal area of NME in the lateral left breast (*long arrow*) and an enlarged axillary lymph node (*short arrow*). Focal NME is also present on T1w axial postcontrast source and subtraction images **(b, c)** and heterogeneous washout kinetics are identified on angiomap **(d)**. Additional axial, sagittal images are shown **(e, f)**. MR-guided biopsy yielded DCIS, intermediate and high nuclear grade, micropapillary and cribriform subtype, with an associated 1-cm IDC grade 2 with LVI, ER/PR (+), HER2/neu (−), one sentinel node was positive for malignancy (1/4).

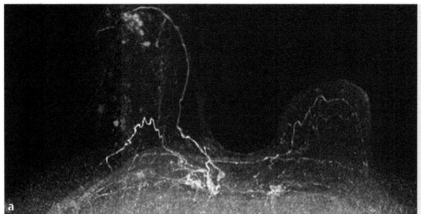

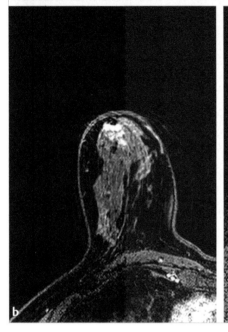

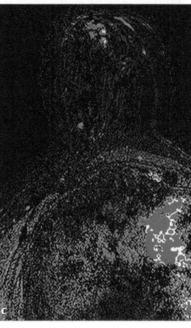

Fig. 4.29 Nonmass enhancement: Focal. High-risk screening: age 76, fifth module. History of left breast IDC grade 3 6 years ago treated with BCS, and right breast DCIS 5 years ago treated with BCS. MIP image **(a)** shows left breast volume loss and decreased BPE, result of prior BCS, and a focal area of NME in the subareolar region of the right breast also present on T1w axial postcontrast source image **(b)**. Heterogeneous, predominantly persistent kinetics are identified on angiomap **(c)**. MR-guided biopsy yielded DCIS, intermediate nuclear grade solid subtype, with cancerization of the lobules. ER/PR (+), Ki67: 10%.

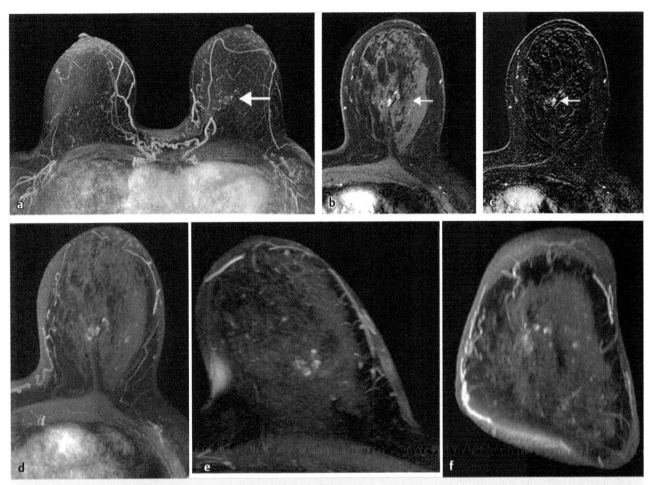

Fig. 4.30 Nonmass enhancement: Focal. Age 59: personal history of right breast DCIS. MIP image **(a)** shows a focal area of NME in the left breast (*arrow*), also seen on T1w axial postcontrast source image **(b)** and subtraction image **(c,** *arrow*). Axial, sagittal, and coronal slab images **(d–f)** are shown. MR-guided biopsy yielded DCIS, intermediate nuclear grade cribriform subtype, ER (+), PR (−), Ki67: 5%.

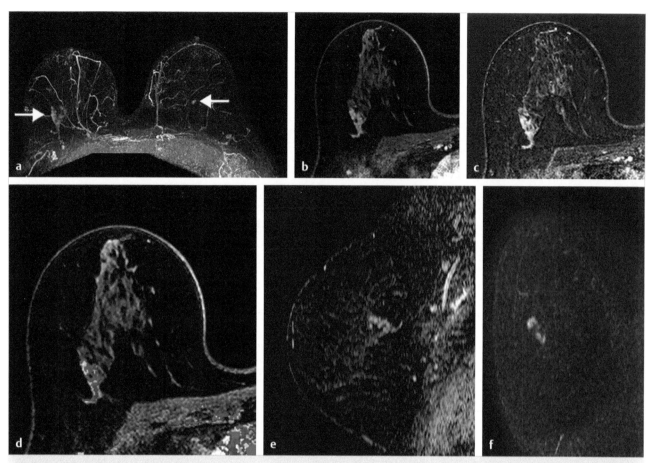

Fig. 4.31 Nonmass enhancement: Segmental. High-risk screening, age 68: MIP image **(a)** shows segmental NME in the posterolateral right breast (*arrow*) and a known fibroadenoma in the central left breast (*arrow*) T1w axial postcontrast source and subtraction images of the right breast **(b, c)** show NME with heterogeneous kinetics, predominantly of the persistent type, identified on angiomap **(d)**. Additional sagittal and coronal reformatted images are shown **(e, f)**. MR-guided biopsy yielded DCIS, 1.5 cm, high nuclear grade solid and cribriform subtype with necrosis and associated LCIS, classic type, ER/PR (+).

Table 4.1 Performance measure for screening and diagnostic breast MRI

	Screening	Diagnostic	Overall
Total number of MRI studies	1,313	1,131	2,444
Total number of MRI studies with positive findings (BI-RADS 0, 4, and 5)	152	194	346
Final BI-RADS 4 or 5			
Biopsies (lesion level)	77	172	249
Cancer diagnoses (lesion)	18	61	79
Cancer detection rate/1,000 examinations	14	47	29
AIR	152/1,313 (12%)	194/1,131 (17%)	346/2,444 (14%)
PPV1	18/152 (12%)	54/194 (28%)	72/346 (21%)
PPV2	18/75 (24%)	53/146 (36%)	71/224 (32%)
PPV3 (examination level)	18/67 (27%)	53/138 (38%)	71/205 (305%)

Abbreviations: AIR, abnormal interpretation rate; MRI, magnetic resonance imaging; PPV, positive predictive value.
Source: Modified from Niell et al.[49]

4.9 Summary

Screening for breast cancer has long been a topic of debate and often a source of high anxiety for women. Over the past four decades, several randomized controlled trials using mammography as a screening tool have clearly shown that early detection can reduce overall mortality from breast cancer. Although there are no long-term outcome studies to date that evaluate the effect of MR screening on breast cancer mortality, the expectation is that the detection of smaller-node negative cancers will improve patient outcomes. Implementation of AB-MR technique as an adjunctive method to screening mammography for women with dense breasts is an innovative and challenging endeavor. The underlying principles of MR interpretation are similar, whether an abbreviated protocol or a full protocol is utilized. Breast imaging facilities will need to reconsider their MRI workflow to allow for efficient throughput of women to be screened, while maintaining technical and interpretive excellence. If successful, AB-MR screening could result in the detection of a significantly larger number of high-grade cancers than other imaging methods while also reducing interval cancers and node positivity.

References

[1] MRI Accreditation—American College of Radiology. Available at: www.acr.org/Quality-Safety/Accreditation/MRI. Accessed January 7, 2015

[2] The Mammography Quality Standards Act Final Regulations: Modifications and Additions to Policy Guidance Help System #9. Available at: www.fda.gov/[Mammography]/[QualitySt.] Oct 8 2014 Accessed January 9, 2016

[3] Heacock L, Melsaether AN, Heller SL, et al. Evaluation of a known breast cancer using an abbreviated breast MRI protocol: Correlation of imaging characteristics and pathology with lesion detection and conspicuity. Eur J Radiol 2016;85:815823

[4] Mango VL, Morris EA, David Dershaw D, et al. Abbreviated protocol for breast MRI: are multiple sequences needed for cancer detection? Eur J Radiol 2015;84:6570. 6. Grimm LJ, Soo MS, Yoon S, Kim C, Ghate SV, Johnson KS. Abbreviated screening protocol for breast MRI: a feasibility study. Acad Radiol 2015; 22:11571162

[5] Harvey SC, Di Carlo PA, Lee B, Obadina E, Sippo D, Mullen L. An abbreviated protocol for high-risk screening breast MRI saves time and resources. J Am Coll Radiol 2016;13:374380

[6] Grimm LJ, Soo MS, Yoon S, Kim C, Ghate SV, Johnson KS. Abbreviated screening protocol for breast MRI: a feasibility study. Acad Radiol 2015; 22:11571162

[7] Kuhl CK, Schrading S, Strobel K, Schild HH, Hilgers RD, Bieling HB. Abbreviated breast magnetic resonance imaging (MRI): first postcontrast subtracted images and maximum-intensity projection-a novel approach to breast cancer screening with MRI. J Clin Oncol. 2014; 32(22):2304–2310

[8] Bird RE, McLelland R. How to initiate and operate a low-cost mammography screening center. Radiology. 1986; 161(1):43–47

[9] van Zelst JCM, Vreemann S, Witt HJ, et al. Multireader study on the diagnostic accuracy of ultrafast breast magnetic resonance imaging for breast cancer screening. Invest Radiol 2018;53:579586

[10] Available at: www.fda.gov/downloads/MedicalDevices/.../ucm094441.pdf. Accessed January 7, 2016

[11] Available at: http://www.acr.org/Quality-Safety/Accreditation/Mammography/Lay-Letters. Accessed January 7, 2015

[12] Bassett LW, Dhaliwal SG, Eradat J, et al. National trends and practices in breast MRI. AJR Am J Roentgenol. 2008; 191(2):332–339

[13] Elsamaloty H, Elzawawi MS, Mohammad S, Herial N. Increasing accuracy of detection of breast cancer with 3-T MRI. AJR Am J Roentgenol. 2009; 192(4):1142–1148

[14] Rahbar H, DeMartini WB, Lee AY, Partridge SC, Peacock S, Lehman CD. Accuracy of 3T versus 1.5 T breast MRI for pre-operative assessment of extent of disease in newly diagnosed DCIS. Eur J Radiol. 2015; 84(4):611–616

[15] Revised 2013 (Resolution 12)* ACR practice parameter for the performance of contrast- enhanced magnetic resonance imaging (MRI) of the breast

[16] Kuhl CK, Bieling HB, Gieseke J, et al. Healthy premenopausal breast parenchyma in dynamic contrast-enhanced MR imaging of the breast: normal contrast medium enhancement and cyclical-phase dependency. Radiology. 1997; 203(1):137–144

[17] DeMartini WB, Liu F, Peacock S, Eby PR, Gutierrez RL, Lehman CD. Background parenchymal enhancement on breast MRI: impact on diagnostic performance. AJR Am J Roentgenol. 2012; 198(4):W373–W380

[18] Kajihara M, Goto M, Hirayama Y, et al. Effect of the menstrual cycle on background parenchymal enhancement in breast MR imaging. Magn Reson Med Sci. 2013; 12(1):39–45

[19] Ellis RL. Optimal timing of breast MRI examinations for premenopausal women who do not have a normal menstrual cycle. AJR Am J Roentgenol. 2009; 193(6):1738–1740

[20] Hegenscheid K, Schmidt CO, Seipel R, et al. Contrast enhancement kinetics of normal breast parenchyma in dynamic MR mammography: effects of menopausal status, oral contraceptives, and postmenopausal hormone therapy. Eur Radiol. 2012; 22(12):2633–2640

[21] Morris EA, Comstock CE, Lee CH, et al. ACR BI-RADS magnetic resonance imaging. In: D'Orsi CJ, ed. ACR BI-RADS Atlas, Breast Imaging Reporting and Data System. 5th ed. Reston, VA: American College of Radiology; 2013

[22] Eshed I, Althoff CE, Hamm B, Hermann KG. Claustrophobia and premature termination of magnetic resonance imaging examinations. J Magn Reson Imaging. 2007; 26(2):401–404

[23] Kanal E, Barkovich AJ, Bell C, et al. Expert Panel on MR Safety. ACR guidance document on MR safe practices: 2013. J Magn Reson Imaging. 2013; 37(3): 501–530

[24] ACR Manual on Contrast Media Version 10 2015. American College of Radiology ISBN: 978-1-55903-012-0

[25] US Food and Drug Administration. Questions and answers on gadolinium-based contrast agents. Updated July 30, 2014. Available at: http://www.fda.gov/Drugs/DrugSafety/DrugSafetyNewsletter/ucm142889.htm. Accessed July 16, 2015

[26] Thomsen HS, Morcos SK, Almén T, et al. ESUR Contrast Medium Safety Committee. Nephrogenic systemic fibrosis and gadolinium-based contrast media: updated ESUR Contrast Medium Safety Committee guidelines. Eur Radiol. 2013; 23(2):307–318

[27] Cova MA, Stacul F, Quaranta R, et al. Radiological contrast media in the breastfeeding woman: a position paper of the Italian Society of Radiology (SIRM), the Italian Society of Paediatrics (SIP), the Italian Society of Neonatology (SIN) and the Task Force on Breastfeeding, Ministry of Health, Italy. Eur Radiol. 2014; 24:2012–2022

[28] Plevritis SK, Kurian AW, Sigal BM, et al. Cost-effectiveness of screening BRCA1/2 mutation carriers with breast magnetic resonance imaging. JAMA. 2006; 295(20):2374–2384

[29] Ahern CH, Shih YC, Dong W, Parmigiani G, Shen Y. Cost-effectiveness of alternative strategies for integrating MRI into breast cancer screening for women at high risk. Br J Cancer. 2014; 111(8):1542–1551

[30] Schnall MD, Blume J, Bluemke DA, et al. Diagnostic architectural and dynamic features at breast MR imaging: multicenter study. Radiology. 2006; 238(1): 42–53

[31] Kuhl CK, Mielcareck P, Klaschik S, et al. Dynamic breast MR imaging: are signal intensity time course data useful for differential diagnosis of enhancing lesions? Radiology. 1999; 211(1):101–110

[32] Bluemke DA, Gatsonis CA, Chen MH, et al. Magnetic resonance imaging of the breast prior to biopsy. JAMA. 2004; 292(22):2735–2742

[33] Kuhl C. The current status of breast MR imaging. Part I. Choice of technique, image interpretation, diagnostic accuracy, and transfer to clinical practice. Radiology. 2007; 244(2):356–378

[34] King V, Brooks JD, Bernstein JL, Reiner AS, Pike MC, Morris EA. Background parenchymal enhancement at breast MR imaging and breast cancer risk. Radiology. 2011; 260(1):50–60

[35] Giess CS, Yeh ED, Raza S, Birdwell RL. Background parenchymal enhancement at breast MR imaging: normal patterns, diagnostic challenges, and potential for false-positive and false-negative interpretation. Radiographics. 2014; 34 (1):234–247

[36] Mousa NA, Eiada R, Crystal P, Nayot D, Casper RF. The effect of acute aromatase inhibition on breast parenchymal enhancement in magnetic resonance imaging: a prospective pilot clinical trial. Menopause. 2012; 19(4):420–425

[37] Delille JP, Slanetz PJ, Yeh ED, Kopans DB, Halpern EF, Garrido L. Hormone replacement therapy in postmenopausal women: breast tissue perfusion

determined with MR imaging—initial observations. Radiology. 2005; 235(1): 36–41

[38] Reichenbach JR, Przetak C, Klinger G, Kaiser WA. Assessment of breast tissue changes on hormonal replacement therapy using MRI: a pilot study. J Comput Assist Tomogr. 1999; 23(3):407–413

[39] Ha R, Sung J, Lee C, Comstock C, Wynn R, Morris E. Characteristics and outcome of enhancing foci followed on breast MRI with management implications. Clin Radiol. 2014; 69(7):715–720

[40] Liberman L, Mason G, Morris EA, Dershaw DD. Does size matter? Positive predictive value of MRI-detected breast lesions as a function of lesion size. AJR Am J Roentgenol. 2006; 186(2):426–430

[41] Eby PR, DeMartini WB, Gutierrez RL, Saini MH, Peacock S, Lehman CD. Characteristics of probably benign breast MRI lesions. AJR Am J Roentgenol. 2009; 193(3):861–867

[42] Raza S, Sekar M, Ong EM, Birdwell RL. Small masses on breast MR: is biopsy necessary? Acad Radiol. 2012; 19(4):412–419

[43] Baltzer PA, Benndorf M, Dietzel M, Gajda M, Runnebaum IB, Kaiser WA. False-positive findings at contrast-enhanced breast MRI: a BI-RADS descriptor study. AJR Am J Roentgenol. 2010; 194(6):1658–1663

[44] Yamaguchi K, Schacht D, Newstead GM, et al. Breast cancer detected on an incident (second or subsequent) round of screening MRI: MRI features of false-negative cases. AJR Am J Roentgenol. 2013; ;201(5):1155-1163

[45] Meissnitzer M, Dershaw DD, Feigin K, Bernard-Davila B, Barra F, Morris EA. MRI appearance of invasive subcentimetre breast carcinoma: benign characteristics are common. Br J Radiol. 2017; 90(1074):20170102

[46] American College of Radiology (ACR) Breast Imaging Reporting and Data System Atlas. (BI-RADS Atlas). Reston, VA: American College of Radiology; 2013. Available at: http://www.acr.org/. Accessed November 22, 2018

[47] Kuhl CK, Schrading S, Leutner CC, et al. Mammography, breast ultrasound, and magnetic resonance imaging for surveillance of women at high familial risk for breast cancer. J Clin Oncol. 2005; 23(33):8469–8476

[48] Morrow M, Waters J, Morris E. MRI for breast cancer screening, diagnosis, and treatment. Lancet. 2011; 378(9805):1804–1811

[49] Warner E. The role of magnetic resonance imaging in screening women at high risk of breast cancer. Top Magn Reson Imaging. 2008; 19(3):163–169

[50] Strigel RM, Rollenhagen J, Burnside ES, et al. Screening breast MRI outcomes in routine clinical practice: comparison to BI-RADS benchmarks. Acad Radiol. 2017; 24(4):411–417

[51] Lee CI, Ichikawa L, Rochelle MC, et al. Breast MRI BI-RADS Assessments and Abnormal Interpretation Rates by Clinical Indication in U.S. Community Practices. Breast MRI BI-RADS assessments and abnormal interpretation rates by clinical indication in US community practices. Acad Radiol. 2014; 21(11): 1370–1376

[52] Dee KE, Sickles EA. Medical audit of diagnostic mammography examinations: comparison with screening outcomes obtained concurrently. AJR Am J Roentgenol. 2001; 176(3):729–733

[53] Sohlich RE, Sickles EA, Burnside ES, Dee KE. Interpreting data from audits when screening and diagnostic mammography outcomes are combined. AJR Am J Roentgenol. 2002; 178(3):681–686

[54] Sickles EA, Miglioretti DL, Ballard-Barbash R, et al. Performance benchmarks for diagnostic mammography. Radiology. 2005; 235(3):775–790

[55] Niell BL, Gavenonis SC, Motazedi T, et al. Auditing a breast MRI practice: performance measures for screening and diagnostic breast MRI. J Am Coll Radiol. 2014; 11(9):883–889

5 Diagnostic MRI: Imaging Protocols and Technical Considerations

Gillian M. Newstead

Abstract

This chapter outlines a practical approach for achieving a standard, high-quality breast MRI examination. Excellent image resolution is a prerequisite for accurate diagnosis. Key components of a high-quality study include a protocol that balances spatial and temporal resolution, achieves homogeneous fat suppression, minimizes artifacts and is consistently applied. Various magnet platforms and breast coils are available for conducting breast MR examinations. Therefore, each facility must tailor their approach to their breast MRI diagnostic protocol accordingly. Shown in this chapter are examples of imaging protocols that include a T2-weighted sequence, a non-fat suppressed T1-weighted sequence and a multi-phase T1-weighted sequence. It is important to recognize that a standard dynamic contrast-enhanced (DCE-MRI) series should be as short as possible and therefore reformatted images (obtained from the initial acquisition plane) rather than multiple acquisitions (obtained in planes other than the initial plane) should be used. A review of patient administration of Gadolinium-based contrast agents and Gadolinium retention in tissue is provided. Also included is a discussion of computer-aided diagnostic (CAD) systems that can improve interpretation and workflow times by organizing and presenting large image datasets and by analyzing lesion kinetic characteristics. Protocols identified as ultra-fast (UF) or accelerated imaging are shown and are now being used in clinical practice. The remainder of the chapter concentrates on the many technical challenges that may occur during the course of achieving optimal DCE-MRI studies, including the identification and review of imaging artifacts that may hamper image quality. The chapter concludes with a discussion of breast MRI accreditation requirements.

Keywords: diagnostic DCE-MRI, technique, ultrafast (UF) (accelerated) sequences, contrast agents, computer-aided analysis, inhomogeneous fat suppression, magnetic susceptibility artifact, motion and misregistration artifact, aliasing (wrap-around) artifact, zebra (moiré) artifact, RF Interference artifact

5.1 Introduction

The imaging protocol for a dynamic contrast-enhanced magnetic resonance imaging (DCE-MRI) study is demanding and should be carefully considered, a practical approach requiring a simple and relatively short (< 20 minutes) standardized acquisition is usually sufficient. There is no single protocol used in clinical practice today, and a variety of acquisitions are employed. Technical requirements for a DCE-MRI acquisition include a magnetic field strength greater than or equal to 1.5 T, a dedicated breast coil, through-plane slice thickness less than or equal to 3 mm, and administration of a gadolinium-based contrast agent (GBCA). Protocols are aimed to balance spatial and temporal resolution in order to exploit maximum sensitivity and specificity, providing analysis of both morphologic and

kinetic lesion features. Studies can be streamlined, by adjusting the T2-weighted (T2w) precontrast and T1w dynamic series so that multiplanar reformatting, obtained at or near isotropic resolution, can replace the need for multiple additional series in various planes. A general approach for a standard DCE-MRI study (including a T2w series) should be to provide a protocol that is completed within 15 to 20 minutes, attains image consistency, minimizes extraneous artifacts, and addresses any other technical challenges. Special acquisitions such as diffusion-weighted imaging (DWI) may be added to the basic protocol as needed.

5.2 Current Standard DCE-MRI Protocols

The American College of Radiology (ACR) and the European Society of Breast Imaging (EUSOBI) have set minimum standards for breast MRI acquisition, these guidelines allowing flexibility regarding acquisition parameters and equipment specification. Essential equipment requirements include access to a high-homogeneity high magnetic field MRI platform (1.5 T or higher), a dedicated bilateral breast receive or transmit-receive coil, and strong magnetic field gradients with short gradient rise times.

5.2.1 Acquisition Plane

Selection of the primary imaging acquisition plane is critical when choosing a breast DCE-MRI protocol and may be the only acquired imaging plane needed. High-resolution multiplanar reformatted images can be reconstructed from the acquired plane, eliminating the need for additional scans and shortening the scanning time. Axial and sagittal acquisition planes are generally preferred to the coronal plane, given that the anatomic segments of the breast are oriented from the nipple to the chest wall and are not aligned segmentally in the coronal plane. Selection of the acquisition plane is particularly important when assessing DCIS, because axial and sagittal imaging may demonstrate linear or segmental enhancement to advantage, whereas coronal imaging may only show cross-section of ducts. Selection of the field-of-view (FOV) depends on the primary acquisition plane and in general should be chosen to be as small as possible, in order to maximize in-plane spatial resolution while also including all breast tissue and axillary regions. Axial acquisition is the most commonly used primary plane in the United States, providing easy bilateral side-by-side assessment of enhancement at identical postcontrast injection time points.

5.2.2 Imaging Protocol

The current standard-of-care breast DCE-MRI protocol consists of a precontrast T2w acquisition followed by a dynamic sequence encompassing a series of T1w acquisitions obtained before and for approximately 5 to 7 minutes after the intravenous administration of a GBCA. In most practices, temporal resolution has remained between 60 and 120 seconds, with a maximum temporal resolution of 240 seconds allowed in the Breast Magnetic Resonance Imaging Accreditation Program.[1] Standard diagnostic imaging protocols capture diffusion rather than perfusion of contrast material into enhancing lesions. The ACR Accreditation Program requires both a T2w (bright fluid) series and a multiphase T1w dynamic series. The dynamic series must include a precontrast T1w series, an early-phase (first) postcontrast T1w series to be completed within 4 minutes of contrast injection, and a late-phase T1w series with features matching the precontrast T1w series.

T2-Weighted Sequence

Inclusion of a precontrast T2w sequence in a breast DCE-MRI protocol allows improved characterization of enhancing lesions visible on the T1w postcontrast sequences. Additionally, the T2w bright fluid sequence identifies fluid collections, breast edema, and benign findings such as lymph nodes, simple cysts, some fibroadenomata, and posttreatment changes. T2w sequences are typically acquired using spin echo (SE), fast spin echo (FSE), or short time inversion recovery (STIR) technique with an inversion time selected to null fat. The long repetition times required for fat-suppressed T2w result in longer scanning times, and the T2w series is usually obtained as a multislice two-dimensional acquisition. Using this protocol, the acquired T2w images are unable to match the higher spatial resolution of the T1w DCE images within a reasonable scan time, thus direct slice-by-slice comparison of the T2w and T1w images is not possible. Some practices choose to acquire T2w images without fat suppression allowing three-dimensional (3D) imaging matching of the spatial resolution of the T2w series with the T1w DCE series. This non–fat-suppressed T2w sequence also allows an overview of breast anatomy, assessment of the amount of fibroglandular tissue (FGT), and improved analysis of lesions identified in the dynamic sequence.

Non–Fat-Suppressed T1-Weighted Sequence

If a fat-suppressed T2w sequence is used, then an additional T1w sequence without fat suppression is recommended prior to acquiring the multiphase T1w sequence. The T1w non–fat-suppressed sequence can provide an overview of anatomy, assess the amount of FGT, and identify fat-containing lesions. This protocol should provide similar parameters and spatial resolution to the subsequent fat-suppressed DCE series. It should be noted that if a non–fat-suppressed T2w series is used in the breast MR protocol, then this sequence is not necessary.

Multiphase T1-Weighted Sequence (DCE-MRI)

This key sequence is used for lesion detection, characterization, and evaluation of lesion contrast enhancement over time. Identical scan parameters must be used for the pre- and postcontrast multiphase T1w series sequences, so that image registration can be performed. A 3D gradient echo (GRE) pulse sequence with a short time of repetition (TR) is commonly used for multiphase T1w imaging. It is also recommended that in order to avoid any confounding T2 contrast, the GRE pulse

sequence should be spoiled.[2] Precontrast images are subtracted from postcontrast images and signal differences between the sequences can be directly compared. Most practices in the United States use fat suppression in the T1w dynamic series, and subtraction images are helpful for highlighting signal from contrast agents. If the dynamic series is performed without fat suppression, then subtraction images are essential for elimination of the fat signal. Knowledge of the k-space sampling pattern is helpful, most Cartesian sequences use rectilinear sampling with the center of the acquisition capturing the high-frequency data providing optimal contrast resolution. When setting up a breast MRI protocol, there is no recommended consensus as to the number of postcontrast acquisitions within a DCE series, or requirements for the total length of the acquisition time. A minimum of at least two postcontrast sequences are needed to provide a basic assessment of kinetic features, and these should include measures of the initial slope of enhancement and of the delayed phase.

Measures of the rate of uptake and washout of contrast media within breast lesions contain diagnostically useful information, and microvascular density is a key factor in determining the initial rate of contrast media uptake and the heterogeneity of enhancement within tumors.[3] The shape of a signal intensity versus time curve (TIC) (or signal time course or kinetic curve) has shown to be useful in the classification of enhancing lesions.[4] Lesions with a fast uptake of contrast followed by a washout phase are more likely to be malignant, while lesions with a slow but persistent uptake are more likely benign. Discrete thresholds are used to classify two parts of the kinetic curve: the initial uptake and the delayed phase (▶ Fig. 5.1).

5.3 Contrast Agents

Although noncontrast MRI techniques are currently under investigation, clinical breast MR examinations currently require the administration of a GBCA. Gadolinium is paramagnetic, shortens the T1 and T2 relaxation times of nearby protons and in most clinical DCE examinations, it is the T1 shortening effect of a GBCA that results in increased signal intensity. Standard DCE-MRI examinations involve injection of a GBCA and subsequent analysis of the kinetic characteristics of any enhancing lesion. Contrast agents should be injected intravenously, ideally using a power injector, and administered as a bolus with a standard dose of 0.1 mmol/kg followed by a saline flush of at least 20 mL. This method ensures rapid arrival at the intravascular space allowing for consistency in contrast enhancement timing across examinations. The paramagnetic properties of chelated gadolinium result in decreased T1, T2, and T2* relaxation times.[5] Acquisitions geared toward fluid detection, such as the T2w series, should be acquired prior to contrast administration. DCE-MRI is performed with T1w because the decrease in relaxation following injection of a GBCA is greatest for T1w sequences. The effect of gadolinium shortening of the T1 (the spin–lattice relaxation time) in its microenvironment results in increased signal in a T1w acquisition. Lesion conspicuity therefore increases after the injection of a GBCA and is highlighted on subtraction (postcontrast minus baseline) images. Relaxivity is the property that is most closely related to differences in signal intensity between enhancing lesions and surrounding parenchyma. In clinical breast imaging, the shorter the T1 (in a

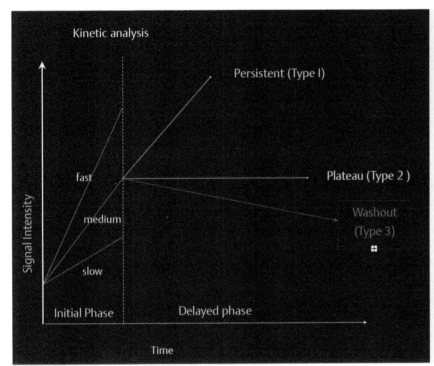

Fig. 5.1 Time-intensity curves. Kinetic analysis of lesion enhancement is shown; signal intensity is plotted over time. The initial phase of enhancement is characterized as fast, medium, or slow, and the delayed phase as persistent plateau and washout.

T1w dynamic sequence), the larger the R1 and the brighter the enhancement and this depends, in part, on the chemical structure of a particular GBCA. A high relaxivity GBCA indicates a greater uptake of contrast in enhancing tissues per unit concentration of contrast agent. The term relaxivity (rl) refers to the change in relaxation rate (R1) per unit concentration of contrast agent describing the effect of a GBCA on T1 and T2 per molar concentration of contrast agent. Regions or lesions with increased blood flow and permeability, such as cancers, will accumulate contrast media to a greater extent than the surrounding tissue.

5.3.1 Deposition of Gadolinium in Tissue

It is well known that not all gadolinium chelates are entirely stable in vivo. There are two structurally distinct categories of commercially available GBCAs: linear and macrocyclic. The structure of a linear GBCA provides a polyamino-carboxyl acid backbone wrapping around the gadolinium ion which is incompletely enclosed, whereas in the macrocyclic structure, the gadolinium ion is "caged" in the ligand. Although patients with normal renal function clear almost all gadolinium from the circulation within a few hours by renal excretion, some free gadolinium may disperse into tissues. Intracranial gadolinium retention has been reported recently showing that trace amounts of gadolinium accumulation, as evidenced by concomitant T1 shortening on MRI, are present in the brains of patients who have received multiple doses of GBCA.[7,8] This effect is seen in patients without renal or hepatic dysfunction and is predominantly found in the globus pallidus, thalamus, pons, and dentate nucleus.[9] The magnitude of the effect is proportional to the cumulative lifetime patient dose. Some research suggests that

this phenomenon occurs more commonly when linear agents with weaker chemical binding to gadolinium are administered, compared to the stronger chemical binding of macrocyclic agents.[10] Visible intracranial changes on T1W images may be present after only four exposures of a GBCA, and these findings often remain for years after the MR studies took place. In 2015, the U.S. Food and Drug Administration (FDA) instituted a review of gadolinium contrast agents to determine whether a safety risk to patients exists. On March 10, 2017, the Pharmacovigilance Risk Assessment Committee (PRAC) of the European Medicines Agency (EMA) formally submitted its recommendation to suspend use of four linear GBCAs due to the potential risk of gadolinium accumulation within humans.[11] The PRAC noted that no clinical diseases or even symptoms have been reported in connection with gadolinium deposition, but the committee decided on a "precautionary approach," noting the paucity of data as well as concern regarding gadolinium's past history of association with nephrogenic systemic fibrosis (NSF) in patients with kidney impairment. A response to the European PRAC recommendations was published by the ACR on April 4, 2017. This report concluded that "after extensive review of the PRAC position and voluminous other materials, the ACR Committee on Drugs and Contrast Media disagrees with the PRAC recommendation." The ACR report concluded that there is abundant evidence that the amount of gadolinium deposited in tissues after a single GBCA dose is incredibly small and found no compelling evidence that any GBCA (including linear agents) pose a safety risk. The ACR additionally endorsed the need for additional research efforts to be directed toward a greater understanding of the mechanisms, cellular effects, and clinical consequences of gadolinium tissue deposition.[12] On September 8, 2017, the Medical Imaging Drugs Advisory Committee (MIDAC) of the U. S. FDA voted to recommend the addition of a warning to labels of GBCAs used during MRI. The new labels will warn that gadolinium may be retained in various organs, including the brain; after use of these agents, linear GBCAs exhibit a greater risk than macrocyclic agents. The warning will also note a greater risk in specific patient populations that include the fetus and children and patients who receive large cumulative doses of GBCAs, such as women undergoing annual GBCA-enhanced MRI because of high risk for breast cancer. At the present time however, although there is clear evidence that residual amounts of gadolinium may be retained in the brain and other parts of the body after administration of GBCA for MRI examinations, there is no definitive evidence that residual gadolinium is associated with adverse health effects. Ongoing research on this topic is underway.

Computer-Aided Analysis

Standard pharmacokinetic models that evaluate lesion enhancement kinetics attempt to replicate the physiology of MRI contrast agent distribution in relationship to normal breast tissue, various parameters describing lesion contrast delivery, accumulation, and washout. Peak lesion enhancement relative to background parenchymal enhancement (BPE) occurs at 1 to 2 minutes after contrast injection for most mass lesions and 2 to 3 minutes after injection for nonmass lesions.[13] Maximum contrast weighting timing of 3D GRE pulse sequences occurs about halfway into the scan for most MRI systems, and absent a time gap between the end of injection and the start of imaging, a postcontrast series of 90-second duration will deliver peak contrast weighting at about 45 seconds from the start of the series. Computer-aided diagnostic (CAD) systems can improve interpretation and workflow times by organizing and presenting large image datasets and by analyzing lesion kinetic characteristics. These systems display color overlays on voxels within enhancing lesions, thereby, demonstrating the kinetics of the delayed phase of lesion enhancement as washout, plateau, or persistent, and the initial rise as slow, medium, or rapid. Implementation of time intensity curves and angiomaps allows a convenient and efficient way for radiologists to assess kinetic enhancement.

A combined assessment of both lesion morphology and kinetics is necessary for diagnosis. MR interpretation may be affected by the variable enhancement of normal tissue (BPE), which usually enhances slowly, generating a persistent kinetic curve. The hormonal response of breast tissue in premenopausal women varies during the menstrual cycle. Marked BPE can limit the sensitivity of the examination,[14,15] and differentiation of enhancing abnormalities from BPE may present a diagnostic challenge.[16] For this reason, it is recommended that screening of premenopausal women should be scheduled preferentially during the second week of the menstrual cycle avoiding week 4 if at all possible. For women undergoing diagnostic applications, including assessment of malignant disease extent, a delay in diagnosis in order to accommodate menstrual cycle scheduling is generally not advisable.

5.4 University of Chicago Protocol

The current routine diagnostic breast MRI protocol at University of Chicago (UC), at field strengths both 1.5 and 3 T, includes a T2w non–fat-suppressed axial sequence followed by a T1w fat-suppressed axial dynamic series, with images acquired before and after intravenous administration of contrast media. The images shown in this book were almost all obtained on a 3-T magnet that was installed in 2010. Although images obtained at both field strengths can provide excellent diagnostic quality, improved contrast and spatial resolution at 3 T reflect the higher signal-to-noise ratio (SNR) per voxel as shown by comparison images of the same lesion obtained at both 1.5 and 3 T (▶ Fig. 5.2; ▶ Fig. 5.3). The UC protocol at 3 T includes five postcontrast acquisitions at a temporal resolution of approximately 70 seconds and spatial resolution of 0.8 × 0.8 × 0.8 cm, obtained for both the T2w and the T1w series. The images from both acquired series are isotropic and are matched spatially, thus allowing multiplanar formatting of both the T2w and the T1w sequences at identical spatial resolution. These protocols both at 1.5 and 3 T are shown in ▶ Table 5.1 and ▶ Table 5.2, respectively. Examples of a benign and a malignant lesion obtained with this protocol at 3 T are shown (▶ Fig. 5.4; ▶ Fig. 5.5).

5.4.1 Ultrafast Techniques for Diagnostic Use

Protocols, referred to as "ultrafast (UF)" or "accelerated" imaging, have been investigated and developed intermittently over the years and are now once again being used in clinical practice. These protocols are aimed toward image sampling of early kinetics within the first minute postcontrast injection at a fast rate (3–8 seconds per time point) for a bilateral scan, as shown in Chapter 3. Current diagnostic DCE-MRI examinations at UC include a high temporal resolution, lower spatial resolution (UF) acquisition during the first minute following contrast injection, followed by a standard, higher spatial resolution acquisition, achieving a total acquisition time of 7 minutes. Lesion conspicuity in UF images is often greatest within the first 30 seconds after contrast media injection, especially when marked BPE is found on later images. UF methods allow measurement of the rate of lesion enhancement with respect to time of initial arterial enhancement in the breast rather than time of injection, thus reducing dependence on global variables such as cardiac output. UF imaging in the first minute postcontrast injection can be incorporated into a standard-length diagnostic protocol, and delayed-phase kinetics can thus also be measured.[17] This approach to UF imaging uses standard Cartesian k-space sampling, which differs from "view-sharing" methods, that are often used in other clinical DCE-MRI high- resolution protocols. Keyhole approaches and other "view-sharing" methods such as "TRICKS" and "TWIST" typically involve scanning the center of k-space at relatively high temporal resolution, and the outer portions of k-space at much lower temporal resolution.[18,19,20] Each image in the dynamic series is then produced from data obtained from different parts of k-space, scanned at different times, resulting in high-quality images, but quantitative analysis of the acquired data with these sequences is difficult. Problems arise when data are analyzed to determine which features are enhancing at what strength and at what rate, particularly in the case of small features (e.g., lesions) with sharp and irregular edges. Information obtained from the initial 10 seconds after uptake initiation is combined with information from other time periods, and the diagnostic utility is thus

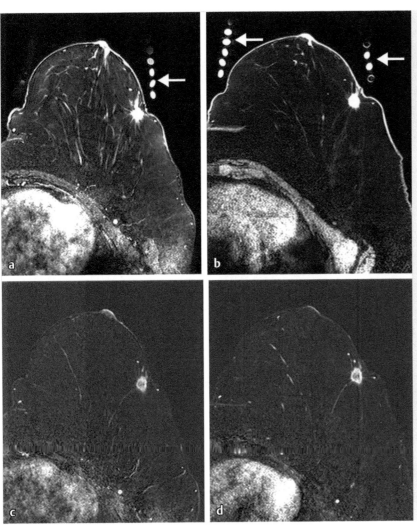

Fig. 5.2 Image quality: 1.5 T versus 3 T. Source and subtraction images of a spiculate cancer are shown at 1.5 T and 3 T. Source images (**a, b**) reveal an IDC in the lateral left breast with a contrast phantom located within the coil surrounding the breast tissue (*arrows*). Higher spatial resolution as evidenced by thinner mass margin spiculation is noted on the 3 T image (**b**). Similar findings are noted on subtraction images (**c, d**), with higher signal and spatial resolution noted on 3 T image (**d**).

diluted. For example, if a narrow blood vessel, the rim of a cancer, or speculations on a suspicious lesion appear to enhance rapidly, it is difficult to determine the true rate of enhancement. Compressed sensing methods have similar problems and produce artifacts.[21,22] Further examples of UF DCE-MRI incorporated into a standard diagnostic acquisition are shown (► Fig. 5.6; ► Fig. 5.7; ► Fig. 5.8; ► Fig. 5.9; ► Fig. 5.10).

UF DCE-MRI allows new approaches to quantitative data analysis, including measurements of the initial rate of lesion enhancement. Time of arrival of the contrast bolus can be accurately measured relative to the initial enhancement in the aorta. This potentially powerful approach can correct for variations in contrast media injection speed and cardiac output, allowing for more standardized measurements. UF imaging may also have other advantages; high temporal resolution protocols allow propagation of the contrast media bolus into a lesion allowing visualization of feeding arteries and draining veins and providing simplified and more accurate measurements of the arterial input function and K_{trans}. Preliminary research suggests that there are significant differences between benign and malignant lesions in parameters that describe contrast media uptake kinetics in the first minute postinjection.

5.4.2 DCE-MRI Technical Requirements

High Signal-to-Noise Ratio

MR acquisitions with adequate SNR are essential for detection and diagnosis of small enhancing masses and ducts (1–3 mm in diameter). It has been shown that high spatial resolution improves diagnostic confidence.[23] Breast MRI should be performed with a magnetic field B_0 strength of 1.5 T or greater. SNR is directly related to B_0 and is nearly double at 3 T than 1.5 T, providing greater SNR per voxel and allowing rapid imaging of both breasts with high in-plane spatial and temporal resolution. Imaging at 3 T also provides improved static magnetic field homogeneity, thus ensuring good fat suppression over the entire imaged volume. High SNR can be obtained by combining a high field strength magnet with a dedicated multichannel breast coil allowing thinner slices and higher spatial and temporal resolution. It is important to note that if the selected matrix is too high (in-plane pixel size is excessively small), or selected slices are too thin, SNR may be compromised, and small enhancing lesions may be difficult to detect. Breast MRI platforms are increasingly moving toward higher field strength, and reports have shown improved sensitivity and specificity

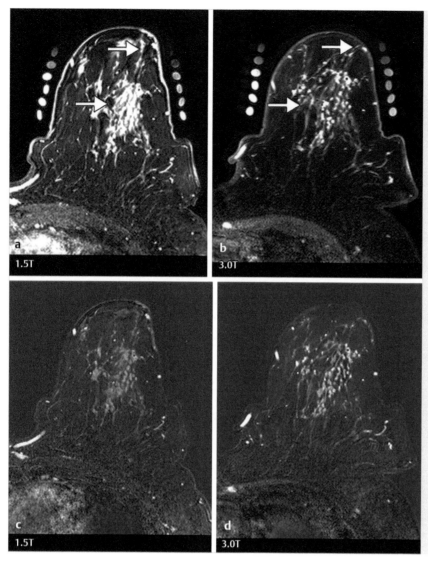

Fig. 5.3 Image quality: 1.5 T versus. 3 T. Source and subtraction images exhibit an extensive left breast segmental NME, representing DCIS, shown at 1.5 T and 3 T (*arrows*). Source images **(a, b)** reveal NME with a contrast phantom located within the coil surrounding the breast tissue. Higher spatial resolution is noted on image **(b)** when compared to image **(a)**. Corresponding subtraction images show higher signal and spatial resolution on the 3 T image **(d)** when compared to the 1.5 T image **(c)**.

with breast MRI at 3 T.[24,25] Ultra high-field MR scanners operating at a field strength of 7 T provide a significantly higher intrinsic SNR and have recently demonstrated feasibility for clinical use. A recent report by Pinker et al studied a cohort of patients with suspicious lesions and showed feasibility of clinical breast MRI at 7 T and the potential for improved diagnostic accuracy.[26]

High Spatial Resolution

High spatial resolution is all about voxel size, high spatial resolution requiring small voxels. Good in-plane spatial resolution of 1 × 1 mm is adequate, and submillimeter isotropic imaging is optimal. Because pixel size is determined by the FOV and the in-plane matrix in each in-plane direction (the frequency-encoding and phase-encoding matrix), it is critical that the FOV be adjusted for each patient according to their body habitus, the goal being to devise the FOV to be as small as possible while including all breast tissue.

Pixel size (frequency) = FOV(frequency)/(number of matrix elements in the frequency-encoding direction).

Pixel size (phase) = FOV(phase)/(number of matrix elements in the phase-encoding direction).

It is useful for technologists to set up separate scanner protocols with optimized FOV for different patient sizes at the magnet console. Although adjustment of the FOV for each patient is important allowing improved spatial resolution, it should not come at the expense of exclusion of critical breast or axillary tissue. Technologists generally keep slice thickness reasonably small to avoid excessive partial volume effects but may have a propensity to exclude tissue at the superior or lateral aspect of the breasts in an effort to reduce scanning times. Slice thickness is the parameter that sets the limit on visibility of the smallest lesions that can be imaged without slice partial volume effects. Decrease in lesion contrast can occur with partial volume effects, and although robustly enhancing lesions may be visible on thicker slices, conspicuity may be compromised for smaller, low-contrast lesions. It should be noted, therefore, that if the selected slice thickness is too small, a reduction in temporal resolution and SNR is likely, whereas if the selected slice thickness is too large, the risk of partial volume artifact is increased.

Table 5.1 AB-MR: Adapted standard protocol at 1.5 T: (Phillips)

Parameters	VISTA	DCE-MRI
Geometry	3D axial	3D axial
FOV (mm)	320–400	320–400
Spatial resolution/interpolated (mm)	0.8/0.8	0.8/0.7
Slice thickness/interpolated (mm)	2/1	2/1
Number of slices	200	175
Slice oversample	Default	1
Slice gap (mm)	N/A	N/A
SENSE acceleration	3 × 2	2.5 × 2
TR (ms)	2,000	5.5
TE (ms)	368	2.7
Flip angle (deg)	90	12
Fast imaging mode	TSE	TFE
Fast imaging factor	120	44
Fat suppression	None	SPAIR
Partial Fourier imaging	No	No
k-space sampling	Cartesian	Cartesian
Number of averages	1	1
Duration (m:s)	2:32	5:24
Temporal resolution (m:s)	N/A	0:54
b values (s/mm^2)	N/A	N/A

Abbreviations: DCE-MRI, dynamic contrast-enhanced magnetic resonance imaging; FOV, field-of-view; SPAIR, spectral attenuated inversion recovery; TE, echo time; TR, time of repetition; TFE, turbo fast echo; TSE, turbo spin echo.
Note: Parameters for VISTA, DCE-MRI are standard clinical parameters, so there is no special consideration to their selection beyond optimization for image quality in given time. VISTA (non–fat-suppressed T2w). DCE-MRI (fat-suppressed T1w): precontrast mask, followed by standard DCE-MRI for two postcontrast acquisitions.

Table 5.2 AB-MR: Adapted standard protocol 3 T scanner: (Phillips)

Parameters	VISTA	DCE-MRI
Geometry	3D axial	3D axial
FOV (mm)	320–400	320–400
Spatial resolution/interpolated (mm)	0.8/0.65	0.8/0.6
Slice thickness/interpolated (mm)	1.6/0.8	1.6/0.8
Number of slices	250	250
Slice oversample	1.33	1
Slice gap (mm)	N/A	N/A
SENSE acceleration	3 × 2	2.5 × 2
TR (ms)	2,000	4.8
TE (ms)	221	2.4
Flip angle (deg)	90	10
Fast imaging mode	TSE	TFE
Fast imaging factor	120	27
Fat suppression	None	SPAIR
Partial Fourier imaging	No	0.85 × 1
k-space sampling	Cartesian	Cartesian
Number of averages	1	1
Duration (m:s)	3:44	2:13
Temporal resolution (m:s)	N/A	1:02
b values (s/mm^2)	N/A	N/A

Abbreviations: DCE-MRI, dynamic contrast-enhanced magnetic resonance imaging; FOV, field-of-view; SPAIR, spectral attenuated inversion recovery; TE, echo time; TFF, turbo fast echo; TR, time of repetition; TSE, turbo spin echo.
Note: Parameters for VISTA and DCE-MRI are standard clinical parameters, so there is no special consideration to their selection beyond optimization. VISTA (non–fat-suppressed T2w). DCE-MRI (fat-suppressed T1w): precontrast mask, followed by standard DCE-MRI for two postcontrast acquisitions.

High Temporal Resolution

Multiphasic enhancement imaging requires both high temporal and spatial resolution. Critical to this effort is homogeneous fat suppression, which can be difficult to achieve with a large FOV. The timing of a selected DCE-MRI protocol should remain the same from patient to patient; however, slice thickness (≤ 3 mm) can be changed according to patient size. Factors used to increase temporal resolution should not include removal of fat suppression, or an increase in slice thickness or a reduction in matrix size. A method of angling the FOV to achieve fewer slices in a given volume can be used to increase spatial resolution. An example of this method is shown in ▸ Fig. 5.11. It should be noted that if the selected FOV is too small, even though all breast tissue is included, the risk of aliasing artifacts is increased and may require an increase in the FOV to correct the problem. Enhancement curves depend on temporal resolution and a slow injection rate or limited cardiac function will delay and dampen peak enhancement.

Robust and Reproducible Fat Suppression

The high signal of fat interferes with the detection of enhancing lesions at MRI, and active fat suppression is widely used in the T1w dynamic sequence for cancer detection. Uniform suppression of the fat signal is challenging at breast imaging because of B_0 inhomogeneity across the FOV, due to the variation in breast tissue types. Different methods for active fat suppression generally rely on differences in resonant frequency between fat and water protons and/or the difference in T1 relaxation times between fat and water. Intermittent fat suppression is commonly employed using a frequency-selective fat saturation pulse to eliminate fat signal in T1w GRE sequences. The chemical shift of water and the methyl group, which is the main component of fat, is 3.5 parts per million (ppm). Fat suppression is accomplished by applying saturation pulses at a frequency of 3.5 ppm (224 Hz at 1.5 T) below the water peak and most MR unit software automatically identifies the water peak as the highest signal peak. In fatty breasts, however, the imaging

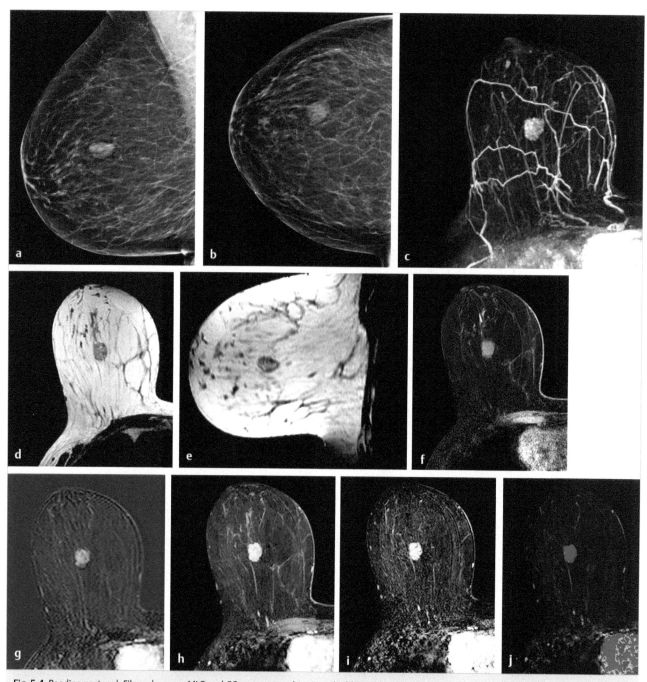

Fig. 5.4 Reading protocol: Fibroadenoma. MLO and CC mammographic views **(a, b)** reveal an oval circumscribed mass in the central right breast with a correlative mass visible on MIP image **(c)**. Axial and sagittal T2w images exhibit circumscribed hyperintense masses **(d, e)**, also seen on precontrast T1w series **(f)** and postcontrast UF series at 47 seconds **(g)**. Source and subtraction images **(h, i)** exhibit an enhancing mass with unenhancing internal septations and homogeneous persistent enhancement, as seen on CAD image **(j)**. (*continued*)

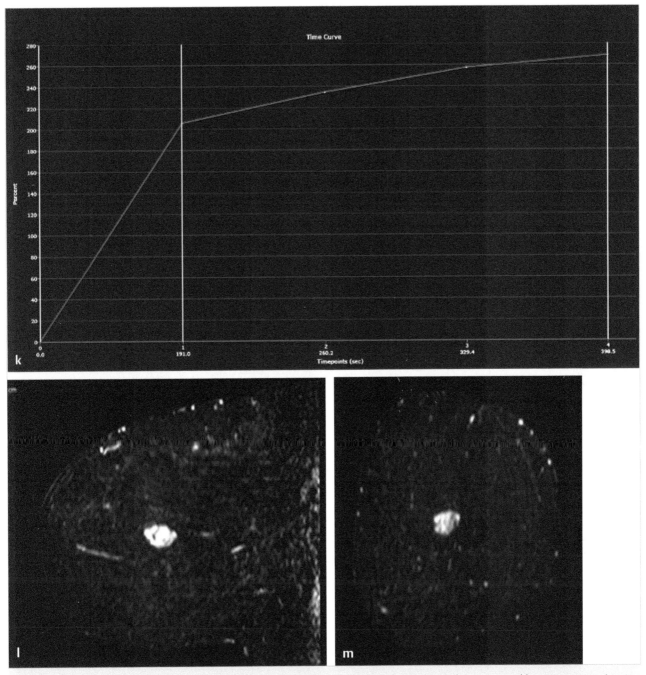

Fig. 5.4 (*continued*) Source and subtraction images exhibit an enhancing mass with unenhancing internal septations and homogeneous persistent enhancement, as seen on TIC (**k**) as well. Sagittal and coronal subtraction images are shown in (**l, m**).

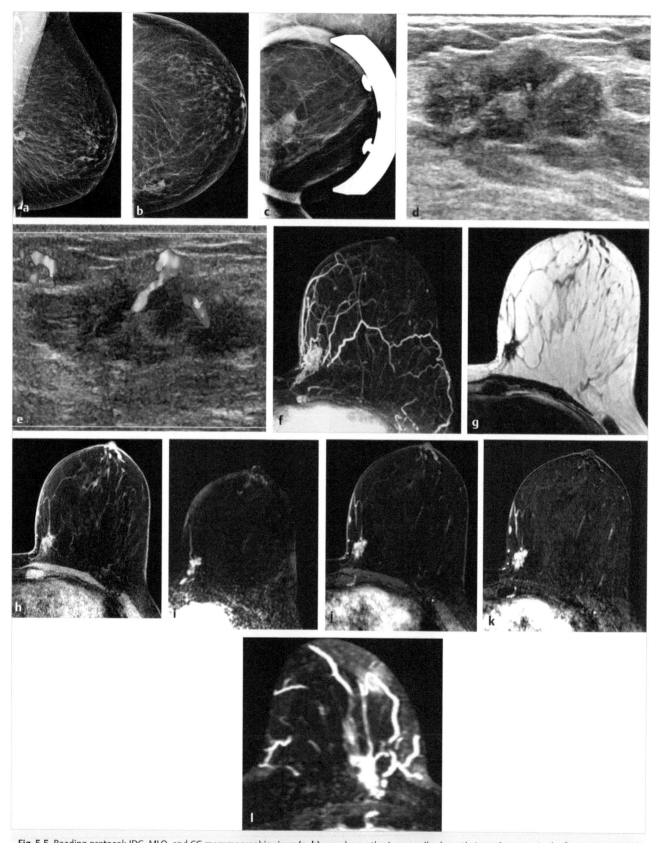

Fig. 5.5 Reading protocol: IDC, MLO, and CC mammographic views (**a, b**) reveal a partly circumscribed, partly irregular, mass in the far posteromedial left breast, seen also on a spot ML view (**c**). Ultrasound images (**d, e**) show an indistinct mass with microlobulation and increased blood flow. A correlative mass is visible on MIP image (**f**). An irregular hypointense mass is present on T2w image (**g**) also visible on precontrast T1w image (**h**) and postcontrast UF series at 21 s (**i**). Source and subtraction images (**j, k**) exhibit heterogeneous enhancement. A sagittal postcontrast source image is shown (**l**). Histology yielded IDC grade 3 with LVI and DCIS intermediate/high grade, solid and cribriform type, ER/PR (+), HER2/neu (−), Ki67: 10%.

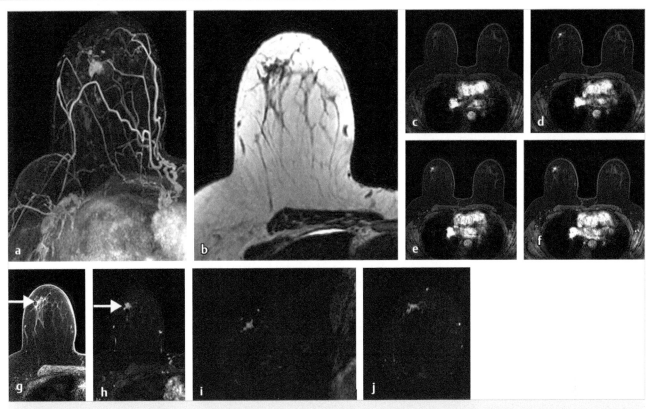

Fig. 5.6 UF technique. MIP image reveals an irregular anterior enhancing mass (**a**) seen as a hypointense mass on T2w image (**b**). UF images: 14 s first visualization of the aorta (**c**), 21 s first visualization of the irregular mass (**d**) also seen at 28 and 35s(**e, f**). Standard postcontrast source and subtraction images obtained at 140 s also show the irregular mass with an adjacent inferior marker clip (**g, h**) (*arrows*). Sagittal and coronal images (**i, j**) are shown. Histology yielded IDC grade 2, ER/PR (−, HER2/neu (+), Ki67: 25%, with DCIS high grade, solid, cribriform with necrosis.

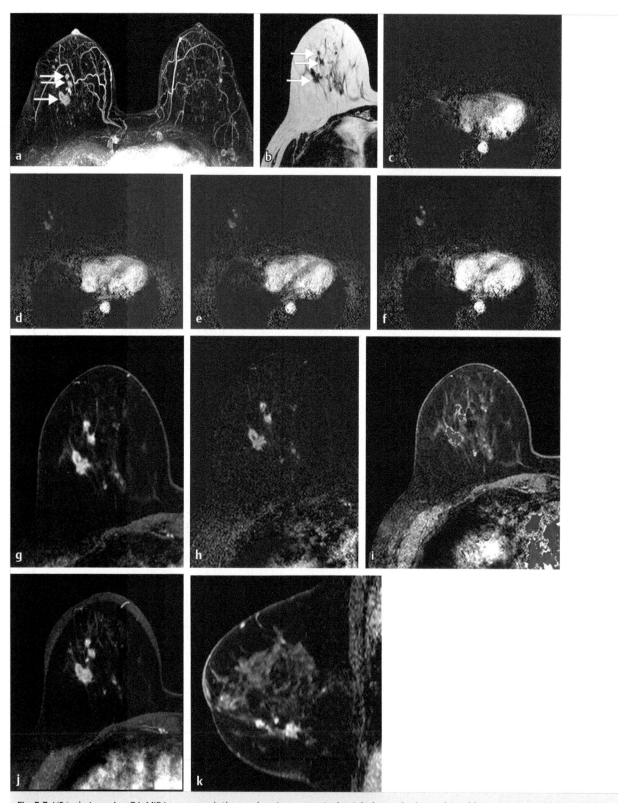

Fig. 5.7 UF technique. Age 74, MIP image reveals three enhancing masses in the right breast (**a**, (*arrows*) in addition to scattered bilateral benign foci, and three correlative low signal masses are visible on T2w image (**b**, *arrows*). UF images: 14 s first visualization of the aorta (**c**) 21 s first visualization of the irregular masses (**d**) also seen at 28 and 35 s (**e, f**). Standard postcontrast source and subtraction images obtained at 140 s show three irregular masses with spiculation (**g, h**), with plateau and persistent kinetics on CAD image (**i**). Slab axial and sagittal images are shown (**j, k**). Histology yielded ILC, ER/PR (+), HER2/neu (−), Ki67: 5 to 9%.

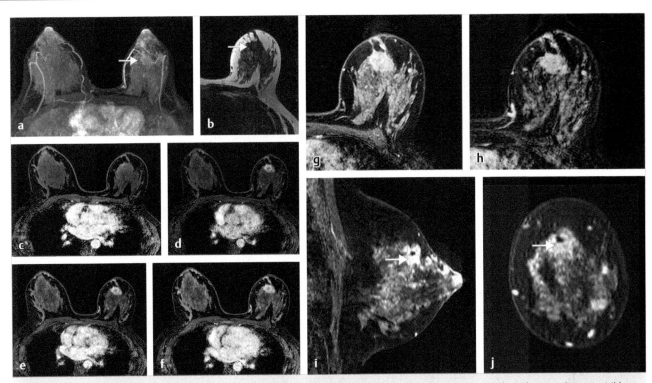

Fig. 5.8 UF technique. MIP image reveals marked BPE and an enhancing mass in the left breast (**a**, *arrow*) with a correlative low-signal mass is visible on T2w image (**b**, *arrow*). UF images: 21 s cardiac and aortic enhancement (**c**) 28 s first visualization of the rim-enhancing mass (**d**) also seen at 35 and 42 s (**e, f**). Postcontrast source and subtraction images obtained at 140 s show the irregular mass (**g, h**). Sagittal and coronal images (**i, j**) are shown with a marker clip seen within the mass (*arrows*). Histology yielded IDC grade 3, ER/PR (+), HER2/neu (−), Ki67: 15 to 20%.

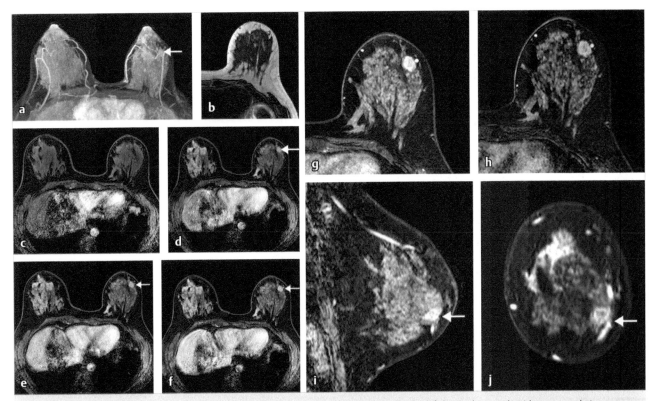

Fig. 5.9 UF technique. MIP image reveals marked BPE and an oval lateral enhancing mass in the left breast (**a**, *arrow*), without a correlative mass on T2w image (**b**). UF images: 28 s cardiac and aortic enhancement (**c**) 35 s first visualization of the oval enhancing mass (**d**, *arrow*) also seen at 42 and 49 s (**e, f**, *arrows*). Post-contrast source and subtraction images obtained at 140 s (**g, h**) show the circumscribed oval mass, also seen on sagittal and coronal reformatted images (**i, J**, *arrows*). Histology: fibroadenoma.

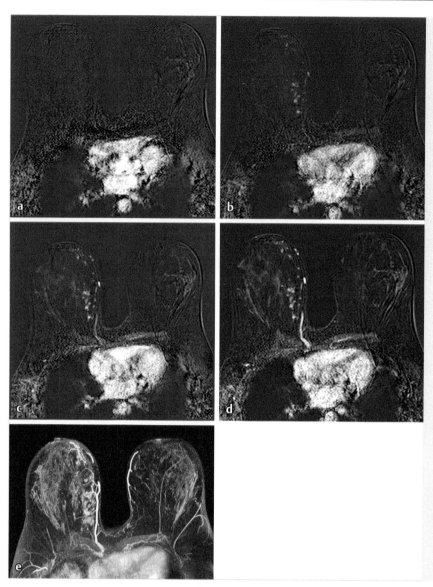

Fig. 5.10 UF technique. Known papillary DCIS in the right breast: UF image at 14 s **(a)** shows cardiac and aortic enhancement. First visualization of NME is seen at 21 s **(b)** with increasing enhancement seen at 28 and 35 s **(c, d)**. The extent of segmental DCIS is shown on slab axial image **(e)** obtained at 120 s.

software may misidentify the fat peak rather than the water peak, applying fat-suppression pulses at the incorrect frequency. In this case, the technologist should manually identify the water peak (▶ Fig. 5.12; ▶ Fig. 5.13).

5.5 Minimization of Artifacts

It is important to recognize imaging artifacts because misinterpretation may result in failure to recognize a suspicious lesion or misidentification of an artifact as an enhancing lesion. Common artifacts seen at breast MRI include inhomogeneous fat suppression, magnetic susceptibility, and motion artifacts, aliasing (wraparound), zebra, and RF-interference artifacts.[27] Once recognized by the radiologist and MR technologist, many artifacts are easily identified; however, on occasion, assistance from a physicist or service engineer may be required for diagnosis and correction of an artifact-related problem. Constant monitoring of the technical quality of MR acquisitions by the technologist and feedback from the interpreting radiologist are

essential for maintaining image quality and for minimizing artifacts.

5.5.1 Inhomogeneous Fat Suppression

Failed fat suppression is also referred to as "chemical shift artifact," because fat tissue saturation is directly related to the difference between the resonance frequencies of fat tissue and water. Inhomogeneous fat suppression is usually caused by inadequate shimming or by incorrect selection of water center frequency, resulting in B_0 inhomogeneity. Poor fat suppression or partial fat suppression failure in the T1w dynamic sequence can lead to misregistration of pre- and postcontrast images and to excessive structured noise in the subtracted images. Achieving good fat suppression can be technically difficult, especially in very fatty breasts. Technologists should review the precontrast T1w series carefully for presence of inhomogeneous fat suppression before injection of contrast, and if fat suppression is compromised, the center frequency should be adjusted. Incorrect selection of the water center frequency can be corrected by adjustment of the automatically selected water center frequency, selected by the system software. Fat-suppressed sequences should exhibit uniform dark fat signal across both breasts (▶ Fig. 5.14) and when fat-suppression failure occurs, fat will appear as a hyperintense signal (▶ Fig. 5.15). Partial fat suppression is frequently encountered in the medial aspect of the breasts and in the region in between the breasts,

as a result of the proximity of the air in the lungs (▶ Fig. 5.16). Nonuniform fat suppression can occur in women with large breasts when some breast tissue is placed very close to coil elements. This artifact is known as "signal flaring" and can be improved by placing MR-compatible sponges between the breast tissue and coil elements (▶ Fig. 5.17). Other techniques to improve fat suppression include reduction of the FOV to limit the amount of air in the regions of interest, and manual adjustment of the shim volume for each patient. When scanning, the technologist is able to shim the magnet at the console once the patient is positioned in the breast coil, adjusting the shim fields according to the individual patient breast size. In the future, development of different sized breast coils to accommodate both small and large breasts could improve focal field homogeneity and image SNR.

5.5.2 Magnetic Susceptibility Artifact

These artifacts appear as bright "spots," signal voids, or signal distortion of tissue, resulting from a signal "mismatch" at the interface of tissues with different local magnetic sensitivities. Metallic objects such as biopsy marker clips, surgical clips chemotherapy ports, etc. can cause disturbances in the main magnetic field resulting in metallic/susceptibility artifacts. Degrees of magnetization vary among breast tissue types and foreign bodies, and these artifacts are found more frequently at high magnetic field strength. Patients with metallic objects, such as breast surgical clips, placed at time of image-guided biopsy may not emit a magnetic resonance signal, thus creating a rapid outphasing of the spins inside the magnetic field with resulting signal loss. Nonferromagnetic titanium biopsy markers are available and cause less distortion than markers made of stainless steel. Postbiopsy marker clips are commonly visible on breast MRI, and the degree of distortion is directly related to the composition of the clip material (▶ Fig. 5.18; ▶ Fig. 5.19).

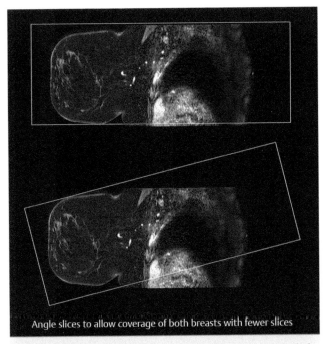

Fig. 5.11 High temporal resolution. This diagram shows a method of angling the FOV, so that entire coverage of the breasts is obtained using fewer slices.

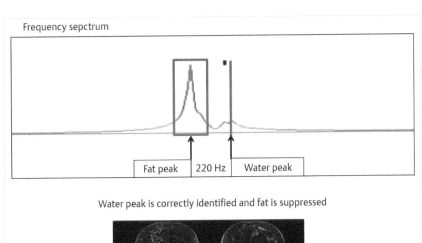

Fig. 5.12 Correct fat-suppression method. The water peak (*red line*) is correctly identified in this diagram, and the frequency-selective fat saturation pulse is therefore correctly positioned to eliminate the fat signal (*red box*).

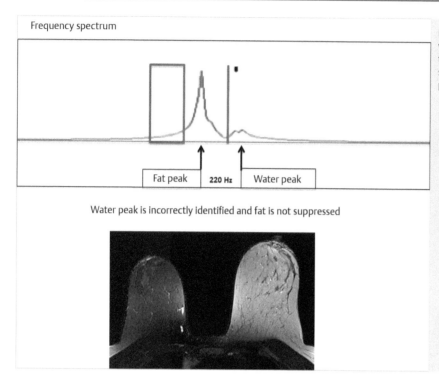

Frequency spectrum

Fat peak · 220 Hz · Water peak

Water peak is incorrectly identified and fat is not suppressed

Fig. 5.13 Incorrect fat-suppression method. The water peak (*red line*) is incorrectly identified in this diagram, and the frequency-selective fat saturation pulse is therefore incorrectly positioned to eliminate the fat signal (*red box*).

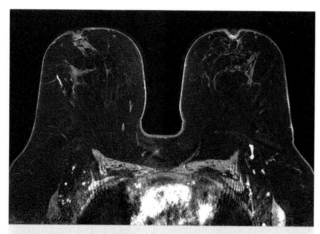

Fig. 5.14 Homogeneous fat suppression. Axial source T1w postcontrast image shows homogeneous fat suppression across both breasts.

Motion, Misregistration Artifact

Physiologic artifacts from cardiac, respiratory, blood flow, and vessel pulsation, as well as patient motion, all propagate in the phase-encoding direction, independent of the direction of the motion. In order to minimize physiologic motion artifacts across the FOV, selection of the phase-encoding gradient should be left-to-right for axial imaging and superior-to-inferior for coronal and sagittal imaging. Patient motion is a common problem and even slight motion can degrade image quality and compromise subtraction and corresponding maximum intensity projection images. Misregistration artifacts are often seen on subtraction imaging and may affect only a few sequences or the entire study. Image blurring and ghosting originating from inconsistencies of phase is caused either by intentional patient movement or physiologic motion from breathing during the acquisition. The periodic movement related to vascular pulsing causes a typical structured noise pattern resulting in "ghosting" of brighter moving tissues in the phase-encoding direction (▶ Fig. 5.20). These artifacts are unrelated to the direction of the movement, and often exhibit a double image of a normal structure or a displacement of the signal coming from the tissues. When motion is severe, repeat examination is often necessary. The small offset between the images obtained from sequences before and after gadolinium injection can generate false images and may even simulate abnormal enhancement by creating "pseudoenhancement" (▶ Fig. 5.21). Most CAD systems have motion correction algorithms that can help to minimize these artifacts. Technologists can alleviate the likelihood of motion by preparing the patient before she enters the magnet and instructing her to remain completely immobile throughout the MR study if at all possible.

Aliasing (Wraparound) Artifact

These artifacts are identified by the appearance of anatomic structures outside the prescribed FOV that are superimposed on images within the selected FOV on the opposite side of the image. Tissue is misplaced from its true anatomic position and outside signal-producing tissue is superimposed on the selected volume. MR manufacturers have established an automatic method to suppress image wrap in the frequency-encoding directions, therefore, this phenomenon is observed in the phase-encoding direction (▶ Fig. 5.22). When imaging in the axial plane, wrap artifacts of the patient's arms may appear, if they are positioned at the patient's sides rather than above her head, because the phase-encoding gradient is typically applied in the left-to-right direction to minimize the effects of cardiac

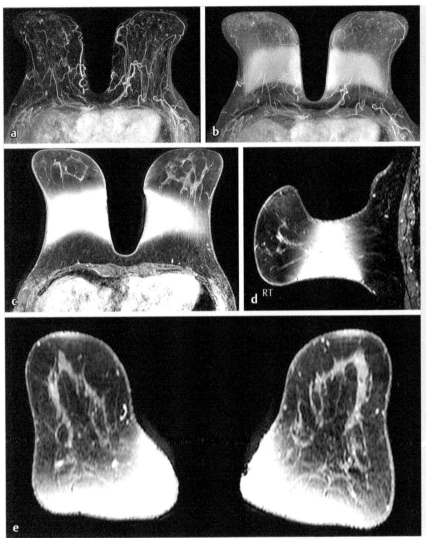

Fig. 5.15 Failed fat suppression. MIP Image (a) reveals large fatty breasts with scattered BPE. Source and subtracted images (b, c) reveal a band of failed fat suppression across both breasts, also shown on sagittal and coronal images (d, e).

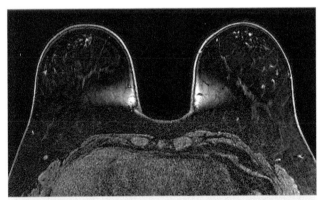

Fig. 5.16 Failed fat suppression. Source precontrast T1w axial image shows medial symmetrical failed fat suppression. This artifact was present on several additional slices (not shown).

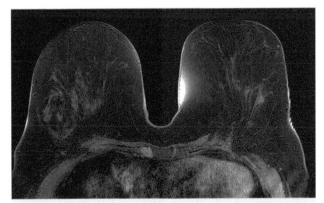

Fig. 5.17 Signal flaring. Axial source precontrast image reveals focal superficial high signal at the medial aspect of the left breast.

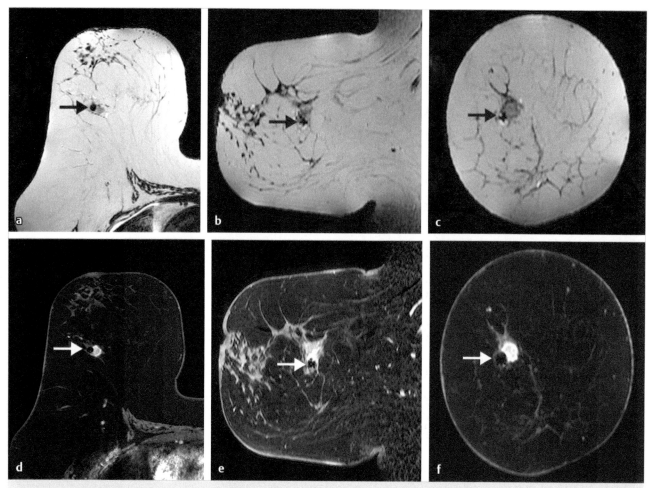

Fig. 5.18 Clip artifact. T2w non–fat-suppressed axial image (**a**) and reformatted sagittal and coronal images (**b, c**) demonstrate a marker clip adjacent to a hyperintense malignant mass (*arrows*). The clip is also visible on T1w source postcontrast axial (**d**, *arrow*) and reformatted sagittal and coronal images (**e, f**, *arrows*).

motion. 3D acquisitions utilize two phase-encoding directions, and therefore, aliasing can also occur in the slice-select direction. 3D "wraparound" appears as ghosting of other sections into the section of interest and is more likely to occur near the end sections of the 3D volume. Aliasing artifacts can be eliminated by increasing the imaging FOV to include all tissue in the phase-encoding direction. Other remedies for phase wrap artifacts include appropriate selection of the phase-encoding direction, application of saturation bands to suppress the signal from outside the FOV, and phase oversampling techniques. These remedies must be carefully monitored in order to avoid increasing the selected acquisition time and prolonging the temporal resolution in the dynamic sequence.

Zebra (Moiré) Artifact

The Zebra artifact is caused by a type of phase interference that affects signal emanating from tissue located outside the selected FOV when poor magnet shimming causes a phase shift between the tissue within, and the tissue outside the selected FOV. Black–white banding is characteristically seen on MRI due to rapid phase shifting as a function of position, causing signals

from the two regions to be out of phase, and therefore to cancel each other. A rapid phase shift can cause a combination or elimination of signal emanating from two different regions, when two diverse signals are in phase or out of phase, respectively. These black and white bands are known as Zebra or *Moiré* artifact (▶ Fig. 5.23). Banding can also occur when the breast coil is not selected, and the body coil is used. The possibility of image wrap or phase shift should be considered when this artifact is found, and the affected sequences should be repeated. Corrections can be made to minimize this artifact, either by eliminating image wrap by enlarging the selected FOV to include all signal-producing tissue, or by applying phase oversampling to minimize phase wrap. Reshimming of the magnet can also reduce phase shift.

Radio Frequency Interference Artifact

MRI rooms are constructed with a radio frequency (RF) shield that completely surrounds the imaging device. RF interference can be caused by an inadvertent source of RF signal located in the room itself, such as faulty fluorescent lights, electronic monitoring systems, or video and music equipment. Other RF

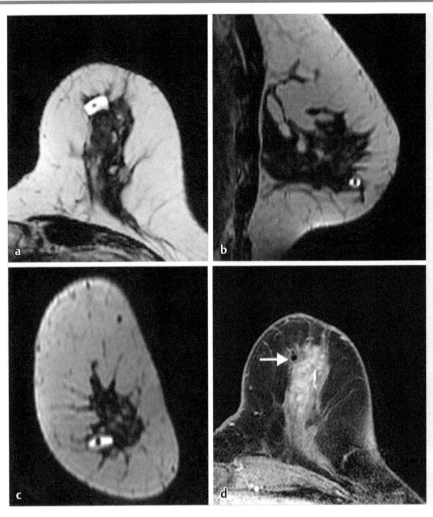

Fig. 5.19 Clip artifact. A Hydromark clip is shown as a high-signal artifact on T2w non–fat-suppressed axial image (**a**) and reformatted sagittal and coronal images (**b, c**). The clip presents as signal loss is on T1w postcontrast axial image (**d**, *arrow*).

interference can occur if there is a "leak" in the RF shield surrounding the imaging unit. This type of RF interference can be due to external causes such as the presence of nearby ongoing construction in the vicinity of the MRI suite. RF interference usually occurs when the technologist fails to close the door to the imaging room before scanning is underway. This artifact can present as either an image with an overall noisy background, or one with bright/dark bands at a fixed location along the frequency-encoding direction that propagate across the image in the phase-encoding direction (▶ Fig. 5.24).

5.6 Patient Positioning

Excellent positioning is key to obtaining good breast MR images. The patient must lie prone without moving for 15 to 20 minutes, and comfort is essential. It is impossible to underestimate the importance of specially trained breast MR technologists who can reassure the patient and manipulate the breasts within the coil so that optimal positioning can be obtained. MR-compatible nipple, scar or mass markers can be applied to the breasts prior to placement in the coil. At the present time only one size breast coil is usually available, and each breast should be symmetrically centered within the aperture of the dedicated coil, and the breasts should be positioned so that a minimum

amount of tissue remains above the coil apertures. Slight flattening of the nipple may occur when positioning a patient with large breasts (▶ Fig. 5.25). Improper positioning can result in asymmetric breast alignment and lateral overlapping of compressed breast tissue between the chest wall and the center partition of the coil. Symmetrical positioning of the breasts in the axial plane is essential for direct side-to-side analysis of image enhancement. An example of poor positioning is shown (▶ Fig. 5.26). A female staff member should be present during positioning, and a radiology nurse or technical assistant can be trained to position the patient. The observation window in the magnet room should be covered during this task to afford patient privacy.

5.7 Accreditation Requirements

The Medicare Improvement for Patients and Providers Act of 2008 (MIPPA) stipulates that all facilities that bill for advanced diagnostic imaging services, such as breast MRI, under the technical component of part B of the Medicare Physician Fee Schedule, must be accredited by a Centers for Medicare and Medicaid Services (CMS) designated accrediting organization to qualify for Medicare reimbursement. The ACR Breast Magnetic Resonance Imaging Accreditation Program[1] requires compliance

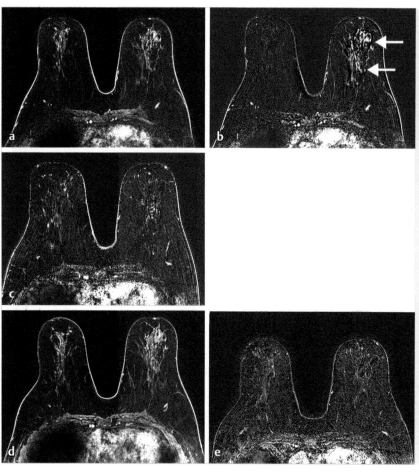

Fig. 5.20 Motion artifact. Screening examination: Axial source and subtraction T1w postcontrast images **(a, b)** reveal slight patient motion as evidenced by ghosting in the left breast originating from inconsistencies of phase *(arrows)*. This finding may be confused with NME, and it is important to recognize the motion artifact. The series was reprocessed using a motion correction algorithm, and the ghosting artifact is decreased as seen on image **(c)**. Repeat examination without motion shows no ghosting artifact, as noted on source and subtraction imaged **(d, e)**; the examination was normal.

with MR safety policies and acceptance testing intending to measure quantifiable MR system parameters, establishment of quality control (QC) measures, and routine QC testing. A technologist must perform a prescribed quality control process weekly. Every MR unit in an MRI department must individually pass accreditation in order to achieve facility accreditation. The ACR specifies certain technical considerations including use of a dedicated bilateral breast coil, simultaneous bilateral imaging capabilities, and compliance with state and federal performance requirements, but does not require minimum field strength for the magnet(s). The in-plane spatial resolution requirement of pixel sizes less than or equal to 1 mm and the slice thickness requirement of less than or equal to 3 mm as specified for dynamic breast MRI are reasonable quality requirements. Professional experience and qualifications are required for all personnel involved in MRI. Interpreting radiologists, MRI technologists, and medical physicists must meet specified qualifications as well as undergo continual clinical experience and education. As part of the accreditation process, submission of clinical images must available for review. Additional requirements include the ability to perform mammographic correlation when interpreting MRI studies and the capacity to perform directed ultrasound of MR-detected abnormalities. Provision of MRI-guided intervention procedures is a requirement and an essential part of any breast MR program and should be available on site, or at an off-site facility that accepts referrals for MR-guided biopsy procedures. The ACR provides all accredited facilities with peer review and constructive feedback on their staff's qualifications, equipment, QC testing, and quality assurance, and can be a helpful resource in all aspects of maintenance of an excellent breast MRI program.

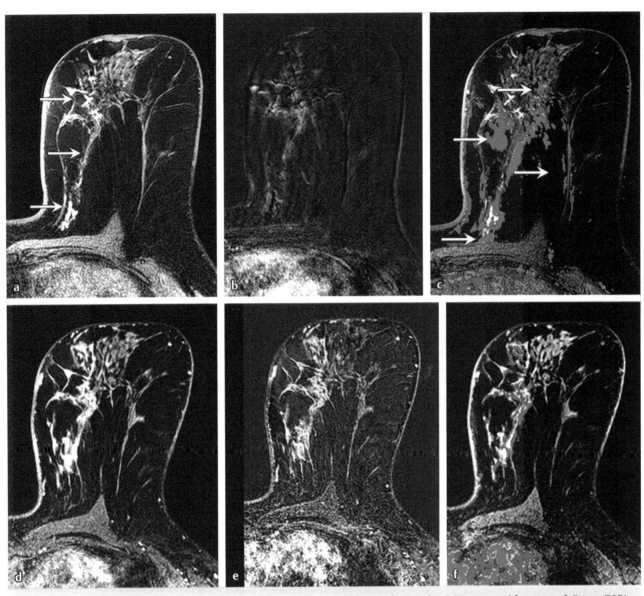

Fig. 5.21 Motion artifact. Patient with mammographic calcifications in the right breast, diagnosed as DCIS, presented for extent of disease (EOD) assessment. Source image **(a)** reveals segmental NME extending from the posterior to the anterior breast (*arrows*). Subtraction image **(b)** exhibits severe motion artifact with blurring and ghosting, false color is also present on angiomap **(c,** *arrows*). Repeat study shows NME with less motion artifact **(d)** but still with some slight motion on subtraction image **(e)**, and diminished blurring is noted on angiomap **(f)**.

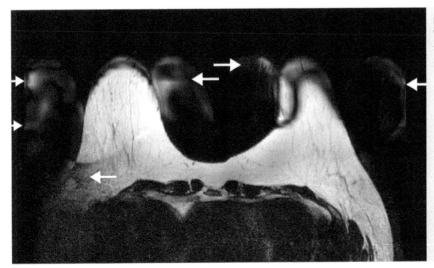

Fig. 5.22 Aliasing (wraparound) artifact. Wraparound artifact is seen on this axial non–fat-suppressed T2w image as shown (*arrows*).

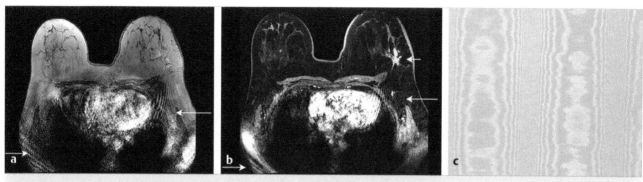

Fig. 5.23 Zebra (moiré) artifact. Newly diagnosed left breast IDC: Skin thickening and an irregular mass (*short arrows*) are shown on postcontrast T1w and T2w images (**a, b**). Black–white banding is noted laterally on both images (**a**) and (**b**) (*long arrows*). The term **moiré** originates from a type of *textile*, traditionally of *silk* with a rippled or "watered" appearance, as shown on image (**c**).

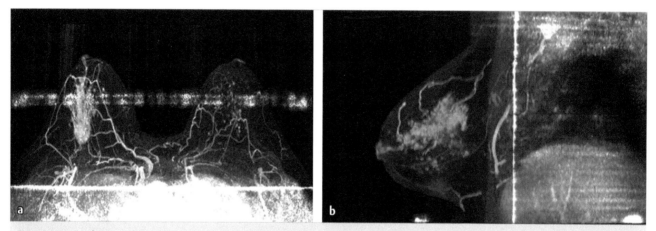

Fig. 5.24 RF interference. Newly diagnosed right breast DCIS: Extensive NME is shown on axial image (**a**) and sagittal image (**b**). RF interference is present as evidenced by bright bands propagating across both images. This interference occurred because the door between the magnet room and the technologist console was not completely closed during scanning.

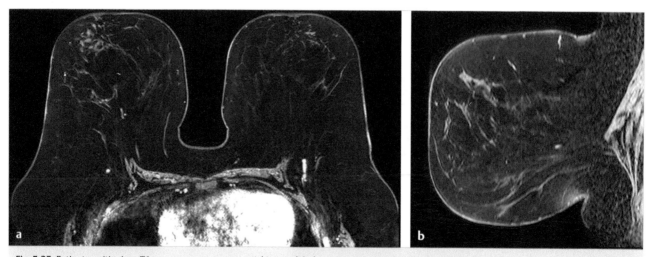

Fig. 5.25 Patient positioning. T1w source postcontrast axial image (**a**) shows a woman with large breasts positioned correctly in the breast coil with slight flattening of the anterior aspect of the breasts. This finding is also noted on right sagittal image (**b**).

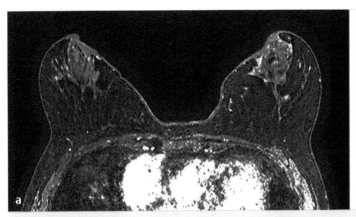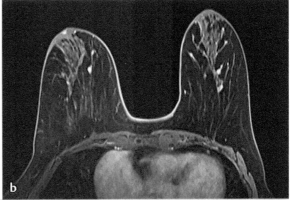

Fig. 5.26 Patient positioning. T1w subtracted postcontrast axial image **(a)** shows a poorly positioned patient with lateral deviation of both breasts, and medially oriented anterior breast tissue with the nipples not in profile. Repeat T1w source postcontrast axial image **(b)** shows improved positioning.

5.8 Summary

Excellent image quality is a prerequisite for accurate diagnosis. Each facility must tailor its approach to a diagnostic protocol according to the equipment available. The series should be as short as possible using reformatted images rather than multiple acquisitions. Key components of a high-quality study include a protocol that balances spatial and temporal resolution, achieves homogeneous fat suppression, minimizes artifacts, and is consistently applied.

References

[1] American College of Radiology Breast MRI Accreditation Program. https://www.acraccreditation.org/modalities/breast-mri. Accessed March 1 2019

[2] Kuhl CK. Current status of breast MR imaging. Part 2. Clinical applications. Radiology. 2007; 244(3):672–691

[3] Buadu LD, Murakami J, Murayama S, et al. Breast lesions: correlation of contrast medium enhancement patterns on MR images with histopathologic findings and tumor angiogenesis. Radiology. 1996; 200(3):639–649

[4] Kuhl CK, Mielcareck P, Klaschik S, et al. Dynamic breast MR imaging: are signal intensity time course data useful for differential diagnosis of enhancing lesions? Radiology. 1999; 211(1):101–110

[5] Hendrick RE, Haacke EM. Basic physics of MR contrast agents and maximization of image contrast. J Magn Reson Imaging. 1993; 3(1):137–148

[6] Kanda T, Ishii K, Kawaguchi H, Kitajima K, Takenaka D. High signal intensity in the dentate nucleus and globus pallidus on unenhanced T1-weighted MR images: relationship with increasing cumulative dose of a gadolinium-based contrast material. Radiology. 2014; 270(3):834–841

[7] McDonald RJ, McDonald JS, Kallmes DF, et al. Intracranial gadolinium deposition after contrast-enhanced MR imaging. Radiology. 2015; 275(3):772–782

[8] Kanda T, Fukusato T, Matsuda M, et al. Gadolinium-based contrast agent accumulates in the brain even in subjects without severe renal dysfunction: evaluation of autopsy brain specimens with inductively coupled plasma mass spectroscopy. Radiology. 2015; 276(1):228–232

[9] Murata N, Murata K, Gonzalez-Cuyar LF, Maravilla KR. Gadolinium tissue deposition in brain and bone. Magn Reson Imaging. 2016; 34(10):1359–1365

[10] EMA's final opinion confirms restrictions on use of linear gadolinium agents in body scans. EMA/457616/201 https://www.ema.europa.eu/en/medicines/.../gadolinium-containing-contrast-agents. Accessed February 10, 2019

[11] American College of Radiology Contrast Media Manual version 10.3, 2018. https://www.acr.org/Quality-Safety/Resources/Contrast-Manual. Accessed January 10, 2019

[12] Kuhl C. The current status of breast MR imaging. Part I. Choice of technique, image interpretation, diagnostic accuracy, and transfer to clinical practice. Radiology. 2007; 244(2):356–378

[13] Delille JP, Slanetz PJ, Yeh ED, Kopans DB, Garrido L. Physiologic changes in breast magnetic resonance imaging during the menstrual cycle: perfusion imaging, signal enhancement, and influence of the T1 relaxation time of breast tissue. Breast J. 2005; 11(4):236–241

[14] Amarosa AR, McKellop J, Klautau Leite AP, et al. Evaluation of the kinetic properties of background parenchymal enhancement throughout the phases of the menstrual cycle. Radiology. 2013; 268(2):356–365

[15] DeMartini WB, Liu F, Peacock S, Eby PR, Gutierrez RL, Lehman CD. Background parenchymal enhancement on breast MRI: impact on diagnostic performance. AJR Am J Roentgenol. 2012; 198(4):W373–W380

[16] Pineda FD, Medved M, Fan X, et al. Comparison of dynamic contrast-enhanced MRI parameters of breast lesions at 1.5 and 3.0 T: a pilot study. Br J Radiol. 2015; 88(1049):20150021

[17] Ramsay E, Causer P, Hill K, Plewes D. Adaptive bilateral breast MRI using projection reconstruction time-resolved imaging of contrast kinetics. J Magn Reson Imaging. 2006; 24(3):617–624

[18] Tudorica LA, Oh KY, Roy N, et al. A feasible high spatiotemporal resolution breast DCE-MRI protocol for clinical settings. Magn Reson Imaging. 2012; 30 (9):1257–1267

[19] Kershaw LE, Cheng HL. A general dual-bolus approach for quantitative DCE-MRI. Magn Reson Imaging. 2011; 29(2):160–166

[20] Chan RW, Ramsay EA, Cheung EY, Plewes DB. The influence of radial undersampling schemes on compressed sensing reconstruction in breast MRI. Magn Reson Med. 2012; 67(2):363–377

[21] Smith DS, Welch EB, Li X, et al. Quantitative effects of using compressed sensing in dynamic contrast enhanced MRI. Phys Med Biol. 2011; 56(15):4933–4946

[22] Kuhl CK. Breast MR imaging at 3T. Magn Reson Imaging Clin N Am. 2007; 15 (3):315–320, vi

[23] Lourenco AP, Donegan L, Khalil H, Mainiero MB. Improving outcomes of screening breast MRI with practice evolution: initial clinical experience with 3 T compared to 1.5 T. J Magn Reson Imaging. 2014; 39(3):535–539

[24] Pinker-Domenig K, Bogner W, Gruber S, et al. High resolution MRI of the breast at 3 T: which BI-RADS® descriptors are most strongly associated with the diagnosis of breast cancer? Eur Radiol. 2012; 22(2):322–330

[25] Pinker K, Baltzer P, Bogner W, et al. Multiparametric MR imaging with high-resolution dynamic contrast-enhanced and diffusion-weighted imaging at 7 T improves the assessment of breast tumors: a feasibility study. Radiology. 2015; 276(2):360–370

[26] Fiaschetti V, Pistolese CA, Funel V, et al. Breast MRI artefacts: evaluation and solutions in 630 consecutive patients. Clin Radiol. 2013; 68(11):e601–e608

[27] Harvey JA, Hendrick RE, Coll JM, Nicholson BT, Burkholder BT, Cohen MA. Breast MR imaging artifacts: how to recognize and fix them. Radiographics. 2007; 27 Suppl 1:S131–S145

6 Diagnostic MRI Interpretation

Gillian M. Newstead and Michael S. Middleton

Abstract

This chapter outlines a standard method for interpretation and reporting of diagnostic MRI examinations and discusses the management of patients with challenging clinical or imaging diagnoses. Included is a structured reading method, providing clarity and uniformity of interpretation across breast MRI practices. Standard reporting includes not only lesion characterization and a final category assessment, but also specifics of the MRI acquisition, type and amount of GBCA administered, volume of fibro-glandular tissue (FGT) and amount of background parenchymal enhancement (BPE). Critical to accurate interpretation is the selection of reading protocols at the workstation which include the T2w Sequence, the MIP Image (First post-contrast T1w Image, both Source and Subtraction), the T1w Dynamic Sequence (Source and Subtracted Images) and the Kinetic Analysis. Sample protocols are shown. A discussion of challenging diagnoses including evaluation of patients with nipple discharge and papillary lesions, are supplemented with 23 case examples. A section on breast MRI Reporting reviews the Breast Imaging Reporting and Data System (BI-RADS®) developed by the American College of Radiology.

An excellent review of breast implants and the MRI findings of breast implants and their associated various abnormalities are further discussed in detail by Dr. Middleton. This section includes a description of the various types of breast implants; the MRI appearances of implant abnormalities including implant rupture; standard reporting of implant cases; and a discussion of methods to deal with challenging cases and pitfalls.

Keywords: diagnostic DCE-MRI interpretation, reading protocol, kinetic classification, interpretation challenges, nipple discharge, papillary lesions, reporting system (BI-RADS), breast implants, implant imaging protocol, implant rupture, implant reporting

6.1 Introduction

In this chapter, we will outline a standard method for interpretation and reporting of diagnostic magnetic resonance (MR) examinations and discuss management of patients with challenging clinical or imaging diagnoses, including evaluation of women with current or prior implants.

6.2 Interpretation Protocol

A standard reading method provides structure and uniformity of interpretation across breast MR practices. The radiology report should include not only lesion characterization and a final category assessment, but also specifics of the MR acquisition, the type and amount of gadolinium-based contrast agent (GBCA) administered, the volume of fibroglandular tissue (FGT), and the amount of background parenchymal enhancement (BPE). A standard interpretation method for diagnostic breast magnetic resonance imaging (MRI) examinations is outlined below, and a standard hanging protocol is illustrated (▸ Fig. 6.1).

6.3 MIP Image (First Postcontrast T1w Image, Source, and Subtraction)

The maximum intensity projection (MIP) images provide a useful overview of breast enhancement. Successful dynamic contrast-enhanced MRI (DCE-MRI) requires a rapid bolus injection of contrast, and this can be evaluated by identifying cardiac and major vascular enhancement on the first postcontrast series. The technologist should always check for the presence of contrast enhancement in the heart and great vessels during scanning. If contrast enhancement is not evident on the first postcontrast images, the technologist should check the injection site. Contrast injection into the subcutaneous tissue of the arm or a break in the tubing delivery mechanism could account for an unsuccessful DCE-MRI study; when this occurs, repeat examination is usually necessary. The radiologist should be certain that the dynamic sequence is acceptable by looking for adequate contrast bolus enhancement in the heart and nearby vasculature. Be aware that low delivery of contrast agent may occur in patients with cardiac failure, resulting in delayed contrast delivery. BPE can be assessed on the first postcontrast MIP image. Enhancing lesions and other findings may also be visible on MIP images (▸ Fig. 6.2) and, if seen, should be further evaluated on source and subtracted images within the complete dynamic series.

6.3.1 T2w Sequence

The T2-weighted (T2w) sequence can be acquired with fat saturation (typically at lower spatial resolution) or without fat saturation (typically at higher spatial resolution). The amount of FGT can be assessed on this series and should be included in the report. This sequence is useful for identification of high-signal fluid, as found in cysts, subareolar ducts, intratumoral necrosis, and subcutaneous/peritumoral edema. Other findings include visualization of normal or abnormal axillary, intramammary and internal mammary lymph nodes, breast masses, skin thickening, and postsurgical changes. The T2w series can also be used for assessment of postsurgical or postbiopsy marker clips and changes resulting from breast reconstruction surgery, and, as will be discussed later in this chapter, can also assist in the assessment of soft-tissue silicone resulting from implant rupture and from breast silicone fluid injections.

The high-spatial-resolution T2w series allows matching of images slice-by-slice with the T1w DCE series. This sequence accomplishes the need for both a T2w series and a non–fat-suppressed T1w precontrast series and incorporates both acquisition requirements into a single acquisition (▸ Fig. 6.3). This high-resolution T2w series provides improved assessment of mass morphology and identification of peritumoral and

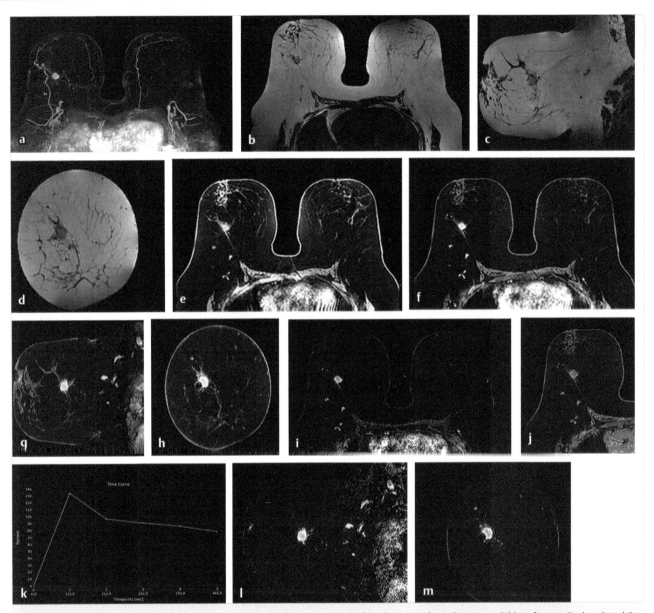

Fig. 6.1 Hanging protocols. This viewing protocol is shown as three separate displays; however, depending on available software, displays 2 and 3 could be condensed into one display for the dynamic sequence. A unifocal IDC is shown in the right breast. Hanging protocol #1 allows a technical assessment of image quality by first viewing of the MIP image (a), providing a series overview with comparison to the T2w images (b–d). Hanging protocol #2 shows the T1w precontrast image (e) and the source T1w postcontrast source images shown in MPR format (f–h). Hanging protocol #3 exhibits T1w postcontrast subtraction images shown in MPR format (i, l, m), with associated angiomap and TIC (j, k). Histology yielded triple negative IDC.

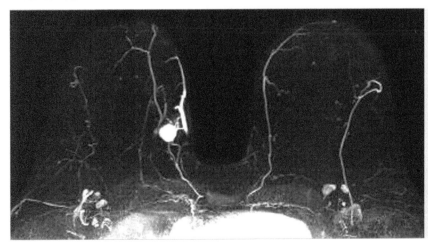

Fig. 6.2 Maximum intensity projection (MIP) image. MIP image (subtracted), obtained at the first postcontrast time point (70 s), reveals a round enhancing mass with associated increased vascularity.

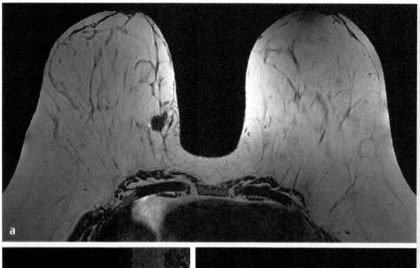

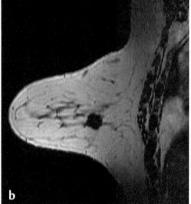
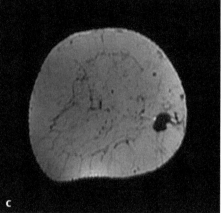

Fig. 6.3 T2w series. T2w series (non–fat suppressed) shows a correlative hypointense mass shown in MPR format (a–c).

prepectoral edema, findings that may not be visualized on the thicker slices that accompany a fat-suppressed T2w acquisition. Although the T2w sequence may not be helpful for evaluation of noninvasive cancer (because NME exhibits very few precontrast findings) it is very useful for characterization of breast masses.

6.3.2 T1w Dynamic Sequence (Source and Subtracted Images)

The pre- and postcontrast source and subtracted series are next reviewed. It is important to check the precontrast images to be sure that the fat saturation is uniform and to check the subtraction images for evidence of motion artifact. Next we search for abnormal enhancement, which is usually seen best at the first and second time points when the enhancement is most intense and is distinct from BPE. Analysis of any enhancing lesion should include a morphologic assessment of shape, margin, internal enhancement, and distribution characteristics; multiplanar reformatting (MPR) and slab images can be useful in this regard (▶ Fig. 6.4; ▶ Fig. 6.5). Lesion size, location, laterality (right or left breast), and breast quadrant (including the appropriate use of "central") and retroareolar and axillary tail should be reported. Lesion distance from the nipple, skin, or chest wall should be measured when appropriate. Although enhancing masses may be visible on the MIP images, careful evaluation of

the first and second postcontrast source and subtraction images is needed for complete diagnosis. If an enhancing lesion is found on the T1w postcontrast series, review of the precontrast T2w series may identify a correlate lesion. Viewing of the later postcontrast sequences is also necessary to ensure identification of certain slowly enhancing cancers and for assessment of treatment response for patients undergoing serial MRI examinations during neoadjuvant chemotherapy; delayed enhancement is the only indication of residual disease in some cases. The ability to compare lesion characteristics on both T2w and T1w sequences with identical spatial resolution can result in improved diagnostic specificity.

6.3.3 Kinetic Classification

DCE-MRI kinetic techniques derived from imaging acquired over a standard time interval following contrast injection (5–7 minutes) include measures of the uptake and washout of contrast in tissues and contain diagnostically useful information. The shape of the signal-intensity-versus-time curve (TIC, or signal time-course, or kinetic curve), which plots signal intensity over time, has been found to be useful in the classification of enhancing lesions. Signal intensity is analyzed on a pixel-by-pixel basis within an enhancing lesion. TIC data can be obtained by using a manual technique, placing a region-of-interest (ROI) of at least 3 pixels on the most suspicious region of enhancement within an enhancing lesion. Changes in signal intensity

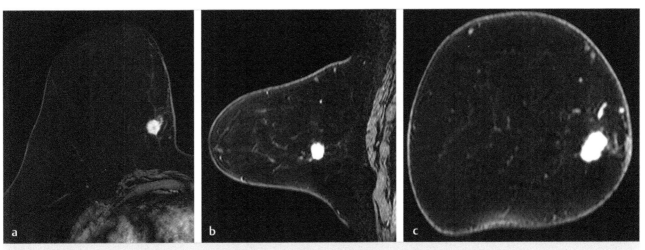

Fig. 6.4 T1w postcontrast source series. T1w postcontrast source images obtained at the first-time point (70 s) are shown in MPR format **(a–c)**.

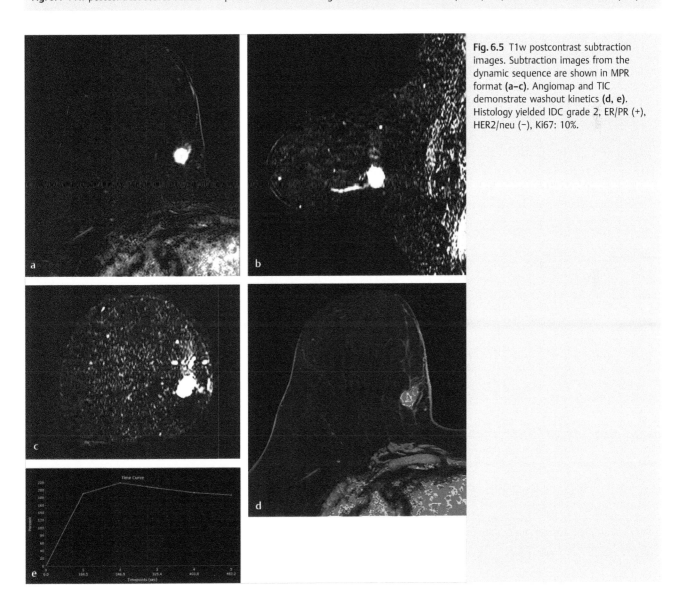

Fig. 6.5 T1w postcontrast subtraction images. Subtraction images from the dynamic sequence are shown in MPR format **(a–c)**. Angiomap and TIC demonstrate washout kinetics **(d, e)**. Histology yielded IDC grade 2, ER/PR (+), HER2/neu (−), Ki67: 10%.

are then monitored over time. Accurate analysis of TIC data strongly depends on predictable delivery of a GBCA using a bolus technique and a dose administered according to patient body weight. Most practices in the United States now utilize computer-aided analysis systems, allowing depiction of kinetic parameters on a pixel-by-pixel basis in parametric images describing intralesional variations in blood flow. These analytic tools can not only automatically display TICs, but also generate color maps of lesions that enhance above a set threshold. Thresholds are usually set between 50% (slow initial rise), 50 to 100% (medium initial rise), and >100% (fast initial rise). The parametric images reflect all lesions or tissues enhancing above a predetermined threshold below which no enhancement is measured, and exhibit "persistent" (continued increasing enhancement >10% above threshold), "plateau" (relatively constant signal intensity), and "washout" (decreasing signal intensity following peak enhancement >10% below threshold). Lesion color-coding of the delayed phase of enhancement can facilitate interpretation of the kinetic data (▶ Fig. 6.6).

Given that MRI is usually the last study in the diagnostic chain to be acquired, knowledge of the patient's medical history and review of all prior imaging studies are essential for optimal interpretation of the breast MR examination.

6.4 Interpretation Challenges

Sources of error in breast MR interpretation may be attributed to technical incidents such as equipment malfunction and artifacts, host-related issues such as marked BPE or motion, and human errors of perception or misinterpretation. As discussed in Chapter 5, breast MRI is technically demanding and requires excellent fat saturation and high spatial and temporal resolution with rapid acquisition of postcontrast sequences. Technical errors in clinical practice that commonly affect interpretation include poor positioning, inadequate contrast injection, and patient motion. Careful assessment of image quality by the technologist and radiologist in routine practice is necessary to avoid these errors. Perception failures at screening account for missed cancers and may be exacerbated by marked BPE, which may mask small malignancies (▶ Fig. 6.7; ▶ Fig. 6.8; ▶ Fig. 6.9; ▶ Fig. 6.10). Appropriate scheduling of the MR examination according to the timing of the patient's menstrual cycle can often alleviate this problem. Small cancers are often best identified on the first postcontrast subtracted series in a standard acquisition, or on an ultrafast sequence where BPE is minimal (▶ Fig. 6.11; ▶ Fig. 6.12). Small or even large in situ cancers may be difficult to detect even in the presence of mild BPE; high

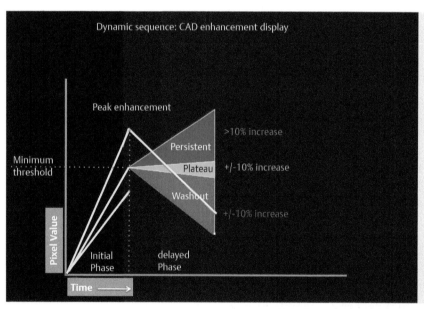

Fig. 6.6 Enhancement kinetics. A display of enhancement kinetics is shown.

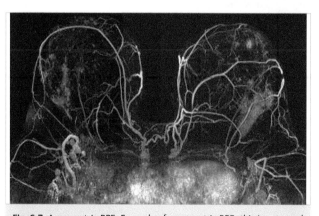

Fig. 6.7 Asymmetric BPE. Example of asymmetric BPE: this is a normal finding.

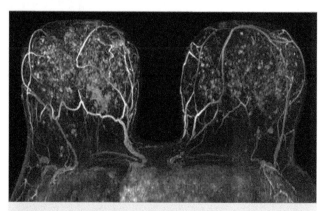

Fig. 6.8 Marked BPE: nodular pattern.

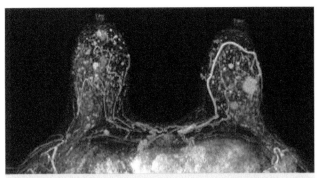

Fig. 6.9 Marked BPE: nodular pattern—multiple bilateral benign enhancing masses representing known fibroadenomata are shown.

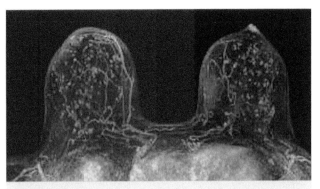

Fig. 6.10 Marked BPE. nodular pattern.

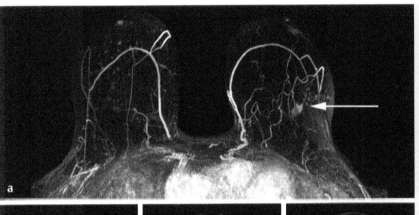

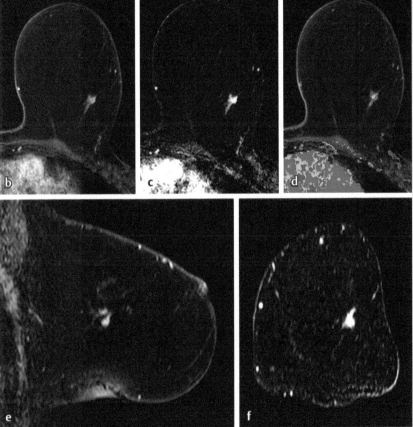

Fig. 6.11 Small IDC with DCIS. High-risk screening (BRCA 2), 4th module: MIP image reveals an irregular enhancing 8-mm mass in the lateral left breast (**a**, *arrow*). T1w postcontrast source and subtracted images show the irregular mass with associated posterior NME (**b, c**). Angiomap shows heterogeneous, washout kinetics (**d**) and sagittal and coronal reformatted images are shown (**e, f**). Histology yielded left breast IDC grade 2, size 8 mm, with DCIS within and adjacent to the mass. ER/PR (+), HER2/neu (–), Ki-67: 15%. Sentinel nodes were negative for malignancy (0/2).

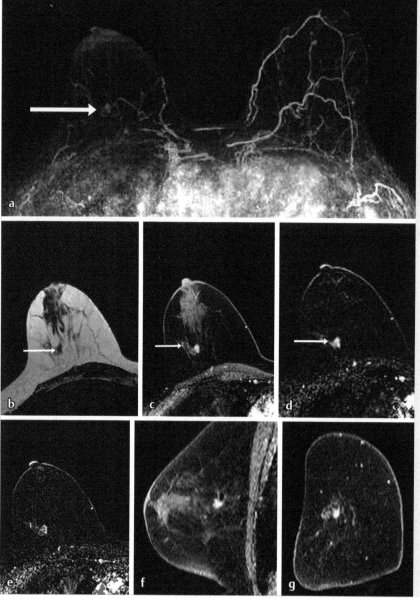

Fig. 6.12 Small ILC with pleomorphic LCIS. MIP image shows an irregular enhancing mass in the posterior aspect of the right breast (**a**, *arrow*), seen as an isointense mass on T2w image (**b**, *arrow*). T1w postcontrast source and subtracted images show mass enhancement with NME extending anterolaterally from the mass (**c, d,** *arrows*). Angiomap shows heterogeneous, washout kinetics (**e**) and sagittal and coronal reformatted images are shown (**f, g**). Histology yielded ILC, 0.9 mm with associated pleomorphic LCIS, ER (+), PR (−), HER2/neu (−), Ki-67: 5–10%. Sentinel nodes were negative for malignancy (0/5).

spatial resolution at 3 T facilitates detection of such cancers (▸ Fig. 6.13; ▸ Fig. 6.14). Benign findings that may cause difficulty in interpretation and affect specificity negatively include certain lymph nodes, papillomata, fat necrosis (▸ Fig. 6.15; ▸ Fig. 6.16; ▸ Fig. 6.17), and fibroadenomata (▸ Fig. 6.18; ▸ Fig. 6.19; ▸ Fig. 6.20). These lesions may exhibit rapid enhancement, often with washout kinetics, careful morphologic analysis being necessary for accurate diagnosis; isotropic or near isotropic, MPR can be useful in these cases.

6.4.1 Skin Enhancement

Skin enhancement may be seen at the site of recent percutaneous biopsy but may also reflect spread of malignancy to the dermis. Malignant skin involvement may be evident remote from the site of a newly diagnosed cancer or may directly involve the dermis. Cowden's syndrome is a rare autosomal dominant inherited disorder characterized by diagnosis of multiple hamartomas and is associated with a predisposition for

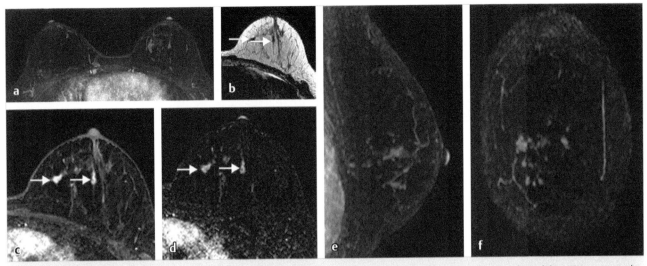

Fig. 6.13 Multifocal IDC and DCIS. A 43-year-old patient, MRI screening, normal mammogram BRCA mutation carrier 5th module: MIP image reveals extensive medial and central NME in the left breast (a). Two irregular masses are seen on T2w and T1w postcontrast source images (b, c *arrows*). Subtracted image (d) exhibits two irregular enhancing masses with surrounding NME low (sub-threshold) enhancement was present. Sagittal and coronal reformatted slab images reveal the extent of NME (e, f). Final histology (following MR-guided biopsy indicating IDC) yielded two IDC lesions 6 and 3 mm in size, grade 3, with associated extensive grade 3 DCIS, ER/PR (+), HER2/neu (–), Ki-67: 50–60%. Sentinel nodes were negative for malignancy (0/5).

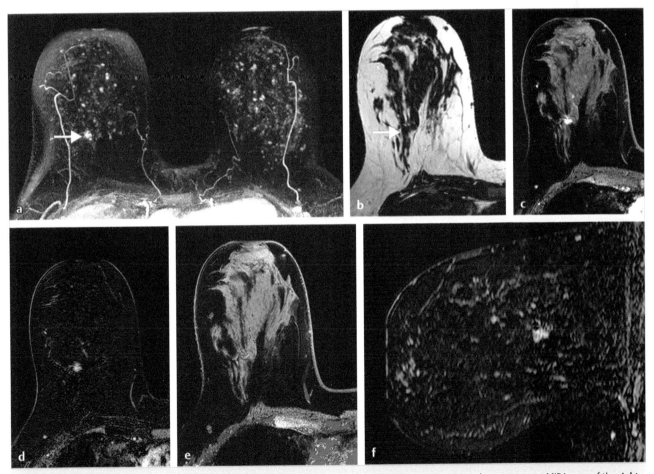

Fig. 6.14 Invasive cancer right breast and in situ cancer left breast. A 47-year-old patient, MRI screening, normal mammogram: MIP image of the **right** breast shows nodular marked BPE with a distinct small irregular mass noted (a, *arrow*). T2w image partially reveals an isointense mass (b, *arrow*), seen with robust enhancement on T1w source postcontrast image (c). Spiculated mass margins are seen on subtracted image (d) and washout kinetics are noted on angiomap (e). Sagittal and coronal reformatted subtraction images are shown (f,g). (*continued*)

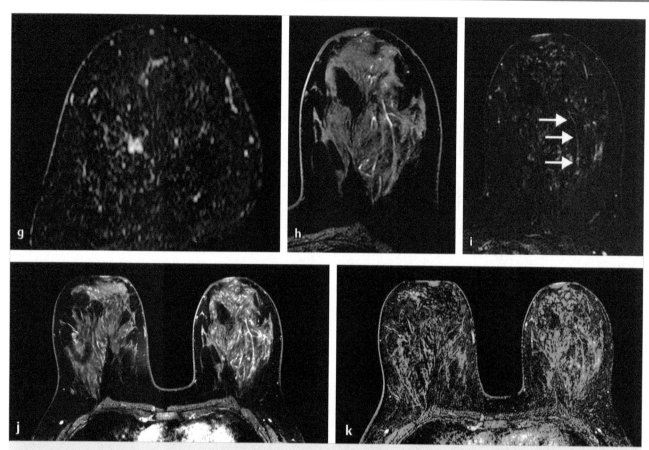

Fig. 6.14 (*continued*) Sagittal and coronal reformatted subtraction images are shown (**f,g**). Histology yielded IDC grade 2, total extent 1.3 cm, with associated DCIS cribriform type and intermediate grade, ER/PR (+), HER2/neu (–). Evaluation of the **left** breast revealed normal MIP and T2w series. Careful review of the dynamic sequence revealed linear branching (ductal) enhancement, visible only on three slices. Precontrast T1w image exhibits segmental ductal fluid (**h**) and correlative postcontrast subtracted image reveals branching linear enhancement (**i**, *arrows*). Similar findings are shown on adjacent postcontrast source image (**j**) and subtracted image (**k** *arrows*). This finding is difficult to perceive, and high spatial resolution is necessary for diagnosis. Histology at simple mastectomy (following MRI-guided biopsy indicating DCIS) yielded low and intermediate DCIS, cribriform and solid type, ER/PR (+).

breast carcinoma. An example of a patient with Cowden's syndrome and an aggressive inflammatory breast cancer (IBC) with direct skin involvement is shown in ▶ Fig. 6.21.

6.4.2 Inflammatory Changes

Inflammation due to mastitis may be focal or diffuse. Detection of segmental NME is usually associated with ductal carcinoma in situ (DCIS); benign diagnoses with this finding and distribution are uncommon. An example of inflammatory changes presenting as segmental NME, mimicking DCIS, is shown in ▶ Fig. 6.22.

6.5 Postsurgical Complications

The T2w series is very helpful for evaluation of the posterior breast and chest wall, particularly when complications from implant augmentation or reconstructive surgery result. An example of postsurgical complications following expander placement for breast reconstruction is shown in ▶ Fig. 6.23.

6.6 The Male Breast

Breast cancer in men is rare, accounting for less than 1% of breast cancers. Physiological gynecomastia occurs in neonates and puberty, and with obesity and ageing. Gynecomastia can be caused by an increased estrogen to testosterone ratio in men treated with estrogen therapy for prostate cancer and by a variety of other medications. Mammography is usually the recommended test when men are referred for imaging. An example of gynecomastia on MRI is shown in ▶ Fig. 6.24.

6.7 Nipple Enhancement

Normal nipple enhancement can mislead the reader because the nipple often enhances with varying intensity due to the rich blood supply of the nipple–areolar complex, and the enhancement may not necessarily be symmetric. The radiologist should be careful when the nipple is inverted because normal nipple enhancement may simulate a subareolar enhancing mass. Abnormal nipple enhancement is found in patients with Paget's disease, IBC, lymphatic obstruction, and inflammation. An

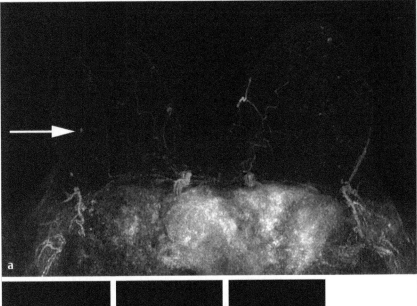

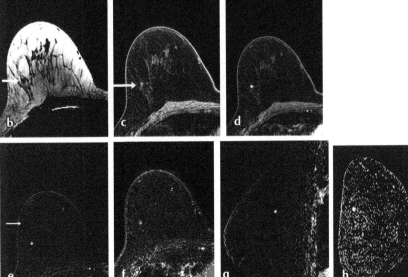

Fig. 6.15 Intramammary lymph node (IMLN). MRI screening, normal mammogram: MIP image reveals mild BPE and a distinct 3-mm circumscribed enhancing mass in the right breast (**a**, *arrow*), seen as isointense on T2w image (**b**, *arrow*) and precontrast T1w image (**c**, *arrow*). Robust enhancement is seen on source postcontrast image (**d**) and subtraction image (**e**) with a minimal hilar notch noted (*arrow*). Washout kinetics are seen on angiomap (**f**) and reformatted sagittal and coronal images are shown (**g, h**). IMLNs usually present with washout kinetics and identification of benign morphology is essential for diagnosis.

example of an epidermal inclusion cyst within the nipple is shown in ▶ Fig. 6.25.

6.8 Breast Carcinoma in Augmented Breasts

Breast implant surgery has been performed routinely for augmentation and reconstruction purposes for over 50 years, employing a large variety of devices including saline, silicone double-lumen types using both saline and silicone, and polyacrylamide gel. Contrast-enhanced MRI is necessary for cancer screening or diagnosis of suspected tumor. A causal relationship between malignancy and implant placement has not been found.[1] Breast carcinomas often contact the implant surface and tumors may spread along the contour of the implant. The use of MR MPR in such cases is particularly helpful for surgical

planning. Examples of two patients with saline implants and associated malignancy are shown in ▶ Fig. 6.26 and ▶ Fig. 6.27.

Breast implant–associated anaplastic large cell lymphoma (BIA-ALCL) is a rare, distinct type of T cell lymphoma which develops around implants, causing pain and breast swelling and, less commonly, a palpable breast mass.[2] The underlying mechanism of this disease is thought to be due to chronic inflammatory change resulting from indolent infections, leading to malignant transformation of T cells that are anaplastic lymphoma kinase (ALK) negative and CD30 positive. Mean time to presentation is about 10 years following augmentation surgery and fluid is shown to develop around the implant. Immunohistochemistry confirms the diagnosis BIA-ALCL with CD30 + and ALK– expression. In most cases, surgical treatment is curative and includes capsulectomy and removal of the implant. When disease is more advanced, chemotherapy, radiotherapy, and lymph node dissection may be necessary.

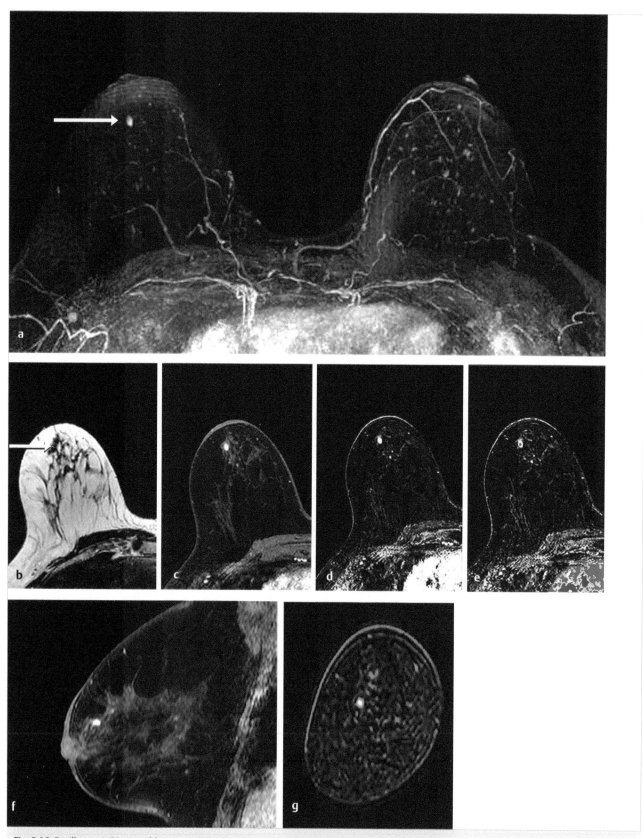

Fig. 6.16 Papilloma. A 71-year-old patient, BRCA 2 carrier MRI screening 10th module: MIP image (**a**) reveals a new distinct 6-mm circumscribed enhancing mass in the right breast, 10 o'clock position anterior depth (**a**, *arrow*), seen as isointense on T2w image (**b** *arrow*). Robust enhancement is seen on source postcontrast image (**c**) and subtraction image (**d**) with persistent kinetics identified on angiomap (**e**). Reformatted sagittal and coronal images are shown (**f**, **g**). Despite benign morphology, MR-guided biopsy was performed with results yielding sclerosing papilloma without atypia.

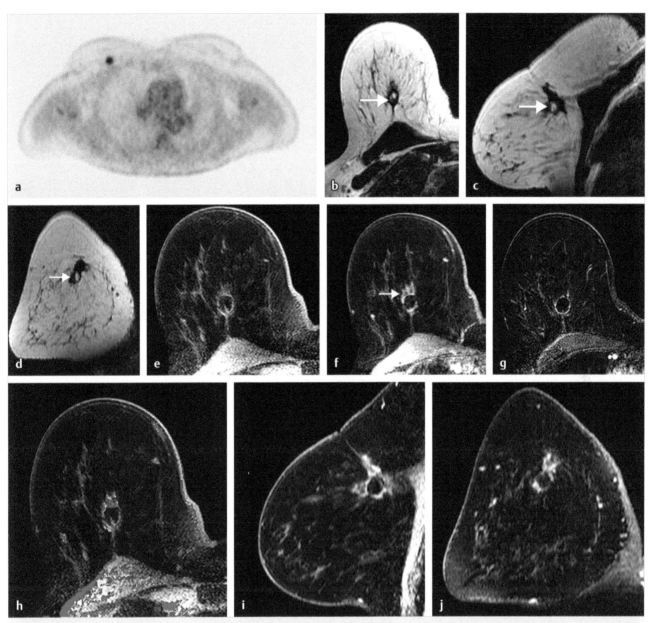

Fig. 6.17 Fat necrosis. Age 65, S/P RT lumpectomy 3 years ago for treatment of IDC grade 3: routine follow-up staging PET examination revealed uptake in the posterior right breast **(a)** at the site of the lumpectomy scar. T2 W axial image with sagittal and coronal reformatting reveals an irregular mass at the scar site with central fat signal **(b–d,** *arrows*). Mass with central fat signal is seen on precontrast image **(e)** and rim enhancement and adjacent anterior NME is noted on postcontrast, source image **(f,** *arrow*) and rim enhancement on adjacent subtraction image **(g)**. Heterogeneous NME with washout kinetics is noted on angiomap **(h)**. Sagittal and coronal images are shown **(i, j)**. MR-guided biopsy yielded fat necrosis. This case emphasizes the importance of multiplanar reformatting for accurate lesion assessment.

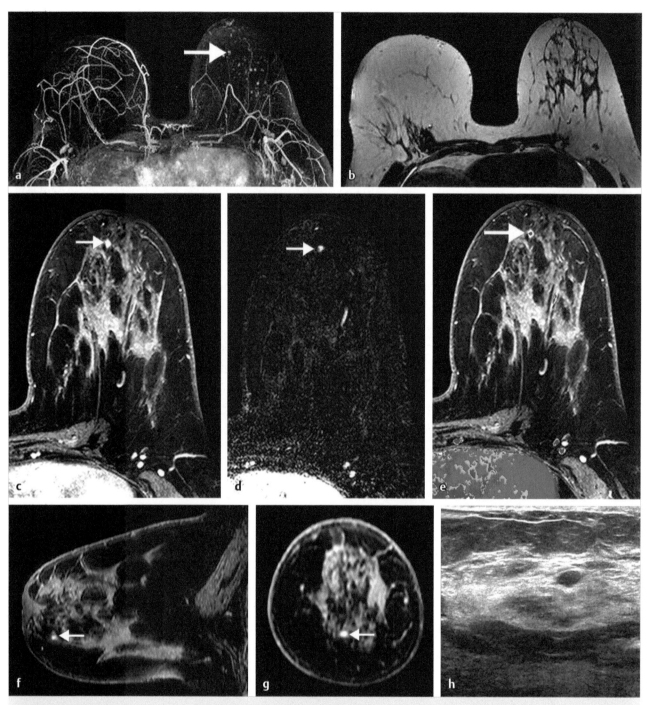

Fig. 6.18 Fibroadenoma. A 37-year-old, personal history of grade 3 DCIS treated with mastectomy 5 years ago. 5th MRI screening module: MIP image reveals autologous reconstruction of the right breast and a new 3-mm mass in the anterior left breast at 6 o'clock position (**a**, *arrow*). T2w image (**b**) shows the reconstructed right breast but no abnormal findings. Source and subtraction postcontrast T1w images identify the 3-mm enhancing mass (**c, d**, *arrows*), also seen with persistent enhancement on angiomap (**e**) and on sagittal and coronal reformatted image (**f, g**, *arrows*). MR-directed ultrasound identified a correlative oval mass, biopsy yielding fibroadenoma (**h**).

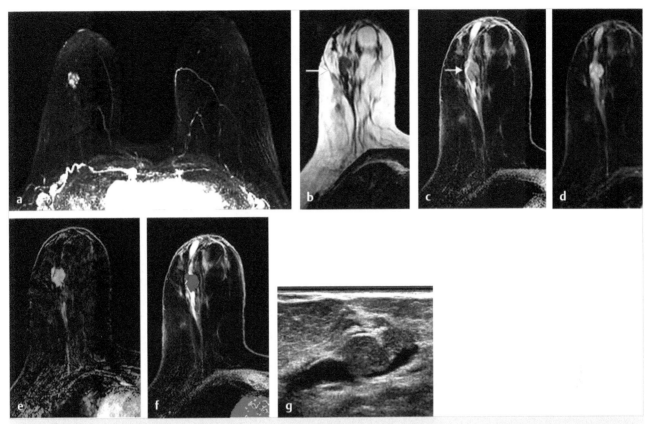

Fig. 6.19 Fibroadenoma. A 55-year-old patient. MIP image (**a**) reveals a circumscribed 13-mm enhancing mass with internal unenhancing septations, seen as isointense on T2w image (**b**, *arrow*). Precontrast T1w image reveals high signal fluid within a dilated duct which is compressed by the mass (**c**, *arrow*). Source postcontrast T1w image (**d**) shows both the high duct signal and the enhancing mass with unenhancing septations. The mass is also shown on subtraction image (**e**), and persistent mass enhancement is seen on angiomap (**f**). MR-directed ultrasound shows the benign mass partially obstructing the dilated duct (**g**). Ultrasound-guided biopsy yielded fibroadenoma.

6.9 Benign Papillary Lesions and Nipple Discharge

Papillary lesions of the breast represent a diverse group of lesions that share a common frond-like growth pattern with epithelium supported by a fibrovascular stroma. These breast lesions include benign papilloma, papillary DCIS, and invasive papillary carcinoma. Myoepithelial cells line the basement membrane in benign papillomata and papillary DCIS lesions, but are absent in invasive papillary carcinoma.

6.9.1 Solitary Intraductal Papillomata

These lesions are usually identified centrally in the large lactiferous subareolar ducts and cause bloody or serous nipple discharge when symptomatic. They are often nonpalpable, ranging from 3 to 5 mm in size, and are frequently mammographically occult.[3] The dominant feature of large duct papilloma is that of a circumscribed mass with or without calcifications on mammography, and a circumscribed hypoechoic mass arising within an ectatic duct or a complex mass with increased blood flow on ultrasound. Papilloma may be associated with a dilated duct on both mammography and ultrasound.[4] MRI features similarly identify a circumscribed subareolar mass smaller than 1 cm,

with rapid homogeneous enhancement and varied kinetics in the delayed phase.[5,6] Dilated ducts exhibiting high T2w and T1w signal caused by hemorrhage may be associated with a papilloma.[7] Although the morphologic characteristics of most papillomata suggest benignity, the kinetic finding of washout in the delayed phase is not uncommon and differentiation from malignancy may require tissue sampling in some cases. Management of large duct papilloma generally depends on whether atypia is associated with the histologic diagnosis.[7,8,9] A diagnosis of papilloma with atypia confers a much higher patient risk (7.5 times) than that of a papilloma without atypia.[10] In clinical practice, most papillomata diagnosed on core biopsy with a finding of associated atypia are excised. There are no consensus recommendations for the management of papilloma without atypia, and in many cases follow-up with clinical examination and imaging is recommended.

6.9.2 Multiple Intraductal Papillomata (Multiple Peripheral Papillomatosis)

These lesions are much less common, arise from the terminal ductal lobular unit, and are usually found in the periphery of the breast. Despite their different site of origin and multiplicity, the imaging findings on MRI are similar to those of solitary

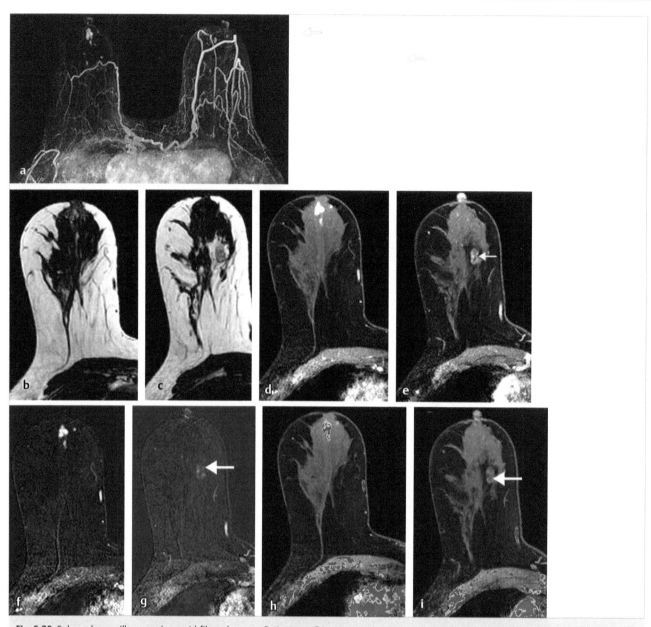

Fig. 6.20 Subareolar papilloma and myxoid fibroadenoma. Patient age 54 years, routine screening. MIP image reveals a multilobulated mass in the right breast subareolar region **(a)**. Two lesions are present in the right breast. T2w image **(b)** reveals hyperintensity in the subareolar region (*arrow*) and a high signal oval mass is seen at 2 o'clock position **(c)**. T1w postcontrast source images show robust subareolar enhancing masses **(d)** and minimal enhancement in the mass at 2 o'clock position **(e,** *arrow*), also seen on subtraction images **(f, g,** *arrow*). Heterogeneous mass enhancement is noted with washout kinetics on angiomap **(h)** and persistent mass enhancement is on angiomap **(i)**. The subareolar location of the multilobulated circumscribed mass with washout kinetics is consistent with the subsequent ultrasound-guided biopsy yielding papilloma. The circumscribed mass at 2 o'clock position with minimal enhancement was also biopsied, yielding myxoid fibroadenoma.

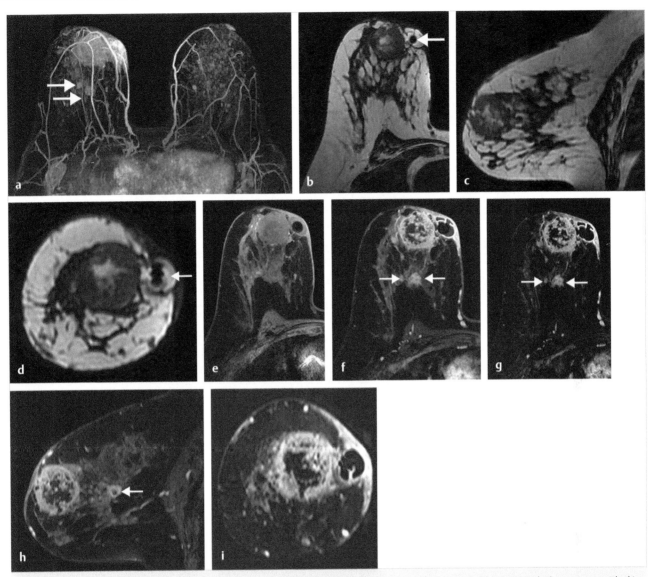

Fig. 6.21 IBC with skin involvement. Patient, age 37, with known Cowden's syndrome presented with a painful anterior right breast mass with skin ulceration: marked BPE and a large anterior enhancing breast mass extending medially to the skin, with two additional small enhancing masses noted posterior to the index lesion, are seen on MIP image (**a**, *arrows*). T2w axial image (**b**) shows a hyperintense subareolar mass with a biopsy marker clip visible just below the skin (*arrow*). Sagittal reformatted T2w image (**c**) demonstrates the mass, also seen on the coronal T2w image, with an extruded marker clip and skin thickening (**d**, *arrow*). Precontrast T1w image reveals heterogeneous isointensity in the mass with an associated medial fluid collection and skin thickening (**e**). Postcontrast image (**f**) shows the mass to enhance with two posterior satellites also identified; similar findings are noted on subtraction image (**g**) where prominent skin enhancement is noted overlying the mass and adjacent fluid collection is also present. Reformatted sagittal image (**h**) reveals rim enhancement in a satellite lesion (*arrow*). Coronal image (**i**) is shown. Final histology yielded IBC grade 3 triple negative, with squamous differentiation and necrotic inflammatory debris, Ki-67: 60%.

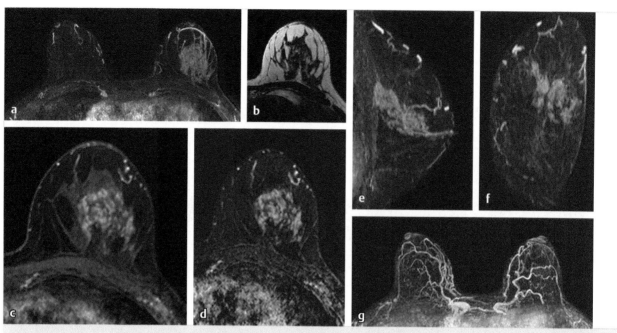

Fig. 6.22 Benign segmental NME (1.5 T). Patient, age 54, presented with pain and a palpable "thickening" in the left breast; mammography and ultrasound were normal. MIP image reveals extensive NME in the central and lateral left breast with increased vascularity **(a)**. T2w image **(b)** is normal; however, diffuse NME is identified on postcontrast T1w source and subtracted images **(c, d)** and on reformatted sagittal and coronal images **(e, f)**. Percutaneous biopsy revealed periductal inflammation with histiocytes and poorly formed granulomas in association with ruptured ductules. Clinical findings subsided and follow-up MRI revealed no abnormal findings, as shown on MIP image **(g)**.

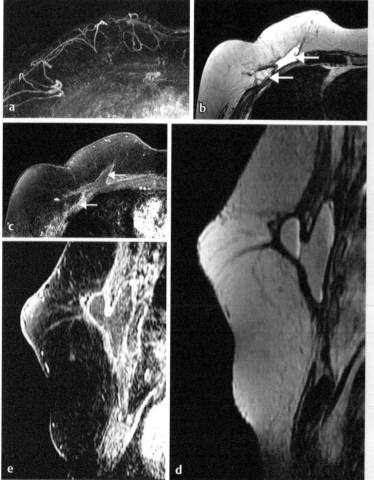

Fig. 6.23 Expander dehiscence; patient aged 50 was diagnosed with right breast DCIS, and was treated with mastectomy and reconstructive surgery. A tissue expander was placed and then removed because of complication with infection. MIP image shows the mastectomy site **(a)**. T2w axial image **(b)** and postcontrast source image **(c)** reveal two fluid collections, also identified on sagittal reformatted images **(d, e)**. The fluid collections were drained and resolved with antibiotic treatment.

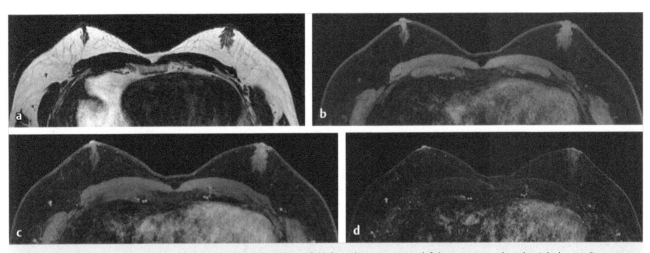

Fig. 6.24 Gynecomastia. Patient aged 62 presented clinically with painful bilateral gynecomastia, left breast greater than the right breast. Precontrast T2w and T1w images **(a, b)** show normal-appearing breast tissue behind the nipple, with a greater amount of tissue noted in the left breast. Postcontrast source and subtraction images reveal minimal enhancement of breast tissue **(c, d)**. No signs of malignancy are present.

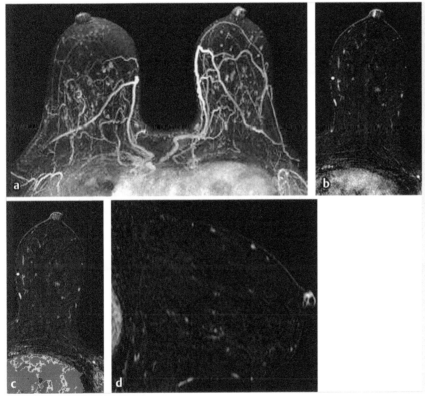

Fig. 6.25 Epidermal inclusion cyst in the nipple. Patient age 41, routine MR screening. MIP image reveals moderate BPE and linear enhancement in the left nipple **(a)**, also seen on T1w subtraction image **(b)**, with persistent kinetics shown on angiomap **(c)**. The finding is also noted on reformatted sagittal image **(d)**.

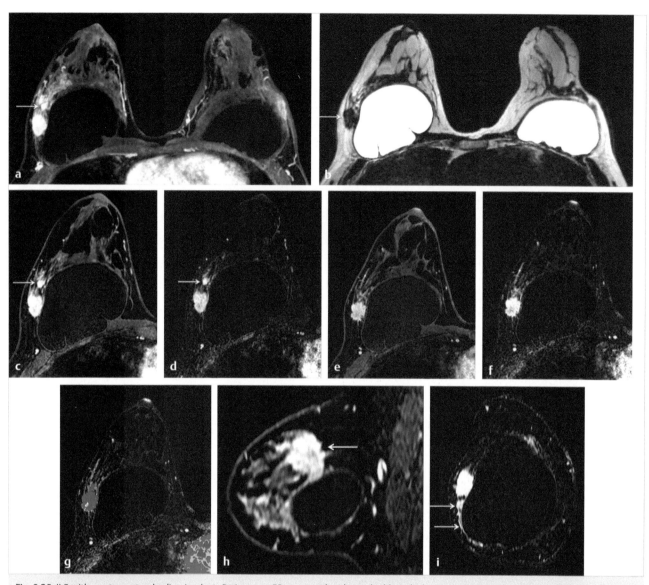

Fig. 6.26 ILC with a retropectoral saline implant. Patient age 52 presented with a palpable right breast mass. Partial MIP image **(a)** reveals an enhancing spiculated mass in the lateral posterior right breast with a second smaller anterior mass (*arrow*) and surrounding NME extending anteriorly. T2w axial image **(b)** exhibits a hypointense mass (*arrow*) and bilateral retropectoral saline implants. Source images **(c, e)** and subtracted images **(d, f)** show to advantage the satellite lesion (*arrows*) and the spiculated index lesion. Angiomap **(g)** demonstrates persistent kinetic mass enhancement, and sagittal source reformatted image **(h)** shows the index mass (*arrow*). Subtracted coronal reformatted image **(i)** reveals enhancing tumor spreading along the implant surface (*arrows*). Final histology yielded ILC grade 2 with associated LCIS, classic type. ER/PR (+), HER2/neu (−), Ki-67: 10%. One sentinel node was positive for malignancy (1/20).

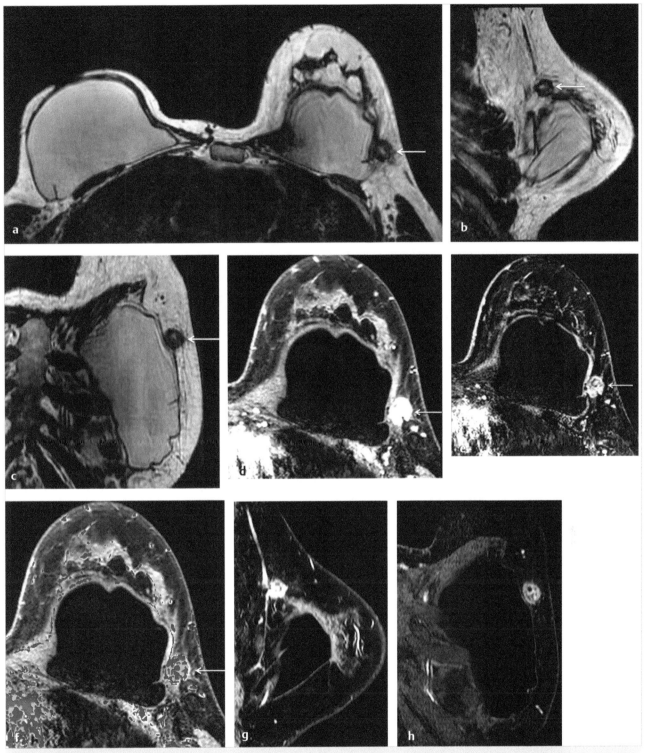

Fig. 6.27 IDC with a retropectoral silicone implant. Patient age 41 with a retropectoral silicone implant presented with a palpable **left** breast mass at 2 o'clock position. She underwent prior **right** breast cancer treatment (IDC and DCIS) with skin-sparing mastectomy, and reconstruction with a silicone implant. T2w axial image **(a)** exhibits bilateral silicone implants and a round hyperintense mass in the left breast corresponding with the palpable mass (*arrow*), also seen on reformatted sagittal and coronal planes **(b, c,** *arrows*). Source and subtracted axial images **(d, e)** show rapid heterogeneous enhancement within the mass (*arrows*), and angiomap **(f)** demonstrates heterogeneous washout mass enhancement (*arrow*), also seen on reformatted sagittal and coronal planes **(g, h)**. Final histology yielded IDC grade 3 with necrosis. ER (+) PR (−), HER2/neu (−). All axillary lymph nodes were negative for malignancy (0/13).

large duct papilloma. A hereditary condition known as juvenile papillomatosis, first described by Rosen in adolescents and young women, confers a slightly higher breast cancer risk, the imaging findings being similar to those of multiple intraductal papillomata.[11]

6.9.3 Clinical Nipple Discharge

The standard-of-care imaging protocol for most women with spontaneous bloody or serous nipple discharge consists of imaging with mammography, ultrasound, and galactography. These studies identify the causative lesion in many, but not all cases, and the gold standard for treatment of patients with nipple discharge and negative imaging findings is surgery with large duct excision.[12,13] Most causes of nipple discharge are benign; a report on 586 patients who underwent surgery for significant nipple discharge stratified the breast pathology as follows: papilloma 48%, fibrocystic change 33%, cancer 14%, and high-risk lesions 7%.[14] Studies have shown that the performance of breast MRI is superior to that of galactography for detection and characterization of papillary lesions,[15,16] and radiologists increasingly use MRI for definitive assessment of women with nipple discharge (▶ Fig. 6.28; ▶ Fig. 6.29). The increased use of MRI for this indication has come into play for two main reasons, both resulting in change of management. Firstly, the addition of MRI to the presurgical imaging protocol results in higher sensitivity than other standard imaging tests and may detect unsuspected malignant disease not associated with the known papilloma, thus affecting patient management (▶ Fig. 6.30). Secondly, absence of significant breast enhance-

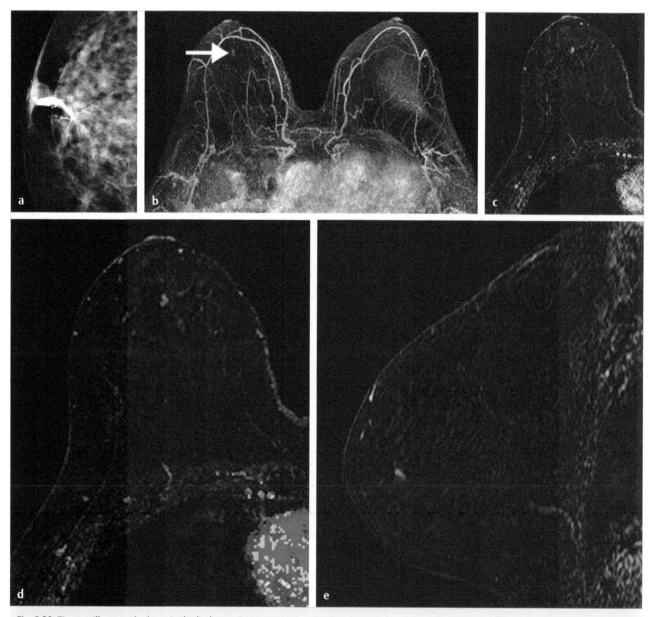

Fig. 6.28 Tiny papilloma with clear nipple discharge. Patient age 71 with new onset of clear nipple discharge. CC view from a galactographic study reveals visualization of the distal portion of the secreting duct but not the peripheral duct system (**a**). MIP image (**b**) reveals a 2 3 mm focus in the right breast behind the nipple (*arrow*). The finding is best seen on T1w postcontrast subtraction image (**c**); washout kinetics is shown on angiomap (**d**). Sagittal reformatted subtraction image is shown (**e**). MR-guided biopsy yielded papilloma.

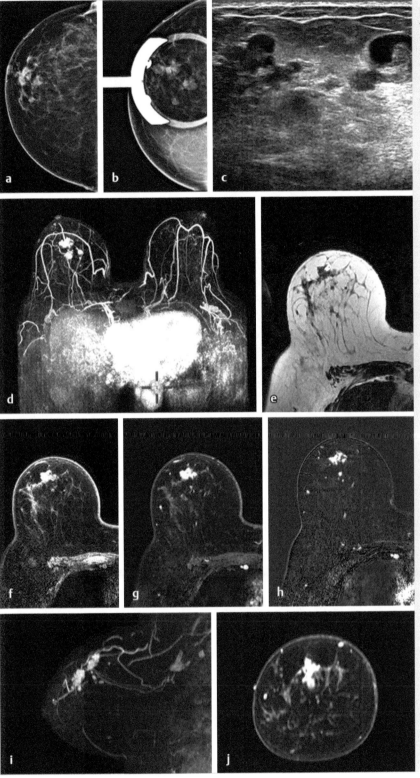

Fig. 6.29 Multiple papillomata. Patient age 40 with new bloody nipple discharge and a palpable subareolar mass. CC mammographic view and spot CC magnified view (**a, b**) reveal multiple circumscribed masses of various sizes in the subareolar region of the right breast. Ultrasound image (**c**) shows dilated ducts with internal solid masses. Needle biopsy of the palpable mass indicated papilloma. MIP image (**d**) reveals multiple robustly enhancing masses, seen as isointense on both T2w image (**e**) and precontrast T1w image (**f**). Source and subtracted T1w postcontrast images (**g, h**) show rapid enhancement, and sagittal and coronal reformatted images are shown (**i, j**). A bracketed needle localization procedure was performed, with histology yielding multiple intraductal papillomata (no atypia) with apocrine metaplasia, the largest papilloma measuring 7 mm.

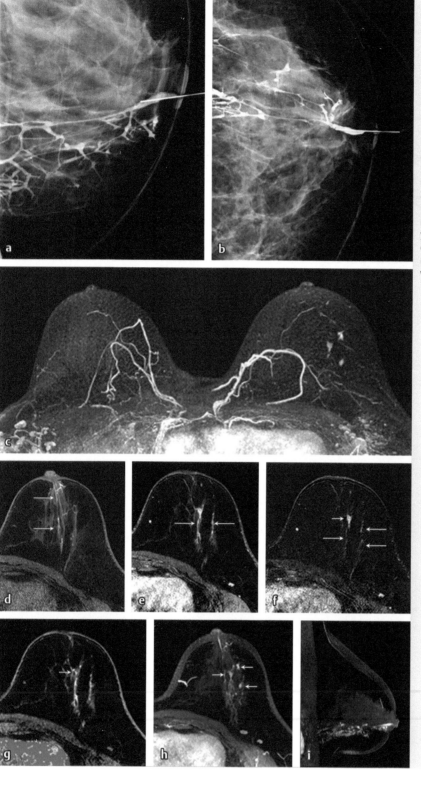

Fig. 6.30 Bloody nipple discharge. Patient, age 57, presented with new bloody discharge; mammography, ultrasound, and galactography (**a, b**) all interpreted as negative. MIP image (**c**) exhibits three irregular small masses in the mid-lateral left breast. Precontrast T2 image reveals duct fluid in a segmental distribution (**d**, *arrows*) and linear enhancement is seen on postcontrast source image (**e**, *arrows*). All three small masses are located within the region of linear enhancement (two not shown) and one is shown on subtracted image (**f**, *short arrow*), *long arrows* identifying linear enhancement. Angiomap (**g**, *arrow*) reveals washout kinetics in the small mass. Slab source axial image (**h**) reveals the three masses located within the segment of ductal fluid and linear enhancement. Sagittal reformatted image is shown (**i**). MR-guided biopsy indicated DCIS. Final histology at simple mastectomy yielded DCIS, low grade, micropapillary, and cribriform type with three solid papillary features measuring 5, 4, and 8 mm. Sentinel lymph node was negative for malignancy.

ment would likely preclude diagnosis of cancer given the high negative predictive value of MRI, and perhaps obviate the need for surgical duct excision, unless the discharge were to be too troublesome for the patient. Further clinical studies are needed; however, thought should be given to the management of women with nipple discharge now that we have a test with exquisite sensitivity and a very high negative predictive value. A reasonable consideration could be to allow a patient the choice of surgery or follow-up when MRI is negative.

6.10 Reporting

Reporting should follow the Breast Imaging Reporting and Data System (BI-RADS) developed by the American College of Radiology (ACR).[17] The indication for the examination, pertinent medical history, the specific MR technique used in summary form, including strength of the magnetic field, type and number of acquisitions, and type and amount of GBCA administered should be incorporated into the report. The report should also include the volume of FGT and the amount of BPE. When abnormal enhancement is detected, the findings should be categorized according to the ACR lexicon descriptors and a final assessment and recommendation should be reported. The radiologist needs to know whether a screening or a diagnostic examination is indicated. Any prior breast imaging studies, including mammography and ultrasound, should be obtained and uploaded onto the departmental PACS ahead of the appointment time. A patient questionnaire provides useful information for the radiologist and it is important to know whether a patient has experienced any new clinical signs or symptoms. A detailed patient history should include knowledge of his/her personal risk for developing breast cancer, any prior biopsies or surgery, or treatment with antiestrogen chemotherapy or radiation therapy.

6.10.1 Assessment Categories

The MRI report should assign an ACR BI-RADS final assessment code indicating the level of suspicion for cancer and follow-up management recommendations (▶ Table 6.1). The final assessment code facilitates patient management by providing the referring physician with an overall summary of the breast MRI findings. This assessment should be made after review of all current breast imaging and extramammary findings, taking into account any clinical findings and prior pathologic and imaging results.

Category 0: Incomplete—Need Additional Imaging Evaluation

This category should be used sparingly. This assessment may be used, for example when a technically unsatisfactory scan is obtained, and an MRI repeat study is recommended, or when additional clinical or other imaging studies are unavailable, but needed in order to provide a complete interpretation of the study. The MR examination is often the last imaging test to be obtained in the diagnostic chain, and the decision to biopsy or not is generally made on analysis of the existing MRI study. On occasion, a final Category 0 assessment may be useful when a finding on MRI is suspicious, such as when a rapidly enhancing

Table 6.1 Assessment category

Assessment	Management	Likelihood of cancer
Category 0 Need additional imaging evaluation	Recommend additional imaging: mammogram or targeted ultrasound	N/A
Category 1 Negative	Routine breast MRI screening if cumulative lifetime risk ≤ 20%	Essentially 0%
Category 2 Benign	Routine breast MRI screening if cumulative lifetime risk ≤ 20%	Essentially 0%
Category 3 Probably benign	Short-interval (6 mo) follow-up	> 0% but ≤ 2%
Category 4 Suspicious	Tissue diagnosis	> 2% but < 95%
Category 5 Highly suggestive of malignancy	Tissue diagnosis	95% or greater
Category 6 Known biopsy-proven malignancy	Surgical excision when clinically appropriate	N/A

Source: Modified from American College of Radiology.[17]

intramammary lymph node with washout kinetics is identified, but a clear demonstration that the finding is benign on ultrasound or mammography would avert a biopsy recommendation. When a Category 0 assessment for additional imaging is rendered, it is essential that clear details in the MRI report describe the level of suspicion of the lesion. If additional imaging does not establish benignity, a final assessment should be rendered in the subsequent imaging report.

Category 1: Negative

This is a normal assessment; no abnormal enhancement is identified, and routine follow-up is advised. If the indication for the MRI examination is for screening, annual follow-up MRI and mammography is recommended in line with established guidelines for high-risk screening.

Category 2: Benign

This is a normal assessment; no abnormal enhancement is identified, and routine follow-up is advised. It is a question of preference as to whether a benign finding on breast MRI is reported, but if it is, a Category 2 designation is appropriate. Specific benign findings such as lymph nodes, implants, cysts, fibroadenomata, or biopsy clips may be reported. If the indication for the MRI examination is for screening, annual follow-up MRI and mammography is recommended in line with established guidelines for high-risk screening.

Category 3: Probably Benign

A Category 3 assessment on MRI requires follow-up MRI instead of biopsy for a lesion judged to have a low probability of malignancy and the expectation of no adverse effect resulting from a short delay in possible cancer diagnosis. Category 3 was initially described as a special mammographic category with detailed descriptors of lesions and a likelihood rate of malignancy ≤ 2%, but greater than the 0% likelihood of malignancy of a characteristically benign finding.[18]

Category 3 lesions are not yet fully elucidated for MRI, and so this assessment should also be used sparingly. For Category 3 MRI findings, the protocol recommends an MRI examination within 6 months from the initial examination, another 1 year later, and then, if the lesion is unchanged, a return to routine imaging. Any Category 3 MRI lesion showing an increase in size or change in morphology on follow-up MRI should undergo tissue sampling.

Although some retrospective studies of Category 3 lesions on MRI, with variable follow-up, have shown an overall malignancy rate of about 4%, other studies report a rate of about 2%.[19,20] Although foci have been described as comprising up to 48% of Category 3 MRI lesions, the likelihood of malignancy is lowest in foci (0.9%) and is highest in NME (4%).[21] Other studies have shown that the imaging characteristics of Category 3 MRI lesions are highly variable.[21,22] A systematic analysis of 15 studies evaluating BI-RADS 3 lesions published in 2018 found that pooled malignancy rates met BI-RADS benchmarks (< 2%) at 1.6% (95% confidence interval [CI]: 0.9–2.3%). Malignancy rates, however, varied, exceeding the 2% rate for nonmass lesions (2.3%; 95% CI, 0.8–3.9%).[23] The prevalence of BI-RADS 3 lesions on breast MRI ranged from 1.2 to 24.3% in this study and malignant lesions were diagnosed at follow-up time points for up to 24 months.

Multiple diffuse bilateral foci are regularly seen in perimenopausal women and should not be considered to be probably benign, but rather should be categorized as benign (Category 2) because they represent a variation of normal BPE. Category 3 on MRI lesions that disappear, decrease, or remain unchanged in size at follow-up without any new sign of malignancy can be downgraded to benign (Category 2) without the need for biopsy. In clinical practice, it is helpful to initiate a meeting with the patient when a Category 3 lesion is recommended. Patients generally welcome a discussion with a physician before deciding whether to be followed or biopsied, and some women prefer a biopsy rather than experience anxiety during the follow-up period. Caution, however, should be applied when applying a Category 3 lesion assessment to women in a high-risk MR screening program because the malignancy risk in this cohort may be greater than 2%.[24,25] A decrease in the frequency of both Category 3 MRI assessments and false-positive outcomes should be possible once radiologist experience is gained and an MR screening program matures; ideally the recall rate should be lower than 10%, and preferably closer to 2 to 3%.

Category 4: Suspicious

The MRI lesions in this category indicate a probability of malignancy of 2 to 95% and constitute a wide variety of findings, all sufficiently suspicious to justify a recommendation for biopsy. Unlike the Category 4 assessments for mammography and ultrasound, the MRI Category 4 is not divided into subcategories 4A, 4B, and 4C. A 2017 report by Strigel et al, however, investigated the outcome of 82 MR screening examinations in a cohort of 860 women with a Category 4 designation on MRI, prospectively subdivided into categories 4A (≥ 2% to ≤ 10%), 4B (> 10% to ≤ 50%), and 4C (> 50% to < 95%), in accordance with Category 4 classification on mammography and ultrasound studies.

Their results indicated that subdivision of Category 4 (4A, 4B, 4C) is feasible, meeting the likely ranges specified for mammography and ultrasound.[26]

Category 4 findings on MRI constitute the vast majority of lesions that require intervention, and MRI guidance for biopsy is often necessary when the target is not visible at either ultrasound or mammography. However, before an MRI-guided biopsy is performed, re-evaluation of prior imaging in order to search for a correlative finding is recommended. An MRI-directed mammogram to search for any correlative subtle calcifications or asymmetries and/or an MRI-directed ultrasound may identify the MRI finding. Biopsy is usually indicated for new or isolated lesions, and it is important to note that 50 to 70% of MRI findings undergoing biopsy prove to be benign.[27] A suspicious abnormality on MRI will be identified as a correlative lesion in about 60% patients undergoing MRI-directed (second-look) ultrasound, allowing ultrasound-guided biopsy.[28] Small lesions such as a mass, focus, or a small area of NME may be difficult to identify at ultrasound and in these cases MRI-guided biopsy is preferable. Practices without the capability of MRI-guided biopsy should refer their patient, when appropriate, to another facility able to perform this procedure under a prearranged practice agreement. Careful correlation of pathology biopsy results with imaging findings is essential for accurate diagnosis.

Category 5: Highly Suggestive of Malignancy

These assessments carry a very high probability (≥ 95%) of malignancy. This category was initially established in an era when preoperative wire localization and subsequent excision was the primary breast interventional procedure, percutaneous biopsy techniques had not been developed, and one-stage surgical treatment was considered without a prior biopsy. Current diagnostic management almost always requires tissue sampling before surgical intervention. In clinical practice today, this assessment is expected to yield a malignant biopsy result at image-guided biopsy, and any nonmalignant diagnosis would be considered discordant, requiring re-biopsy or excision.

Category 6: Known Biopsy-Proven Malignancy

This category is reserved for patients with a known breast cancer, the MRI examination being performed prior to surgical intervention or neoadjuvant chemotherapy. If the examination to evaluate extent of disease depicts the known malignant lesion and no additional findings, then a Category 6 assessment is appropriate until treatment is accomplished. In the event that a new suspicious MRI finding is found in the ipsilateral or contralateral breast, a Category 4 or 5 assessment should be rendered and further tissue sampling obtained. Following successful treatment, the Category 6 assessment should revert to a benign Category 1 or 2. Category 6 is a temporary assessment and should not be included in breast imaging audits, because the diagnosis of malignancy has already has been established.

6.11 Breast Implants

The many normal and abnormal appearances of breast implants have been described.[29,30,31,32,33,34] For a detailed description of the physical, mammographic, and imaging appearances of the many types of conventional (silicone- and saline-filled) breast implants that have been used over the last ~58 years, as well as the appearances of the early sponge implants that preceded them, the interested reader is referred in particular to two of those publications.[31,32]

Early breast implant publications appeared almost exclusively in the plastic surgery literature. However, with reports of complications in the 1970s, the medical literature and implant-related terminology became multidisciplinary, and in some cases duplicative and even ambiguous. To avoid and perhaps to help resolve this ambiguity, we will first briefly provide an overview of that terminology and of the different implant types that have been used.

We will then review and discuss what we require of a breast implant-related MRI protocol, the advantages and disadvantages of the sequences that may be used in that protocol, and the signs and categories of breast implant rupture and of soft-tissue silicone.

Finally, the types of information that should be reported will be discussed, and several current interpretation pitfalls and common clinical scenarios will be described.

6.11.1 Terminology and Types of Implants

A variety of implant types and tissue planes of placement are shown in ▸ Fig. 6.31.

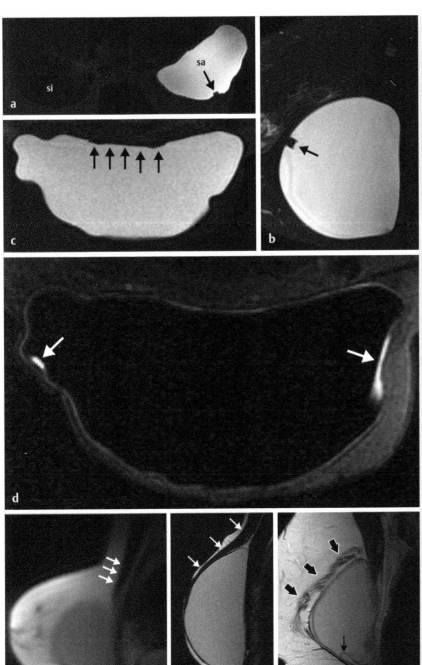

Fig. 6.31 **(a)** Left implant is saline-filled (sa); *arrow* marks diaphragm valve anteriorly. Note that right implant is silicone gel–filled (si) and is dark due to applied silicone suppression (*T2-weighted, silicone suppressed*). **(b)** Saline-filled implant; *arrow* marks another style of diaphragm valve anteriorly (*T2-weighted, no suppression*). **(c)** Single-lumen silicone gel–filled implant. *Arrows* mark location of shell patch posteriorly (*T2-weighted, inversion recovery fat nulled, water suppression*). **(d)** Single-lumen silicone gel–filled implant. Silicone is dark due to applied silicone suppression. *Arrows* marks small amounts of bright intracapsular water-like fluid, outside the implant (*T2-weighted, silicone suppression*). **(e)** Scout image. Subglandular single-lumen silicone gel–filled implant. *Arrows* mark pectoralis major muscle, behind implant (*T1-weighted, no suppression*.) **(f)** Submuscular single-lumen silicone gel–filled implant. *Arrows* mark pectoralis major muscle anterior to implant (*T2-weighted, no suppression*). **(g)** Single-lumen silicone gel–filled implant placed in a submuscular plane. *Wide anterior arrows* mark latissimus dorsi muscle. Note appearance of the laterally oriented muscle fibers on this sagittal image. This implant is in a state of fully collapsed rupture; *posterior narrow arrow* identifies a portion of the collapsed implant shell (*T2-weighted, no suppression*).

Types of Implants

Fourteen breast implant types have been described.[31,32] The most common types have always been single-lumen silicone gel–filled, and single-lumen saline-filled. Both of these implant types have characteristic appearances and are usually easily distinguishable from each other. However, one cannot assume that one will see only these two implant types in a clinical setting; other implant types are still used today, and older implants of other types are still in place, some of which are highly prone to rupture.

Plane of Placement

Breast implants are usually placed in front of the pectoralis major muscle (*subglandular*, or *prepectoral*) or behind it (*submuscular*, or *subpectoral*); in each case, we prefer the first of these alternative terms, but rarely are any of them misunderstood. Less commonly, especially in reconstructive settings, implants can be placed behind pectoralis minor or deep to a latissimus dorsi or a serratus flap in order to provide adequate muscular coverage; these are all formally also submuscular placements.

Silicon and Silicone

Silicon (Si) is an atom of atomic number 14; it has a most common atomic weight of 28 and is the eighth most common element in the universe, by weight. After early work by others, it was given its current name in 1817 by Thomas Thomson.[35] It sits just below carbon in the periodic table, and so can form long-chain molecules. *Silicone* is such a long-chain molecule consisting of multiple *siloxane* (–Si(CH$_3$)$_2$–O–) subunits, typically with –Si-(CH$_3$)$_3$ end units. These silicone chains are often chemically linked to each other at multiple locations along their lengths to form a *matrix*; non-crosslinked silicone chains are viscous *fluids*.

Shells

Nearly all breast implants consist of a silicone elastomer *shell* consisting of highly crosslinked silicone, and one to three compartments that contain silicone gel, saline, or both. These silicone rubber *shells* have been called *capsules* by some, but we avoid that term because we reserve the term *capsule* for the tissue layer (the *fibrous capsule*) that forms around all breast implants, beginning within hours of the time they are placed. Implant *shells* are also referred to by some as *bags*, and some double-lumen implants indeed do have a "bag-in-a-bag'" construction, but many others do not. In general, we prefer the term *shell*, rather than *bag*.

Bleed and Rupture

Let us deal with *rupture* first. It is a bad term; it implies some kind of violent process, and implants do not behave like that. They do not burst in any kind of explosive way. The shell can split in a variety of settings, sometimes suddenly, and then the silicone gel within the implant will bulge out and slowly spread around the implant inside the fibrous capsule, and if there is a defect in the fibrous capsule, silicone gel can then ooze or bulge into the breast and other tissues outside the fibrous capsule. The term rupture was coined early and used often, so I am afraid we are stuck with it. Just do not think it typically implies

a violent burst or explosion, although failure can be rapid, for example, when there is trauma to the breast.

Now let us deal with *bleed*. The *silicone gel* filling most implants consists of *silicone matrix* (~ 20%) mixed with *silicone fluid* (~ 80%). Silicone *fluid* diffuses through the implant shell, even when the implant is new, even before it is placed into a patient; this is *silicone fluid bleed*, and its presence does not in any way indicate that an implant is ruptured. All silicone gel–filled implants do it—they always have done it. Some do it more ("high-bleed" implants), and some do it less ("low-bleed" implants), but there are no "no-bleed" implants. In the 1970s, implants with very thin shells tended to develop small, focal defects allowing silicone *gel* (i.e., matrix + fluid) to ooze into the space around the implant, but still inside the fibrous capsule. That process was called *gel bleed* because the amount of silicone gel that got out was often small; oozing of silicone gel out of the implant was typically slow, and at the time of removal (explantation) these implants were still filled with almost all of their silicone gel, except for the thin layer of silicone gel outside the implant, usually inside the fibrous capsule. If examined carefully, one could usually find the small hole, crease, or defect in the shell through which silicone gel was seen to ooze, so these implants were considered to be "ruptured" because there was a defect in the implant shell. However, when true *silicone fluid bleed* (from truly intact implants) was equated with, or called *silicone gel bleed*, implants were incorrectly considered to be ruptured; and if silicone *gel bleed* (from ruptured implants) was equated with, or called *silicone fluid bleed*, implants were incorrectly considered to be "only bleeding" and thus not ruptured. To avoid these misunderstandings, we suggest only using the term *bleed* to refer to the normal process of diffusion of silicone fluid through the shell of an intact implant (i.e., *silicone fluid bleed*), and not using the term *bleed* to mean or imply rupture, and not using the term *gel bleed* at all.

Intracapsular, Capsular, and Extracapsular

Intracapsular rupture refers to the rupture of a silicone gel–filled implant, where there is no evident silicone gel outside the fibrous capsule. The implant can be in any degree of collapse, from uncollapsed to fully collapsed (more on those terms below; see Section 6.11.3). *Intracapsular rupture* thus implies only that the implant is ruptured, and that silicone gel is not seen, or is not otherwise evident (as on an MRI scan) outside the fibrous capsule.

Extracapsular rupture refers to rupture (again, any degree of collapse, from uncollapsed to fully collapsed), where silicone gel that has escaped the implant has also gotten through a defect in the fibrous capsule into the tissues outside the fibrous capsule. The term *extracapsular rupture* thus only means that an implant is ruptured, and that silicone is seen, or is otherwise evident (as on an MRI scan) outside the fibrous capsule, no matter what form it is in (silicone gel, silicone granuloma, or both; see Section 6.11.4).

Capsular silicone (i.e., silicone in any form, fluid or gel) refers only to the deposition of silicone within the substance of the fibrous capsule. It can occur in normal, intact implants (from silicone fluid bleed), or from ruptured implants (from silicone gel) embedded within the fibrous capsule. Thus, capsular silicone can be present in the fibrous capsules of intact or ruptured implants.

6.11.2 Imaging Protocol

Depending on the clinical presentation, one or more of the following capabilities is required of an implant integrity-related MRI protocol:
- Adequate **resolution** to visualize the implant shell(s).
- Adequate **contrast** to distinguish silicone, and silicone-containing tissue from breast fatty and water-like tissues.
- Adequate ability to distinguish problems related to **cancer** in the breast, from problems related to implant integrity.

Resolution

To determine whether an implant is ruptured, the slice thickness and the slice gap should be low/thin enough, and the matrix high enough so that the implant shell can be adequately visualized and followed across sequential acquired images. If this requirement is met, silicone gel within folds (if it is present) and silicone gel between the (outer) implant shell and the fibrous capsule (if it is present) can be identified so that rupture (if it is present) may be recognized. Thus, the resolution should be sufficient to recognize the *shell fold pattern* (from normal, through to fully collapsed rupture; see Section 6.11.3 on "Rupture"). A related requirement is that the implant type should be identifiable so that rupture (if present) fold patterns specific to that implant type may be recognized.

Contrast

Breasts with silicone gel–filled implants or soft-tissue silicone can be thought of as consisting of only three MRI signal moieties: silicone, fat, and water. To determine whether silicone gel is present in a pattern indicating rupture (i.e., silicone gel outside the implant; see Section 6.11.3 on "Rupture"), or whether soft-tissue silicone is present in one or more of its various forms; see Section 6.11.4 on "Soft-Tissue Silicone"), the relative intensities of silicone, water, and fat should be distinguishable.

Cancer

The requirement to distinguish implant integrity-related from cancer-related problems can be fulfilled by simply adding one or more implant-related sequences to a standard breast cancer protocol. Implant integrity-related problems are sometimes evident on cancer-related sequences, but usually they cannot be adequately understood given the varied presentations and appearances of cancer in the breast and the limited ability of cancer-related sequences to show implant integrity-related problems.

Several types of MRI sequence can accomplish one or more of these requirements—some better than others. One particular sequence, a fast spin-echo inversion-recovery (FSE-IR) sequence, with fat nulling and water suppression, stands out as being most helpful to detect both implant rupture and soft-tissue silicone. In that sequence, fat signal is nulled (i.e., reduced), water-like signal is suppressed (thus also reduced), and silicone signal compared to that of fat and water is high (bright). Typical parameter settings for that sequence are given in ▶ Table 6.2. The main advantages and disadvantages of this and other sequences are listed in ▶ Table 6.3; note that T1w and T2w sequences with no suppression are useful adjunct sequences to the FSE-IR sequence.

Table 6.2 T2-weighted fast spin-echo inversion-recovery sequence parameters

Parameter	Value(s)	Notes
Sequence type	2D fast spin-echo inversion recovery (IR)	This sequence is available on most, if not all, scanners
Imaging plane	Axial	Sagittal imaging is also adequate in most cases, but implant shell-fold patterns and most other implant-related problems are evaluated better more often in the axial plane
Number sequences	Two; one for each breast	Imaging one breast at a time takes longer but gives more consistent and better results because automated shimming is more likely to be successful for single-breast imaging, and higher resolution is more easily attained
TR	>2,000 ms	A long TR value helps achieve adequate SNR
TE	Minimum	Not a critical factor since TE is not being used to derive contrast, and lower TE values give higher signal
TI	160–190 ms	This is the approximate "nulling time" for fat
ETL	~10	Any higher value of ETL will save time, and still provide good SNR
BW	Any	Not a critical factor; higher BW may be used to shorten scanning time
NEX	1	This NEX value provides adequate signal at the above-noted slice thickness and FOV
Flip angle	Default	For spin echo sequences, this value is usually about 180 degrees
FOV	~200 mm	This is adequate for most single-breast imaging.
Slice thickness	4 mm	4-mm slice thickness is a good value. Even at 5-mm slice thickness, the ability to discern fold patterns is decreased. 3-mm slice thickness would be better but can necessitate NEX = 2 to obtain adequate signal, and so takes longer. The fold pattern for most modern implants placed since the mid-1980s can be discerned at 4-mm slice thickness
Slice gap	0 mm	Ability to discern fold patterns decreases if slice gaps are used.
Matrix	At least 256 × 160	Lower matrix values than this for single-breast imaging can impair ability to discern shell fold patterns
Suppression	Water	Reduces water-like signal
Phase-encoding direction	Right-left	Helps avoid motion artifact from the heart.
Saturation bands	Off	Saturation is not usually needed.

Table 6.3 Advantages and disadvantages of various types of pulse sequence

	Sequence	Advantages	Disadvantages
1	T2-weighted fast spin-echo inversion recovery (IR) with fat nulling and water suppression	1. Allows best identification of signs of rupture and of soft-tissue silicone because silicone is bright, and fat and water are dark 2. Most useful if used together with unsuppressed T1-weighted and T2-weighted sequences (#2 and #3, below)	1. MRI technologist needs to have experience in shimming and setting of operating frequency so that water is adequately suppressed 2. Reader needs to be able to recognize the appearance of failure of water suppression 3. Can be difficult to determine relationship of implant and any soft-tissue silicone that may be present from adjacent muscles
2	T1-weighted gradient-echo with no suppression	Useful as an adjunct sequence to #1 (above) to show relationship to adjacent muscles	1. Not sensitive alone to detect implant rupture 2. Not sensitive alone to detect soft-tissue silicone
3	T2-weighted fast spin-echo with no suppression	Useful as an adjunct sequence to #1 (above) to help resolve ambiguities that may result from failed water suppression	1. Images partially compromised by fat–water and silicone–water chemical-shift artifact 2. Silicone and water will both be bright, and so identifying soft-tissue silicone may be difficult 3. Ability to distinguish soft-tissue silicone is reduced because fat remains moderately bright
4	T2-weighted fast spin-echo with fat suppression only	Silicone gel is bright, so good for recognition of implant rupture	1. MRI technologist needs to have experience in shimming and setting of operating frequency so that fat is adequately suppressed 2. Reader needs to be able to recognize the appearance of failure of fat suppression 3. With suboptimal shimming, fat suppression can turn into silicone suppression 4. Silicone and water will both be bright, and so identifying soft-tissue silicone may be difficult 5. Images may be compromised by silicone–water chemical-shift artifact
5	T2-weighted fast spin-echo with water suppression only	Silicone gel is bright, so good for recognition of implant rupture	1. MRI technologist needs to have experience in shimming and setting of operating frequency so that water is adequately suppressed 2. Reader needs to be able to recognize the appearance of failure of water suppression 3. Ability to distinguish soft-tissue silicone is reduced because fat remains moderately bright
6	T1-weighted gradient-echo with silicone suppression	This can be useful to confirm the presence of silicone in soft tissues, but usually that is already evident on sequence #1 (above)	1. MRI technologist needs to have experience in shimming and setting of operating frequency so that silicone is adequately suppressed 2. With suboptimal shimming, silicone suppression can change to fat suppression 3. Not sensitive to detect implant rupture 4. Not sensitive to detect soft-tissue silicone

6.11.3 Rupture

The term *rupture* on a breast implant MRI scan describes the situation where a hole, tear, or other defect of any size has developed in the outer implant shell of a silicone gel–filled breast implant, and silicone gel from inside the implant is evident on that scan, outside the implant.

As noted above, the term *intracapsular rupture* denotes that silicone gel from a ruptured implant is seen (i.e., on MRI) to be contained within the fibrous capsule, and the term *extracapsular rupture* denotes that silicone gel from a ruptured implant is seen (i.e., on MRI) not to be contained within the fibrous capsule. These terms do not describe how much silicone has escaped from the implant, the degree of collapse of the implant, how much silicone is present outside the fibrous capsule, or the state/form/amount of any silicone that may be present outside the fibrous capsule. We make the distinction here "on MRI" because we are focusing specifically on the MRI appearances of breast implants in their various possible states; however, these terms may also be applicable in other settings.

If the shell of a saline-filled implant develops a hole, tear, or other defect, unless detected very early, it tends to deflate, and the saline is absorbed by the body. Thus, we do not refer to failed saline-filled implants as being *ruptured*, but as being *deflated*. Deflations can be slow or rapid, so early deflation may not be evident on any kind of imaging. Also, almost all saline-filled implants are filled through a self-sealing value when they are placed. That valve can leak, sometimes very slowly, and so some deflated saline-filled implants do not in fact have any shell hole, tear, or other defect—they just have a leaky valve.

Knowledge of whether an implant is ruptured (or deflated) can help patients and their physicians decide whether it should be removed. If a silicone gel–filled implant is known to be ruptured, information provided by an MRI scan can be helpful to the surgeon in planning the operation and removing the implant. Rupture of an implant can occur during its removal, and if an implant is already in a ruptured state before surgery, not infrequently the rupture may be exacerbated during the removal operation. Thus, the condition of a silicone gel–filled implant before surgery often cannot definitively be determined from the description of its condition during or after surgery.

Four "categories" of silicone gel–filled breast implant rupture have been described: *uncollapsed*, *minimally collapsed*, *partially collapsed*, and *fully collapsed*.[29,30,32,33,34] As noted above, silicone gel that has escaped from an implant may be contained within or not contained within the fibrous capsule, for any degree of collapse.

Examples of normal shell fold patterns are shown in ▶ Fig. 6.32. Examples of shell fold patterns for a variety of ruptured implants are shown in ▶ Fig. 6.33.

Normal Appearance of a Silicone Gel–Filled Implant

The key to understanding the various MRI appearances of silicone gel-filled breast implant rupture is to consider the degree of filling of the implant, the implant shell itself, and the implant shell infolding that develops when the implant is in a patient. Implants are manufactured to be round, oval, or anatomically shaped ("taller" at the lower end than the upper end), and can be low profile (quite markedly underfilled), moderate profile (underfilled), or high profile (less underfilled). All implants are underfilled because they are intended to be naturally soft, and overfilling them would make them less soft, and perhaps also less naturally shaped when in the patient. Higher profile implants tend to be used in reconstructive settings, when both form and bulk are being provided by the implant.

A fibrous tissue capsule begins to form around implants within hours of the time they are placed; hereinafter we will refer to this just as a *fibrous capsule*. When an implant is placed into a patient's breast, it almost always undergoes some infolding of the implant shell, within the fibrous capsule, just like a soft pillow would undergo some infolding if you crunched it up in your hands. When shell folds are present they may have an undulating appearance, or they may be well formed. The perceived undetectability, softness, firmness, or hardness of a breast containing an implant is subjective, but as a general rule

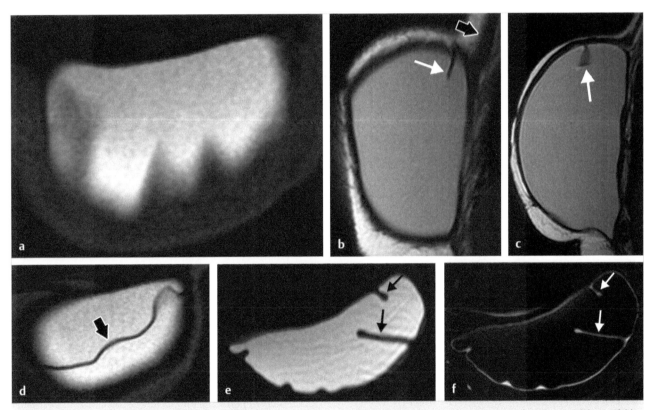

Fig. 6.32 Typical MRI appearances of implant folds. (a) Single-lumen silicone gel–filled implant; *arrows* mark appearance of anterior "undulating" folds (*arrows*). This is the normal appearance of an implant that probably is perceived as being "soft" by the patient (*T2-weighted, inversion recovery fat nulled, water suppression*). (b) Single-lumen silicone gel–filled implant (not ruptured); *narrow arrow* marks a typical, normal appearance of a simple shell fold. The implant is placed in the submuscular plane (under pectoralis major), but on this image only the pectoralis minor muscle is seen (*wide arrow*, behind the implant) (*T2-weighted, no suppression*). (c) Single-lumen silicone gel–filled implant (not ruptured) placed in the submuscular plane; *arrow* marks a typical, normal appearance of a "travelling" fold. The fold has this appearance due to volume averaging; it "slants" from a relatively anterior position at one edge of this acquired slice (4-mm slice thickness) to a more posterior position at the other edge of this slice (*T2-weighted, no suppression*). (d) Single-lumen silicone gel–filled implant (not ruptured); *wide arrow* marks a typical, normal appearance of a "bisecting fold." Think of the implant, which is not ruptured, as being folded in upon itself within the fibrous capsule, and then visualize this axial image as capturing a cross-sectional view of that normal fold (*T2-weighted, inversion recovery fat nulled, water suppression*). (e, f) Textured single-lumen silicone gel–filled implant (not ruptured); *arrows* mark typical, normal folds. They appear wider than usual in (e) because suppressed water (dark signal) is present within the fold. In (f), the silicone gel of the implant has dark signal due to silicone suppression being applied, and the water in the folds is bright because the sequence is T2-weighted (e: *T2-weighted, inversion recovery fat nulled, water suppression*; f: *same slice location, T2-weighted, silicone suppression*).

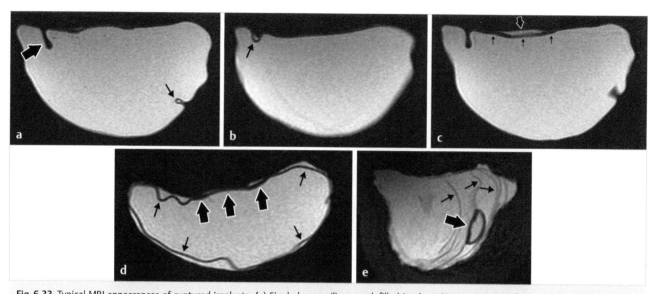

Fig. 6.33 Typical MRI appearances of ruptured implants. (**a**) Single-lumen silicone gel–filled implant. *Narrow arrow* marks appearance of an anterior fold with silicone (bright signal) evident outside the implant shell, "within" the fold (and inside the fibrous capsule) indicating with a very high of degree of confidence that this implant is in a state of *uncollapsed rupture*; this is a *keyhole* sign. A posterior fold is dark (*wide arrow*) but appears thicker because water-suppressed water-like fluid is in the fold (*T2-weighted, inversion recovery fat nulled, water suppression*). (**b**) Single-lumen silicone gel–filled implant. *Arrow* marks a location where the posterior implant shell appears to be slightly "pulled" inward from the surrounding fibrous capsule (hence, the *pull-away* sign). The small amount of silicone gel posterior to the implant shell at that location is outside the implant, and inside the fibrous capsule, indicating with a very high of degree of confidence that this implant is in a state of *uncollapsed rupture* (*T2-weighted, inversion recovery fat nulled, water suppression*). (**c**) Single-lumen silicone gel–filled implant. *Arrows* mark the (dark) shell patch, posteriorly. The shell patch is thicker than the rest of the implant shell, which can be appreciated by looking through all the other (not shown here) slices. Note the presence of bright silicone (*wide arrow*) outside (posterior to) the shell patch, indicating that this implant is in a state of *minimally collapsed rupture*. This is called the *back-patch* sign because the shell patch is almost always located on the posterior surface of the implant. The shell patch can be seen elsewhere than posteriorly in MR images if the implant has rotated in position. Note also the normal-appearing travelling fold anteriorly, and the normal-appearing thicker fold posteriorly due to water-suppressed water-like fluid in the fold (*T2-weighted, inversion recovery fat nulled, water suppression*). (**d**) Single-lumen silicone gel–filled implant. *Narrow arrows* mark the implant shell, surrounded in many places by a thin but easily and definitively identified layer of bright silicone gel, indicating that this implant is in a state of *minimally collapsed rupture*. Note the location of the shell patch, marked by wide arrows, slightly thicker at its edges where implant shell overlaps with shell patch (*T2-weighted, inversion recovery fat nulled, water suppression*). (**e**) Standard double-lumen silicone gel–filled implant (originally, silicone gel in the inner lumen, saline in the outer lumen). *Thin arrows* mark several of the many layered segments of implant shell that are part of this fully collapsed implant. For this implant, we say that "the shell is in the gel," which is a classic appearance of *fully collapsed rupture* (as opposed to the "gel being in the shell" for a normal, intact implant). The wide arrow marks a type of "button" valve which was used in some standard double-lumen (and some other types of) implants, mostly in the 1970s. The "button" is itself actually a separate small ovoid silicone elastomer shell (set just inside the outer implant shell) which is filled with thicker silicone gel and was intended to self-seal after saline was injected through it into the outer lumen; thus, it is a kind of "valve." Note the absence of dark water bubbles inside this implant, which indicates that either saline was never added to this implant (less likely) or that it escaped from the outer lumen before the inner silicone gel–filled lumen ruptured (more likely). Thus, silicone gel is present in this implant in the inner lumen (its original location), in the outer lumen (where the saline probably used to be), and outside the implant as a whole within the fibrous capsule (*T2-weighted, inversion recovery fat nulled, water suppression*).

undulating shell folds suggest softer perceived breast firmness, and well-formed folds suggest greater perceived breast firmness. Capsular contracture is said to be present when the fibrous capsule contracts around the implant. Although different amounts of breast implant filling can make a difference in perceived breast softness, true breast hardness is more a consequence capsular contracture, thickening, and sometimes capsular calcification.

If you could see into the fibrous capsule, and we can of course do that with MRI, you would see implant shell just under and parallel to the fibrous capsule in many places, and in one or more places the shell would appear to be "going into" the gel of the implant. The places where the shell appears to dip "into" the implant are called *folds*. The tip of each fold forms a rounded loop because the implant shell has some thickness, and it does not fold "flat" (at its tip) unless placed under high pressure. Now we can visualize what happens when an implant ruptures.

Uncollapsed Rupture

If a hole, tear, or other defect develops, say, deep within a fold, or anywhere else on the implant shell, silicone gel starts to seep out and to spread around the implant, inside the fibrous capsule. Now go back to that loop at the tip of the infolded shell described in the last paragraph; that, as it turns out, is the most easily evident (i.e., on MRI) place where silicone gel may collect during early implant rupture. The shell forming the fold is seen as a dark, smooth line/loop on MRI, with bright silicone (signal) inside the implant on one side of it and a tiny amount of bright silicone (signal) outside the implant at the tip of the fold. This appearance, indicating *uncollapsed rupture*, has been variously called the *keyhole, inverted keyhole, noose, pull-away* and *loop* signs—they are all the same thing: just a little bit of silicone gel outside the implant shell evident on MRI, collecting in, or at the tip of an infolded shell fold. If more silicone gel escapes the implant, bright silicone can start to be seen in the rest of the fold, as well as at its tip. Going back to the section above on the MRI protocol, if the imaging slice thickness is too thick or the matrix is too low, these appearances of early rupture may not be evident.

Minimally Collapsed Rupture

As more silicone gel escapes a ruptured implant, in addition to the above locations within folds, silicone gel starts to collect in large enough amounts between the implant shell and the fibrous capsule where they run parallel to each other, and then it starts to become evident on MRI scans. That has been called the *parallel-line sign* (where the two lines are the adjacent dark fibrous capsule, and the dark implant shell are parallel to each other with bright silicone gel being seen between them). Bright silicone can also be seen outside the (often thicker) "shell patch" at the back of the implant that was used to close the several-centimeters-diameter hole in the implant shell at the time that the shell was manufactured, before it was filled with silicone gel; this has been called the *back-patch sign*. These two appearances are signs of *minimally collapsed rupture*.

Partially and Fully Collapsed Rupture

If more silicone gel escapes, the implant still looks "like an implant" on MRI, but the bases of the folds start to grossly move inwards, away from the fibrous capsule. This is *partially collapsed rupture*. As more silicone gel escapes, as long as the implant continues to look "like an implant," albeit even a markedly underfilled one, it is still called partially collapsed rupture. When sections of shell from one side of the implant approach closely to or contact sections of shell from the other side of the implant, and segments of implant shell appear to start layering upon each other, and the implant no longer has even a "partially filled implant" appearance, it is called *fully collapsed rupture*. This last stage has also been called the *linguini sign*; we suggest avoiding that term, however, because there are appearances of very underfilled, intact implants that, to a less experienced reader, may suggest "linguini." An example of that pitfall is shown below in the "Common Interpretation Challenges and Pitfalls" section (6.11.6).

6.11.4 Soft-Tissue Silicone

Soft-tissue silicone (i.e., silicone that is evident on MRI outside the fibrous capsule) is seen mainly in four forms: *silicone gel*, *silicone granuloma*, *infiltrated silicone*, and *silicone adenopathy*. The form that silicone takes in soft tissue probably depends, in part, on whether the silicone gel is highly cohesive (very early breast implants from the 1960s and early 1970s), minimally cohesive (many implants from the mid-1970s to the mid-1980s, when the silicone gel was most often a viscous, sticky, runny fluid), or moderately cohesive (many modern implants; mid-1980s and onwards; branded as having a cohesive gel, but not nearly as cohesive as the very early implants). The best MRI pulse sequence to detect soft-tissue silicone is Sequence #1 in ▶ Table 6.3 (fast spin-echo, inversion recovery, fat nulled, water suppressed).

Soft-tissue silicone gel has the same appearance (i.e., the same homogeneity and brightness) as silicone gel within implants. It has this appearance just after it has extruded through a hole or defect in the fibrous capsule immediately adjacent to and just

outside the fibrous capsule, where it may remain for a long time or even indefinitely. Extruded silicone gel also may migrate outward as a single, or as separated smaller collections away from the outer surface of the implant fibrous capsule into breast tissues, and in rare cases superiorly into the axilla and even into the arm. Pathways of migration differ depending on the tissue plane into which the implant has been placed (i.e., subglandular, submuscular). Migrated silicone gel collections have a globular appearance with the same homogeneity and brightness as silicone gel inside the implant, and may develop their own fibrous capsules, as one might expect for any foreign body. Soft-tissue silicone gel globules may remain in that state for a long time or even indefinitely.

Soft-tissue silicone granuloma results from tissue ingrowth and scar formation in silicone-laden tissue, whether the silicone is in the form of a silicone gel collection/globule or of silicone-infiltrated tissue. Silicone granuloma on T2w, fat-nulled, water-suppressed pulse sequences is generally heterogeneous in texture and variably dark depending on exactly whether the subvoxel, microscopic "mix" is of (bright) silicone, (dark) water-like tissue, and (dark) scar tissue (▶ Fig. 6.34). Silicone

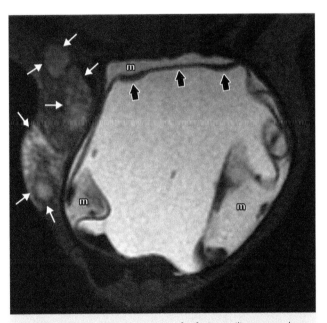

Fig. 6.34 The typical MRI appearance of soft-tissue silicone granuloma (main outlines marked with *narrow arrows*) which is typically inhomogeneous in appearance, with darker and brighter areas, and which is located outside the implant fibrous capsule. Silicone granuloma results when soft-tissue silicone from a ruptured implant incites scar tissue formation, with ingrowth of fibrous tissue into the silicone gel that has escaped from the implant. The implant here itself is in a state of minimally collapsed rupture, and since we know in this case that silicone is outside the fibrous capsule, we call this *extracapsular rupture*. Note the clearly identifiable back-patch, again seen to be thicker at its edges due to overlap, as was also seen, for example, in ▶ Fig. 6.33 **d** (*wide arrows*). Note also that intracapsular silicone gel outside the implant and inside the fibrous capsule appears darker than silicone gel inside the implant; this is probably due to intravoxel micromixing (m) where silicone gel that has escaped from the implant is mixing with water-suppressed water-like fluid that probably originally accumulated because this is a textured implant (see ▶ Fig. 6.37 for further discussion) (*T2-weighted, inversion recovery fat nulled, water suppression*).

granuloma heterogeneity may not be evident if image slices are too thick, or the matrix is too low, and silicone granuloma may not be evident at all on sequences where fat is bright (or not nulled, or not suppressed), or water is not suppressed.

Silicone adenopathy occurs when soft-tissue silicone collects in lymph nodes, most often axillary and internal mammary, and less frequently, infraclavicular and supraclavicular. Some silicone-containing lymph nodes are enlarged, and others are not, but the presence of silicone in a node is usually accompanied by some degree of node enlargement. MRI identification of silicone adenopathy depends on two things: a determination that the structure is a lymph node based on usual anatomic criteria, and a determination that silicone is evident on MRI in the node. Many sequences will allow anatomic identification of a lymph node, but detection of an observable amount of silicone in a lymph node on MRI is best accomplished using the same sequence that is used to detect silicone granulomas (Sequence #1 in ▶ Table 6.3; fast spin-echo, inversion recovery, fat nulled, water suppressed). An example of silicone adenopathy is shown in ▶ Fig. 6.35. Because nodes start out containing no silicone, and silicone accumulation in them (when it occurs) is gradual, lower amounts of silicone in nodes will not be detectable by MRI. At higher amounts, when the additional brightness in the node on silicone-bright sequences becomes discernable on MRI compared to the normal appearance of nodes, one may say that silicone adenopathy is present. Extracapsular silicone resulting from rupture of any silicone gel–filled implant can result in silicone adenopathy. However, some older implants, especially if they are polyurethane-coated,

tend to have high silicone fluid bleed rates, and escaped silicone fluid alone from those types of implants, even if the implants are intact, can cause silicone adenopathy. The French PIP implants especially are known to cause both marked lymph node enlargement and silicone deposition in nodes. The presence of silicone in a node is not itself a reason to remove it, especially because the benefits of doing so are not established, and because there are significant risks of doing so, especially for axillary and higher nodes.

Infiltrated silicone from breast implants is rarely identifiable as such on MRI but is essentially universally present for silicone fluid breast injections.[29,30,32,33,34] In that setting, typically there is scar tissue formation which is firm to palpation, and extensively silicone-infiltrated tissue that may not be evident to palpation; thus, the extent of silicone-containing soft tissue is almost always underestimated on palpation for cases of silicone fluid breast injections.

6.11.5 Reporting

The portion of a breast MRI report relating to implants should include, at minimum:

- The indication for the examination.
- Pertinent medical implant-related history (including the reason why implants were placed [cosmetic augmentation, reconstruction after breast cancer–related surgery, or for other reasons], whether there were previous implants placed or prior implant rupture, etc., and whether there were ever silicone fluid breast injections).

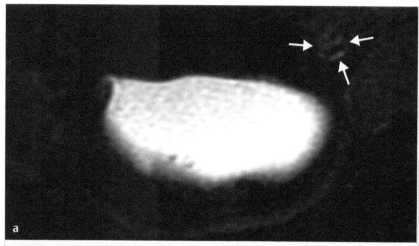

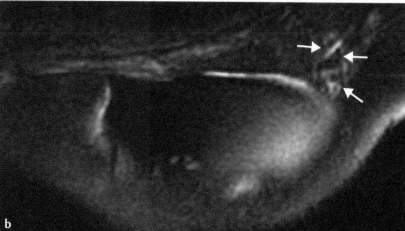

Fig. 6.35 The typical MRI appearance of silicone adenopathy. (a) Single-lumen silicone gel–filled implant, minimally collapsed rupture (signs of rupture not shown on this image), showing subtle but definite silicone adenopathy on this water-suppressed image. This implant is from a non-U.S. manufacturer, of a type that is known to rupture frequently and to be associated with flagrant silicone adenopathy (*T2-weighted, inversion recovery fat nulled, water suppression*). (b) Same implant, same slice location as (a) showing water-like fluid associated with the silicone adenopathy (*arrows*). Note that the implant in this image, and parts of the lymph node are dark because of silicone suppression, and that water-like fluid around the implant (another common finding for these implants), and associated with the lymph node, are bright (*T2-weighted, silicone suppression*).

- The pulse sequence(s) used.
- The general implant type for (each) implant (silicone gel–filled, saline-filled, double-lumen, etc.).
- The tissue plane of placement for (each) implant (subglandular or submuscular).
- The state of (each) implant (no evidence of rupture, or ruptured for implants containing silicone gel; deflated or not, for implants filled only with saline).
- For silicone gel–filled implants that are ruptured, the degree of implant collapse.
- A description of the amount, location, and form (silicone gel collection, silicone granuloma, infiltrated silicone or silicone adenopathy) of any soft-tissue silicone that may be present.

If the implants were imaged on other modalities, MRI findings should be correlated with findings from those other modalities. For example, it may be clear from prior mammograms that an implant is of the standard double-lumen type (silicone gel in the inner lumen, saline in the outer lumen); this information may be helpful in the interpretation of the MRI.

If the MRI was also obtained in part to detect or characterize breast cancer, an assessment should be made as to how the breast implant–related findings relate to any breast (or other) cancer–related findings, including their proximity to each other, and their relation to findings on other modalities. If an intravenous contrast agent was administered, the soft-tissue enhancement pattern of any soft-tissue implant-relating findings should be described. Note that silicone granulomas may enhance slowly, and mildly.

If implant placement or other medical records are available, it could be helpful to state the manufacturer, model, type, and volume of each implant. This information can be obtained from so-called implant "tags," or "stickers," that are added to medical records when implants are placed.

It is not appropriate to suggest treatment on the basis of MRI breast implant integrity–related findings alone; that decision should rest with the patient and their treating physician because breast implant integrity–related findings often form only a part of what should be considered in those decisions.

6.11.6 Common Interpretation Challenges and Pitfalls

We will discuss here several common interpretation challenges and pitfalls frequently encountered in breast implant and soft-tissue silicone MRI.

Fully Collapsed Rupture versus Complex Folds in an Intact Implant

Very underfilled silicone gel–filled implants develop numerous shell infoldings, some of which may appear to bisect (▶ Fig. 6.32d) or even trisect the implant. This complex-fold appearance can be confused with the multiply-layered fold pattern seen in fully collapsed, ruptured implants (▶ Fig. 6.33e). The key to distinguishing these appearances is that shell folds in intact implants extend all the way to the edge of the implant, whereas they do not for ruptured, fully collapsed implants; it can be helpful to follow the folds, running through all of the

images rapidly on an image viewer. Identifying the back-patch also can help distinguish these appearances; if (bright) silicone is seen on both sides of the back-patch (on silicone-bright sequences), then the implant is ruptured (▶ Fig. 6.33c). For further examples of these appearances, please see Middleton and McNamara.[32]

Mixed Intracapsular Silicone–Water Appearance of Ruptured Textured-Surface Silicone Gel–Filled Implants

Until the mid-1980s, breast implants were manufactured with a smooth outer surface; after that, implants could have smooth or textured outer surfaces. Textured-surface implants tend to develop small, sterile, water-like fluid collections outside the implant, within the fibrous capsule. These are easily spotted on standard, unsuppressed (and non-water-nulled) T2w sequences. If an implant ruptures when surrounded by such an intracapsular water-like fluid layer, silicone gel from the ruptured implant will mix with the water-like fluid over time. The resulting fold pattern is still that of a ruptured implant, but the intracapsular silicone gel outside the implant consists of highly mixed silicone gel and water bubbles, instead of "pure" silicone gel (▶ Fig. 6.36). This mixture usually has an inhomogeneous appearance but can appear homogeneous if slices are too thick or resolution is too coarse. Water bubbles in the mixture will be dark on T2w, water-suppressed images, and when those dark water bubbles are micro-mixed with bright silicone bubbles within each voxel, the overall mixture will have intermediate brightness, less than the brightness of the silicone gel within the implant.

Soft-Tissue Silicone versus Failed Water Suppression

Identification of soft-tissue silicone often depends on the success of water suppression, so that on T2w fat-nulled, water-suppressed images, any tissue with bright signal can be inferred to contain or to consist of silicone. If water suppression fails, that inference is no longer valid. The three main ways that water suppression may fail are failure to shim adequately, failure to correctly set the scanner operating frequency, and presence of sufficient magnetic field inhomogeneity locally due to susceptibility effects, such as nearby metal, magnetic material, air, or even calcification. The MRI technologist, with assistance and training as needed from an applications specialist from the MRI scanner manufacturer, is responsible for ensuring adequate shimming and for correctly setting the scanner operating frequency before a scan is undertaken. There are known methods available to accomplish these tasks, but discussion of those methods is beyond the intended scope of this work. The third source of failed water suppression, local susceptibility effects, is usually patient-related and so may be unavoidable. The radiologist should be able to identify failed water suppression if known blood vessels are bright, other known water-like material is bright (such as saline within a saline-filled breast implant or within a double- or a triple-lumen implant), or intracapsular water-like fluid water is visible around a textured implant. An example of inadequate water suppression are shown in ▶ Fig. 6.37.

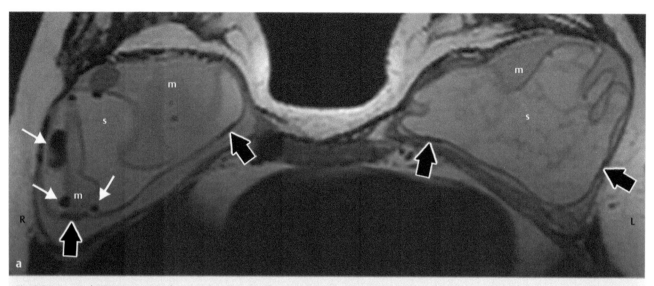

Fig. 6.36 A typical MRI appearance of ruptured, textured-surface, single-lumen silicone gel–filled breast implants. The mechanism here is that, first, a layer of water-like fluid originally surrounded each of these implants because they have textured outer surfaces and, then later, the implants ruptured, and silicone gel escaped into the intracapsular space around the implants where it micro-mixed over time with the intracapsular water-like fluid that was already there. **(a)** Normally on a T2-weighted image, water-like fluid in the intracapsular space around an intact silicone gel–filled implant will be very bright, and silicone gel inside the implant will be less bright. When water suppression is applied, as in this image of ruptured implants, the signal intensity of the silicone gel would be relatively unchanged (s), and any remaining larger collections of water-like fluid would become dark, as seen in the several bubbles of un-mixed water-like fluid present here in the right implant (e.g., see *narrow arrows*). Areas of micro-mixed silicone gel and water are darker than silicone gel but brighter than water because very small dark (water-suppressed) water bubbles are volume averaged with bright silicone gel within each voxel, resulting in the observed middle intensity (m). Another helpful observation here is that the relatively wide (in this case, about 105 mm diameter) posterior shell patches can be identified by the slightly thicker shell appearance where implant shell overlaps with shell patch (*wide arrows*). These images are of sufficient resolution to also note that the shell patches of these implants are set just inside the implant shell, which helps to definitively identify areas of overlap between shell and patch. The appearance of intravoxel volume-averaged mixed silicone gel and suppressed-signal water outside of the shell patches tells us that that the mixed-signal material is indeed outside of the implants and inside the fibrous capsules. This distinguishes the appearance of these implants from standard double-lumen implants where the silicone gel-containing inner lumen has ruptured into the saline-containing outer lumen, but the outer implant shell is still intact. Note the stringy-appearing inhomogeneity within the left implant; this is probably due to small amounts of intracapsular water-like fluid that have infiltrated into that implant. This appearance is also seen in **(b)** and **(c)** (*T2-weighted, water suppression*). (*Continued*)

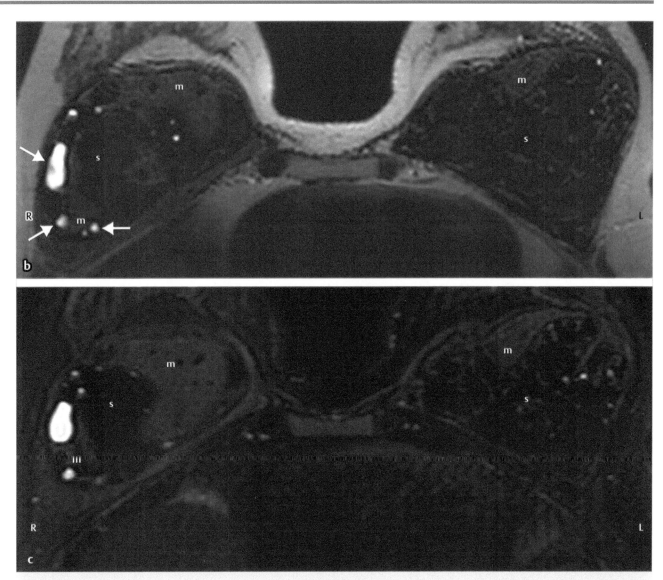

Fig. 6.36 (*continued*) (**b**) In this image (same implants, same slice location as (**a**), silicone suppression results in the silicone gel inside the implants (s) now being dark. The mixed-signal material (m) outside the implants is again of a middle intensity, but this time the suppressed-signal silicone is mixed with full-signal water, within each voxel. The larger bubbles of water-like fluid in the right implant (*arrows*) are bright on this image, which is the same intensity they would have on an un-suppressed T2-weighted image (*T2-weighted, silicone suppression*). (**c**) This image (same implants, same slice location as (**a**) and (**b**)) conveys almost the same information as was shown in those figures; silicone suppression results in silicone gel inside the implants (s) being dark, mixed-signal material (m) outside the implants is again of middle intensity, and the remaining larger water-like bubbles are again bright (*arrows*). The only difference in this image from (**b**) is that inversion-recovery fat nulling has been applied, resulting in breast fat having dark signal. However, the main purpose of nulling fat signal is so that any extracapsular silicone that may be present outside the fibrous capsule can be detected, but with both silicone suppression and fat nulling applied here, that would be difficult or not possible. Using inversion-recovery fat nulling together with water suppression would have been a better sequence to use, so that any extracapsular silicone (which would have had brighter signal) could be detected against a background of dark breast fat (*T2-weighted, inversion recovery fat nulled, silicone suppression*).

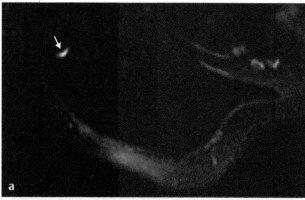

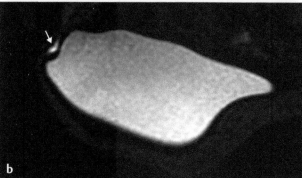

Fig. 6.37 The typical MRI appearance of failure of water suppression for a textured-surface, intact, gel–gel double-lumen implant (for which silicone gel is present in both the inner and the outer lumen). These images are through a part of the implant where the inner silicone gel–filled lumen is not present. **(a)** This T2-weighted image in which silicone suppression was applied shows dark silicone gel inside the (outer lumen of the) implant and a small amount of bright intracapsular water-like fluid (*arrow*) in the intracapsular space outside the implant (*T2-weighted, silicone suppression*). **(b)** This T2-weighted image (same implant, same slice location as (a)), in which inversion-recovery fat nulling and water suppression were applied, shows a small amount of bright signal outside the implant (*arrow*). If water suppression were adequate, this would indicate that silicone gel was outside the implant, and thus that the implant was ruptured. However, at this same location on the silicone-suppressed image **(a)** there is also bright signal, and so it definitely represents water-like fluid. Thus, there is no implant rupture, and the bright signal on this image (*arrow*) just represents failed water suppression. In this case, the failure of water suppression is probably due an inadequate shim which may be related to the location of this slice, which is through the upper breast where shimming is occasionally less than optimal (*T2-weighted, inversion recovery fat nulled, water suppression*).

6.12 Summary

The terminology of breast implant MRI and pulse sequences to image breast implants and soft-tissue silicone were described. Normal and abnormal appearances of breast implants and soft-tissue silicone were described and explained. Common interpretation challenges and pitfalls were reviewed including: complex folds versus collapsed rupture; an appearance of ruptured, textured-surface silicone gel-filled implants; and the importance and appearance of failed water suppression.

References

[1] Noels EC, Lapid O, Lindeman JH, Bastiaannet E. Breast implants and the risk of breast cancer: a meta-analysis of cohort studies. Aesthet Surg J. 2015; 35(1): 55–62

[2] Leberfinger AN, Behar BJ, Williams NC, et al. Breast implant-associated anaplastic large cell lymphoma: a systematic review. JAMA Surg. 2017; 152 (12):1161–1168

[3] O'Malley FP, Pinder SE, eds. Breast Pathology. Philadelphia, PA: Churchill Livingston; 2006

[4] Brookes MJ, Bourke AG. Radiological appearances of papillary breast lesions. Clin Radiol. 2008; 63(11):1265–1273

[5] Bhattarai N, Kanemaki Y, Kurihara Y, Nakajima Y, Fukuda M, Maeda I. Intraductal papilloma: features on MR ductography using a microscopic coil. AJR Am J Roentgenol. 2006; 186(1):44–47

[6] Daniel BL, Gardner RW, Birdwell RL, Nowels KW, Johnson D. Magnetic resonance imaging of intraductal papilloma of the breast. Magn Reson Imaging. 2003; 21(8):887–892

[7] Tominaga J, Hama H, Kimura N, Takahashi S. Magnetic resonance imaging of intraductal papillomas of the breast. J Comput Assist Tomogr. 2011; 35(1): 153–157

[8] Kurz KD, Roy S, Saleh A, Diallo-Danebrock R, Skaane P. MRI features of intraductal papilloma of the breast: sheep in wolf's clothing? Acta Radiol. 2011; 52(3):264–272

[9] Rosen PP. Rosen's Breast Pathology. 3rd ed. Philadelphia, PA: Lippincott Williams and Wilkins; 2009

[10] Mulligan AM, O'Malley FP. Papillary lesions of the breast: a review. Adv Anat Pathol. 2007; 14(2):108–119

[11] Rosen PP, Cantrell B, Mullen DL, DePalo A. Juvenile papillomatosis (Swiss cheese disease) of the breast. Am J Surg Pathol. 1980; 4(1):3–12

[12] Sanders LM, Daigle M. The rightful role of MRI after negative conventional imaging in the management of bloody nipple discharge. Breast J. 2016; 22(2): 209–212

[13] Morrogh M, Park A, Elkin EB, King TA. Lessons learned from 416 cases of nipple discharge of the breast. Am J Surg. 2010; 200(1):73–80

[14] Leis HP , Jr. Management of nipple discharge. World J Surg. 1989; 13(6):736–742

[15] Morrogh M, Morris EA, Liberman L, Borgen PI, King TA. The predictive value of ductography and magnetic resonance imaging in the management of nipple discharge. Ann Surg Oncol. 2007; 14(12):3369–3377

[16] Nakahara H, Namba K, Watanabe R, et al. A comparison of MR imaging, galactography and ultrasonography in patients with nipple discharge. Breast Cancer. 2003; 10(4):320–329

[17] American College of Radiology. Breast Imaging Reporting and Data System (BI-RADS). 5th ed. Reston, VA: American College of Radiology; 2013

[18] Sickles EA. Probably benign breast lesions: when should follow-up be recommended and what is the optimal follow-up protocol? Radiology. 1999; 213 (1):11–14

[19] Spick C, Szolar DH, Baltzer PA, et al. Rate of malignancy in MRI-detected probably benign (BI-RADS 3) lesions. AJR Am J Roentgenol. 2014; 202(3): 684–689

[20] Bahrs SD, Baur A, Hattermann V, et al. BI-RADS® 3 lesions at contrast-enhanced breast MRI: is an initial short-interval follow-up necessary? Acta Radiol. 2014; 55(3):260–265

[21] Gutierrez RL, DeMartini WB, Eby PR, Kurland BF, Peacock S, Lehman CD. BI-RADS lesion characteristics predict likelihood of malignancy in breast MRI for masses but not for nonmasslike enhancement. AJR Am J Roentgenol. 2009; 193(4):994–1000

[22] Eby PR, DeMartini WB, Gutierrez RL, Saini MH, Peacock S, Lehman CD. Characteristics of probably benign breast MRI lesions. AJR Am J Roentgenol. 2009; 193(3):861–867

[23] Spick C, Bickel H, Polanec SH, Baltzer PA. Breast lesions classified as probably benign (BI-RADS 3) on magnetic resonance imaging: a systematic review and meta-analysis. Eur Radiol. 2018; 28(5):1919–1928

[24] Kuhl CK, Schrading S, Bieling HB, et al. MRI for diagnosis of pure ductal carcinoma in situ: a prospective observational study. Lancet. 2007; 370(9586): 485–492

[25] Lehman CD, Gatsonis C, Kuhl CK, et al. ACRIN Trial 6667 Investigators Group. MRI evaluation of the contralateral breast in women with recently diagnosed breast cancer. N Engl J Med. 2007; 356(13):1295–1303

[26] Strigel RM, Burnside ES, Elezaby M, et al. Utility of BI-RADS assessment category 4 subdivisions for screening breast MRI. AJR Am J Roentgenol. 2017; 208 (6):1392–1399

[27] Abe H, Schmidt RA, Shah RN, et al. MR-directed ("second-look") ultrasound examination for breast lesions detected initially on MRI: MR and sonographic findings. AJR Am J Roentgenol. 2010; 194(2):370–377

[28] Spick C, Baltzer PA. Diagnostic utility of second-look US for breast lesions identified at MR imaging: systematic review and meta-analysis. Radiology. 2014; 273(2):401–409

[29] Middleton MS. Magnetic resonance evaluation of breast implants and soft-tissue silicone. Top Magn Reson Imaging. 1998; 9(2):92–137

[30] Middleton MS. Breast implant and soft tissue silicone evaluation. In: Stark DD, Bradley W, eds. Magnetic Resonance Imaging. 3rd ed. St. Louis, MO: Mosby; 1998:337–353

[31] Middleton MS, McNamara MP , Jr. Breast implant classification with MR imaging correlation: (CME available on RSNA link). Radiographics. 2000; 20(3):E1

[32] Middleton MS, McNamara MP Jr. Breast Implant Imaging. Philadelphia, PA: Lippincott, Williams, and Wilkins; 2003

[33] Middleton MS, McNamara MP Jr. Breast Implant MR Imaging. In: Edelman RR, Hesselink JR, Zlatkin MB, eds. Clinical Magnetic Resonance Imaging. 3rd ed. New York, NY: Elsevier; 2005:2455–2482

[34] Middleton MS. MR evaluation of breast implants. Radiol Clin North Am. 2014; 52(3):591–608

[35] Thomson T. A System of Chemistry in Four Volumes. 5th ed. Vol. 1. London: Baldwin, Cradock, and Joy; 1817, p252

7 Image Interpretation: Noninvasive Cancer

Gillian M. Newstead

Abstract

The focus of this chapter is to review the imaging characteristics of non-invasive cancer (ductal carcinoma in situ [DCIS]) and the MRI appearance of this lesion which often presents as non-mass enhancement. The increased sensitivity for MRI detection of DCIS in recent years, above and beyond the sensitivity of mammography, is likely due to improved spatial and temporal resolution made possible with use of modern higher field strength magnets and newer acquisition protocols. Reported MRI sensitivities for DCIS in the more recent literature are significantly higher than those of mammography and range from 79% to 97%. Ultrafast perfusion imaging is also able to detect non-mass enhancement (NME) reliably even at lower spatial resolution, with the advantage that absence of BPE in these 1-30 second images greatly improves lesion conspicuity. In this chapter we discuss not only the biology and the distinct molecular and genetic expression profiles of DCIS, but also the salient features of this diagnosis which can be challenging because NME is not generally seen on precontrast imaging and lacks a clear lesion interface and distinct margins. The focus on the imaging findings in this chapter is exemplified by 37 case examples of normal ducts, ductal pathology and DCIS. A discussion of MRI investigations of DCIS and the clinical management of patients with a DCIS diagnosis, is also included in this chapter.

Keywords: biology of DCIS, molecular markers, gene expression profiles, MR imaging of DCIS, Paget's disease, interpretation challenges, MRI investigations of DCIS, clinical management of DCIS

7.1 Background

Ductal carcinoma in situ (DCIS) has been known for many years as a "mammographic disease." This diagnosis, rarely identified before the advent of mammographic screening, has increased dramatically over the years, with 63,410 new DCIS cases diagnosed in women in 2017 in the United States. The increasing rate of DCIS is strongly associated with a concurrent increase in rates of mammography screening and is similar to the increasing incidence of DCIS in other developed countries where breast screening programs are conducted. Early reports in the 1930s of a precursor lesion that could progress to invasion led to first use of the term *carcinoma in situ*. In the era before breast screening, most *in situ* lesions were detected clinically as a palpable mass, Paget's disease, or nipple discharge. Incidence in the United States has increased sevenfold, from 1973 through the late 1990s, with the most rapid increase found among women older than 50 years. As of January 1, 2005, an estimated 500,000 women were living with a diagnosis of DCIS in the United States and this number is estimated to increase to more than one million women by 2020 assuming constant incidence and survival rates.

DCIS is defined as a preinvasive form of breast cancer whereby a clonal proliferation of malignant epithelial cells originating in the terminal ductal lobular unit (TDLU) remain confined to ducts and do not invade beyond the basement membrane into the surrounding breast tissue. Evidence suggests that approximately 30 to 50% of DCIS lesions will progress to invasion over time if left untreated.[1,2] The important question is, of course, whether advanced imaging can not only improve identification of DCIS but also select those lesions that are most likely to invade. DCIS is generally found as microcalcifications on mammography and nonmass enhancement (NME) on magnetic resonance imaging (MRI). Both methods exhibit morphologic and distribution characteristics, which reflect a spectrum of heterogeneous lesions with diverse histological, molecular, and genetic characteristics. MRI, although not as widely used clinically as mammography, is a functional imaging technique and has the highest sensitivity for DCIS of all imaging modalities.[3]

7.2 Mammography

DCIS typically presents as a nonpalpable, 10- to 20-mm, calcified lesion detected at mammography, usually exhibiting calcifications in a grouped, linear, or segmental distribution. Calcifications with suspicious morphology on mammography include amorphous, course heterogeneous, fine pleomorphic, and fine linear or fine linear-branching subtypes. The typical fine linear malignant calcifications contained within lobules and ducts are probably caused by central necrosis occurring as a result of hypoxia, because blood supply by diffusion from extraductal vessels becomes inadequate due to rapid tumor growth. DCIS may involve multiple sites contained within the same ductal system separated by normal tissue ("skip lesions"), involving adjacent or even remote ductal systems which may occupy an entire breast lobe.[4] Although calcified necrotic tumor is a frequent mammographic presentation of DCIS, other findings such as mass, asymmetry (associated with fluid in the micropapillary subtype), or architectural distortion are seen in approximately 10 to 20% of cases.

7.3 Biology of Ductal Carcinoma In Situ

Noninvasive cancers comprise a heterogeneous group of lesions with variable histopathologic, biologic, and genetic features. Lesions that are heterogeneous in grade are assigned the highest grade; standard histologic assessment of DCIS typically involves assessment of both qualitative and quantitative features. Qualitative features include assessment of the architectural growth pattern, nuclear grade (high-, intermediate-, and low-grade cytologic features), and presence or absence of central necrosis. High-grade noninvasive lesions with high mitotic indices generally exhibit rapid growth rates and will almost invariably progress to invasion, whereas low-grade lesions may remain quiescent, never invade, and, if they do invade, will progress to low-grade invasive cancer. Tabar and colleagues have postulated that certain morphologic characteristics of calcifications represent a *duct-forming* invasive cancer rather than an *in situ* lesion and therefore patients with this type of presentation may require more aggressive treatment. Careful mammographic and pathologic evaluation with correlation of magnified mammographic imaging and large section histology specimens has informed this opinion.[5]

Few studies have focused on risk factors for DCIS; however, it is generally agreed that the risk factors for *in situ* disease are the same as those for invasive breast cancer. These indicators include increasing age, family history of breast cancer, genetic predisposition, high mammographic density, late age at menopause, and nulliparity. The natural history of DCIS, and of breast cancer overall, is still poorly understood and it makes sense therefore to focus research efforts on this earliest stage of breast cancer in order to gain knowledge about its origins and the mechanisms responsible for progression from noninvasive to invasive disease. In order to achieve this goal, we must improve our understanding of the biology of DCIS and the key events responsible for its transition to invasion. Invasive tumors require a vascular supply for continued growth and depend on angiogenesis, which is the term describing the complex process leading to the formation of new blood vessels from a preexisting vascular network, and this is likely also true for DCIS lesions.[6] Neoangiogenesis in invasive cancer is mediated not only by vascular endothelial growth factor (VEGF), a potent angiogenic factor, but also by other angiogenic and antiangiogenic factors. Tumor angiogenesis is an independent prognostic factor in invasive cancer, and is correlated with VEGF, microvessel density (MVD), and contrast enhancement in breast MRI. It is reasonable therefore to expect that the kinetic behavior of DCIS enhancement would also reflect DCIS biology. Expression of VEGF has been found in approximately 85% of DCIS lesions.[7] Angiogenesis in preinvasive cancer may not necessarily be associated with the typical dense, leaky neovasculature seen with invasive cancers. Studies of the vascular distribution associated with DCIS have shown two patterns: (1) vascular cuffing forming a ring, wherein blood vessels pack densely around neoplastic ducts immediately underlying the basement membrane,[8] or (2) a more diffusely dispersed pattern with scattered permeating blood vessels located in the surrounding stroma. These patterns of microvasculature are reflected in the enhancement patterns at high-resolution MRI, presenting often as clustered ring or diffuse (heterogeneous/homogeneous) enhancement. The diffuse enhancement pattern is often associated with high histologic grade and necrosis.

7.3.1 Molecular Markers

Cancer is a genetic disease wherein malignant transformation is driven by changes in DNA. In the larger context of tumor biology, the molecular profiles of DCIS and invasive breast cancer are similar, supporting a common origin. The distinct molecular characteristics of DCIS mirror those of invasive breast cancer by tumor grade.[9] Molecular pathways are altered in DCIS, and characterization by DNA, RNA, and protein can not only elucidate the molecular pathways critical for cancer etiology but also identify disease subtypes that have the potential to correlate with prognosis and therapeutic prediction. Surprisingly, few differences on a genomic or gene-expression level exist

between DCIS and invasive disease, and DCIS breast lesions are considered to be nonobligate precursors of invasive cancer. This general understanding has not resulted from tracking the natural history of this disease and following women with DCIS over time without treatment, but rather by acknowledgment of a large body of indirect evidence linking the precursor status of *in situ* disease to invasion. For example, considerable evidence points to the increased risk of invasive ductal carcinoma (IDC) recurrence at the resection site in women with prior DCIS diagnosis and treatment, and the frequent coexistence of invasive and noninvasive disease in the same lesion, sharing of many of the same molecular and genetic abnormalities in both.[10,11]

Protein expression in DCIS is usually assessed via immunohistochemistry (IHC) obtained on tissue sections. Estrogen receptor (ER) status is a proven prognostic marker in breast cancer; its main clinical value is its ability to predict response to hormonal therapy. Most laboratories in the United States use IHC to determine ER and progesterone receptor (PR) results on primary breast carcinoma. Approximately 70 to 80% of DCIS lesions are ER-positive and are less likely to be associated with high nuclear grade, human epidermal growth factor (HER-2/neu) or p53 positivity, or a high proliferative rate (Ki-67). Only 20 to 30% of DCIS patients exhibit HER-2/neu overexpression[12] by measuring *ErbB2* gene amplification, as assessed by IHC or fluorescence in situ hybridization (FISH). HER-2/neu-positive DCIS is more likely to be ER–, PR–, and have high nuclear grade. The proportion of HER-2/neu-positive DCIS is similar to IDC; however, the triple-negative phenotype (ER–, PR–, HER-2/neu-negative) is less common in DCIS.[13]

7.3.2 Gene Expression Profiles

Microarray analysis, identifying specific gene expression profiles, yields prognostic and predictive information that may be useful for indicating the likelihood of response to therapy. In the past few years, there have been several commercially available prognostic gene expression profile assays developed for clinical breast cancer assessment, Oncotype DX and MammaPrint among them. These companies provide a commercial assay designed to assess tumor recurrence probability and have developed a prognostic indicator for DCIS, providing treatment decision support for patients with newly diagnosed breast cancer. The onco*type* DX method utilizes quantitative reverse transcription-polymerase chain reaction to analyze the expression of 21 genes (16 cancer-related and 5 control genes) and to provide an estimated distant disease recurrence score ranging from 0 to 100. Further understanding of the genesis of aggressive forms of DCIS and how these lesions transform themselves and progress to invasion is needed before confident therapeutic management of women with this diagnosis can be determined.

7.4 MRI of Ductal Carcinoma In Situ

Reported MRI sensitivities for DCIS in the more recent literature are significantly higher than mammography and range from 79 to 97%. Optimal technique is a prerequisite for improved identification of NME, and when achieved, individual ducts are discernable and tumor is readily identified in both ducts and lobules. We know that DCIS exhibits heterogeneous findings on both mammography and MRI, with each modality exhibiting some features that are associated with lesion aggressiveness. The histologic classification of DCIS was initially based on metrics developed for IDC: invasive cancers classified as grade I, II, or III, and noninvasive cancers categorized as low, intermediate, or high grade based on nuclear features such as size and mitotic activity. Mixed histologic subtypes are found in more than one-half of DCIS cases.[14] DCIS, however, unlike IDC, exhibits singular architectural growth patterns that reflect cell distribution within the duct lumen; these patterns of tumor growth are often visualized on mammography as calcium distribution in ducts and lobules and on MRI as internal enhancement patterns of NME. The nuclear grading and histologic growth patterns of in situ lesions are classified as solid, papillary, micropapillary, cribriform, and presence or absence of necrosis. Studies have shown that imaging can reflect tumor biology, for example, fine linear/fine linear-branching patterns of calcifications at mammography show considerably worse survival outcome than amorphous or round calcifications,[15] and higher-grade *in situ* lesions at MRI exhibit increased contrast enhancement compared with low-grade DCIS.[3,8]

Accurate diagnosis of DCIS may be challenging because NME is not generally seen on precontrast imaging and lacks a clear lesion interface and distinct margins. However, modern MRI methods obtained at higher spatial and temporal resolution show excellent visualization of involved ducts and lobules.[16] Typical signs include a distinctive nonmass morphology, clumped or clustered ring internal enhancement, in a segmental, linear, or regional distribution. Unlike mammography where the DCIS finding is often that of calcified necrotic tumor, MRI detects intermediate- and high-grade DCIS and associated foci of invasive cancer that is often occult at mammography and ultrasound.

7.4.1 Terminal Ductal Lobular Units and Ducts

Normal TDLUs measure about 1 mm in diameter, enhance in varying degrees, and represent normal background parenchymal enhancement (BPE) on MRI. The entire TDLU complex including surrounding fat and fibrous tissue measures about 5 mm. High-resolution MRI can visualize normal (nonenhancing) central ducts measuring 0.1 mm in diameter, seen best in fatty breasts (▶ Fig. 7.1). Abnormal enhancing ducts containing DCIS (▶ Fig. 7.2) may be visible not only in the subareolar region but also with variable distribution throughout the affected breast; these diseased ducts enlarge up to about 1.0 mm in diameter and are visible in any type of FGT.

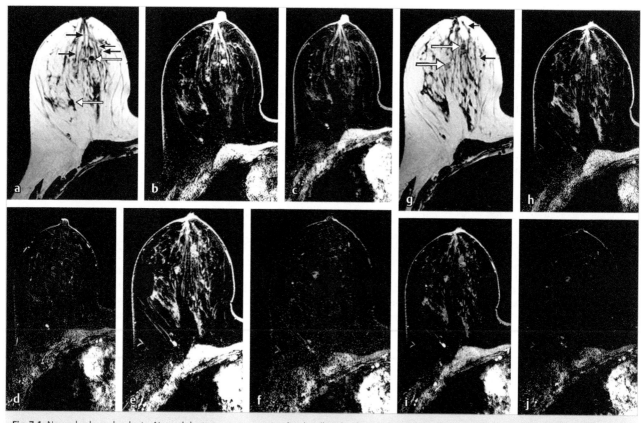

Fig. 7.1 Normal subareolar ducts. Normal duct structures are visualized well in this fatty breast on the T2w non-fat-sat image (a) (*short arrows*); small cysts are also seen (*long arrows*). These findings are also visible on T1w fat-sat precontrast image (b), seen without enhancement on postcontrast T1w image (c), and subtraction image (d). Similar findings are seen on an adjacent slice showing normal ducts on T2w image (e, *short arrows*), cysts (e, *long arrows*), and T1w precontrast image (f). No enhancement is seen on postcontrast T1w image (g) or subtracted image (h). Nonenhancing ducts are benign.

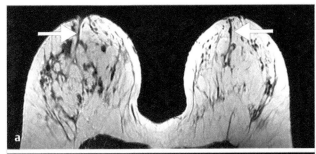

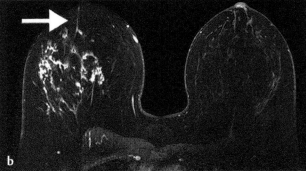

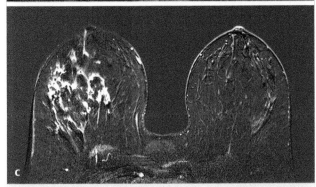

Fig. 7.2 Enhancing duct containing high-grade DCIS. Subareolar ducts are seen bilaterally on T2w non-fat-sat image (**a**, *arrows*). T1w postcontrast image (**b**) and correlative subtraction image (**c**) show enhancement of an abnormal right subareolar duct, but no enhancement of a normal left duct. Extensive segmental right breast NME is shown with visible peripheral enhancing ducts. Histology: DCIS, high grade, solid with necrosis. ER (–), PR (+).

Benign, nonenhancing, dilated ducts are often identified in the subareolar region in women of all ages and may contain fluid or debris with signal intensities similar to water: hyperintense on T2-weighted (T2w) and hypointense on T1w series (▶ Fig. 7.3). Other ectatic ducts may contain proteinaceous or hemorrhagic intraductal material exhibiting variable signal on T2w and T1w series: the higher the protein content, the lower the signal intensity on T2w series and the higher the intensity on T1w series (▶ Fig. 7.4; ▶ Fig. 7.5). Infrequently, benign ectatic ducts may become inflamed exhibiting duct wall and periductal enhancement separated by nonenhancing duct contents. These ducts can be differentiated from enhancing malignant ducts by their typical "tram-track" appearance on MRI (▶ Fig. 7.6; ▶ Fig. 7.7). Ducts with a linear enhancement distribution are clearly visible at high-resolution MRI and should be considered to be suspicious, whether visible centrally or elsewhere in the

Table 7.1 Descriptors for nonmass enhancement

Distribution	a. Focal
	b. Linear
	c. Segmental
	d. Regional
	e. Multiple regions
	f. Diffuse
Internal enhancement patterns	a. Homogeneous
	b. Heterogeneous
	c. Clumped
	d. Clustered ring

Source: American College of Radiology.[17]

breast. This pattern of enhancement generally indicates a high-risk lesion, such as atypical duct hyperplasia (ADH) and lobular neoplasia, or DCIS. Examples of high-risk lesions are shown: pleomorphic LCIS (▶ Fig. 7.8), ▶ Fig. 7.9; ▶ Fig. 7.10), flat epithelial atypia (FEA) (▶ Fig. 7.11), and ADH (▶ Fig. 7.12). High-risk lesions exhibit MR findings which may be very similar in morphology and internal enhancement characteristics to DCIS lesions (▶ Fig. 7.13), with the exception that the enhancement is generally lower and detection is more difficult at lower field strength.

7.5 Morphology of Ductal Carcinoma In Situ

NME is described in the ACR Breast Imaging Reporting and Data System (BIRADS) MRI Lexicon[17] as enhancement that is not a mass or focus but is still discrete from normal, surrounding BPE. This definition includes enhancement patterns that may extend over small or large regions and may exhibit normal fibroglandular tissue or fat interspersed between the abnormally enhancing components. NME is characterized by its distribution and pattern of internal enhancement (▶ Table 7.1), and is the reported lesion type in the majority of DCIS cases.[18,19] Although any distribution pattern can be seen in DCIS lesions, segmental and linear enhancement is most commonly found.[10,19,20] The lexicon descriptors for NME are discussed below.

7.5.1 Distribution of Enhancement

Focal enhancement is defined as a small, confined area whose internal enhancement may be characterized as a nonmass internal enhancement pattern, occupying less than a breast quadrant volume and may exhibit fat or normal glandular tissue interspersed between the abnormally enhancing components (▶ Fig. 7.14). Linear enhancement is arrayed in a line (not necessarily a straight line) or a line that branches (▶ Fig. 7.15). This distribution may elevate suspicion for malignancy as it suggests enhancement within or around a duct. Segmental enhancement is defined as triangular or cone shaped with the apex at the nipple, suggesting enhancement within or around a duct or ducts and their branches, thus increasing the likelihood of malignancy (▶ Fig. 7.16; ▶ Fig. 7.17; ▶ Fig. 7.18; ▶ Fig. 7.19). Regional enhancement encompasses more than a single duct system and is used for enhancement that occupies a large portion of breast tissue, at a minimum 25% of a quadrant. This

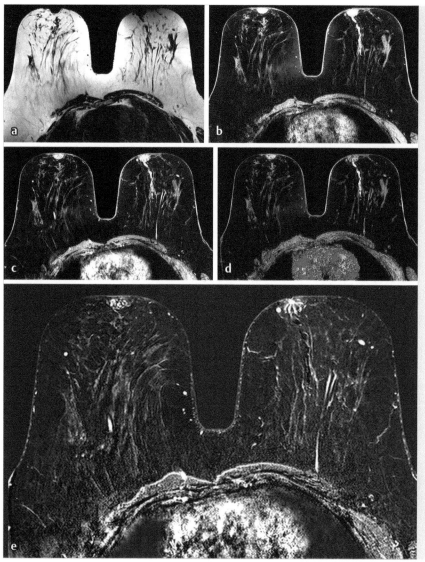

Fig. 7.3 Ectatic duct. Dilated subareolar duct is seen in the left breast on T2w non-fat-sat image (a), exhibits high signal on T1w precontrast image (b) and postcontrast image (c), and shows no abnormal enhancement on angiomap (d). The duct is not visible on subtraction image (e). The high duct signal represents intraductal fluid or proteinaceous material.

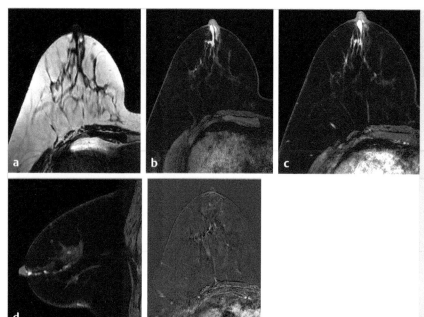

Fig. 7.4 Ectatic duct. A low-signal dilated subareolar duct is seen in the right breast on T2w non-fat-sat image (a), with several dilated ducts exhibiting high signal, visible on T1w precontrast image (b) and postcontrast source image (c). Sagittal reformatted source image (d) shows the largest duct to advantage. Absence of linear enhancement on subtracted image (e) confirms a benign diagnosis.

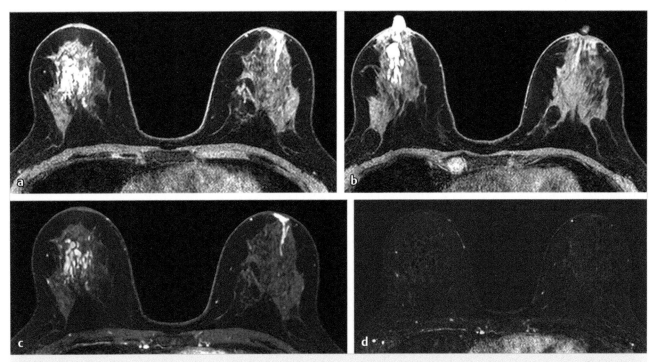

Fig. 7.5 Ectatic ducts. Precontrast T1w images **(a, b)** show bilateral ectatic high-signal subareolar ducts with dilated ducts extending into the central right breast. Postcontrast image **(c)** shows similar findings; however, no linear enhancement is seen on subtraction image **(d)**.

distribution pattern can be seen in invasive cancers such as lobular or HER2-enriched lesions in addition to DCIS lesions, bearing in mind that lack of orientation toward the nipple might suggest an invasive process (► Fig. 7.20). Enhancement of multiple regions, by definition, does not conform to a segmental distribution and can be seen as two large volumes of tissue (► Fig. 7.21). Diffuse categorization is defined as enhancement being distributed randomly throughout the breast (► Fig. 7.22).

7.5.2 Internal Enhancement Patterns

Lexicon descriptors for internal enhancement patterns are classified as homogeneous, heterogeneous, clumped, and clustered ring. Homogeneous enhancement is defined as confluent and uniform (► Fig. 7.23), whereas heterogeneous enhancement is nonuniform and variable in signal intensity, with a random pattern separated by areas of normal breast parenchyma or fat (► Fig. 7.24). Clumped, also described as "cobblestone" enhancement of varying shapes and sizes with occasional confluent areas, may look beaded or like a "string of pearls" if it is in a line. This finding is suspicious for DCIS and tissue sampling is usually required (► Fig. 7.25). Clustered ring enhancement consists of thin enhancing rings clustered together around the ducts and periductal stroma (► Fig. 7.26). This suspicious finding is best seen on high-resolution images and was first described in a report by Tozaki and colleagues who reported on 61 patients with clustered ring enhancement, histology yielding 63% (22/35) malignant lesions and only 4% of benign lesions (1/26).[21] The ring pattern of enhancement as seen in these cases is likely a reflection of contrast medium accumulation in the periductal stroma or ductal wall, associated with an abundant blood supply and a washout enhancement pattern. This internal

enhancement pattern is more frequently observed today, because of the improved spatial and temporal resolution made available in recent years. The micropapillary-cribriform subtype of DCIS is a fluid-producing lesion that may present with nipple discharge. This tumor is often high-grade and mammographically occult in its early stages. The fluid produced by this tumor can enlarge the affected breast ducts and may involve an entire breast lobe, resulting in a segmental asymmetry with or without associated calcification at mammography. Micropapillary-cribriform DCIS is easily diagnosed on MRI, ductal fluid is sometimes visible on T2w series, and the tumor generally enhances rapidly in a segmental distribution, often with washout kinetics in the delayed phase (► Fig. 7.27; ► Fig. 7.28). Papillary DCIS may also present as NME with small peripheral papillomata identified within a segmental distribution of enhancement (► Fig. 7.29).

MRI Kinetic Features of DCIS

Although identification of DCIS lesions in clinical practice is usually based on morphology, quantitative assessment of kinetic behavior may provide important biologic information because lesion enhancement is related to angiogenesis and MVD. DCIS often exhibits kinetic curves that persistently rise or plateau over time, a pattern not often seen with invasive malignancy. In routine practice, the kinetic parameters and criteria that work best to distinguish benign and malignant mass lesions may not work as well with nonmass lesions.[22] DCIS enhancement rates will often remain below the typical enhancement thresholds of invasive cancers; computer-aided design (CAD) software systems calibrated to the enhancement pattern of invasive cancers, typically 80% or thereabouts, will likely

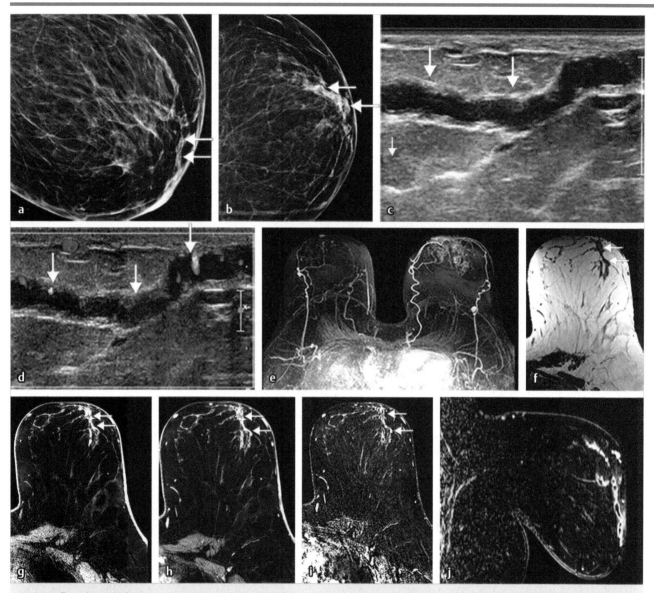

Fig. 7.6 Inflamed ectatic duct. Patient presents with anterior left breast pain. MLO and CC cropped images of the anterior-central left breast **(a, b)** show a solitary dilated subareolar duct, also visible on ultrasound, exhibiting increased blood flow on color Doppler **(c, d)**. MRI shows left subareolar enhancement on MIP image **(e)**. A correlative dilated duct is visible on T2w non-fat-sat image **(f)** with a high duct signal seen on T1w precontrast image **(g)**, likely representing intraductal fluid or proteinaceous material. Postcontrast source and subtracted images **(h, i)** exhibit duct wall enhancement with a classic "tram-track" appearance. The duct wall enhancement is seen to advantage on subtracted sagittal image **(j)**. Clinical symptoms resolved within 2 months.

consistently fail to highlight many cases of DCIS, particularly the lower grade lesions. The limitations of the current CAD systems could be overcome and diagnostic accuracy improved if kinetic classifiers could be trained separately to accommodate various lesion types based on enhancement morphology (mass or nonmass). At present, radiologists rely mostly on the morphologic characteristics of DCIS for diagnosis rather than the standard kinetic analysis using time intensity course curves.

7.6 Paget's Disease

Paget's disease of the breast is an uncommon presentation of breast malignancy, accounting for 1 to 3% of all breast tumors,

first described in 1856 by Velpeau, followed by the description of Sir James Paget in 1874.[23] The presentation is clinical, with nipple or areolar changes that include erythema, eczema, and ulceration with bleeding and itching. Delay in diagnosis is not infrequent because the clinical findings may be mistaken for a benign dermatologic condition. The histopathology of Paget's disease presents as infiltration of the nipple epidermis with large round and ovoid tumor cells, associated with an underlying invasive or noninvasive carcinoma. It is widely accepted that these cells are ductal carcinoma cells that have migrated from the underlying mammary ducts to the epidermis of the nipple. This theory on the pathogenesis of Paget's disease is supported by the presence of associated underlying breast carcinoma in

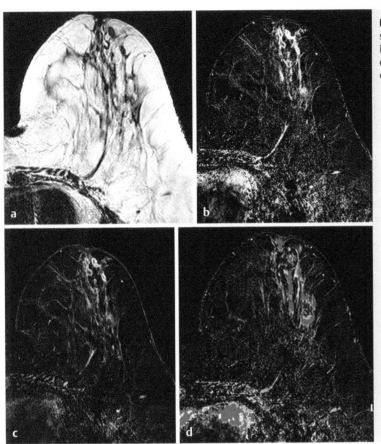

Fig. 7.7 Inflamed ectatic duct. T2w image does not show significant duct dilation (a), but postcontrast subtracted images at 1 minute and 2 minutes (b, c) exhibit duct wall enhancement with persistent enhancement pattern shown on the angiomap image (d).

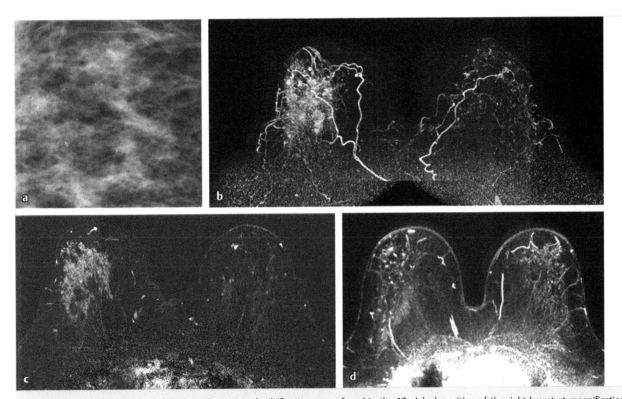

Fig. 7.8 Pleomorphic and classic LCIS. Loosely scattered calcifications were found in the 12 o'clock position of the right breast at magnification mammography, stereotaxic biopsy yielding LCIS (a). MIP image (b) shows diffuse NME with heterogeneous enhancement, also seen on subtracted image (c) and slab image (d). Subsequent wide surgical excision yielded pleomorphic and classic LCIS.

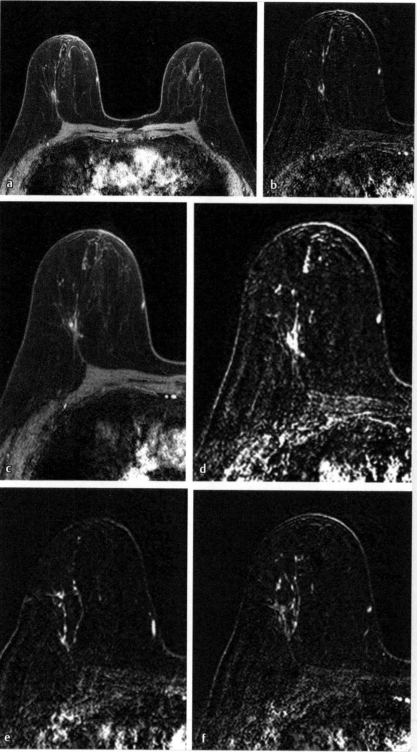

Fig. 7.9 Pleomorphic LCIS. Screening MRI identified linear nonmass enhancement in the left breast (negative mammogram). Two adjacent slices, each showing a source and a correlative subtraction image, are shown (a–d). Linear enhancement is noted extending from the posterior breast toward the nipple. A central enhancing duct and more lateral enhancing ducts are visible. Two inferior subtraction images (e, f) exhibit multiple areas of linear enhancement likely representing additional enhancing ducts. It should be noted that the duct enhancement is low, below standard thresholds on CAD systems. MR-guided biopsy yielded pleomorphic LCIS with pagetoid extension. High spatial resolution is necessary for visualization of these subtle findings.

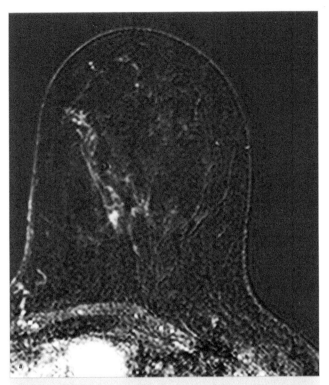

Fig. 7.10 Pleomorphic LCIS and ALH. Screening MRI identified a focus in the lateral left breast, with associated linear enhancement extending anteriorly toward the nipple. This lesion was only identified on T1w postcontrast subtraction imaging, in part because of low initial enhancement. MR-guided biopsy yielded pleomorphic LCIS and ALH.

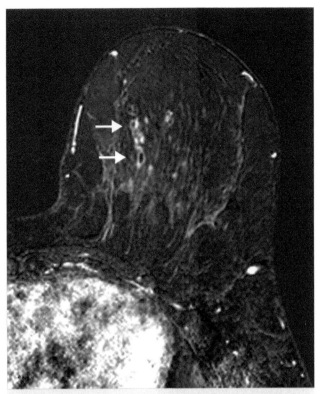

Fig. 7.11 FEA, columnar cell change. Screening MRI identified linear distribution with a clustered ring internal enhancement pattern (*arrows*) on T1w postcontrast subtraction image. This lesion was seen well on one subtraction slice only. MR-guided biopsy yielded FEA and columnar cell change.

nearly all patients; the diagnosis is confirmed with a full-thickness biopsy of the nipple and areola. The imaging presentation of Paget's disease is varied, and mammography may be normal because of the late appearance of microcalcification. MRI is the imaging procedure of choice for women with Paget's disease, allowing accurate identification of underlying invasive and/or noninvasive disease (▶ Fig. 7.30; ▶ Fig. 7.31; ▶ Fig. 7.32; ▶ Fig. 7.33; ▶ Fig. 7.34).

7.6.1 Interpretation Challenges

Recognition of DCIS lesions at MRI may present a diagnostic challenge because the findings of NME are not usually visible on T2w sequences, with or without fat suppression, nor on unenhanced T1w images, because the lesions may be indistinguishable from normal breast parenchyma. Review of the postcontrast source (nonsubtracted) datasets, where both enhancing and nonenhancing parenchyma is visible, may help the radiologist to distinguish segmental distribution of DCIS from patchy, often peripheral BPE. Subtraction images usually show NME to advantage and radiologists usually rely on morphology for initial diagnosis of DCIS because, as already noted, kinetic features most commonly show a range of initial contrast uptake with plateau, persistent, or washout kinetics seen in the delayed postcontrast phase. Identification of segmental enhancement, commonly seen in DCIS, is an important diagnostic

finding. Software that allows the radiologist to create a slab image (or thin maximum intensity projection [MIP]) of an area in question at the reading workstation is often very useful, because if NME (rather than focal BPE) is present, the segmental distribution pattern will be accentuated (▶ Fig. 7.35). Postimage processing with multiplanar reformatting may increase the confidence of diagnosis and assist in determination of the extent of disease.

The distinctive morphology of DCIS and the variable kinetic patterns discussed here may prompt some to suggest that MR acquisitions that emphasize spatial over temporal resolution are more sensitive to DCIS. Although spatial resolution is important, sufficient temporal resolution is also needed in order to distinguish the more slowly and moderately enhancing pure DCIS lesions from enhancing parenchyma (▶ Fig. 7.36; ▶ Fig. 7.37). Recognition and understanding of the unique morphology and kinetic characteristics of pure DCIS on MRI allows improved detection of early noninvasive disease.

7.6.2 MRI Investigations of DCIS

An important study of 167 women with pure DCIS imaged with mammography and dynamic contrast-enhanced MRI (DCE-MRI), published in 2007 by Kuhl and colleagues,[3] reported that the sensitivity of MRI was vastly superior to mammography in the detection of DCIS: 92% for MRI versus 56% for mammogra-

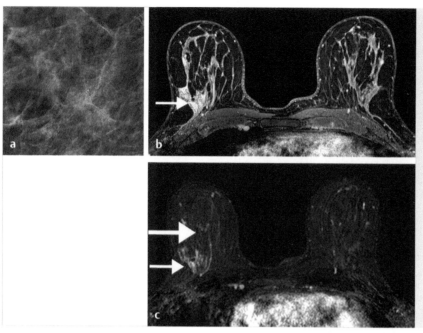

Fig. 7.12 ADH; spot magnification mammographic image (**a**) shows a faint, 5-mm, cluster of calcifications in the posterior 4 o'clock position of the right breast. Stereotactic biopsy yielded ADH. Biopsy clip (*arrow*) is seen on the T1w postcontrast source image (**b**) and subtracted image (**c**). NME is noted surrounding the clip-on images (**b**, **c**) and an anterior focus is also noted (*long arrow*). MRI-guided biopsy of the anterior focus yielded ADH.

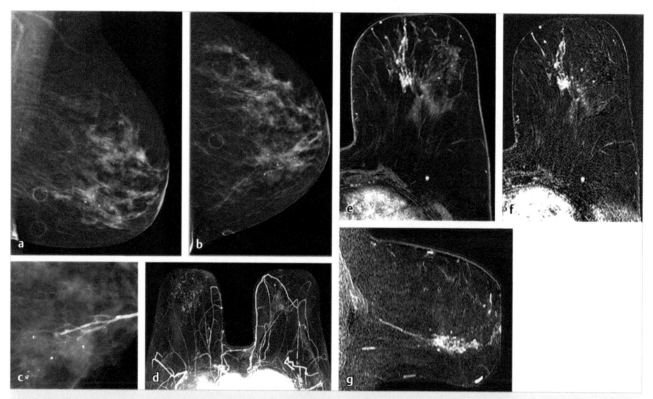

Fig. 7.13 Low-grade DCIS. Patient presented with left breast intermittent clear nipple discharge. Loosely scattered dense punctate and pleomorphic calcifications, within an area of asymmetry, were noted in the inferomedial left breast at mammography (**a, b**). Galactography identified a normal secreting duct leading to an area of mammographic asymmetry (**c**). Stereotaxic biopsy of the mammographic calcifications yielded low-grade DCIS. MRI shows mild BPE on MIP image (**d**) but no other findings. Postcontrast T1w source images (**e**) and subtracted image (**f**) exhibit clumped central enhancement measuring 11 mm with anterior, linear (ductal), and branching enhancement extending to the nipple. Sagittal reformatted image (**g**) is shown. Histology: low-grade DCIS, cribriform, and micropapillary, scattered within 7.0 cm of background ADH.

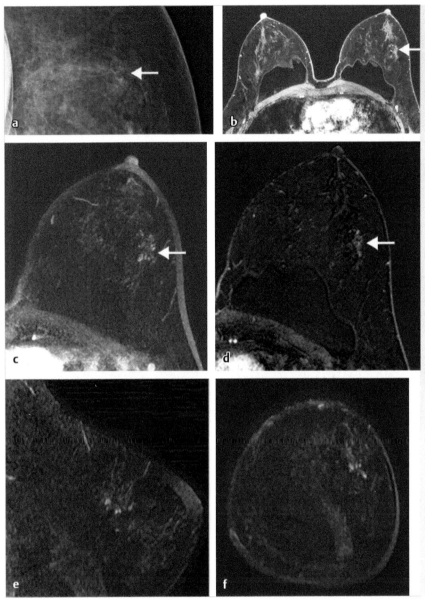

Fig. 7.14 NME distribution: focal enhancement. Magnified image of the left breast LMCC shows a posterior saline implant and a cluster of punctate calcifications at 2 o'clock position mid-depth (**a**, *arrow*). Axial postcontrast T1w image shows bilateral saline implants and a correlative focal NME (**b**), seen also on slab image (thin MIP) (**c**) and subtraction image (**d**). Reformatted slab images, sagittal (**e**) and coronal (**f**), show the extent of this focal area of enhancement to advantage. Histology: 1-mm tubular carcinoma associated with 7-mm low-grade DCIS, ER/PR (+), HER-2/neu (–).

phy. This study also showed a strong MRI sensitivity for high-grade lesions, 98%, compared with only 52% sensitivity for these lesions on mammography. Among the DCIS lesions depicted only by mammography, 83% were either low or intermediate grade. The sensitivity of mammography decreased as nuclear grade increased, while MRI tended to detect fast-growing high-grade lesions with or without necrosis.

Jansen and colleagues used an empirical mathematical model to analyze kinetic curves of NME versus mass enhancement in 34 benign and 79 malignant lesions.[24] They found that NME lesions exhibited significantly lower contrast uptake and slower washout compared with mass lesions (▶ Fig. 7.38). Furthermore, sensitivity and specificity of kinetic analysis was reduced in NME lesions compared with mass lesions. Another study compared the kinetic features of benign and malignant masses and NME in 552 women, including 396 malignant lesions and 156 benign lesions.[25] Malignant masses significantly showed shorter time to peak enhancement and stronger washout

curves than benign masses. However, when benign and malignant nonmass lesions were compared, washout measures of signal enhancement ratio (SER) were the only statistically significant different findings. Reports correlating in situ lesions and their relationship to nuclear grade enhancement characteristics at MRI and mammographic findings are rare. A report on 82 consecutively diagnosed pure DCIS lesions on DCE-MRI classified the MRI results according to nuclear grade and X-ray mammographic presentation.[26] In general, nonmass clumped enhancement in a segmental or linear distribution predominated, with most (68%) exhibiting rapid initial phase enhancement. Delayed phase curves were variable, demonstrating 28% persistent, 27% plateau, and 45% washout behavior. DCIS lesions with fine pleomorphic, fine linear, or fine linear-branching calcifications and masses on mammography were more suspicious by conventional kinetic standards on MRI than lesions with amorphous or indistinct calcifications, showing variable delayed phase curves. Among cases with linear or linear-

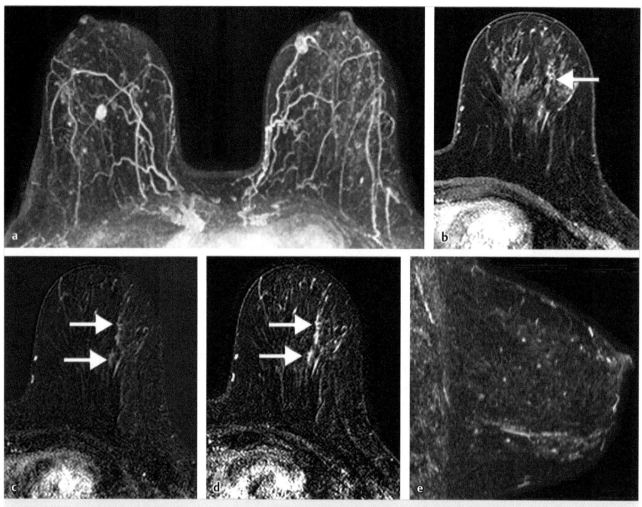

Fig. 7.15 NME distribution: linear enhancement. High-risk screening MRI shows enhancing masses in the central right breast and anteromedial left breast, both representing known fibroadenomata, seen on MIP image **(a)**. Source postcontrast T1w image **(b)** shows possible linear enhancement (*arrow*), confirmed on subtraction images **(c, d)** (*arrows*), where multiple linear (ductal) areas of enhancement are identified. When multiple enhancing ducts are identified, segmental enhancement could also be described as linear, as shown on the sagittal reformatted image **(e)**. MR-guided biopsy yielded high-grade DCIS, solid, ER (+), PR (–).

branching calcifications, 45% exhibited washout kinetics and an average time to peak enhancement just below 3.5 minutes, in contradistinction to cases with amorphous or indistinct calcifications where only 22% showed washout curves and the average time to peak enhancement was 4.4 minutes. DCIS cases presenting as mammographic masses reached peak enhancement earlier than cases presenting as calcifications, the majority exhibiting washout curves (90%).

Reports by Viehweg and colleagues[27] suggest that the mammographic appearance of pure DCIS may be related to its underlying physiology and vasculature in a way that traditional nuclear grading is not, and other investigators have reported that perfusion rates increase when comparing benign, in situ, and invasive lesions and that perfusion rates are correlated with MVD in DCIS lesions. Other reports have shown an increase in vessel density around ducts with DCIS, although with variable patterns,[28] and found that the expression of angiogenic growth factors such as VEGF increases from hyperplasia to DCIS.[29,30] Esserman and colleagues studied the relationship between SER values of invasive tumors and tumor vascularity and histologic grade, and found that higher SER values correlate with higher vascularity and higher pathologic grade.[31]

A study by Jansen et al[32] using a transgenic mouse model has shown that gadolinium crosses the basement membrane and accumulates within ducts in DCIS. The authors hypothesize that protease secretion of cancer cells may cause increased permeability of the basement membrane, allowing contrast to enter the ducts. The importance of ongoing research into the biology of DCIS was highlighted at the National Institutes of Health State of the Science Conference Statement in 2009. The participants concluded that the primary task for research going forward is to identify subsets of DCIS patients, based on their risk of progression to invasive carcinoma.[18]

7.6.3 Clinical Management of DCIS

Indirect evidence suggests that approximately 50% of DCIS lesions will not progress to life-threatening disease.[13,18,19]

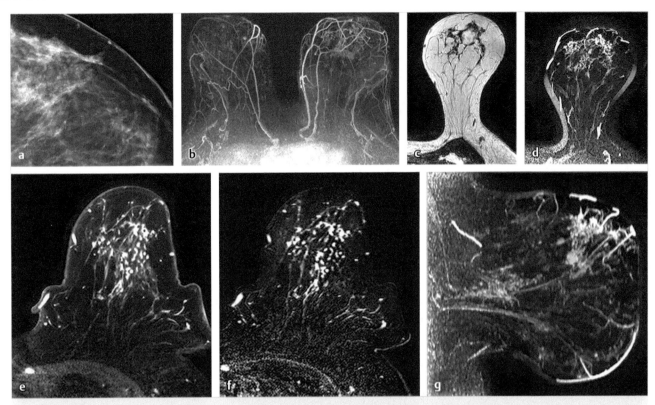

Fig. 7.16 NME distribution: segmental enhancement. Screening mammogram identified pleomorphic microcalcifications, segmentally distributed, in the upper outer quadrant of the left breast, with calcifications extending to the skin as shown in magnified CC image **(a)**. MRI shows anterior left breast NME on the MIP image **(b)** with asymmetry on T2w image **(c)** and correlative NME on slab postcontrast subtracted image **(d)**. Postcontrast source subtraction images **(d–f)** show segmental enhancement from the anterior to the posterior breast, with individual ducts visible, and associated clumped enhancement. Sagittal reformatted image **(g)** is shown. Histology: DCIS, intermediate and high nuclear grade, associated with necrosis and microcalcifications, ER/PR (–).

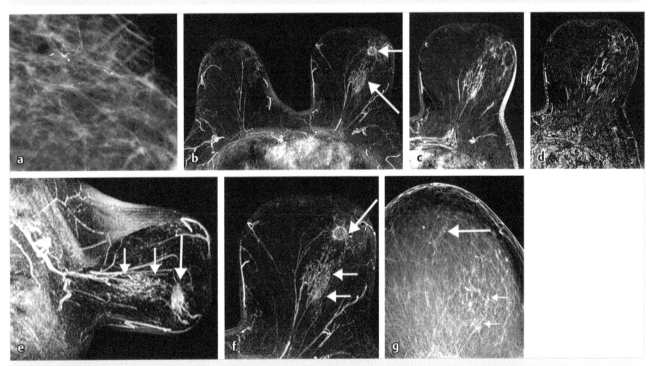

Fig. 7.17 NME distribution: segmental enhancement. Screening mammogram identified pleomorphic linear calcifications in the anterolateral left breast on LMCC image **(a)**. Stereotactic biopsy yielded carcinoma in situ, high-grade, solid type with central necrosis and associated microcalcifications. MRI shows a seroma at the site of stereotactic biopsy (*short arrow*) and linear (ductal) NME (*long arrow*) within a region of segmental enhancement extending from the central breast toward the nipple, on postcontrast thin MIP image **(b)**. T1w postcontrast subtraction image **(c)** shows ducts enhancing below the CAD threshold, as seen on image **(d)**. Sagittal slab reformatted source image **(e)** shows the distribution of NME (*short arrows*) and an anterior (postbiopsy) enhancing seroma (*long arrow*). **(f, g)** A correlation between NME in the central left breast on MRI and a region of asymmetry and distortion without calcification on the cropped CC mammogram. Histology: ductal carcinoma in situ, intermediate grade, solid type with associated central necrosis and microcalcifications.

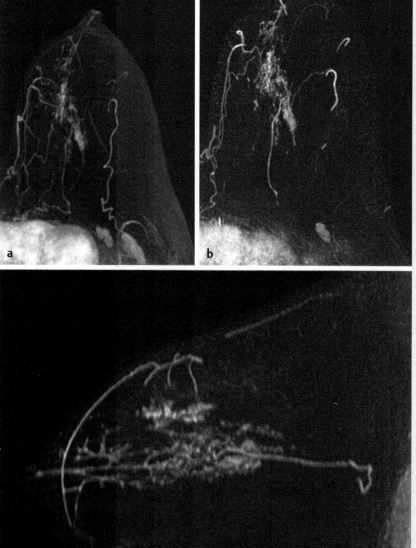

Fig. 7.18 NME distribution: segmental enhancement. MRI screening of the left breast at time of a newly diagnosed right breast ILC is shown. Left breast mammogram was normal. A segmental NME occupying an entire breast lobe is seen on postcontrast T1w axial source image (a) and subtraction image (b). Extensive NME, extending from the posterior breast to the nipple, exhibits clumped and linear enhancement. The main lactiferous duct is shown to enhance to the nipple, seen well on sagittal reformatted image (c). Histology: ductal carcinoma in situ, high nuclear grade, solid type, with atypical lobular hyperplasia and DCIS focally extending into lactiferous duct of the nipple.

Although direct evidence is scant, there are some temporal reports linking DCIS to IDC resulting from studies of women with DCIS who were initially misdiagnosed as a benign lesion, were followed, and eventually developed IDC in 14 to 59%.[19] Further support for this evidence can be found in ongoing work in animal models, where direct observations can be made of preneoplastic lesions as they progress over time.[33,34,35]

Despite the fact that mammography has proved to be uniquely successful in the detection of preinvasive cancer, early detection, and effective treatments yielding excellent cure rates, there is considerable concern that a significant portion of DCIS patients are *overdiagnosed* and *overtreated*. Nearly all cases of DCIS are now treated with some combination of surgery, radiation, and systemic therapy, an approach that invariably results in *overtreatment* of many women. This topic was highlighted in early 2015 when numerous articles in the media focused on the treatment of DCIS and questioned whether women with this disease were *overdiagnosed* because they would never develop a life-threatening breast cancer, and therefore could be subjected to unnecessary treatment.

In this context, Narod and colleagues investigated breast cancer mortality in a cohort of 108,000 DCIS patients identified in the Epidemiology and End Results (SEER) database from 1988 to 2011.[36] These patients were treated with a variety of therapeutic protocols; results yielded an estimated breast cancer–specific mortality rate of 1.1% at 10 years and 3.3% at 20 years. This study showed that the risk of death from breast cancer for women who had received a diagnosis of DCIS was increased by 1.8 times, compared with that of women in the U.S. general population. Those women who developed an ipsilateral invasive in-breast recurrence were 18.1 times more likely to die of breast cancer than women who did not develop a recurrence.

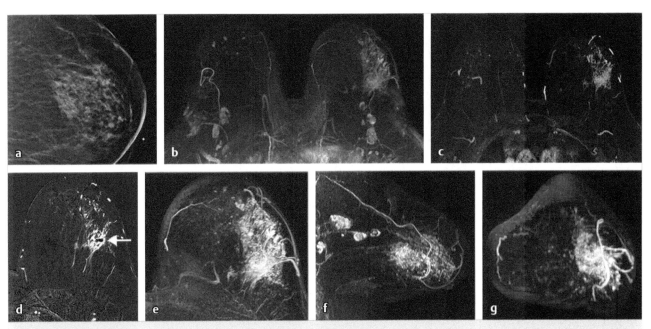

Fig. 7.19 NME distribution: segmental enhancement. Screening mammography identified a slight increase in the number of loosely scattered faint punctate and pleomorphic calcifications seen in the lateral left breast on cropped LMMLO view. (a) Biopsy of these calcifications revealed ADH and LCIS. MRI was requested for further assessment. Extensive segmental non-mass-like enhancement in the lateral left breast is noted on postcontrast MIP image (b) corresponding to the region of mammographic calcification. Several benign foci are also noted in the right breast. (c) Homogeneous enhancement and clumped NME, and (d) a seroma (arrow) from prior biopsy. Axial (e), sagittal (f), and coronal (g) slab reformatted images show the extent of enhancement. Histology: mammary carcinoma in situ, intermediate grade with mixed ductal and lobular features, associated with necrosis and calcification, ER/PR (+) with three foci of microinvasion.

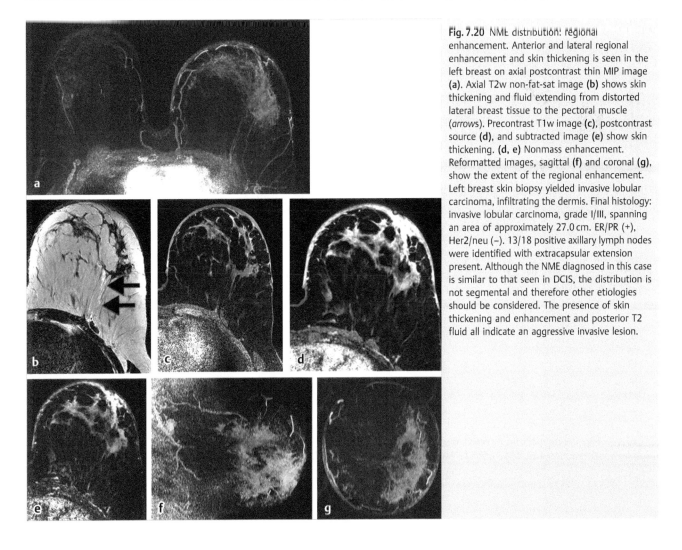

Fig. 7.20 NME distribution: regional enhancement. Anterior and lateral regional enhancement and skin thickening is seen in the left breast on axial postcontrast thin MIP image (a). Axial T2w non-fat-sat image (b) shows skin thickening and fluid extending from distorted lateral breast tissue to the pectoral muscle (arrows). Precontrast T1w image (c), postcontrast source (d), and subtracted image (e) show skin thickening. (d, e) Nonmass enhancement. Reformatted images, sagittal (f) and coronal (g), show the extent of the regional enhancement. Left breast skin biopsy yielded invasive lobular carcinoma, infiltrating the dermis. Final histology: invasive lobular carcinoma, grade I/III, spanning an area of approximately 27.0 cm. ER/PR (+), Her2/neu (–). 13/18 positive axillary lymph nodes were identified with extracapsular extension present. Although the NME diagnosed in this case is similar to that seen in DCIS, the distribution is not segmental and therefore other etiologies should be considered. The presence of skin thickening and enhancement and posterior T2 fluid all indicate an aggressive invasive lesion.

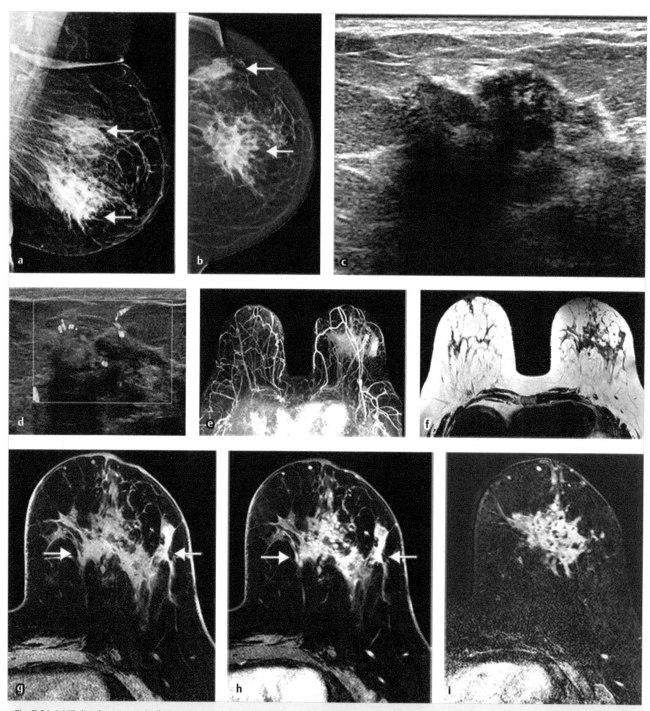

Fig. 7.21 NME distribution: multiple regions enhancement. Mammography identifies two regions of developing asymmetry in the left breast (**a**, **b**, *arrows*). Correlative ultrasound of the medial asymmetry shows a hypoechoic irregular lesion (**c**) with increased blood flow on color Doppler (**d**). Postcontrast MIP image (**e**) exhibits nonmass enhancement in the central, lateral, and medial left breast. Diffuse distortion in the central left breast is seen on T2w non-fat-sat image (**f**, *arrows*) and precontrast T1w image (**g**, *arrows*). Postcontrast axial source image (**h**) and subtracted image (**i**) exhibit heterogeneous enhancement with predominantly persistent enhancement, seen on the angiomap image (**j**). (*continued*)

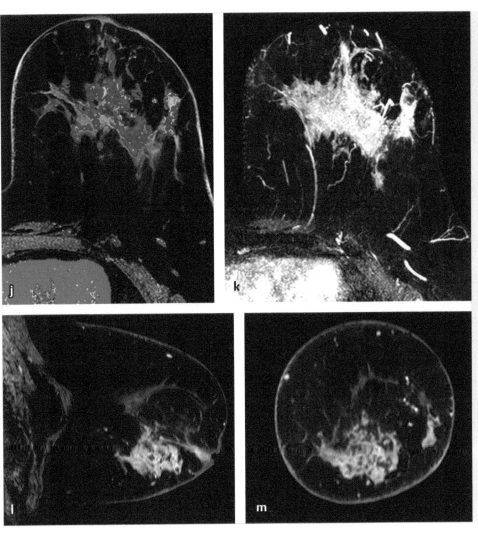

Fig. 7.21 (*continued*) Postcontrast axial source image (**h**) and subtracted image (**i**) exhibit heterogeneous enhancement with predominantly persistent enhancement, seen on the angiomap image (**j**). Thin MIP axial image (**k**) demonstrates the extent of nonmass enhancement, whereas sagittal and coronal reformatted images (**l,m**) additionally exhibit "ring-like" areas of tumor necrosis. Histology: triple-negative IDC grade 3 with associated DCIS. One positive sentinel node (1/3).

Use of radiotherapy for patients undergoing BCS reduced the risk of developing an ipsilateral invasive recurrence from 4.9 to 2.5% but did not reduce breast cancer–specific mortality at 10 years (0.9 vs. 0.8%). An accompanying editorial by Esserman and Yau[37] made the case that given the low breast cancer mortality risk found in this study, much of DCIS should be considered to be a "risk factor" for invasive breast cancer and an opportunity for targeted preventive measures. Additionally, these authors proposed that radiation therapy should not be routinely offered after lumpectomy for non-high-risk patients, because mortality is not affected, and further recommended that low- and intermediate-grade DCIS (calcifications) need not be a target for screening or early detection. The editorial concluded by recommending further research to improve understanding of the biological characteristics of the highest-risk DCIS lesions.

On the other hand, a report on the long-term results from the UK/ANZ DCIS trial[38] showed that women with DCIS who had received treatment with wide local excision only had a 10-year rate of subsequent breast cancer events of more than 30%, suggesting a serious potential for DCIS to progress. Adding to the discussion on these issues, a recent paper by Duffy and colleagues, using data from the UK National Health Service Breast Screening Programme, with a 3-year screening interval,[39] investigated the association between the detection of DCIS and the number of invasive interval cancers subsequent to the relevant screen. They found a negative association between screen detection of DCIS and subsequent invasive interval cancer incidence and found that for every three screen-detected cases of DCIS, there was one fewer invasive interval cancer detected in the next 3 years. This association remained after adjustment for numbers of small screen-detected invasive cancers and for numbers of grade 3 invasive screen-detected cancers. The authors concluded that detection and treatment of DCIS is worthwhile for prevention of future invasive disease, but also point out that these findings cannot give definitive proof of the progressive potential or otherwise of individual DCIS cases, and that only measures of leaving DCIS untreated and followed could give such evidence.

An ongoing DCIS trial in the United Kingdom, the "Surgery versus Active Monitoring for Low-Risk DCIS (LORIS)" trial, might provide some additional insights into management of DCIS patients by using an experimental therapeutic approach. The LORIS trial is investigating the safety of patient outcome by monitoring women with core-biopsy diagnosed low-risk DCIS treated without a subsequent surgical excision. Women meet-

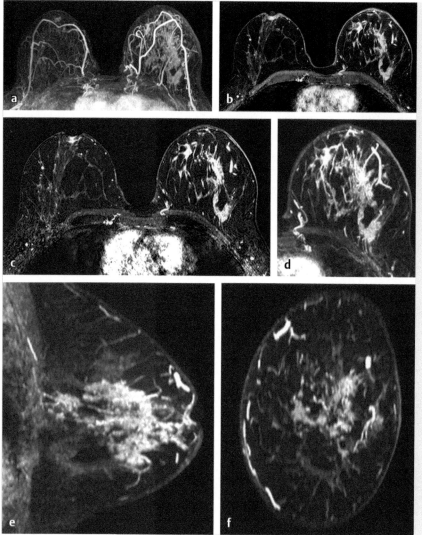

Fig. 7.22 NME distribution: diffuse enhancement. Diffuse pleomorphic calcifications were found in the left breast on mammography, with stereotactic biopsy yielding DCIS. MRI was requested for assessment of disease extent. Postcontrast MIP image (**a**) shows diffuse NME throughout the left breast with associated increased vascularity. Postcontrast source image (**b**) and subtraction image (**c**) show diffuse left breast enhancement. Slab reformatted images; axial (**d**), sagittal (**e**), and coronal (**f**) show the extent of disease with the sagittal image demonstrating orientation of enhancement toward the nipple. Histology: widespread high-grade solid DCIS with scattered foci of microinvasion.

ing LORIS eligibility criteria include those aged ≥ 46 years, with screen-detected calcifications yielding non-high-grade DCIS diagnosed by core biopsy, absent nipple discharge, or strong family history of breast cancer. There is a requirement for central pathology oversight confirming the grade of DCIS for patient eligibility; however, MRI assessment for DCIS characterization and disease extent is not an entry criterion. The trial is currently enrolling patients at about 60 centers in the United Kingdom, and has a noninferiority design aiming to show that in this group of women, active monitoring is not inferior to standard surgery. The primary end point is the outcome of ipsilateral invasive breast cancer–free survival at 5 years.[40]

The important clinical question to be decided therefore is whether favorable cases of DCIS can be watched rather than immediately treated (core biopsy followed by imaging surveillance) or treated with excision without radiation therapy. Although for some women a conservative approach may be appropriate, this treatment may not be suitable for all patients. Current knowledge does not allow us to identify reliably which DCIS lesion, if left untreated, will progress to invasive breast cancer and how long that progression might take. Moreover, the fact remains that for any individual DCIS patient who receives treatment, it is not known with certainty what would have happened if the treatment had not taken place. This debate has led many oncologists and surgeons to question the efficacy of current standard therapeutic protocols and instead focus on treatment based on individual prognostic indicators. Indeed, some advocates for tailored intervention recommend surgical approaches that are guided by advanced imaging methods such as MRI and molecular assessment of tumor biology.

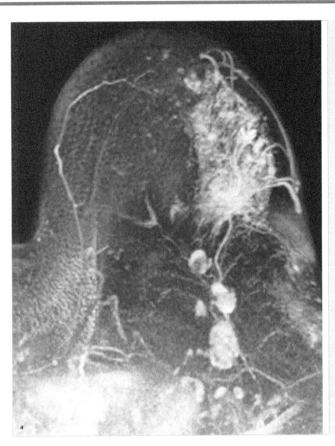

Fig. 7.23 Internal enhancement patterns: homogeneous. Homogeneous nonmass enhancement is seen in the lateral left breast on postcontrast MIP image.

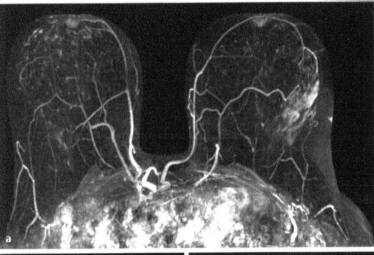

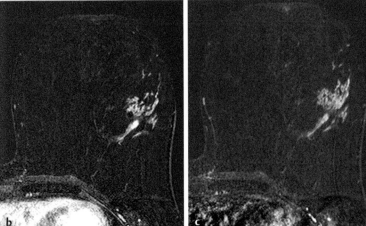

Fig. 7.24 Internal enhancement patterns: heterogeneous (and clustered ring). NME is seen in the central and lateral left breast, on MIP image (a). Postcontrast T1w source (b) and subtracted image (c) exhibit NME with a heterogeneous enhancement pattern with clustered ring enhancement also shown. Histology: DCIS, intermediate grade, cribriform and micropapillary types, with associated central necrosis and calcifications and cancerization of lobules at least 4 cm in extent.

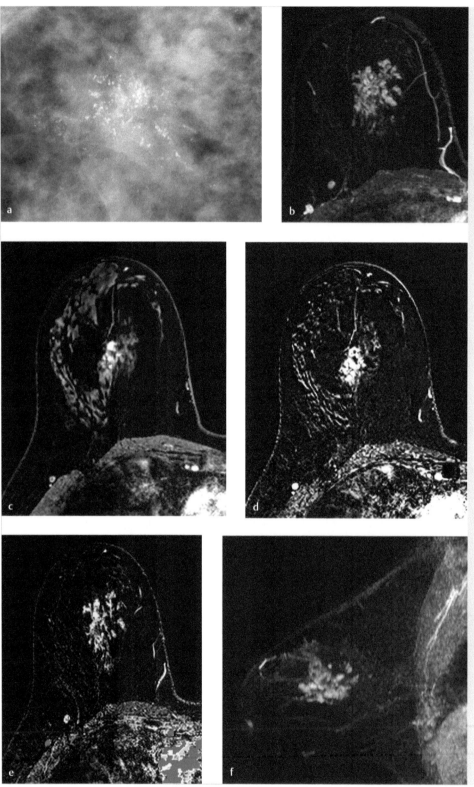

Fig. 7.25 Internal enhancement patterns: clumped. Mammographic screening identified a cluster of pleomorphic calcifications in the central right breast, as seen on magnified CC spot view (a). Postcontrast T1w thin MIP image (b) shows clumped NME, correlating in location with the mammographic microcalcification. Source and subtraction images (c, d) show a classic clumped enhancement pattern with predominantly persistent and plateau late phase enhancement seen on angiomap (e). Sagittal reformatted image (f) shows disease extent. Histology: DCIS, high-grade with necrosis.

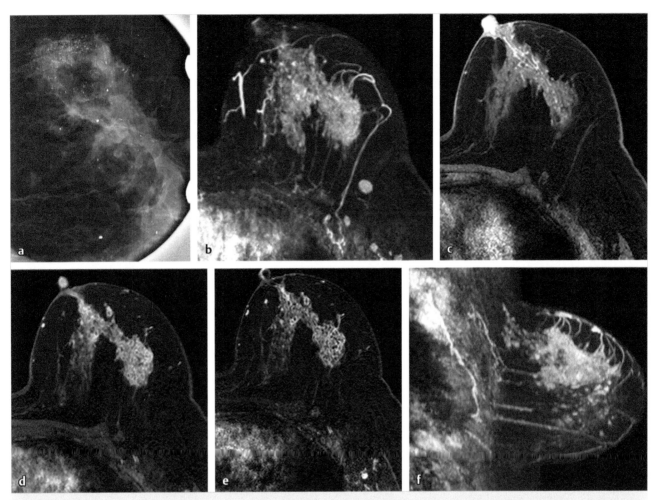

Fig. 7.26 Internal enhancement patterns: clustered ring. Screening mammography identified extensive pleomorphic and linear microcalcifications in a segmental-distribution in the superolateral left breast (**a**). Postcontrast MIP image (**b**) shows increased vascularity and NME, correlating in location with the mammographic calcifications. Source postcontrast T1w image (**c**) shows high signal within the ductal system leading to the NME, representing fluid. Source image (**d**) and subtracted image (**e**) show classic clustered ring enhancement. Sagittal reformatted slab image (**f**) shows the disease extent. Histology: highgrade DCIS, solid with necrosis and rare microinvasion: ER/PR (–), HER-2/neu (+).

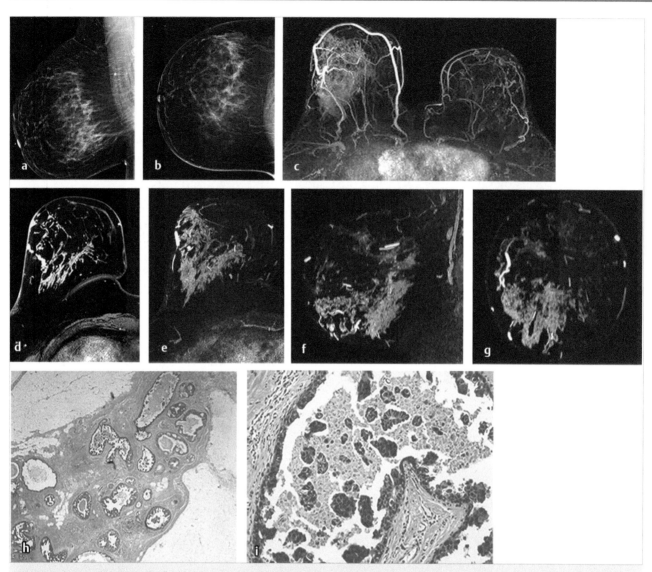

Fig. 7.27 Micropapillary DCIS. The fluid produced by this tumor can enlarge the affected breast ducts and may result in a finding of asymmetry at mammography as seen on right MLO and CC views (**a, b**) without calcifications. Associated calcifications may be occur but usually become visible later in the disease process. MIP image (**c**) shows extensive NME in the central and lateral right breast, also seen on postcontrast T1w image (**d**) and subtraction slab image (**e**) reformatted images (**f, g**) are shown. Histology: ductal carcinoma in situ, intermediate to high nuclear grade, clinging and micropapillary patterns, with apocrine features and focal necrosis, images (**h, i**).

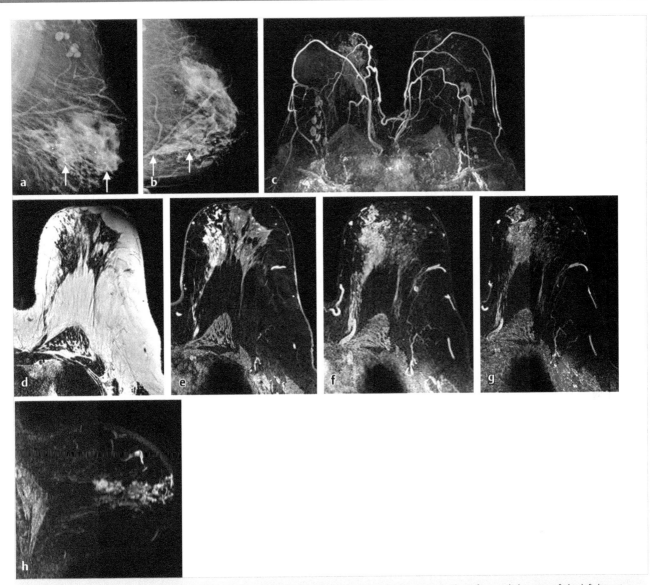

Fig. 7.28 Micropapillary DCIS (1.5 T). Screening mammography identified a segmental asymmetry in the inferomedial aspect of the left breast as shown on MLO and CC views (**a, b**; *arrows*). No calcifications are visible. Postcontrast MIP image reveals a segmental distribution of NME, correlating in location and extent with the mammographic asymmetry (**c**). T2w non-fat-sat image (**d**) is shown; postcontrast source and subtracted T1w image (**e, f**) reveal segmental clumped enhancement extending from the pectoral muscle to the nipple. Angiomap (**g**) exhibits persistent kinetics, and a sagittal reformatted image (**h**) is shown. Histology: DCIS, intermediate grade, micropapillary, papillary, and cribriform subtype.

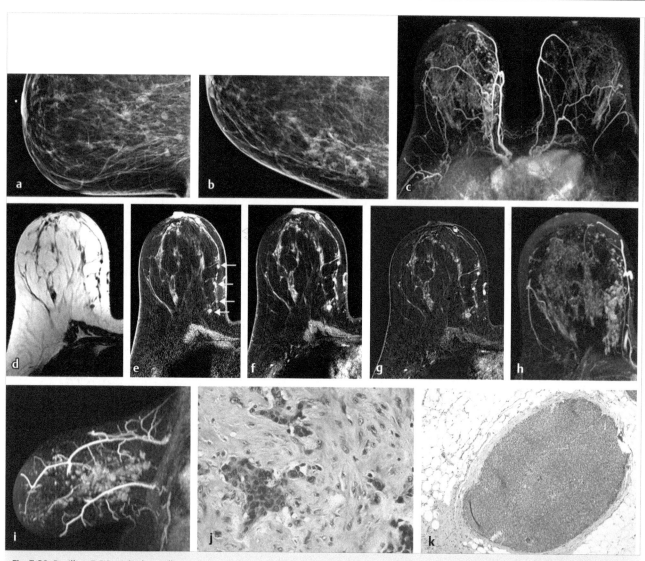

Fig. 7.29 Papillary DCIS. Multiple small round masses are seen in the central, posterior, and inferior right breast on spot MLO view (**a**) and CC view (**b**). Axial MIP image (**c**) exhibits NME with multiple small masses noted within the segmental enhancement, which extends from the far posterior breast to the nipple. Axial T2w non-fat-sat image (**d**) and precontrast T1w image (**e**) both also demonstrate multiple small round masses in the medial right breast (*arrows*). These masses are seen to advantage on postcontrast source image (**f**) and subtraction image (**g**). Thin MIP axial image (**h**) and sagittal image (**i**) show the extent of disease. Histology: DCIS, intermediate/high-grade solid and papillary types ER/PR (+) (**j, k**).

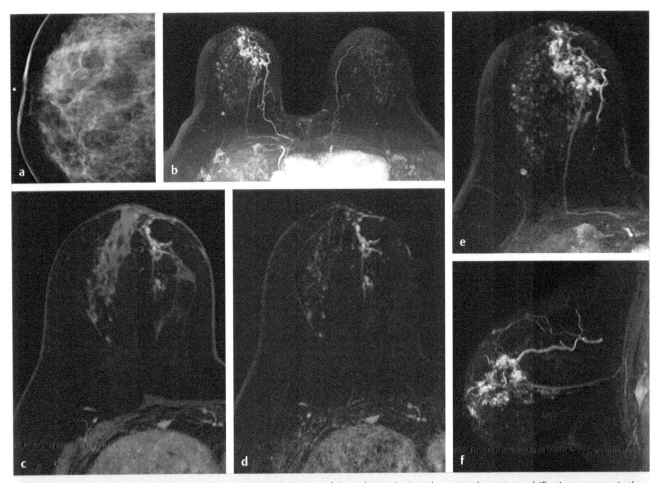

Fig. 7.30 Paget's disease. Patient presents with erythema and crusting of the right nipple. Loosely scattered punctate calcifications are seen in the anterior right breast (**a**). MIP image demonstrates increased vascularity in the right breast, with NME in the anteromedial aspect extending to the nipple (**b**). Source and subtracted postcontrast images (**c, d**) show linear-branching enhancing ducts in the subareolar region. Slab reformatted images; axial (**e**) and sagittal (**f**) show disease extent. Histology: ductal carcinoma in situ, high nuclear grade, solid type, with necrosis, Paget's disease of the nipple.

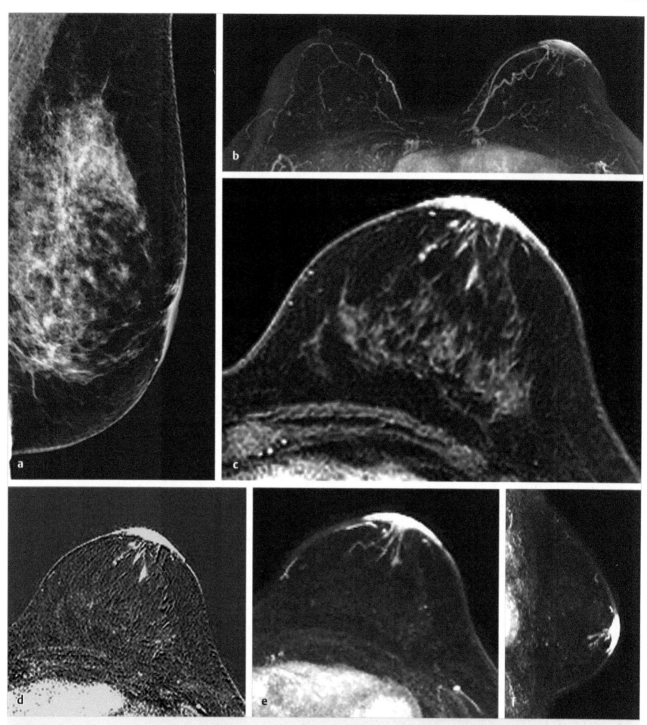

Fig. 7.31 Paget's disease. MLO view of the left breast **(a)** shows no finding in this patient with a red ulcerated nipple. MIP image **(b)** shows enhancement of the nipple–areolar complex. Source and subtracted postcontrast images **(c, d)** show enhancing lactiferous ducts behind the nipple, also noted on subtracted slab axial **(e)** and sagittal image **(f)**. No additional enhancing lesions are identified. Histology: DCIS high grade, involving tissue underneath the lactiferous sinuses, 3.2 cm in extent with involvement of the epidermis: ER/PR (–). The sentinel node was negative for malignancy (0/1).

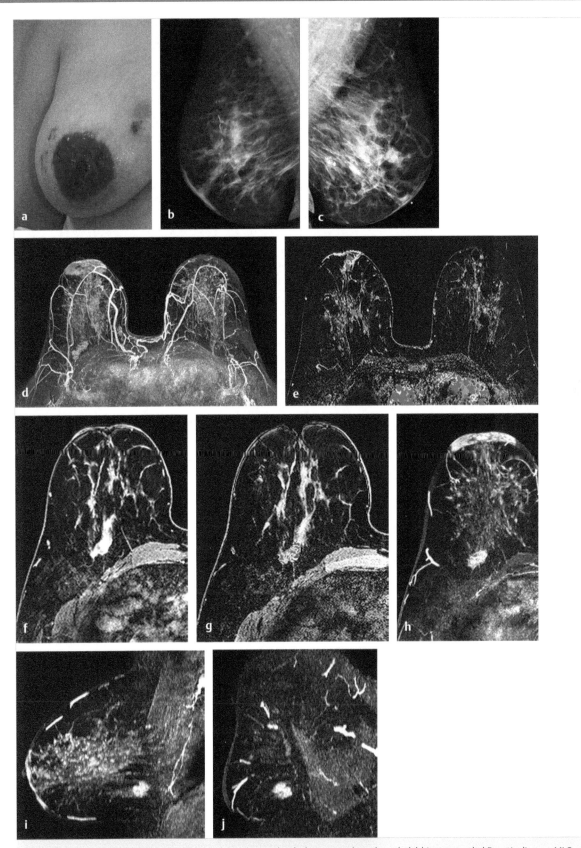

Fig. 7.32 Paget's disease. Patient presented with an ulcerated right breast nipple and areola **(a)** biopsy revealed Paget's disease. MLO mammographic views of both breasts **(b, c)** show skin thickening in the right areola and subareolar asymmetry. Benign scattered calcifications are visible in both breasts. MRI shows enhancement of the right nipple and areola with additional NME localized to the subareolar region on MIP image **(d)**, also seen well with washout kinetics shown on angiomap **(e)**. Source postcontrast images **(f, g)** show an enhancing right irregular mass at the posterior 6 o'clock position with washout enhancement. Thin MIP reformatted images, axial **(h)**, sagittal **(g)**, and coronal **(i)**, all demonstrate a spiculated 1.5-cm mass at 6 o'clock position, suspicious for invasive cancer. Marked BPE and multiple bilateral benign foci are also noted in both breasts. Histology: extensive high-grade DCIS in the anterior right breast, solid and cribriform with a 2-mm focus of invasion. ER /PR (–), HER-2/neu (+). Invasive duct carcinoma identified at 6 o'clock position: IDC grade 2.

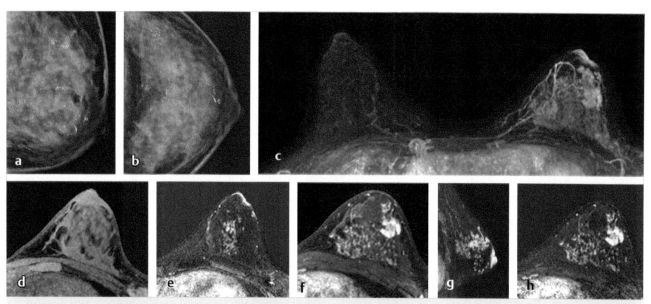

Fig. 7.33 Paget's disease. Patient age 28 years with a clinical presentation of Paget's disease in the left breast. Cropped ML and CC views of the left breast **(a, b)** show diffuse pleomorphic calcifications, high-grade type, throughout the left breast with associated skin thickening of the nipple and areola. MRI reveals enhancement of the nipple–areolar complex, diffuse NME throughout the breast, and an irregular mass at 2 o'clock position, seen on MIP image (1.5T) **(c)**. Precontrast T1w axial image **(d)** taken at the level of the nipple shows skin thickening, and postcontrast subtracted image **(e)** exhibits nipple enhancement and central clumped NME. Subtracted images **(f, g)** show an irregular enhancing mass and diffuse clumped NME, also seen on sagittal reformatted image **(h, i)**. Histology: IDC grade 3 with diffuse DCIS, solid with necrosis, ER/PR (+) HER-2/neu (−) Ki-67: 25%.

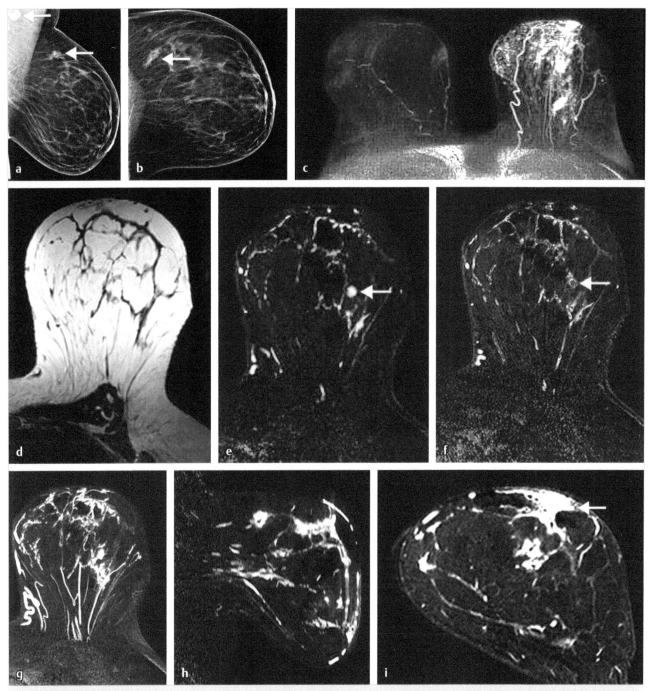

Fig. 7.34 Paget's disease. Patient, age 31 years, presented with erythema of the left areola. This high-risk patient is known to have Li–Fraumeni syndrome; no palpable masses were found on clinical examination. Mammographic views exhibit a focal asymmetry, in the superolateral posterior aspect of the left breast, and an enlarged left axillary lymph node (**a, b,** *arrows*). The breast composition is predominantly fatty. Postcontrast MIP image demonstrates increased vascularity and diffuse NME in the left breast with enhancement of the nipple–areolar complex and a focal NME corresponding with the mammography finding of asymmetry (**c**). T2w image (**d**) reveals a fatty breast without abnormal findings, and T1w postcontrast subtracted image reveals enhancement of all of the sparsely distributed breast tissue, which is asymmetric when compared to the right breast (**e**). Persistent enhancement is shown on angiomap (**f**); incidental note is made of a benign mass (**e, f,** *arrows*). Slab axial and sagittal images show the extent of enhancement well (**g, h**). Coronal subtracted image at the level of the nipple (**i**) shows nipple and subareolar enhancement (*arrow*). This interesting case demonstrates enhancement of all visible breast tissue and represents diffuse DCIS. Histology: DCIS spanning 15 cm, high nuclear grade with Paget's disease of the nipple. One < 0.5-mm focus of microinvasive ductal carcinoma, ER/PR (–), HER-2/neu (+). One positive sentinel node was identified (1/1).

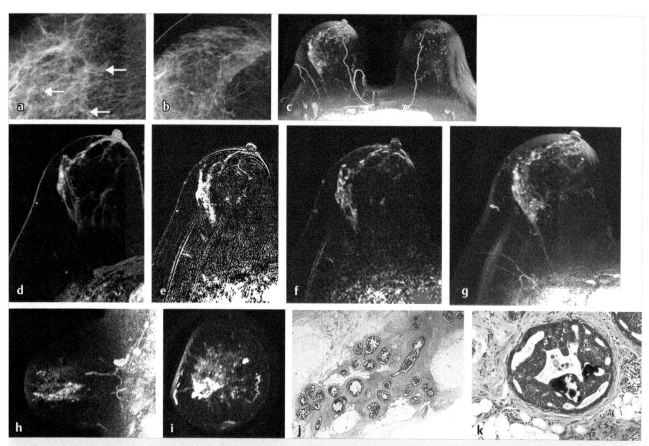

Fig. 7.35 Slab technique. Screening mammography identified multiple clustered, punctate, calcifications in the lateral right breast, as seen on RMML and RMCC images (**a, b**). Stereotactic biopsy yielded DCIS, low and intermediate nuclear grade. MIP image (**c**) shows segmental clumped NME extending from the posterior breast to the subareolar region. Postcontrast T1w source and subtracted images (**d, e**) identify NME with an enhancing lactiferous duct visible to the nipple. Persistent late-phase enhancement is seen on CAD image (**f**). Slab reformatted images; axial (**g**), sagittal (**h**), and coronal (**i**) demonstrate NME extent. Final histology: DCIS, intermediate grade, cribriform, papillary, and micropapillary type, associated with microcalcifications and necrosis, ER/PR (+) two pathology slides show the classic micropapillary pattern (**j, k**).

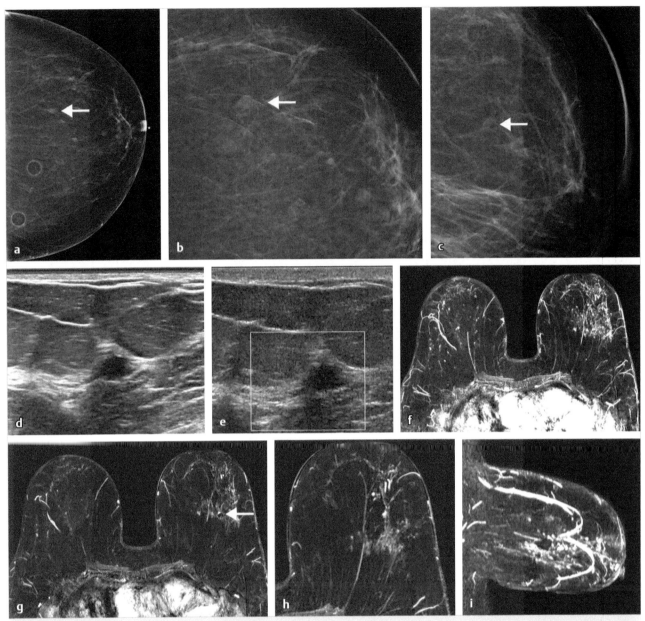

Fig. 7.36 High-resolution technique. Mammography screening identified a new asymmetry in the central lateral left breast (**a**; *arrow*), also shown on LMCC and LMML views (**b, c**; *arrows*). Ultrasound correlate (**d, e**) reveals an irregular hypoechoic lesion measuring 6 × 4 × 9 mm, biopsy yielding DCIS, solid and micropapillary. Subtracted T1w image (**f**) exhibits segmental NME with linear enhancing ducts visible in the left breast, and adjacent slice (**g**) shows a marker clip at site of prior ultrasound-guided biopsy (*arrow*). Multiple enhancing ducts are seen on axial image (**h**), and sagittal reformatted slab image (**i**) showing segmental distribution of enhancement to the nipple. Final histology: DCIS, low and intermediate grade, cribriform with apocrine features.

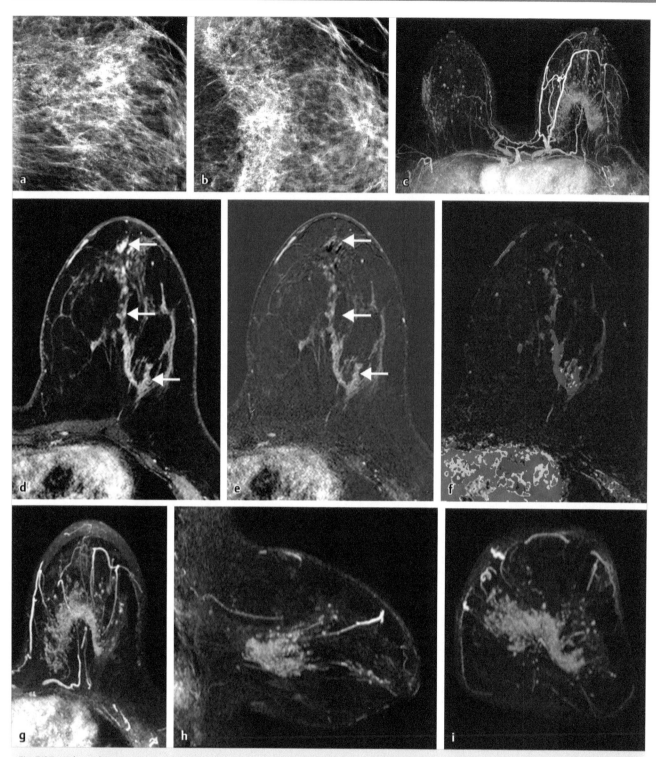

Fig. 7.37 High-resolution technique. Multiple cluster pleomorphic calcifications are identified in the central and lateral left breast at screening, and shown on LMML and LMCC views (**a, b**). Stereotactic biopsy yielded high-grade DCIS. MRI was recommended for further assessment. Postcontrast MIP image (**c**) shows increased vascularity and confluent NME in the left breast at the posterior fibroglandular–fat junction. Source and subtraction T1w postcontrast images reveal linear NME extending from the central and posterior breast to the nipple (**d, e**, *arrows*). Angiomap (**f**) exhibits persistent kinetics involving the anterior NME component extending to the nipple. Slab reformatted images (**g–i**) are shown. Final histology: DCIS high and intermediate grade, cribriform with calcification and necrosis spanning 14 cm, involving the lactiferous ducts. Rare foci of microinvasion < 1 mm present, sentinel node surgery negative for axillary metastases, ER/PR (+), HER-2/neu (–). This case illustrates the importance of high contrast and spatial resolution imaging for detection of linear (ductal) enhancement, and the benefit of slab reformatting for assessing the extent of NME.

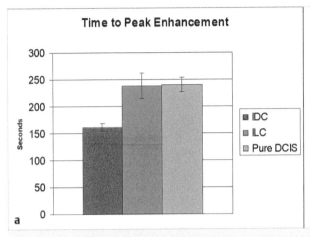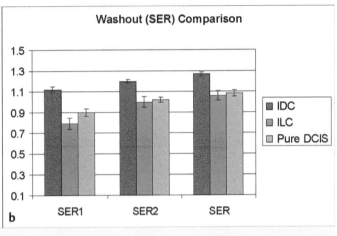

Fig. 7.38 (a, b) Kinetic analysis: cancer by histologic type.

7.7 Summary

Multiple studies have shown that only about 20-30% of the cancers diagnosed at mammography screening are detected at the noninvasive stage; therefore, there is room for improvement in early diagnosis. The increased sensitivity for MRI detection of DCIS in recent years is likely due to improved spatial and temporal resolution, made possible with use of modern higher field strength magnets and newer acquisition protocols. Ultrafast (UF) perfusion imaging is able to detect NME even at lower spatial resolution, with the advantage that absence of BPE in these 1- to 30-second images greatly improves lesion conspicuity. Despite important gains in improved detection of DCIS, important questions remain: What is the precise mechanism for DCIS enhancement at MRI? How can we confidently identify indolent subsets of DCIS and thus select a subset of patients who might benefit from less aggressive therapy?

The central question for clinical management of all women with a DCIS diagnosis concerns risk prediction for invasion. Studies of the biology of DCIS lesions have shown us that the marked inter- and intralesion heterogeneity found in DCIS is governed by alteration of molecular pathways responsible for regulating cellular proliferation, apoptosis, and genome integrity. The significance of molecular signatures in this context is not fully understood; the microenvironment likely plays an important role and it is reasonable to expect that some preinvasive breast cancer progression is predetermined and some progression is governed by stochastic events occurring over time. Quantitative mathematical modeling of high temporal resolution kinetic data, unlike the typical qualitative or semi-quantitative measures that are used currently in clinical practice, could provide further insight into DCIS biology and ultimately improve diagnosis and treatment. There is the intriguing possibility that by use of high-resolution MR techniques, correlations could be established between lesion biomarkers such as MVD, ER status, and quantitative MR enhancement characteristics. Such profiles could yield surrogate imaging parameters that could provide prognostic and predictive markers for both preinvasive and invasive disease.

Providing answers to these questions could help guide physicians toward individual treatment for patients and spare some women with less aggressive disease from "*overtreatment.*" In the context of a general concern about *overdiagnosis*, understanding the biology of DCIS is critical step toward achieving the important clinical goal of risk stratification and confident identification of low-risk subsets of women. Although not every woman undergoes routine breast cancer screening, those who do might benefit from the higher overall increased sensitivity obtained by MRI. It is possible the detection of small aggressive DCIS lesions at MR screening will improve overall patient outcome beyond the current clinical practice that relies primarily on the proven benefits of mammography.

References

[1] Leonard GD, Swain SM. Ductal carcinoma in situ, complexities and challenges. J Natl Cancer Inst. 2004; 96(12):906–920

[2] Page DL, Dupont WD, Rogers LW, Landenberger M. Intraductal carcinoma of the breast: follow-up after biopsy only. Cancer. 1982; 49(4):751–758

[3] Kuhl CK, Schrading S, Bieling HB, et al. MRI for diagnosis of pure ductal carcinoma in situ: a prospective observational study. Lancet. 2007; 370(9586): 485–492

[4] Tot T. Subgross morphology, the sick lobe hypothesis, and the success of breast conservation. Int J Breast Cancer. 2011; 2011:634021

[5] Tabar L, Tot T, Dean PB. Breast Cancer: Early Detection with Mammography. Stuttgart: Georg Thieme Verlag; 2007:129–172

[6] Fitzgibbons PL, Page DL, Weaver D, et al. Prognostic factors in breast cancer. College of American Pathologists Consensus Statement 1999. Arch Pathol Lab Med. 2000; 124(7):966–978

[7] Hieken TJ, Farolan M, D'Alessandro S, Velasco JM. Predicting the biologic behavior of ductal carcinoma in situ: an analysis of molecular markers. Surgery. 2001; 130(4):593–600, discussion 600–601

[8] Guidi AJ, Fischer L, Harris JR, Schnitt SJ. Microvessel density and distribution in ductal carcinoma in situ of the breast. J Natl Cancer Inst. 1994; 86(8):614–619

[9] Kerlikowske K, Molinaro AM, Gauthier ML, et al. Biomarker expression and risk of subsequent tumors after initial ductal carcinoma in situ diagnosis. J Natl Cancer Inst. 2010; 102(9):627–637

[10] Allred DC, Wu Y, Mao S, et al. Ductal carcinoma in situ and the emergence of diversity during breast cancer evolution. Clin Cancer Res. 2008; 14(2):370–378

[11] Polyak K. Molecular markers for the diagnosis and management of ductal carcinoma in situ. J Natl Cancer Inst Monogr. 2010; 2010(41):210–213

[12] Tamimi RM, Baer HJ, Marotti J, et al. Comparison of molecular phenotypes of ductal carcinoma in situ and invasive breast cancer. Breast Cancer Res. 2008; 10(4):R67

[13] Kuerer HM, Albarracin CT, Yang WT, et al. Ductal carcinoma in situ: state of the science and roadmap to advance the field. J Clin Oncol. 2009; 27(2):279–288

[14] James JJ, Evans AJ, Pinder SE, Macmillan RD, Wilson AR, Ellis IO. Is the presence of mammographic comedo calcification really a prognostic factor for small screen-detected invasive breast cancers? Clin Radiol. 2003; 58(1):54–62

[15] Lodato RF, Maguire HC , Jr, Greene MI, Weiner DB, LiVolsi VA. Immunohisto-chemical evaluation of c-erbB-2 oncogene expression in ductal carcinoma in situ and atypical ductal hyperplasia of the breast. Mod Pathol. 1990; 3(4):449–454

[16] Pickles MD, Gibbs P, Hubbard A, Rahman A, Wieczorek J, Turnbull LW. Comparison of 3.0 T magnetic resonance imaging and X-ray mammography in the measurement of ductal carcinoma in situ: a comparison with histopathology. Eur J Radiol. 2015; 84(4):603–610

[17] American College of Radiology. Breast Imaging Reporting and Data System. 2nd ed. https://www.acr.org/Clinical-Resources/Reporting-and-Data-Systems/Bi-Rads

[18] Allegra CJ, Aberle DR, Ganschow P, et al. National Institutes of Health State-of-the-Science Conference statement: Diagnosis and Management of Ductal Carcinoma In Situ September 22–24, 2009. J Natl Cancer Inst. 201 0; 102(3):161–169

[19] Erbas B, Provenzano E, Armes J, Gertig D. The natural history of ductal carcinoma in situ of the breast: a review. Breast Cancer Res Treat. 2006; 97(2):135–144

[20] Holland R, Hendriks JH, Vebeek AL, Mravunac M, Schuurmans Stekhoven JH. Extent, distribution, and mammographic/histological correlations of breast ductal carcinoma in situ. Lancet. 1990; 335(8688):519–522

[21] Tozaki M, Igarashi T, Fukuda K. Breast MRI using the VIBE sequence: clustered ring enhancement in the differential diagnosis of lesions showing non-mass-like enhancement. AJR Am J Roentgenol. 2006; 187(2):313–321

[22] Jansen SA, Shimauchi A, Zak L, et al. Kinetic curves of malignant lesions are not consistent across MRI systems: need for improved standardization of breast dynamic contrast-enhanced MRI acquisition. AJR Am J Roentgenol. 2009; 193(3):832–839

[23] Caliskan M, Gatti G, Sosnovskikh I, et al. Paget's disease of the breast: the experience of the European Institute of Oncology and review of the literature. Breast Cancer Res Treat. 2008; 112(3):513–521

[24] Jansen SA, Fan X, Karczmar GS, et al. DCEMRI of breast lesions: is kinetic analysis equally effective for both mass and nonmass-like enhancement? Med Phys. 2008; 35(7):3102–3109

[25] Jansen SA, Shimauchi A, Zak L, Fan X, Karczmar GS, Newstead GM. The diverse pathology and kinetics of mass, nonmass, and focus enhancement on MR imaging of the breast. J Magn Reson Imaging. 2011; 33(6):1382–1389

[26] Jansen SA, Newstead GM, Abe H, Shimauchi A, Schmidt RA, Karczmar GS. Pure ductal carcinoma in situ: kinetic and morphologic MR characteristics compared with mammographic appearance and nuclear grade. Radiology. 2007; 245(3):684–691

[27] Viehweg P, Lampe D, Buchmann J, Heywang-Köbrunner SH. In situ and minimally invasive breast cancer: morphologic and kinetic features on contrast-enhanced MR imaging. MAGMA. 2000; 11(3):129–137

[28] Guidi AJ, Schnitt SJ, Fischer L, et al. Vascular permeability factor (vascular endothelial growth factor) expression and angiogenesis in patients with ductal carcinoma in situ of the breast. Cancer. 1997; 80(10):1945–1953

[29] Heffelfinger SC, Miller MA, Yassin R, Gear R. Angiogenic growth factors in preinvasive breast disease. Clin Cancer Res. 1999; 5(10):2867–2876.m

[30] Heffelfinger SC, Yassin R, Miller MA, Lower E. Vascularity of proliferative breast disease and carcinoma in situ correlates with histological features. Clin Cancer Res. 1996; 2(11):1873–1878

[31] Esserman L, Hylton N, George T, Weidner N. Contrast-enhanced magnetic resonance imaging to assess tumor histopathology and angiogenesis in breast carcinoma. Breast J. 1999; 5(1):13–21

[32] Jansen SA, Paunesku T, Fan X, et al. Ductal carcinoma in situ: X-ray fluorescence microscopy and dynamic contrast-enhanced MR imaging reveals gadolinium uptake within neoplastic mammary ducts in a murine model. Radiology. 2009; 253(2):399–406

[33] Damonte P, Hodgson JG, Chen JQ, Young LJ, Cardiff RD, Borowsky AD. Mammary carcinoma behavior is programmed in the precancer stem cell. Breast Cancer Res. 2008; 10(3):R50

[34] Namba R, Maglione JE, Davis RR, et al. Heterogeneity of mammary lesions represent molecular differences. BMC Cancer. 2006; 6:275

[35] Namba R, Maglione JE, Young LJ, et al. Molecular characterization of the transition to malignancy in a genetically engineered mouse-based model of ductal carcinoma in situ. Mol Cancer Res. 2004; 2(8):453–463

[36] Narod SA, Iqbal J, Giannakeas V, Sopik V, Sun P. Breast cancer mortality after a diagnosis of ductal carcinoma in situ. JAMA Oncol. 2015; 1(7):888–896

[37] Esserman L, Yau C. Rethinking the standard for ductal carcinoma in situ treatment. JAMA Oncol. 2015; 1(7):881–883

[38] Cuzick J, Sestak I, Pinder SE, et al. Effect of tamoxifen and radiotherapy in women with locally excised ductal carcinoma in situ: long-term results from the UK/ANZ DCIS trial. Lancet Oncol. 2011; 12(1):21–29

[39] Duffy SW, Dibden A, Michalopoulos D, et al. Screen detection of ductal carcinoma in situ and subsequent incidence of invasive interval breast cancers: a retrospective population-based study. Lancet Oncol. 2016; 17 (1):109–114

[40] Francis A, Fallowfield L, Rea D. The LORIS Trial: Addressing overtreatment of ductal carcinoma in situ. Clin Oncol (R Coll Radiol). 2015; 27(1):6–8

8 Image Interpretation: Invasive Cancer

Gillian M. Newstead

Abstract

In this chapter, we review the imaging characteristics of invasive breast cancer, focusing primarily on their various morphologic and kinetic findings on MRI. Additionally, we discuss the heterogeneous nature not only of the imaging findings, but also the clinical, histologic and molecular characteristics of invasive breast cancer as they apply to patient outcome. Microarray-based, high-throughput gene expression profiling methods have been applied to the investigation of breast cancer. These efforts are aimed towards improved understanding of the molecular basis of tumor biological features such as histologic grade, metastatic propensity, and identification of tumor genetic signatures that are associated with prognosis and therapeutic response. We show the imaging characteristics of invasive breast cancer and characterize their findings on MRI according to the BI-RADS Atlas-MRI. The most common histologic type of invasive breast cancer is now classified as Invasive Breast Carcinoma of No Special Type (IBC-NST), a change from the prior edition of the WHO Classification of Tumors of the Breast where it was designated Invasive Ductal Carcinoma Not Otherwise Specified (IDC-NOS). We review the MR imaging findings for invasive cancers grouped by both histology and their molecular signatures. These findings are shown in the 86 case examples that accompany this chapter.

As future research unfolds, it is possible that the imaging phenotype of invasive breast cancer, particularly as applied to DCE-MRI with associated advanced computer analysis, may well provide even more independent prognostic and predictive markers, complementing existing biomarkers, and thus improving patient care.

Keywords: MR Imaging of invasive cancer, molecular signatures of breast cancer, invasive carcinoma no special type (NST), invasive lobular carcinoma, histologic subtypes of invasive cancer, tubular subtype, mucinous subtype, medullary subtype, papillary subtype, luminal A subtype, luminal B subtype, HER2/neu-enriched subtype, triple-negative and basal-like sub-type, inflammatory breast cancer (IBC), uncommon tumor subtypes

8.1 Introduction

In this chapter, we will review the magnetic resonance imaging (MRI) characteristics of the various subtypes of invasive cancer and correlate the MR lesion phenotype and kinetic characteristics with histology and established biomarkers.

8.2 Background

Invasive breast cancer is a heterogeneous disease often harboring various histologic subtypes within a main tumor mass (intratumoral heterogeneity) or within separate tumor satellite lesions (intertumoral heterogeneity). Histologic heterogeneity may be found even within the morphologic types of invasive cancer, such as ductal, lobular, and other less common

subtypes.[1] For many decades, breast cancer treatment has been primarily guided by the histologic classification of cancers using tumor grade, morphology, and the tumor–node–metastasis (TNM) staging method, based on cancer size, nodal status, and the presence or absence of distant metastases. The TNM classification predates the era of modern imaging and identifies the size of the largest invasive tumor focus as the main descriptive factor, discounting tumor multifocality in the overall assessment.[3] Tumors vary in both grade and histopathology. Grade is based on cellular differentiation: the higher the grade, the more "poorly differentiated" the cancer cells. It is well known that imaging phenotypes based on morphologic analysis of invasive cancers seen on mammography, ultrasound, and MRI can provide prognostic information.

In recent years, molecular subtyping of breast cancer has complemented the standard histologic classification to encompass treatment stratification based on prognostic indicators.[3,4] Microarray-based, high-throughput gene expression profiling methods have been applied to the investigation of breast cancer. These efforts are aimed toward improved understanding of the molecular basis of tumor biological features such as histologic grade, metastatic propensity, and identification of tumor genetic signatures that are associated with prognosis and therapeutic response. Although molecular subtyping for every patient with breast cancer could potentially enable clinicians to guide therapy more effectively, the costs of genetic analysis are high because of the need for technical expertise, and specialized equipment for individual sample processing. Molecular subtype analysis is not currently feasible for all patients and other markers have been established. Immunohistochemical (IHC) analyses are used to substitute for genetic profiling and are widely used in clinical practice. IHC markers of breast cancer include estrogen (ER) and progesterone (PR) receptors, and HER-2/neu overexpression. They have the advantage of rapid testing at a lower cost than formal genetic analysis; however, their results have been less robustly predictive of patient outcomes. A report by the IMPAKT 2012 Working Group on molecular subclasses of breast cancer showed that concordance for molecular subtype classification, between IHC and formal genetic analysis, ranges from 41 to 100% within varying subtypes.[5] Despite increased costs, tumor stratification based on tumor biology and gene expression profiles derived from DNA microarrays can now be made available to patients and are slowly being integrated into clinical practice.

The original influential studies published by Perou et al[6,7] defined a molecular subtype classification of breast cancer into four main categories: luminal A, luminal B, HER-2/neu positive, and basal-like. These groups are distinguished by distinct patterns of genomic additions and deletions, providing prognostic information and influencing systemic treatment decisions. The main distinction between these molecular subtypes is at the ER level and secondarily on the level of HER-2/neu. Of these molecular subtypes, two are ER positive, the luminal A (human epidermal growth factor receptor 2 negative [HER2–]) and luminal B (HER2+) groups, and two are ER negative, the basal (HER2–) and ERBB2 (HER2+) groups. These transcriptome-

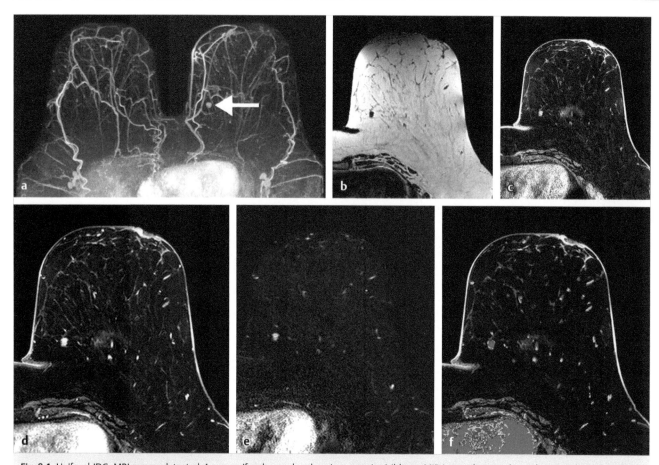

Fig. 8.1 Unifocal IDC. MRI screen-detected 4-mm unifocal, round, enhancing mass is visible on MIP image (**a**, *arrow*) as a low signal mass on T2w image (**b**) and on precontrast T1w image (**c**). Postcontrast source and subtracted images (**d,e**) show margin irregularity and angiomap (**f**) shows washout enhancement within the mass. Histology: IDC grade 3, with apocrine features. ER/PR (+), HER-2/neu (–).

based subtypes[1] correlate well with other histological and clinical features; luminal A and B lesions generally are of a lower grade with a more favorable prognosis when compared to basal and ERBB2 subtypes, which are often higher grade with a worse prognosis. Additionally, rapidly growing tumors overexpress genes such as Ki-67, a marker of cellular proliferation known to correlate with increased mitotic indices at histopathology. Prognostic information, obtained from the tumor of each individual patient using tumor genetic signatures, or IHC markers, can guide therapy and provide selected treatment for each individual patient. Why are imaging biomarkers important? Imaging is quantitative, can sample the entire cancer, measure intratumoral heterogeneity, and complement other predictive and prognostic indicators. Serial imaging is noninvasive and can monitor tumor response during therapy.

8.3 MRI of Invasive Cancer

The vast majority of invasive cancers present as masses, noting that only a small subset of invasive cancers exhibit non–mass

enhancement as the primary imaging finding. The most common histologic type of invasive breast cancer is now classified as invasive breast carcinoma of no special type (IBC-NST), changed in the fourth edition of the World Health Organization (WHO) Classification of tumors of the breast from invasive ductal carcinoma not otherwise specified (IDC-NOS).[1] The term "ductal" is no longer included in the new definition, the rationale being that the term "ductal" conveys unproven histogenetic assumptions, and that IDC-NOS does not comprise a uniform group of cancers. The IBC-NST lesions constitute about 75 to 80% of all breast cancers; invasive lobular carcinomas (ILCs) contribute another 10 to 15%; and special subtypes, tubular, medullary, papillary, and mucinous constitute the majority of the remaining malignant lesions. Invasive tumors may be further defined by their distribution and extent and are categorized as unifocal (► Fig. 8.1; ► Fig. 8.2), multifocal/multicentric (► Fig. 8.3; ► Fig. 8.4; ► Fig. 8.5; ► Fig. 8.6), and diffuse (► Fig. 8.7).

Multifocal cancer is usually defined as disease confined to one quadrant, whereas multicentric disease may involve more than one quadrant. This distinction may be difficult to apply in clinical practice, whereas confluent tumor involvement of most of the breast tissue is easily defined as diffuse disease. Inflammatory carcinoma is distinguished by its clinical presentation rather than by a distinct histologic subtype.

[a] **Transcriptome** is the set of all messenger RNA molecules in one cell or a population of cells.

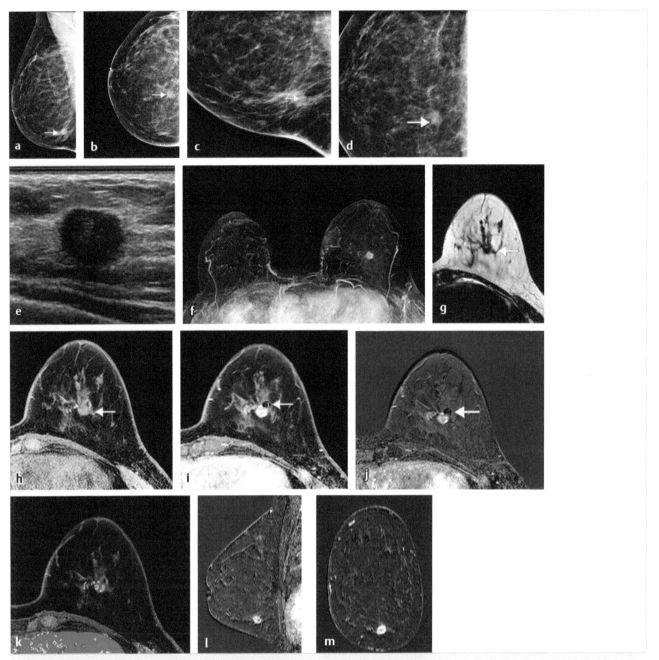

Fig. 8.2 Unifocal IDC. MLO, CC views (**a,b**, *arrows*) and spot ML and CC views (**c, d**, arrows) demonstrate a 9-mm, round, indistinct mass with an ultrasound correlate (**e**). MIP image (**f**) demonstrates a unifocal round mass, visible on precontrast series, hypointense on T2w (**g**, *arrow*) and isointense on T1w (**h**, *arrow*). Postcontrast source and subtracted images (**i, j**) show the mass to exhibit rim enhancement and an adjacent postbiopsy marker clip is present (*arrows*). Angiomap with washout kinetics (**k**) and sagittal and coronal reconstructed images (**l, m**) are also shown. Histology: IDC grade 2. ER/PR (+), HER-2/neu (−).

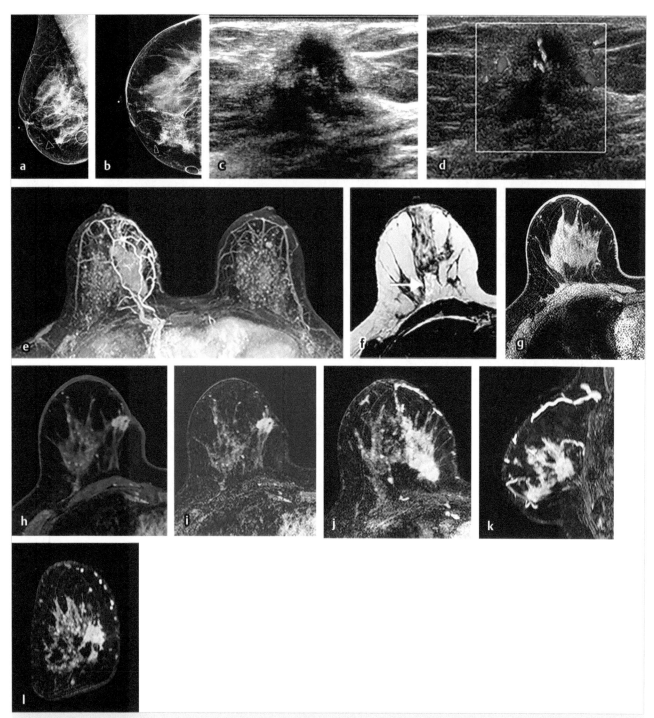

Fig. 8.3 Multicentric ID. A 43-year-old patient presented with a 4-cm palpable mass in the inferomedial right breast, visible on MLO and CC views (**a, b**) as an irregular, spiculated mass with fine pleomorphic internal calcifications. Ultrasound correlate (**c, d**) shows an irregular shadowing mass with internal vascularity. MIP image (**e**) demonstrates confluent abnormal enhancement throughout the right medial breast with increased vascularity and marked bilateral BPE. T2w image exhibits anterior skin thickening and fluid is seen posterior to the mass extending to the pectoral muscle indicating an aggressive lesion (**f**, *arrow*). Precontrast image (**g**) shows anterior skin thickening. Postcontrast source and subtracted images (**h, i**) show diffuse skin thickening without skin enhancement and an irregular mass with heterogeneous internal enhancement, and linear enhancement extending to the nipple. MPR slab images (**j-l**) show the extent of malignant involvement. Histology: IDC (tubulo-lobular) grade 2, focally associated with DCIS, low and intermediate nuclear grade, cribriform, micropapillary and solid type, ER/PR (+), HER-2/neu (−), blood vessel and lymphatic invasion. 20/29 axillary lymph nodes were confirmed positive for malignancy.

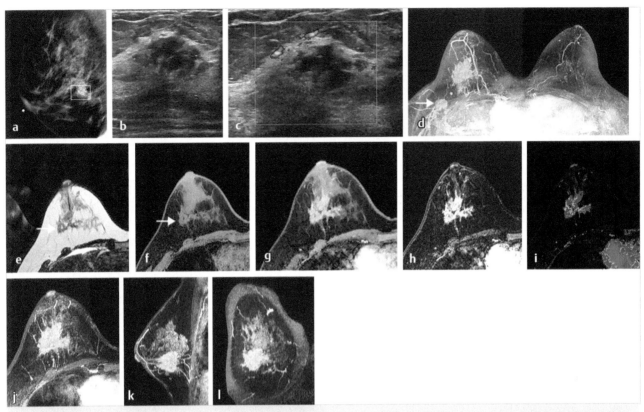

Fig. 8.4 Multifocal IDC. A partly obscured right breast mass with internal pleomorphic calcifications is seen on a cropped MLO MG view (**a**). Correlative ultrasound shows an irregular hypoechoic mass with rim vessels (**b, c**). An irregular enhancing mass is found on MIP image (**d**) with associated increased breast vascularity and an enlarged axillary lymph node (*arrow*). The mass is hypointense on T2 (**e**, *arrow*) and isointense on T1 precontrast (**f**, *arrow*), and exhibits heterogeneous internal enhancement and increased size, on postcontrast source and subtracted images (**g, h**). Angiomap (**i**) exhibits heterogeneous enhancement with washout and slab MPR images (**j-l**) are shown. Histology: IDC grade 2 with lymphovascular invasion and DCIS, high nuclear grade, comedo type and solid type. ER/PR (+), HER-2/neu (−). Six axillary lymph nodes were positive for malignancy (6/21).

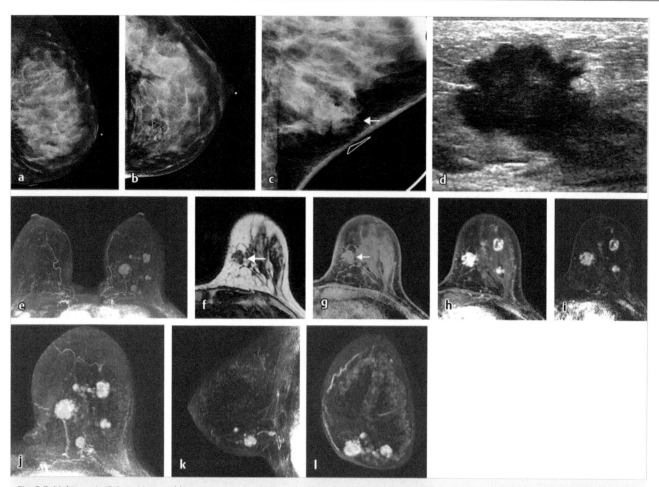

Fig. 8.5 Multicentric IDC. A 44-year-old woman presents with a palpable mass in the inferior, posterior, and medial left breast, identified with a skin marker, but obscured on MLO and CC views (**a,b**) and visible on a spot MG view (**c**). Correlative ultrasound demonstrates an irregular spiculated mass (**d**). MIP image (**e**) shows multiple irregular masses in the mid and posterior left breast. The largest palpable mass exhibits hypointensity on T2w (**f**), isointensity on T1 precontrast (**g**), and multiple homogeneous enhancing masses of various sizes on postcontrast series (**h, i**). Slab MPR images (**j-l**) demonstrate to advantage the overall lesion sizes and location. Histology: IDC grade 2, ER (+), PR (−), HER-2/neu (+).

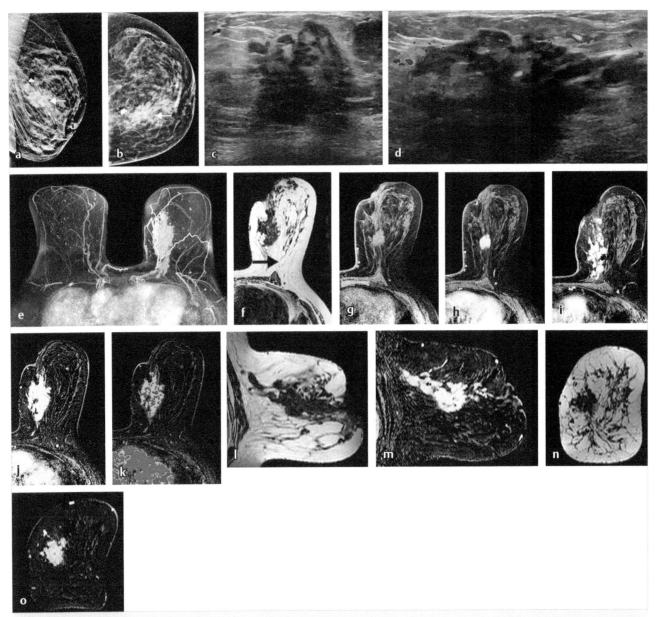

Fig. 8.6 Multicentric IDC. Screen-detected asymmetry is seen at 9:00 on LT MG- MLO/CC views (**a,b,** *arrows*) just inferior and anterior to an incidental calcified fibroadenoma. Correlative ultrasound reveals an irregular heterogeneous mass with internal vascularity (**c,d**). MIP image (**e**) shows extensive confluent enhancement in the medial left breast. T2w image (**f**) demonstrates a correlative area of hypointensity and posterior fluid extending to the pectoral muscle (*arrow*), a sign of tumor aggressiveness. The primary mass is isointense on precontrast T1w image (**g**) and enhances robustly on the source image (**h**). Adjacent slice (**i**) shows the extent of tumor involvement with multiple additional masses of various sizes demonstrated. Confluent enhancement, with internal focal areas of necrosis, is seen on source image (**j**) with heterogeneous kinetics, including washout, seen on angiomap (**k**). Reformatted T2w and T1w images, in the sagittal and coronal planes are shown (**l-o**). Histology: IDC grade 3, ER (+), PR (–), HER-2/neu (+), Ki-67: 20%.

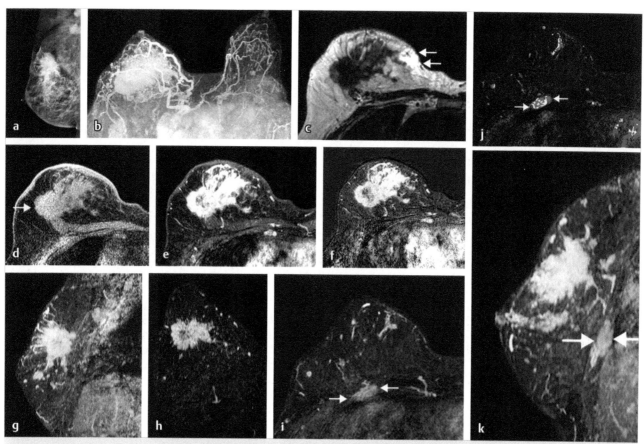

Fig. 8.7 Diffuse IDC. A large palpable right breast mass with skin marker and lymphadenopathy is seen on MG image (**a**) and MIP image (**b**). The mass is hypointense on T2w (**c**) and medial fluid is present (*arrows*). Precontrast image (**d**) identifies the isointense mass (*arrow*) which enhances robustly and heterogeneously, with spiculation noted on postcontrast source and subtracted images (**e, f**). Diffuse skin thickening, but no skin enhancement, is present. Sagittal and coronal slab images (**g, h**) show extent of disease. Enhancement of the pectoral muscle on axial, angiomap, and sagittal images (**i-k**, *arrows*) denote pectoral muscle invasion. Histology: inflammatory carcinoma, IDC grade 2, with malignant involvement of dermal lymphatics. ER/PR (+), HER-2/neu (–), LVN. Sixteen axillary lymph nodes were positive for malignancy (16/25).

Table 8.1 Mass descriptors

Shape	Margin	Internal enhancement characteristics
Oval	Circumscribed	Homogeneous
Round	Not circumscribed	Heterogeneous
Irregular	- Irregular	Rim enhancement
	- Spiculated	Dark internal septations

American College of Radiology ACR BI-RADS. Magnetic resonance imaging. Source: ACR Breast Imaging Reporting and Data System, Breast Imaging Atlas. Reston, VA: American College of Radiology; 2013:1-178

Table 8.2 Nonenhancing findings

Ductal high-contrast signal on T1w	Posttherapy skin thickening and trabecular thickening
Cyst	Architectural distortion
Postoperative collections (seroma, hematoma)	Signal void from foreign bodies, clips, etc.
Nonenhancing mass	

American College of Radiology ACR BI-RADS. Magnetic resonance imaging. Source: ACR Breast Imaging Reporting and Data System, Breast Imaging Atlas. Reston, VA: American College of Radiology; 2013:1-178

8.3.1 BI-RADS Atlas—MRI

The BI-RADS Atlas[8] defines a mass as a three-dimensional space-occupying structure, with a convex-outward contour and is further categorized by shape, margin, and internal enhancement characteristics. High spatial resolution techniques allow optimal morphologic analysis with superior definition of both shape and margins. A mass may or may not displace or otherwise affect the surrounding normal breast tissue, and may be associated with other enhancing or nonenhancing findings (► Table 8.1; ► Table 8.2).

Shape Descriptors

An oval mass is elliptical or egg-shaped and includes lobulation, with two or three undulations (► Fig. 8.8; ► Fig. 8.9; ► Fig. 8.10). A round mass is spherical, ball-shaped, circular, or globular in shape (► Fig. 8.11) and an irregular lesion's shape is neither round nor oval and usually implies a suspicious finding (► Fig. 8.12).

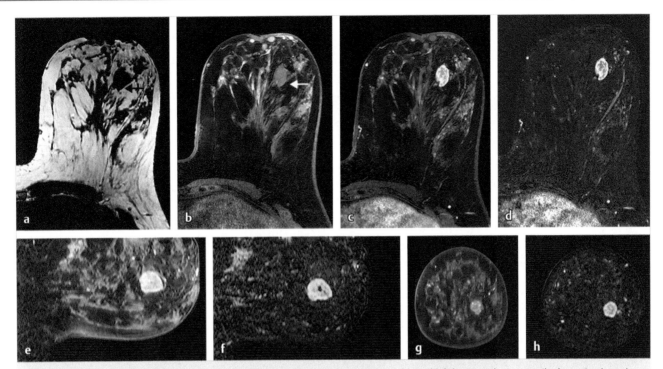

Fig. 8.8 Oval mass. Tubular adenoma. **(a)** T2w: hypointense oval mass in the anterior and lateral left breast with circumscribed margins (*arrow*). **(b)** T1w precontrast: isointense oval mass (*arrow*). **(c)** T1w postcontrast 120s: heterogeneously enhancing oval mass with circumscribed margins. **(d)** Subtraction image. **(e-h)**. Source and subtraction reformatted sagittal and coronal images.

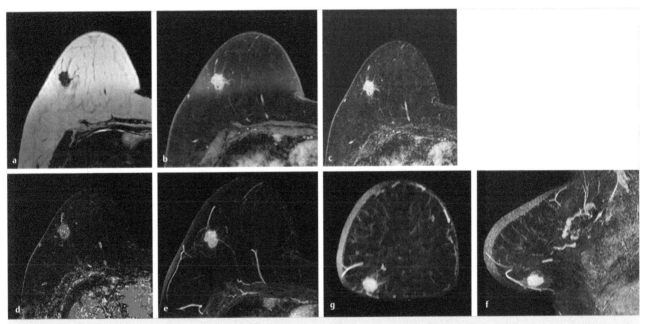

Fig. 8.9 Oval mass: IDC grade 2. **(a)** T2w: hypointense oval mass with spiculation. **(b)** T1w precontrast: hyperintense irregular mass. **(c)** T1w postcontrast: heterogeneous enhancement and spiculated margins. **(d)** Subtraction image. **(e)** Angiomap shows washout enhancement. **(f, g)** Multiplanar slab images.

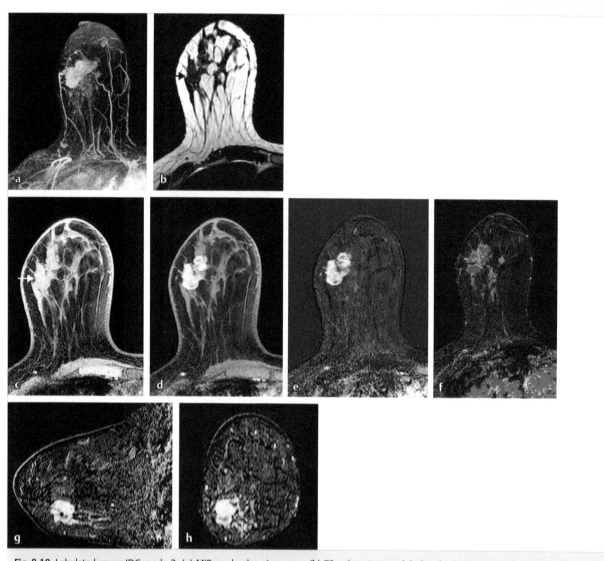

Fig. 8.10 Lobulated mass: IDC grade 2. (**a**) MIP: oval enhancing mass. (**b**) T2w: hypointense lobulated mass (*arrow*). (**c**) T1w precontrast: isointense mass (*arrow*). (**d**) T1w postcontrast: lobulated mass with heterogeneous internal enhancement. (**e**) Subtraction image. (**f**) Angiomap: predominantly persistent enhancement with some washout. (**g, h**) Sagittal and coronal reformatted images.

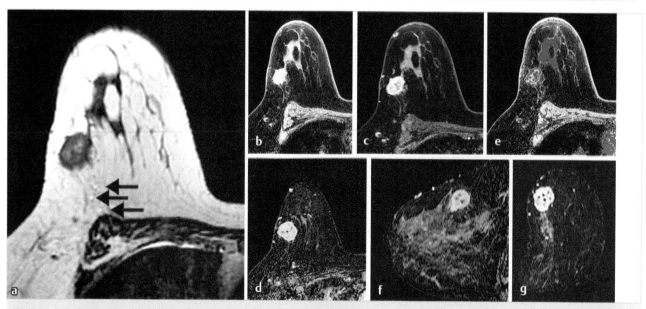

Fig. 8.11 Round mass: IDC triple negative. (**a**) T2w: hyperintense round mass with irregular margins. Note: linear fluid posterior to the cancer, sign of an aggressive tumor (*arrows*). (**b**) T1w precontrast: hyperintense round mass. (**c**) T1w postcontrast: heterogeneous internal enhancement, irregular margins. (**d**) Subtraction image. (**e**) Angiomap: washout kinetics. (**f, g**) Reformatted sagittal and coronal images.

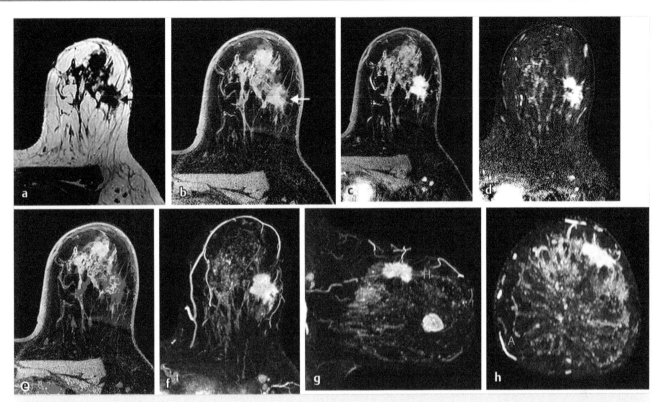

Fig. 8.12 Irregular mass: IDC. (**a**) T2w: hypointense irregular mass with irregular margins (*arrow*). (**b**) T1w precontrast: isointense irregular mass (*arrow*). (**c**) T1w postcontrast: homogeneous internal enhancement, with spiculation. (**d**) Subtraction image. (**e**) Angiomap: heterogeneous uptake with washout kinetics. (**f-h**) MPR slab images.

Margin Descriptors

The margin is the edge or border of a lesion. The descriptors of margin, in addition to the descriptors of shape, are important predictors of benignity or malignancy. A circumscribed margin (changed from smooth in the prior lexicon) is sharply demarcated with an abrupt transition between the lesion and surrounding tissue (▶ Fig. 8.13). The entire margin must be well defined in its entirety to be qualified as "circumscribed." A not circumscribed margin may be categorized as irregular, edges that are either uneven or jagged (▶ Fig. 8.14), or spiculated, lines radiating from a mass implying a suspicious finding (▶ Fig. 8.15; ▶ Fig. 8.16; ▶ Fig. 8.17; ▶ Fig. 8.18). When reporting a mass with both irregular shape and margin, the MRI report should indicate that there is "a mass of irregular shape and margin." In general, circumscribed masses are indicative of benign lesions in all imaging methods in contradistinction to noncircumscribed masses, which are suspicious for carcinoma. Margin analysis is highly dependent on optimal spatial and temporal resolution for accurate diagnosis at MRI.

Internal Enhancement Characteristics

Internal enhancement describes the enhancement pattern within an abnormally enhancing structure, and is an important reflection of lesion biology.[9] Enhancement patterns are characterized as homogeneous, a confluent uniform enhancement of a mass, and heterogeneous, a nonuniform enhancement of a mass with variable signal intensity. Homogeneous enhancement is suggestive of a benign process; however, some small cancers can exhibit homogeneous enhancement, and careful margin assessment with high spatial and temporal resolution is essential for an accurate diagnosis of benignity (▶ Fig. 8.19). Heterogeneous enhancement is generally more characteristic of malignant lesions (▶ Fig. 8.20).[9] Rim enhancement is more pronounced at the periphery of a mass, and is commonly seen in high-grade malignancies. Cysts can become inflamed and enhance peripherally, but are usually bright on T2-weighted (T2w) sequences confirming internal fluid, unless they are very small or contain proteinaceous material (▶ Fig. 8.21). Fat necrosis (oil cysts) and normal postoperative seromata may

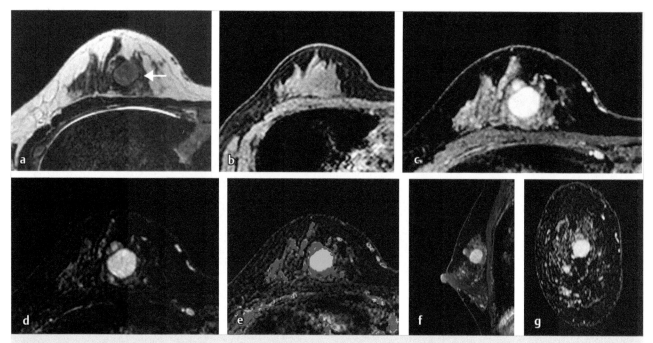

Fig. 8.13 Circumscribed margin: fibroadenoma. (**a**) T2w: hyperintense circumscribed round mass (*arrow*). (**b**) T1w precontrast: no findings. (**c**) T1w postcontrast: homogeneously enhancing mass with circumscribed margins. (**d**) Subtraction image. (**e**) Angiomap: plateau kinetics. (**f, g**) MPR slab images.

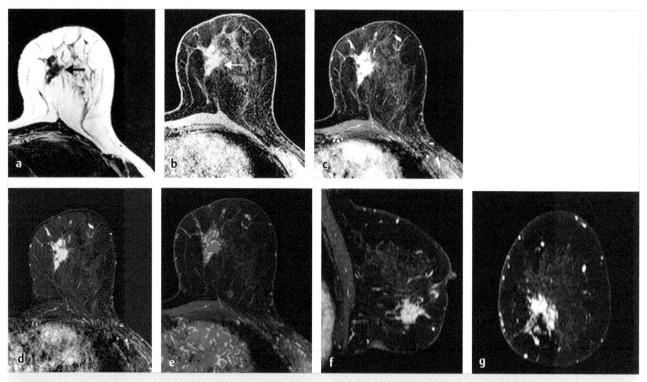

Fig. 8.14 Irregular margin: IDC grade 2, HER-2/neu +, (**a**) T2w: hypointense irregular mass and margin (*arrow*). (**b**) T1w precontrast: hyperintense irregular mass and margin (*arrow*). (**c**) T1w postcontrast: heterogeneously enhancing mass with irregular margins. (**d**) Subtraction image. (**e**) Angiomap: heterogeneous washout kinetics. (**f, g**) MPR slab images: sagittal and coronal images.

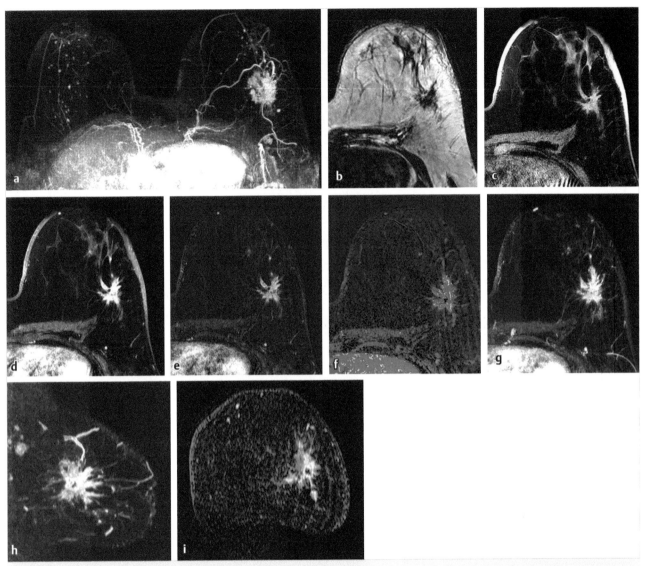

Fig. 8.15 Spiculated margin: IDC grade2. (**a**) Subtraction MIP: spiculated mass left breast with increased vascularity. (**b**) T2w: hypointense irregular mass with spiculated margins. Note subcutaneous edema and diffuse skin thickening. (**c**) T1w precontrast: isointense irregular mass with spiculated margins. Note diffuse skin thickening. (**d**) T1w postcontrast: heterogeneously enhancing mass with spiculated margins. (**e**) Subtraction image. (**f**) Angiomap: heterogeneous enhancement with washout kinetics. (**g-i**) MPR images.

exhibit smooth peripheral enhancement. Rim enhancement of a solid mass is a suspicious finding (▶ Fig. 8.22; ▶ Fig. 8.23). The MRI features with the highest predictive value for malignancy are lesion mass types with irregular shape, irregular or spiculated margins, and marked enhancement.[10] Dark internal septations are seen as nonenhancing lines within an enhancing mass. These dark septations are seen more frequently at higher spatial resolution (3.0 Tesla) on either T2w precontrast or T1-weighted (T1w) postcontrast series and are suggestive of a fibroadenoma if other morphologic and kinetic characteristics

support benignity (▶ Fig. 8.24; ▶ Fig. 8.25). Myxoid fibroadenomata are highly cellular with moderate internal mucoid material exhibiting hyperintense signal on T2 in some cases. These circumscribed masses usually show dark internal septations and heterogeneous enhancement on T1w series (▶ Fig. 8.26, ▶ Fig. 8.27). Fibroadenomata are frequently seen on breast MR studies, often occult at mammography, and must be confidently recognized as benign lesions whenever possible. Nonenhancing masses with benign morphology are benign.

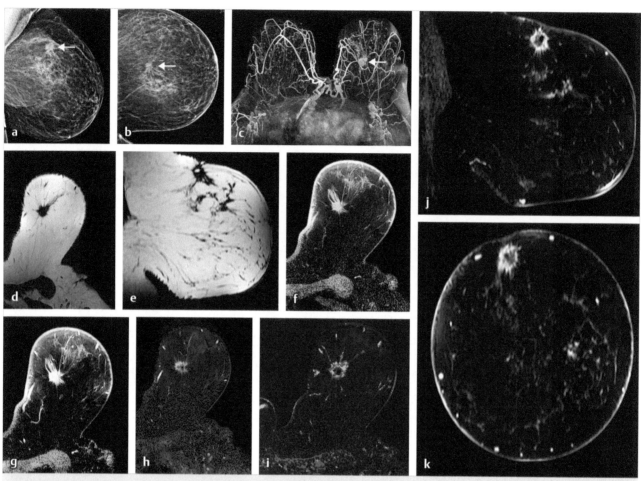

Fig. 8.16 Spiculated margin: IDC grade 2. (**a, b**) ML and CC MG views: spiculated mass at 12:00. (**c**) MIP: correlative mass (*arrow*). (**d**) T2w: hypointense irregular mass with spiculated margins. (**e**) T2w: sagittal view shows a superficial spiculated mass. (**f**) T1w precontrast: isointense small spiculated mass. (**g**) T1w postcontrast: homogeneously enhancing mass with spiculation. (**h**) Subtraction image. (**i**) Angiomap: heterogeneous washout enhancement. (**j, k**) MPR images.

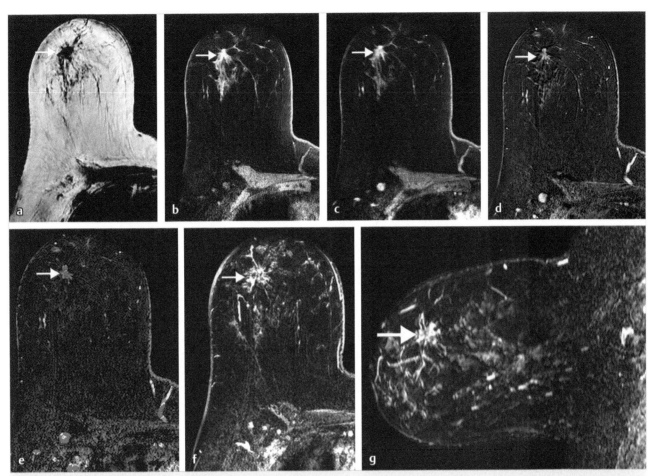

Fig. 8.17 Spiculated margin: ILC grade 2. (**a**) T2w: spiculated mass (*arrow*). (**b**) T1w precontrast: hyperintense small spiculated mass (*arrow*). (**c**) T1w postcontrast: heterogeneously enhancing mass with spiculated margins (*arrow*). (**d**) Subtraction image shows a small enhancing spiculated mass (*arrow*). (**e**) Angiomap: heterogeneous enhancement with persistent kinetics (*arrow*). (**f, g**) Axial/sagittal reformatted image (*arrows*).

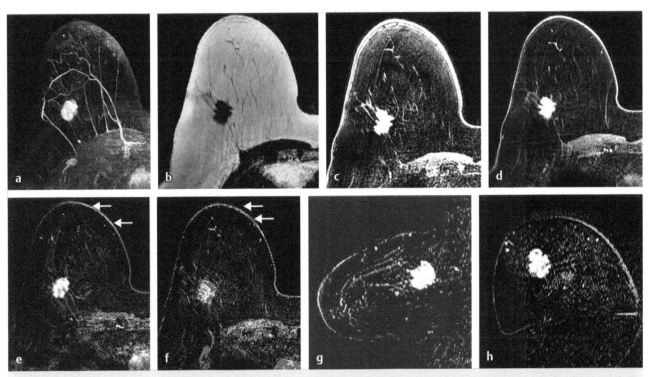

Fig. 8.18 Spiculated margin: IDC grade 2. (**a**) MIP image. (**b**) T2w: hypointense spiculated mass. (**c**) T1w precontrast: isointense spiculated mass. (**d**) T1w postcontrast: homogeneously enhancing mass with spiculated margins. (**e**) Subtraction image: note the focal medial skin enhancement from an incidental focal skin infection (*arrows*). (**f**) Angiomap: homogeneous enhancement with washout kinetics and medial skin enhancement (*arrows*). (**g, h**) Reformatted sagittal and coronal images.

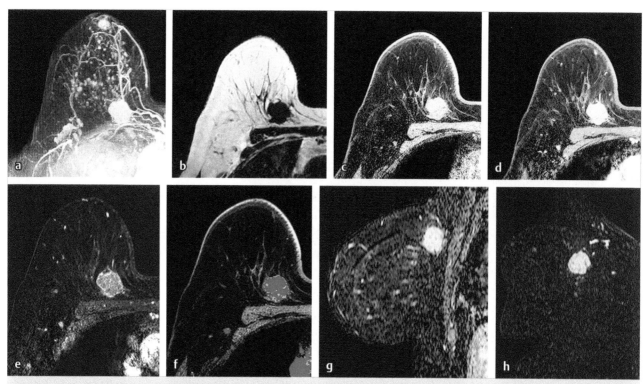

Fig. 8.19 Homogeneous enhancement. IDC grade 3: triple negative. (**a**) MIP image: homogeneously enhancing posteromedial mass. (**b**) T2w: hypointense irregular mass. (**c**) T1w precontrast: isointense mass. (**d**) T1w postcontrast source: homogeneously enhancing mass. (**e**) T1w postcontrast subtraction: thin rim and central homogeneous enhancement. (**f**) Angiomap: homogeneous internal enhancement with washout kinetics. (**g, h**) Reformatted sagittal and coronal images.

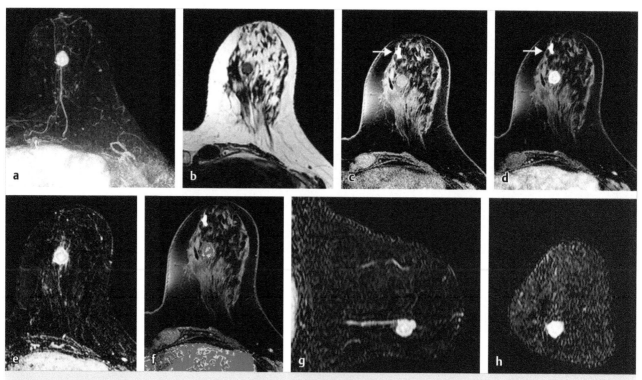

Fig. 8.20 Heterogeneous enhancement. IDC grade 3: HER2 enriched. (**a**) MIP image: heterogeneously enhancing mass with central enhancing nidus. (**b**) T2w: hypointense, round, circumscribed mass. (**c**) T1w precontrast: isointense mass with anterior ductal fluid (*arrow*). (**d**) T1w postcontrast source: heterogeneously enhancing mass with anterior ductal fluid (*arrow*). (**e**) T1w postcontrast subtraction: heterogeneously enhancing mass with central enhancing nidus (note: benign ductal fluid subtracted out). (**f**) Angiomap: heterogeneous internal enhancement with washout kinetics. (**g, h**) Reformatted sagittal and coronal images. Note focal failed fat suppression medially on source T1w images.

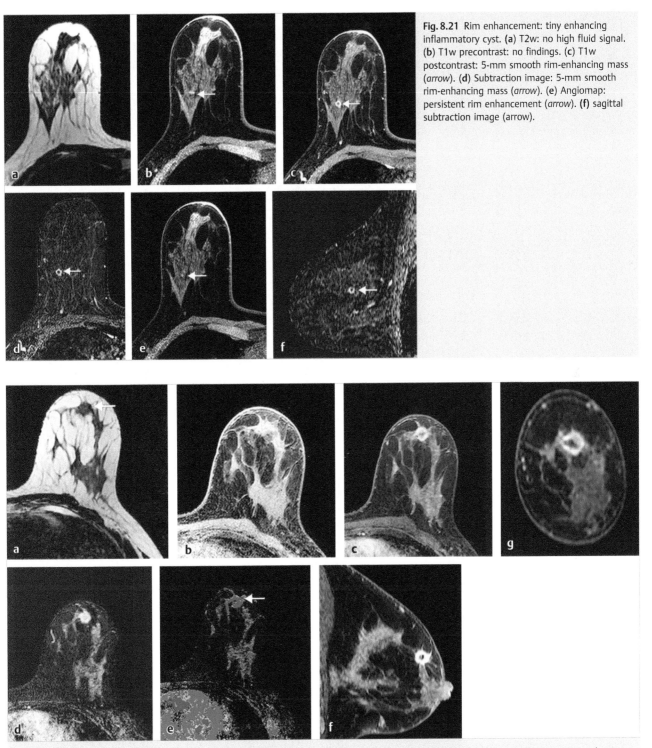

Fig. 8.21 Rim enhancement: tiny enhancing inflammatory cyst. **(a)** T2w: no high fluid signal. **(b)** T1w precontrast: no findings. **(c)** T1w postcontrast: 5-mm smooth rim-enhancing mass (*arrow*). **(d)** Subtraction image: 5-mm smooth rim-enhancing mass (*arrow*). **(e)** Angiomap: persistent rim enhancement (*arrow*). **(f)** sagittal subtraction image (arrow).

Fig. 8.22 Rim enhancement: IDC grade 2. **(a)** T2w: isointense mass (*arrow*). **(b)** T1w precontrast: no findings. **(c)** T1w postcontrast: irregular rim-enhancing mass. **(d)** Subtraction image. **(e)** Angiomap: predominantly persistent kinetics. **(f)** Sagittal image: rim enhancement with spiculation noted. **(g)** Coronal image: rim enhancement with spiculation noted.

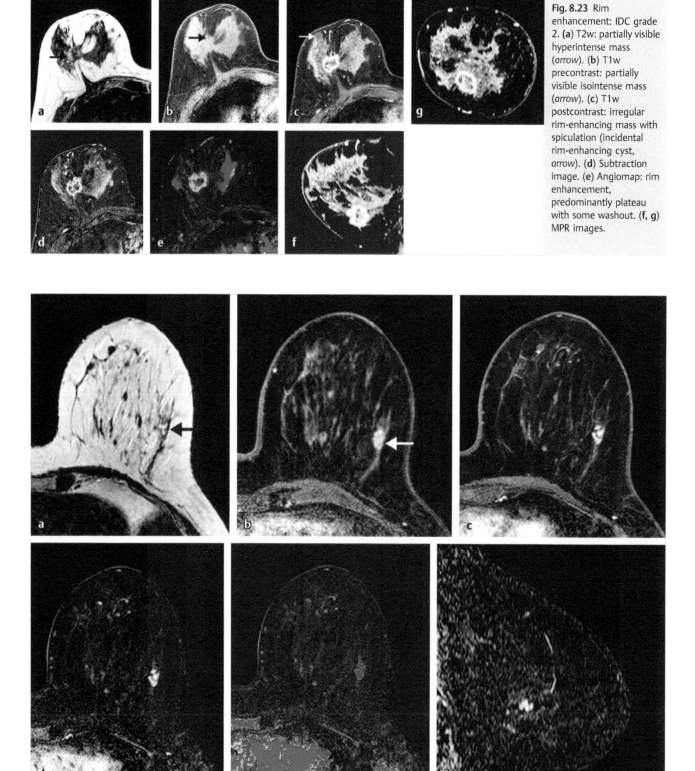

Fig. 8.23 Rim enhancement: IDC grade 2. (a) T2w: partially visible hyperintense mass (*arrow*). (b) T1w precontrast: partially visible isointense mass (*arrow*). (c) T1w postcontrast: irregular rim-enhancing mass with spiculation (incidental rim-enhancing cyst, *arrow*). (d) Subtraction image. (e) Angiomap: rim enhancement, predominantly plateau with some washout. (f, g) MPR images.

Fig. 8.24 Unenhancing internal septations: small fibroadenoma. (a) T2w: hyperintense mass (*arrow*). (b) T1w precontrast: oval mass, circumscribed margins (*arrow*). (c) T1w postcontrast: enhancing mass with unenhancing internal septations. (d) Subtraction image. (e) Angiomap: homogeneous persistent enhancement. (f) Sagittal image.

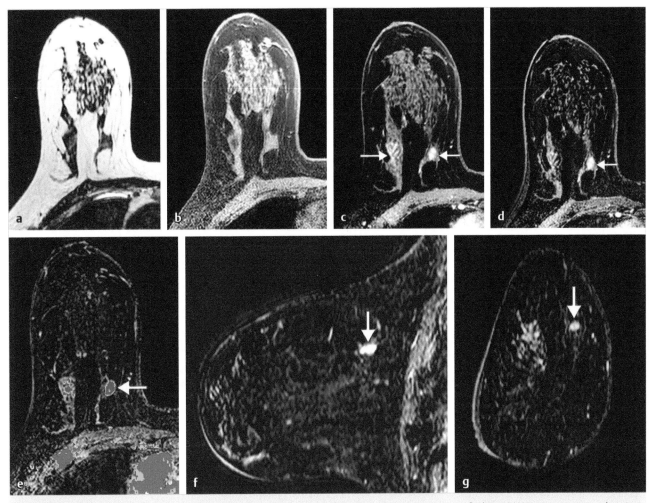

Fig. 8.25 Unenhancing internal septations: tiny fibroadenoma. **(a)** T2w: no findings. **(b)** T1w precontrast: no findings. **(c)** T1w postcontrast: enhancing mass with a transverse unenhancing internal septation (*short arrow*). Note: Focal BPE lateral to the lesion (*long arrow*). **(d)** Subtraction image: enhancing mass with a transverse unenhancing internal septation (*arrow*). **(e)** Angiomap: predominant persistent enhancement. **(f, g)** MPR images: mass with transverse septation (*arrows*).

Fat-Containing Lesions

These masses are generally benign and include lesions such as lipomata, fibroadenolipomata (hamartoma) (▶ Fig. 8.28; ▶ Fig. 8.29), and lymph nodes (▶ Fig. 8.30; ▶ Fig. 8.31). The key to accurate diagnosis is identification of fat signal within the lesion on a non–fat-suppressed high-resolution T2w or T1w series. Fat necrosis may present as a rim-enhancing mass exhibiting varying enhancement (▶ Fig. 8.32). History of prior trauma or surgery may explain the enhancing finding, and verified central fat content on non–fat-suppressed images may confirm the diagnosis (▶ Table 8.3).

T2w Precontrast Mass Findings

High-resolution T2w sequences provide important information and, when evaluating breast masses, can improve specificity of diagnosis. Comparing the morphology and signal intensity on T2w and T1w images can be helpful. High T2w signal may signify extensive necrosis seen most frequently in high-grade lesions, or in mucinous/loose myxoid stroma seen in mucinous carcinoma. Cystic or microcystic tumor components are rare and can be found most frequently in papillary cancers. Intratumoral fat-containing tissue usually indicates a benign diagnosis. The presence of peritumoral, stromal, subcutaneous, or prepectoral edema augurs an aggressive malignancy type.

Table 8.3 Fat-containing lesions

Lymph nodes: normal or abnormal	Hamartoma/Fibroadenolipoma
Fat necrosis	Postoperative seroma/hematoma with fat

Source: American College of Radiology ACR BI-RADS. Magnetic resonance imaging. Source: ACR Breast Imaging Reporting and Data System, Breast Imaging Atlas. Reston, VA: American College of Radiology; 2013:1–178.

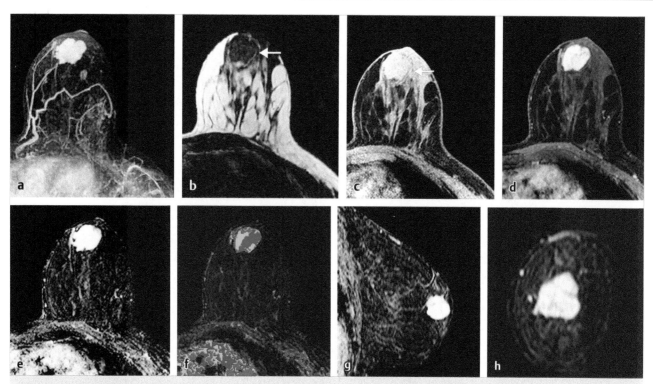

Fig. 8.26 Unenhancing internal septations: myxoid fibroadenoma. MIP Image (**a**) reveals a lobulated subareolar enhancing mass, seen as isointense on T2w (**b**) (*arrow*) and isointense on T1w precontrast image (**c**). Post contrast source and subtraction images (**d, e**) reveal robust enhancement with unenhancing internal septations and heterogeneous washout kinetics on angiomap (**f**). (**g, h**) MPR images.

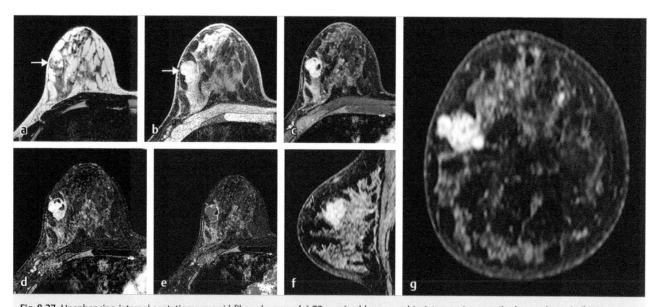

Fig. 8.27 Unenhancing internal septations: myxoid fibroadenoma. (**a**) T2w: mixed hyper- and isointense circumscribed mass (*arrow*). (**b**) T1w precontrast: isointense circumscribed mass (*arrow*). (**c**) T1w postcontrast: heterogeneously enhancing mass with unenhancing internal septations. (**d**) Subtraction image. (**e**) Angiomap: uniform persistent enhancement. (**f, g**) MPR images.

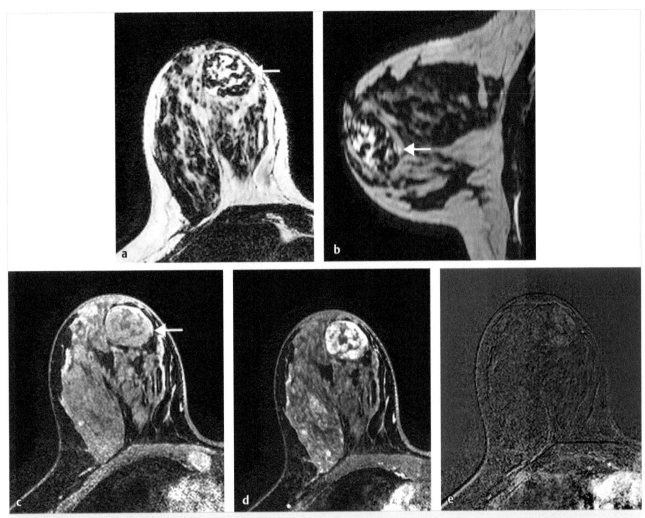

Fig. 8.28 Fat-containing lesion: fibroadenolipoma. (**a**) T2w: oval, fat-containing, circumscribed subareolar mass (*arrow*). (**b**) T2w: sagittal view (*arrow*). (**c**) T1w precontrast: thin capsule with breast tissue and internal fat signal (*arrow*). (**d**) T1w postcontrast: selective enhancement of breast tissue within the thin capsule. (**e**) Subtraction image: no findings.

8.4 Kinetic Curve Assessment

Kinetic analysis of suspect lesions should be assessed after complete evaluation of the MRI findings. The first postcontrast series is generally selected for kinetic analysis because abnormal tissue is usually most intense and distinct from normal background parenchymal enhancement at this time point. Kinetic information is typically expressed as a time intensity curve (TIC), plotting the signal intensity of the most suspicious enhancement finding on a pixel-by-pixel basis, depicting the enhancement rate over time. The TIC can be manually calculated by placing a region of interest (ROI) of at least three pixels within a lesion or can be automatically created by CAD systems (dedicated software generating lesion color maps and TIC graphs). The TIC depicts the initial phase of enhancement within the first 2 minutes following injection or until peak enhancement is reached, and the delayed phase of enhancement depicts the TIC after 2 minutes or after the peak enhancement is reached and is used to describe the curve shape. Malignancies generally enhance rapidly in the initial phase of contrast enhancement with contrast washout in the delayed phase. Evaluation of both morphologic and kinetic data is essential for diagnosis.

8.4.1 Initial Phase

Initial enhancement is determined by comparing signal intensity in the precontrast image to the first postcontrast image acquired. An intensity increase of less than 50% is classified as "slow," 50 to 100% is classified as "medium," and greater than 100% enhancement is classified as "fast."

8.4.2 Delayed Phase

Delayed enhancement is divided into three main categories:
• Persistent curves (type 1) are defined as showing ≥ 10% of the initial enhancement with continuously increasing enhancement throughout the delayed phase.

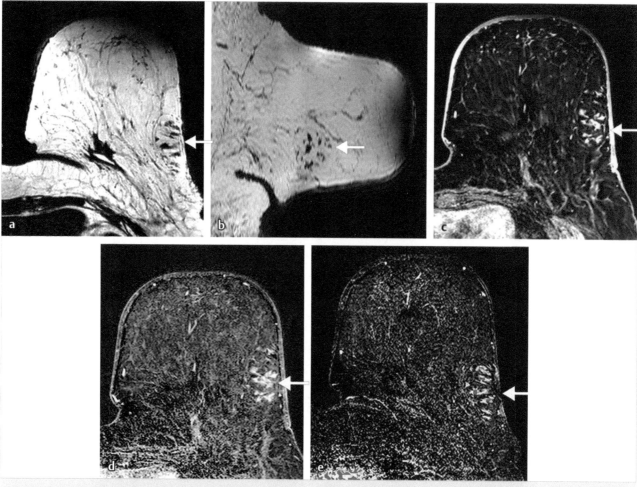

Fig. 8.29 Fat-containing lesion: fibroadenolipoma. (**a**) T2w: oval, fat-containing mass with thin capsule (*arrow*). (**b**) T2w sagittal view: (*arrow*). (**c**) T1w precontrast: oval mass with internal fat signal (*arrow*). Note skin thickening resulting from BCS 5 years previously. (**d**) T1w subtraction: selective enhancement of breast tissue within the thin capsule (*arrow*). (**e**) Angiomap: persistent parenchymal enhancement within the lesion (*arrow*).

- Plateau curves (type 2) are equal to the initial enhancement and remain constant in their signal intensity once peak enhancement is reached, usually after 2 to 3 minutes.
- Washout curves (type 3) are defined as showing ≤ 10% of the initial enhancement with continuous decreasing signal intensity after peak enhancement is reached (▶ Fig. 8.33).

Kinetic Curve Assessment

In general, benign lesions exhibit persistent curves, and malignant lesions exhibit washout curves, although there is considerable overlap between the kinetic curves that depict malignant and benign lesions. Diagnosis should only be made after consideration of both the morphologic and kinetic features of an enhancing lesion. Kinetic features reflect underlying lesion biology and the efficacy of advanced computerized analytic methods, using both morphologic and kinetic data, will be discussed in Chapters 12 and 13.

8.5 Histologic Subtypes of Invasive Cancer

As previously noted, the most common type of invasive breast carcinoma (75–80%) is classified as IBC-NST. This category incorporates all breast adenocarcinomas that fail to exhibit specific histologic characteristics that would warrant classification as one of the special types. The WHO classification recognizes the existence of at least 17 distinct histological special types.[1] Invasive malignancies exhibit distinctive morphologic, kinetic, and molecular characteristics that are reflected on mammography, ultrasound, and MRI. The imaging characteristics of the most common special types of invasive cancer will be reviewed.

8.5.1 Invasive Lobular Carcinoma

Invasive lobular carcinoma accounts for 10 to 15% of all invasive cancers, is known to be difficult to diagnose both on clinical

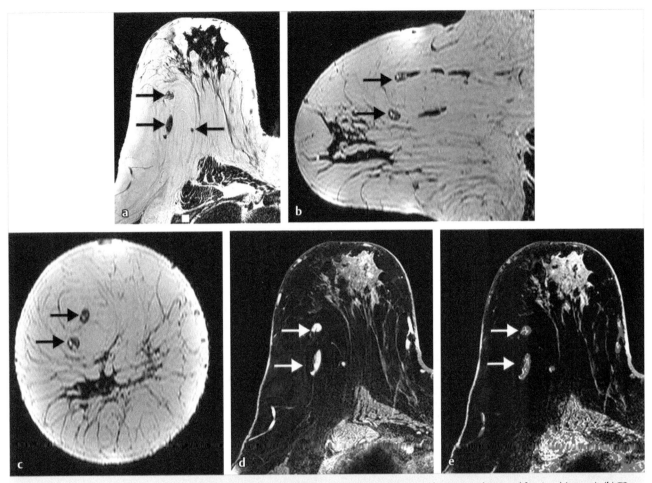

Fig. 8.30 Fat-containing lesion: intramammary lymph nodes (IMLN). (**a**) T2w: several oval and round masses with internal fat signal (*arrows*). (**b**) T2w: sagittal image (*arrows*). (**c**) T2w: coronal image (*arrows*). (**d**) T1w precontrast: circumscribed masses (*arrows*). (**e**) Angiomap: washout kinetics (*arrows*).

examination and on mammography, and is usually larger at initial presentation, more frequently exhibiting multifocal/multicentricity than IDC. Palpable thickening and skin or nipple retraction may be the most common clinical findings rather than detection of a discrete breast mass. The growth pattern of uniform, small, round tumor cells, typically infiltrating in a single file without mass formation, may limit conspicuity at mammography. The reported sensitivity of mammography ranges from 34 to 92%[11]; however, even when detected, size underestimation is common. Lack of desmoplastic reaction and absence of associated ductal carcinoma in situ (DCIS) with visible microcalcification also contribute to difficulties in lesion perception. ILC is diagnosed, in part, by absence of e-cadherin expression, a gene involved in cell–cell cohesion, thought to account for the singular growth pattern.

The most common presentation on mammography is that of a spiculated or ill-defined mass; however, findings of asymmetry and architectural distortion are more commonly found in ILC lesions than in IDC lesions. In some cases, a sheet-like infiltrating pattern of the tumor may result in decreased natural breast elasticity in the affected breast, limiting breast compression at mammography so that the breast appears to be smaller than the contralateral breast. This finding is known as the "shrinking breast" sign. The affected breast may appear to be of normal size, however, on clinical examination thickening of the breast may be evident.[11,12,13] Ultrasound has a higher sensitivity for ILC than mammography (68–98%) and findings usually present as an irregular, hypoechoic mass with indistinct or spiculated margins and acoustic shadowing.[14]

Histology

The heterogeneous nature of ILC is well established, and histologic subtypes of ILC lesions have been described. In 1982, Dixon and colleagues categorized 103 ILC lesions as classical, solid variant, alveolar variant, or mixed histologic subtypes, the classic and mixed types being the most common.[15] The classic type of ILC is described as a single filing growth pattern, with "peri-parenchymal" distribution and diffuse multifocal invasion. The solid variant consists of a "sheet-like" pattern or irregular-shape nests of cells, whereas the alveolar type is described as globular aggregates of 20 or more cells. These three subgroups exhibit small noncohesive regular cells with round or oval nuclei, whereas the fourth mixed type demonstrates cohesive cells with nuclear pleomorphism. Recently, subclassification has been reported using histological features and IHC[16];

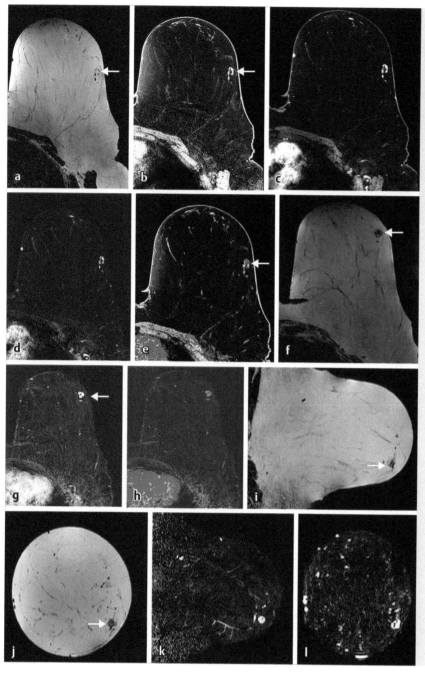

Fig. 8.31 Fat-containing lesion: intramammary lymph node (IMLN). IMLN no. 1: **(a)** T2w: oval circumscribed mass with fatty hilum (*arrow*). **(b)** T1w precontrast: oval circumscribed mass with fatty hilum (*arrow*). **(c)** T1w postcontrast: oval circumscribed mass with fatty hilum (*arrow*). **(d)** Subtraction image: (*arrow*). **(e)** Angiomap: washout kinetics, typically present in IML nodes. Identification of a fatty hilum is helpful for a confident benign diagnosis. IMLN no. 2: **(f)** T2w: round circumscribed mass with fatty hilum (*arrow*). **(g)** T1w subtraction: round circumscribed mass with fatty hilum (*arrow*). **(h)** Angiomap: washout kinetics, **(i, j)** reformatted: T2w sagittal and coronal images (*arrows*). **(k, l)** reformatted: T1w subtraction sagittal and coronal images.

however, no clear differences in long-term patient outcome between the different histologic subtypes was found in either study.[15,16]

Two studies have reported on the mammographic imaging appearance of ILC subtypes and histopathology.[17,18] In 2014, Tabar and colleagues[17] reported on 428 consecutive cases of ILC, diagnosed in the screening era, from 1996 through 2010, and compared patient outcome of these cases with a cohort of ILC cases diagnosed and treated in the prescreening era 25 to 30 years earlier.[8] A classification of the mammographic features of ILC lesions was made with an approximate correlation to the earlier histologic classification of Dixon and colleagues[15] (▶ Table 8.4). ILC subtypes vary in their imaging characteristics and lesion size at diagnosis. The alveolar subtype is often

extremely difficult to detect at mammography even though it is often palpable and multifocal, because it consists of many individual, tiny, scattered 2- to 3-mm cancer foci, often involving an entire quadrant but without a discrete tumor mass. Tumor sizes differed significantly in this study according to

Table 8.4 Mammographic features of ILC subtypes

Classical	Architectural distortion
Solid variant pattern	Round- or oval-shape mass
Alveolar	Equivocal asymmetries
Mixed pattern	Solitary or multifocal spiculated mass

Abbreviation: ILC, invasive lobular carcinoma.

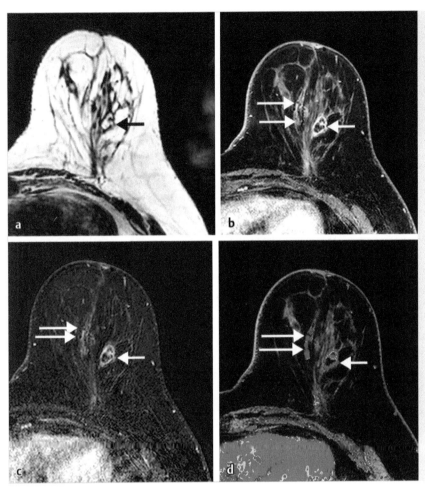

Fig. 8.32 Fat-containing lesion: fat necrosis 6 months post-BCS. (**a**) T2w: irregular mass with internal fat signal (*arrow*). (**b**) T1w postcontrast: irregular rim-enhancing mass with internal fat signal (*short arrow*). Note: adjacent nonmass enhancement with tiny foci of internal fat signal represents an additional region of fat necrosis (*long arrows*). (**c**) Subtraction image: (*arrows*). (**d**) Angiomap: washout enhancement is noted in the main mass (*short arrow*). Persistent enhancement is noted in the additional region of fat necrosis (*long arrows*).

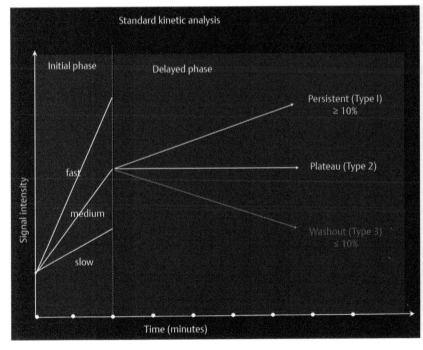

Fig. 8.33 Kinetic analysis graph.

195

their mammographic subtypes ($p < 0.001$). Large tumor sizes (≥ 30 mm) were overwhelmingly more likely to be found in architectural distortion cases (76%) than in spiculated masses (21%), round masses (25%), and equivocal asymmetric densities (34%). Patient outcome was shown to be related to mammographic appearance when long-term survival of women with ILC lesions was compared in the two groups (1960–1970 vs. 1996–2010). Outcome for women with spiculated and circular/oval-shape lesions diagnosed during the screening era was dramatically improved; however, no change in survival was found in women with the classical architectural distortion subtype, despite the advent of screening mammography in the latter group and the introduction of new therapeutic regimens.

Magnetic Resonance Imaging

The MRI findings of ILC reflect the morphologic findings seen on mammography and ultrasound; however, determination of disease extent is more accurate at MRI, and ILC lesions, found to be occult on mammography and ultrasound, are almost always visible on MRI. An irregular or spiculated-shape mass, with heterogenous internal enhancement, is a common presentation of ILC, although focal and "sheet-like" regional nonmass enhancement may also be found.[13,19,20,21] ILC rarely presents as a round mass, an important distinction compared to IDC lesions, which may often present as round masses with not circumscribed margins, and are generally grade 2 lesions. Mann and colleagues reported that a round-shape mass was identified in only 1 of 143 ILC lesions.[19] ILC has been described as a "stranding" pattern of tumor enhancement, associated with multiple, small, enhancing foci, by some investigators, possibly reflecting the single-file pattern of tumor growth.[15,22] Reports on the kinetic features of ILC generally conclude that in the initial phase of enhancement, ILC enhances more slowly than IDC, although peak enhancement measures may be similar. In the delayed phase of enhancement, ILC exhibits washout curves less frequently and a larger proportion of the tumor shows persistent delayed-phase curves than are seen in IDC.[23]

Multimodal images of the four main presentations of ILC are shown.

1. The classical subgroup of ILC: architectural distortion (▶ Fig. 8.34).

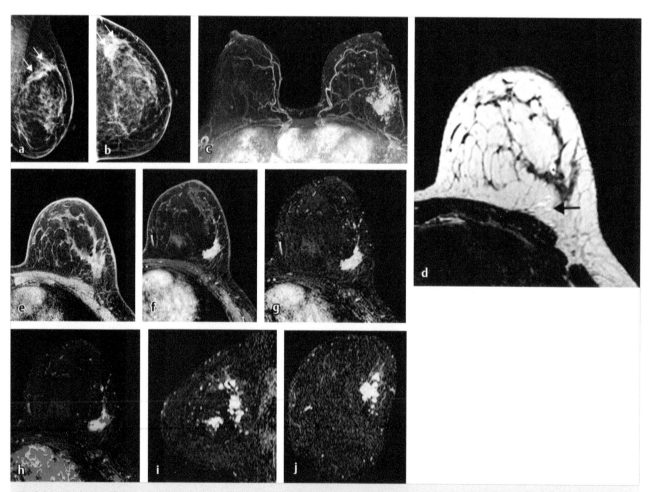

Fig. 8.34 ILC: classic subtype. A triangular sebaceous marker indicates the site a palpable architectural distortion in the superolateral left breast on MLO and CC mammographic views (**a,b**, *arrows*). MIP image (**c**) shows increased vascularity and multiple enhancing masses of variable sizes, the aggregate extending beyond the mammographic extent. T2w image (**d**) reveals a low signal lesion on T2w image with fluid posterior to the lesion, indicating aggressive histology (*arrow*). T1w, pre- and postcontrast, and subtraction images (**e, f, g,**) reveals multiple enhancing masses. Angiomap shows robust, mostly plateau, enhancement (**h**). Reformatted sagittal and coronal images (**i, j**) are shown. Histology: ILC classic-type grade 2 with LCIS. ER/PR (+), HER-2/neu (–), Ki-67: 15%.

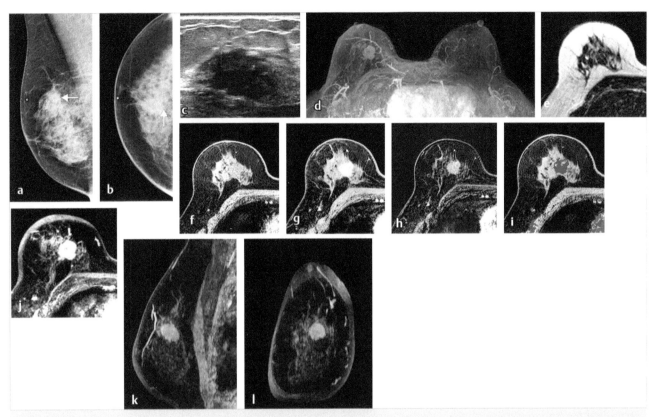

Fig. 8.35 ILC: solid variant pattern. A mass with obscured margins is seen on MLO and CC mammographic views (**a,b**, *arrows*; note the palpable skin markers). Multilobulated mass is identified on ultrasound (**c**). MIP image (**d**) shows a round enhancing mass with irregular margins with low signal on T2W image (**e**). T1w, pre- and postcontrast, and subtraction images (**f h**) show a unifocal mass with heterogeneous internal enhancement. Washout enhancement is seen within a predominantly persistently enhancing mass (**i**). MPR images (**j-l**). Histology: ILC grade 2, ER/PR (+), HER-2/neu (+).

2. The solid variant pattern subgroup of ILC: round/oval mass (▶ Fig. 8.35; ▶ Fig. 8.36).
3. The alveolar subtype of ILC: asymmetric density/NME (▶ Fig. 8.37; ▶ Fig. 8.38; ▶ Fig. 8.39; ▶ Fig. 8.40; ▶ Fig. 8.41).
4. The mixed pattern of ILC: spiculated mass(s): (▶ Fig. 8.42; ▶ Fig. 8.43; ▶ Fig. 8.44).

Additional ipsilateral malignant lesions detected only on MRI were found in 32% of patients, in a study of preoperative assessment of ILC extent, resulting in changed management in 28% of cases.[19] Another study of preoperative assessment of ILC showed management change in 49% women, 40% needing more extensive surgery and 9% needing less extensive surgery (▶ Fig. 8.43, ▶ Fig. 8.44).[24] Patients with an ILC diagnosis are more likely to have positive surgical margins after lumpectomy than patients with IDC lesions. Reduction in reexcision rates of ILC lesions by use of preoperative MRI has been shown in a study of 267 patients undergoing breast conserving surgery (BCS). Investigators reported a 9% reexcision rate in the MRI group compared to a 27% reexcision rate in the group without preoperative MRI.[25] MRI has been shown to be an essential imaging method in the preoperative assessment of women with a new diagnosis of ILC.

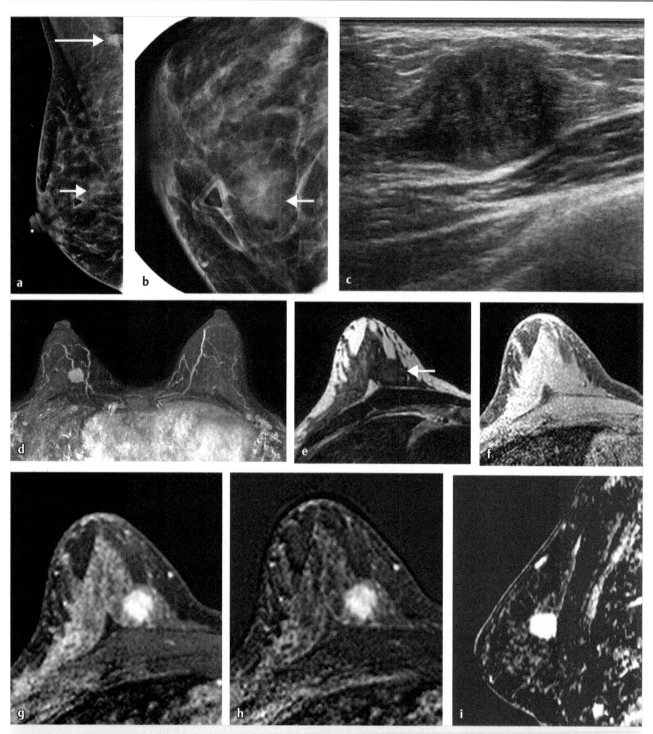

Fig. 8.36 ILC: solid variant pattern (1.5 T). A partially obscured mass, identified by a palpable skin marker, is visible in the right breast MLO and spot CC views (**a**, **b**, *short arrows*) and a suspicious lymph node is seen in the axilla (**a**, *long arrow*). A round isoechoic mass is seen on ultrasound (**c**) presenting as a unifocal, homogeneously enhancing mass on MIP image (**d**). The mass is isointense and partly outlined on T2w image (**e**) but not visible on precontrast image (**f**). T1w postcontrast source, subtracted and sagittal images (**g-i**) demonstrate homogeneous enhancement. Histology: ILC grade 2, ER/PR (+), HER-2/neu (−). One axillary lymph node was positive for malignancy (1/10).

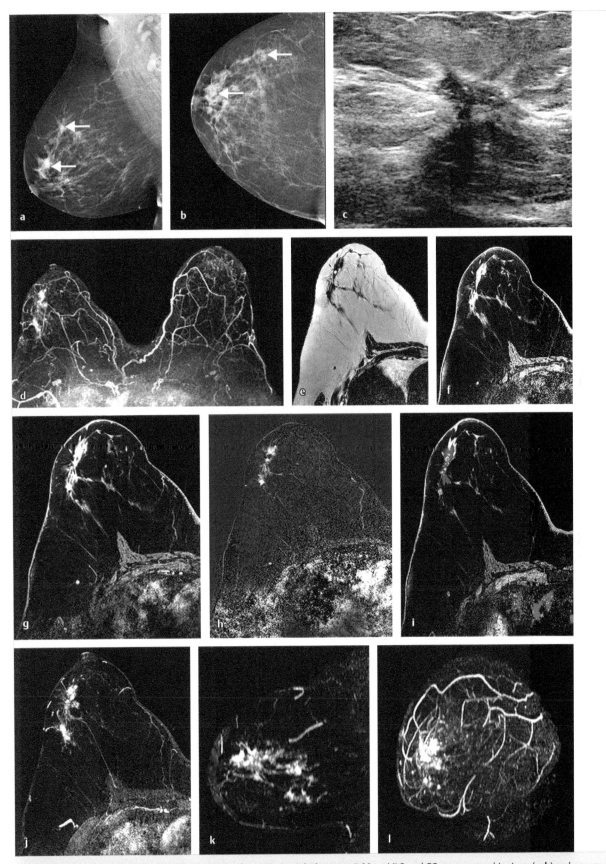

Fig. 8.37 ILC: classic subtype. A distortion is seen in the posterior right breast at 9:00 on MLO and CC mammographic views (**a, b**) and a second area of distortion with intervening asymmetry is noted in the subareolar region (*arrows*). An irregular shadowing mass is seen at 9:00 on ultrasound (**c**). MIP image (**d**); T2w (**e**); and T1w, pre-, postcontrast and subtraction images (**f, g, h**) demonstrate two irregular masses with some distortion, spiculation, and intervening NME. Angiomap exhibits some washout within an area of predominantly persistent enhancement (**i**) and MPR slab images (**j-l**) show disease extent to advantage. Histology: ILC classic-type grade 2, 6.5 cm, with focal pleomorphic features, ER/PR (+), HER-2/neu (−), Ki67: 10%. One axillary node was positive for malignancy (1/14).

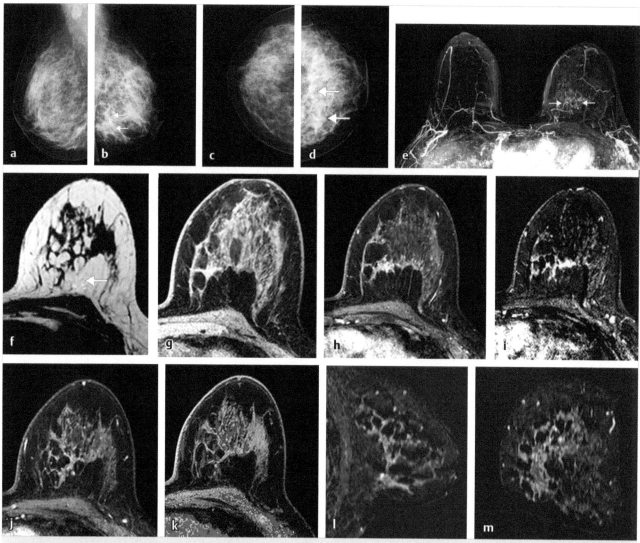

Fig. 8.38 (a–m) ILC. Alveolar subtype "shrinking" left breast. The left breast appears smaller than the right, and a diffuse asymmetry is noted in the posterior left breast at the fibroglandular/fat junction on bilateral mammographic views (**a-d** *arrows*). Regional NME is seen in the posterior left breast on MIP image (**e**) and posterior fluid indicating an aggressive lesion is seen on T2w image (**f**) (*arrows*). T1w precontrast image (**g**) shows no findings; however, postcontrast source and subtracted images (**h, i**) and adjacent slice (**j**) show NME predominantly in the medial posterior breast, correlating in location with the mammographic findings. Histology: ILC grade 2, alveolar subtype: ER/PR (+), HER-2/neu (−). 27/30 axillary lymph nodes were positive for malignancy.

8.5.2 Invasive Duct Carcinoma

Tubular Subtype

Tubular carcinoma is an uncommon, low-grade subtype of invasive carcinoma accounting for fewer than 2% of all invasive breast cancers, its incidence increasing with the use of screening mammography. These cancers are generally small and node negative with a favorable prognosis, the overall 10-year disease-free survival rate for tubular cancer being greater than 90%. Tubular carcinoma contains a central fibroelastotic core that entraps glandular proliferating elements, exhibiting round, ovoid, or angulated tubules formed by a single layer of small, regular cells with little nuclear pleomorphism. A tubular component greater than 90% is a requirement for a histologic diagnosis of tubular carcinoma.[26,27]

Imaging Findings

The hallmark finding, on all modalities, is that of spiculation, which corresponds to reactive stroma surrounding the tumoral mass, seen on ultrasound as an echogenic "halo." Small tubular cancers usually present on MRI as spiculated or irregular masses, with heterogeneous enhancement and persistent

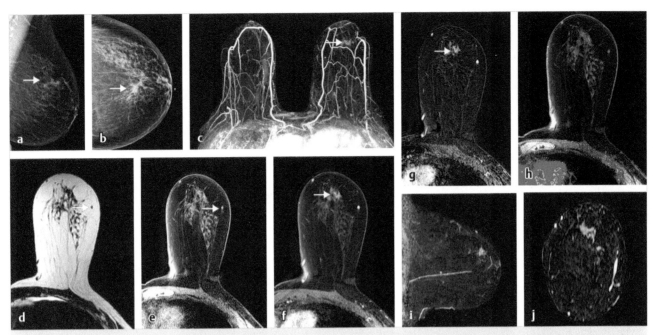

Fig. 8.39 ILC. Alveolar subtype. A developing asymmetry is noted in the left breast at 12.00 on mammographic views (**a, b,** *arrows*). A correlative focal NME is seen on MIP image (**c,** *arrow*). T2w and T1w precontrast images (**d, e**) show no abnormal findings; however, a small round mass (*arrows*) indicate a transverse section of a blood vessel, confirmed when adjacent slices are viewed. Postcontrast source and subtracted images (**f, g**) exhibit NME, correlating in location and size with the mammographic findings. Persistent enhancement is noted within the lesion on angiomap (**h**). MPR views (**i, j**) are shown. Histology: ILC grade 1, alveolar subtype, with ALH. ER/PR (+), HER-2/neu (–). The sentinel node was negative for malignancy (0/1).

kinetics (▶ Fig. 8.45; ▶ Fig. 8.46; ▶ Fig. 8.47). Minimal enhancement or initial enhancement rates less than 100% are commonly found. This enhancement pattern can be explained by the slow progression of the contrast material within the dense fibrous and elastotic stromal components. The morphologic features of radial scar (complex sclerosing lesion) often mimic those of tubular carcinoma and their kinetic behavior is often variable. Although visible on MRI, the distinction between these two lesions is usually not possible if lesion enhancement is present, and pathologic examination of the surgically excised tumor is generally needed.

Mucinous Subtype

Mucinous carcinoma can be divided into two histologic categories with varying imaging findings and differing patient prognoses: the pure mucinous type and the mixed mucinous type.

Pure mucinous carcinoma is an uncommon variety of invasive breast cancer accounting for 1 to 7% of all breast cancers and typically seen in older women. The term "pure mucinous carcinoma" is used when the tumor comprises less than 10% in volume of an associated IBC-NST. This subtype has an excellent prognosis and is characterized as a luminal A molecular subtype, with a 10-year survival rate of 87 to 90%. The dominant histologic feature of this lesion is the production of extracellular mucin, where islands of tumor cells float on pools of mucin.

Imaging Findings

The mammographic findings usually appear as a mass, with circumscribed or microlobulated margins. Complex mixed cystic

and solid masses are frequently seen at ultrasound; they may be isoechoic or hypoechoic, with associated with acoustic enhancement. Mucinous carcinoma presents as a lobular, round, or oval mass with smooth or irregular margins on MRI. A characteristic of high-signal intensity region within the mass is seen on the T2w series, caused by the high water content of the mucin. Areas of isointense T2 signal may be visible internally, demonstrating fibrous septations or areas of hemorrhage and necrosis—the solid tumor components showing lower T2 signal intensity. Internal enhancement patterns are often heterogeneous, reflecting the distribution of the internal cellular elements and mucin.[28,29,30] Kinetic features usually exhibit a slow initial rise and persistent enhancement in the delayed phase. These lesions are generally lower grade, the slow diffusion of contrast through mucin accounting for the slower enhancement in the initial phase (▶ Fig. 8.48; ▶ Fig. 8.49; ▶ Fig. 8.50; ▶ Fig. 8.51; ▶ Fig. 8.52; ▶ Fig. 8.53).

Mixed Mucinous Carcinoma

This cancer comprises variable amounts of IBC-NST in addition to a mucinous component. These tumors have an increased likelihood of axillary lymph node metastases and an overall worse prognosis than the pure type. The 10-year survival rate for mixed mucinous carcinoma is 54 to 66%.

Imaging Findings

The imaging features are directly related to the amount of extracellular mucin versus solid tumor within the mass. Mixed mucinous tumors may be of higher grade, exhibit noncircumscribed margins, and exhibit rapid rim enhancement with

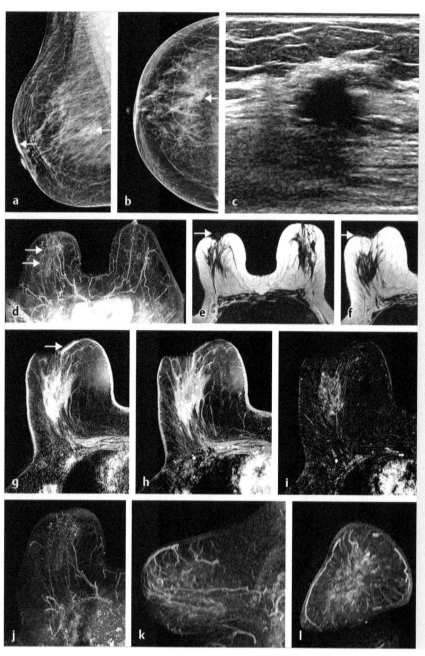

Fig. 8.40 ILC. Alveolar subtype. Example of a challenging diagnosis: a developing posterior asymmetry and periareolar skin thickening is noted in the right breast on mammographic views (**a, b**, *arrows*). Ultrasound image (**c**) demonstrates an irregular mass, and MIP shows minimal NME in the right breast (**d**, *arrows*). T2w images (**e, f**, *arrows*) and T1w precontrast images (**g**, *arrow*) show nipple retraction and associated skin thickening. Postcontrast source and subtracted images (**h, i**) show regional NME, larger in extent than the mammographic findings. Subthreshold enhancement in the lesion is noted by absence of color on angiomap (**j**). Reformatted sagittal and coronal images are shown (**k, l**). Histology: ILC grade 2, with LCIS. ER/PR (+), HER-2/neu (−), Ki-67: 5%. Sentinel nodes were negative for malignancy (0/2).

washout kinetics in the delayed phase. Studies have shown that the apparent diffusion coefficient (ADC) of pure mucinous tumors, at diffusion weighted imaging (DWI), is higher than that of IDC-NST and also of benign lesion such as fibroadenomata. DWI findings may thus be helpful in distinguishing between these lesions and in improving diagnostic specificity.[31,32] It is important to note, however, that not all malignant masses with high T2w signal represent mucinous carcinoma. Many rapidly growing, aggressive, invasive ductal carcinomas also exhibit high signal intensity on T2w images, reflecting fluid within areas of intratumoral necrosis.

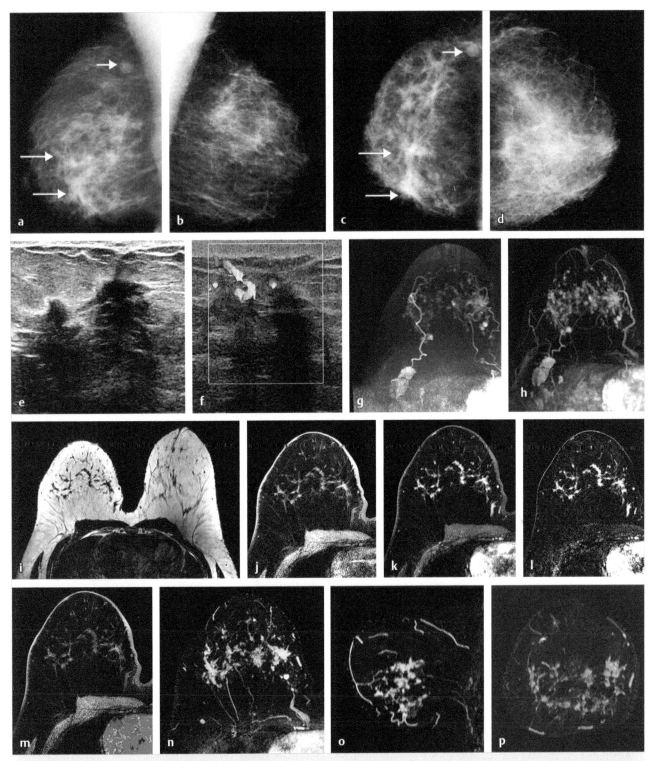

Fig. 8.41 ILC. Alveolar subtype. Bilateral MLO and CC views (**a–d**) are shown. The right breast is less compressible and thus appears smaller than the left, due to presence of a diffuse infiltrative malignancy. A palpable right inferomedial architectural distortion (*long arrows*) and an enlarged right intramammary lymph node (*short arrows*) are identified. Ultrasound image (**e**) demonstrates two irregular masses with increased vascularity (**f**). 70 s postcontrast MIP image (**g**) shows diffuse NME, increasing in degree and extent as shown on 210 s MIP image (**h**). T2w images of both breasts show decrease in right breast size with distorted breast tissue (**i**). T1w precontrast image (**j**) shows skin thickening, postcontrast source, and subtracted images (**k, l**) show regional NME with persistent kinetics on angiomap (**m**). MPR slab views are shown (**n-p**). Histology: ILC grade 2 with blood vessel and lymphatic invasion present at mastectomy. ER/PR (+), HER-2/neu (−). Twelve axillary lymph nodes were positive for malignancy (12/13).

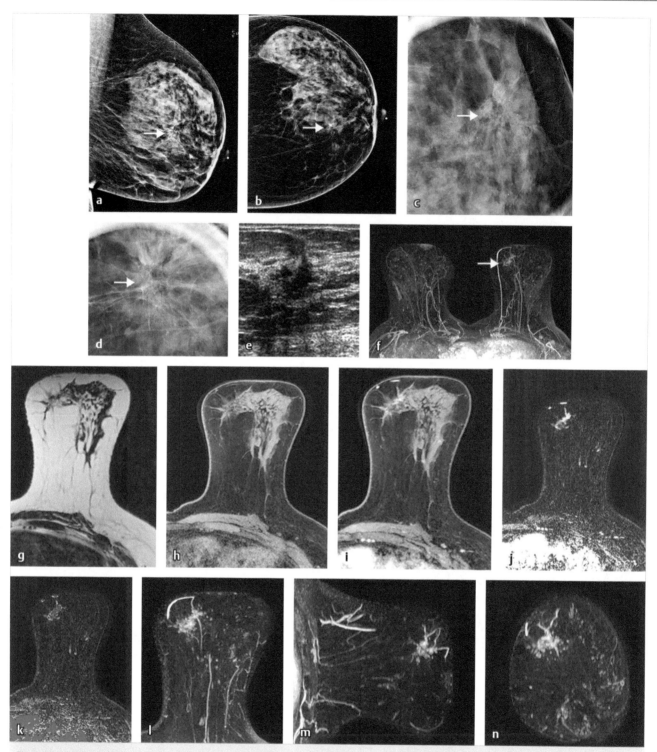

Fig. 8.42 ILC. Mixed pattern subtype. Spiculation and distortion is noted in the left breast at 9:00 on mammographic views (**a, b,** *arrows*) and spot magnification views (**c, d,** *arrows*). Ultrasound image (**e**) demonstrates an irregular mass with spiculation, and MIP image shows enhancement correlating with the location of the MG and ultrasound findings (**f,** *arrow*). T2w image (**g**) and T1w precontrast images (**h**) show no abnormal findings. Postcontrast source and subtracted images (**i, j**) show enhancement of the spiculated mass and surrounding foci with persistent kinetics on angiomap (**k**). MPR slab views are shown (**l-n**). Histology: ILC grade 1, total lesion size 4.3 cm. ER/PR (+), HER-2/neu (–). Sentinel nodes were negative for malignancy (0/3).

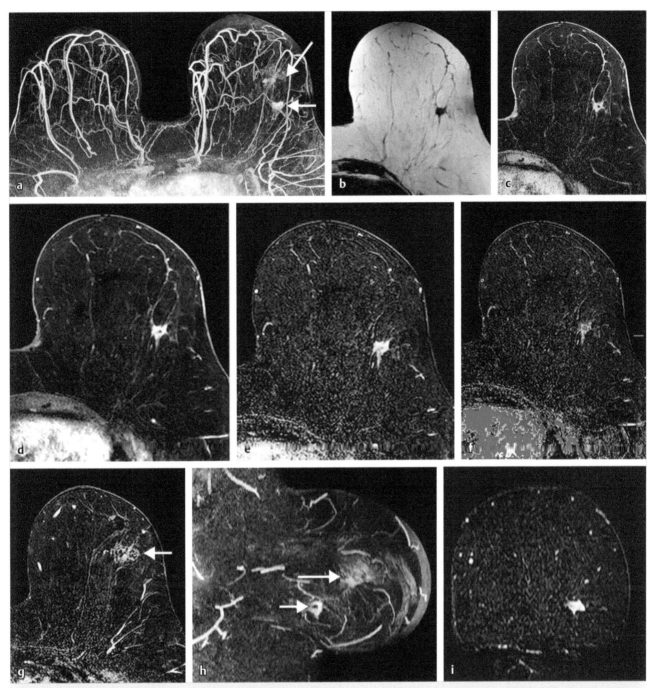

Fig. 8.43 ILC. Mixed pattern subtype. MIP image (**a**) shows an irregular, spiculated mass in the lateral left breast (*short arrow*) and a focal area of NME anterior to the mass (*long arrow*). The previously biopsied index mass is visible on precontrast T2w and T1w images (**b,c**). Postcontrast source (**d**), subtraction (**e**), and angiomap images (**f**) show internal enhancement with a postbiopsy marker clip and heterogeneous kinetics including washout. Axial subtraction image (**h**) shows NME located anterior to the mass, representing additional malignancy (*long arrow*). Sagittal image (**h**) shows both the mass (*short arrow*) and anterior NME (*long arrow*). A coronal image of the index mass (**i**) is also shown. Histology: extensive ILC grade 2 representing the index lesion and the focal anterior NME, both associated with LCIS classic type. ER/PR (+), HER-2/neu (−), Ki-67: 5%. One axillary node was positive for malignancy.

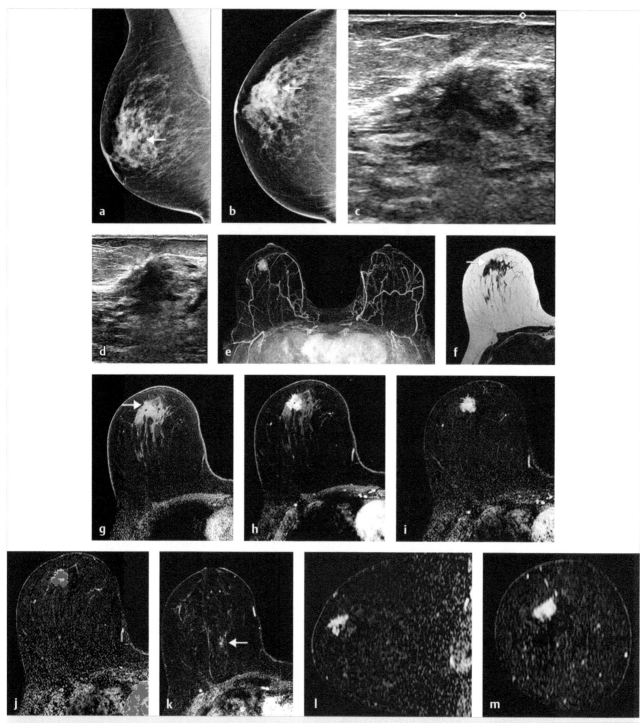

Fig. 8.44 ILC. Mixed pattern subtype. Screening MLO and CC MG views (**a,b**) show a partly obscured mass in the anterior right breast (*arrows*) and correlative ultrasound (**c,d**) demonstrating an irregular spiculated mass with hypoechogenicity, which is also seen on MIP image (**e**). The index spiculated mass is seen well on precontrast image T2w (**f**, *arrow*) and a marker clip from prior biopsy is seen within the mass on T1w image (**g**, *arrow*). Postcontrast images, source (**h**), subtraction (**i**), and angiomap (**j**) show relatively homogeneous internal mass enhancement with predominantly persistent kinetics. A focal area of minimal NME was also found on an additional slice, in the posteromedial breast on image (**k**, *arrow*), suggesting additional malignant involvement and confirmed with MR BX. Sagittal and coronal images (**l,m**) are shown. Histology: ILC grade 2, >6 cm, with associated LCIS classic type: ER (+), PR (−), HER-2/neu (−), Ki-67: 5%. 28/28 axillary lymph nodes were positive for malignancy with extranodal extension.

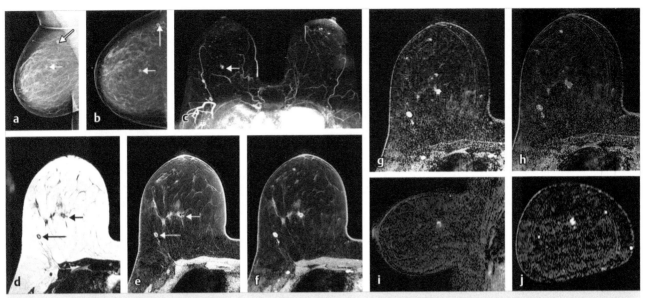

Fig. 8.45 IDC. Tubular subtype. Screening MG views of the right breast (**a, b**) show a 4-mm irregular mass, centrally located at 12:00 and a lateral, normal IMLN incidentally noted (*long arrows*). MIP image (**c**) shows a correlative irregular enhancing mass, also seen well on precontrast T2w image (**d**) (*short arrow*) and a fat-containing IMLN (*long arrow*). Marker clip from prior biopsy is seen on precontrast T1w image (**e**) (*short arrow*), and the IMLN (*long arrow*). Postcontrast images, source (**f**), subtraction (**g**), and angiomap (**h**) show homogeneous persistent enhancement in the index mass. Sagittal and coronal images (**i, j**) are shown. Histology: IDC grade 1 with tubular features. ER/PR (+), HER-2/neu (–), Ki-67: 6%. Sentinel nodes negative for malignancy (0/4).

Medullary Subtype

Medullary cancer accounts for 5 to 7% of all breast cancers; unlike mucinous carcinoma, which is typically found in older women, there is an increased incidence in women aged 35 or younger (11%), and in women with a genetic predisposition for breast cancer. The fourth edition of the WHO Classification of Tumours of the Breast (2012) advocates abandoning the terms "true medullary carcinoma," "atypical medullary carcinoma," and "invasive carcinoma NST with medullary features," and recommends using the term "carcinoma with medullary features" for this group of tumors, because morphological and IHC features may overlap and interobserver reproducibility may be variable. Women diagnosed with medullary carcinoma have a 10-year survival rate of 92%.[33] These lesions present as a mass and must exhibit specific histologic features described as, a "syncytial" growth pattern (> 75%), diffuse moderate to marked lymphocytoplasmacytic infiltrate, moderate to marked nuclear pleomorphism, and complete histologic circumscription.[1] The growth pattern of medullary carcinoma has been characterized as that of a "pushing" margin, with volumetric increase in mass size, a circumscribed margin, and absence of infiltration of the surrounding tissue. Histologic evidence of lymphocytoplasmacytic infiltration within and around the tumor is an essential diagnostic feature. Carcinomas with medullary features are more common in patients with BRCA1 germ-line mutations.

Imaging Findings

Although medullary carcinoma is characterized as circumscribed at histology, the presence of surrounding lymphocyto-plasmacytic infiltration may account for the imaging finding of an indistinct margin.[33] These lesions generally present as a non-calcified high-density mass at mammography with circumscribed or indistinct margins. Ultrasound features include a hypoechoic mass with lobular, circumscribed, or indistinct margins and variable posterior acoustic findings. Most medullary carcinomas exhibit oval or lobular masses with smooth margins on MRI, with findings of isointensity or hyperintensity on T2 W series, and isointensity or hypointensity on precontrast T1w series. Central necrosis and rim enhancement patterns predominate and kinetic features generally exhibit plateau or washout curves (▶ Fig. 8.54; ▶ Fig. 8.55). Internal septations are thought to represent fibroepithelial septations at histology, and delayed-phase peripheral enhancement possibly representing peritumoral inflammatory changes has been reported.[34,35] Some lesions may not exhibit all of the features of medullary carcinoma as described previously, and may not experience the same good prognosis. These lesions may more frequently be associated with calcifications indicating associated DCIS.[33]

Papillary Subtype

Papillary carcinomas are rare, accounting for fewer than 2% of all breast carcinomas, are found most frequently in an older patient population, and are usually associated with a good prognosis. The histologic hallmark of both benign and malignant papillary tumors is a singular epithelial frond-forming growth pattern supported by a fibrovascular stalk. Papillary carcinomas can be categorized as intraductal, encapsulated, and invasive. (An example of intraductal papillary carcinoma is shown in Chapter 7, Fig. 7.29.)

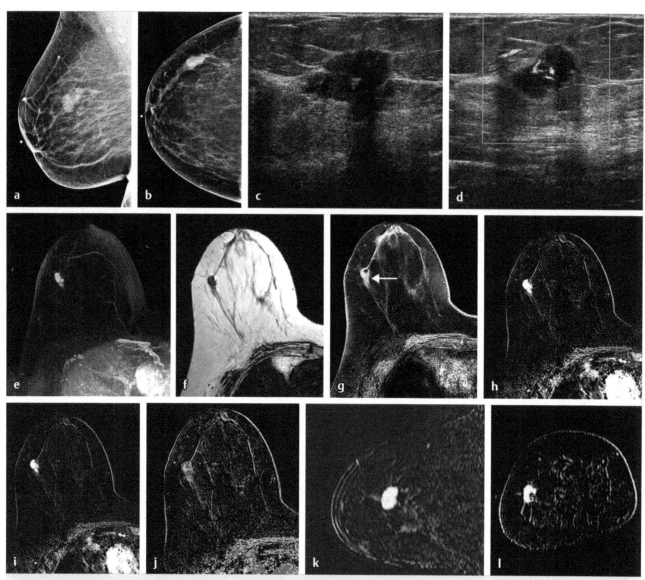

Fig. 8.46 IDC. Tubular subtype. Screening MG views of the right breast (**a, b**) show an 11-mm, partly obscured, irregular mass at 10:00 with correlative ultrasound images (**c, d**) and increased blood flow shown on image (**d**). MIP image (**e**) shows a lobulated, irregular, enhancing mass, also seen well on precontrast T2w image (**f**). Marker clip from prior biopsy is seen in the mass on precontrast T1w image (**g**) (*arrow*). Postcontrast images, source (**h**), subtraction (**i**), and angiomap (**j**) exhibit robust mass enhancement with heterogeneous washout kinetics. Sagittal and coronal images (**k, l**) are shown. Histology: IDC grade 1 with tubular features and low grade, solid DCIS. ER/PR (+), HER-2/neu (–). Sentinel nodes were negative for malignancy (0/3).

Encapsulated Papillary Carcinoma

Bloody nipple discharge is often the presenting clinical sign of encapsulated papillary carcinoma, found in 5 to 25% of cases.[36] This lesion is thought to represent an obstructed and cyst-like dilated duct containing a central mass encased by a thickened fibrous wall. Encapsulated carcinomas are generally thought to be noninvasive if myoepithelial cells are identified within the duct wall; however, in 85% of cases, myoepithelial cells may be absent, suggesting an indolent invasive histology. Additional foci of IBC-NST may be identified causing infiltration of the fibrous capsule in some cases.[36,37] Encapsulated papillary carcinoma usually presents mammographically as a round, oval, or lobulated mass with circumscribed or indistinct margins,

located in the retroareolar region (▶ Fig. 8.56). Associated calcifications may be present. Ultrasound findings consist of single or multiple hypoechoic complex masses with a cystic component and posterior acoustic enhancement.[38,39] Hemorrhage within the cyst fluid in papillary lesions may be caused by stalk torsion, and infarction of the solid components.

Imaging Findings

There is scant information in the literature regarding the MRI findings of encapsulated papillary carcinoma; however, a few reports describe complex masses visible on T2w images with high signal representing the fluid component. Hemorrhage may present as fluid–fluid levels within the cystic component on

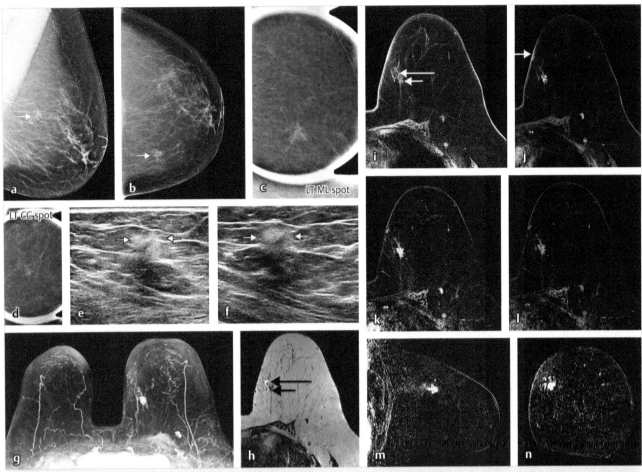

Fig. 8.47 IDC. Tubular subtype. Screening MG views of the left breast (**a,b** *arrows*) and spot compression views (**c,d**) demonstrate a 7-mm irregular indistinct mass at 10:00, with correlative ultrasound images (**e,f**) showing an irregular mass, with a surrounding echogenic halo representing dense surrounding fibrous tissue (*arrows*). MIP image (**g**) shows robust enhancement in the mass, which is visible on precontrast T2w and T1w images (**h,i**, *short arrows*). A biopsy-placed marker clip artifact is also seen (*long arrows*). Postcontrast images, source (**j**) shows the enhancing mass with spiculation and postbiopsy focal skin enhancement (*arrow*). Subtraction image (**k**) and angiomap (**l**) exhibit enhancement with heterogeneous washout kinetics. Sagittal and coronal images (**m, n**) are shown. Histology: IDC grade 2 with tubular features and low grade, solid DCIS. ER/PR (+), HER-2/neu (−). The sentinel node was negative for malignancy (0/1).

T2w series and may be identified as high precontrast signal on T1w series. These tumors exhibit variable morphology, usually present as round- or oval-shape masses with inconsistent marginal findings and low enhancement (▶ Fig. 8.56, ▶ Fig. 8.57).[40]

Invasive Papillary Carcinoma

Invasive papillary carcinoma is infrequently found, as either an intracystic papillary carcinoma with small foci of stromal invasion extending beyond the fibrous capsule (intracystic invasive papillary carcinoma)[38] or as a tumor composed predominantly of papillae containing a central fibrovascular core lined by neoplastic cells (solid invasive papillary carcinoma).[41]

Imaging Findings

Invasive papillary carcinomas typically exhibit round, ovoid, or lobulated shapes and circumscribed margins at MRI that correlate well with the circumscribed macroscopic appearance revealed at gross examination (▶ Fig. 8.58). The invasive component may be small, and this is particularly true in the case of encapsulated papillary carcinoma. Solid tumors and the solid portions of intracystic carcinomas usually demonstrate washout kinetic curves and a maximum initial enhancement rate greater than 100%.

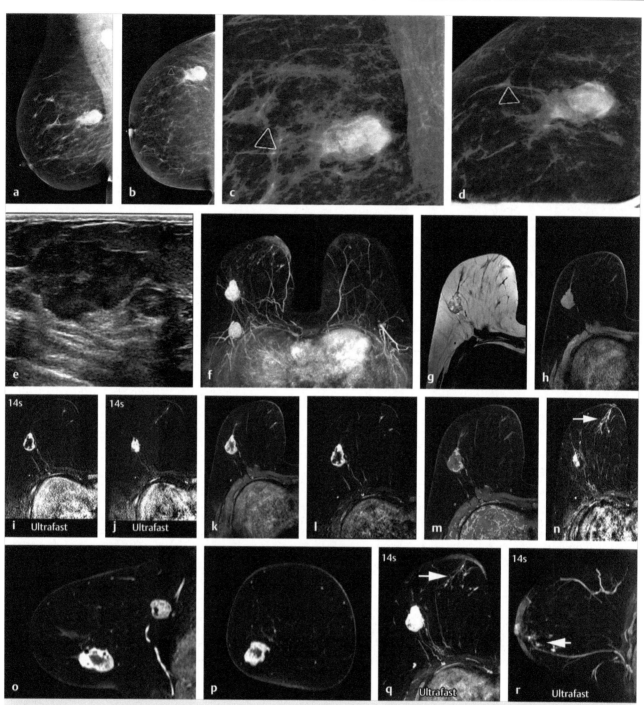

Fig. 8.48 IDC. Mucinous subtype. Age 37. Diagnostic MG–MLO/CC views of the right breast (**a, b**) and spot compression views (**c, d**) show a palpable, oval, high-density mass at 9:00, identified with a triangular skin marker. Ultrasound image (**e**) demonstrates a correlative mixed density microlobulated mass. MIP image (**f**) shows 3.0-cm mass with enhancement and an enlarged right axillary mass representing a metastatic lymph node. T2w image (**g**) shows high signal intensity within the lobulated mass, representing a classic finding of mucinous cancer. T1w precontrast image (**h**) exhibits isointensity and ultrafast postcontrast subtraction images obtained at 14 s (**i, j**) show rim enhancement in the index cancer (**i**) and NME, slice at the level of the nipple, suggests DCIS extending to the nipple (**j**, *arrow*). T1w source and subtraction images obtained at 70 s (**k, l**) show rim enhancement of the index cancer, exhibiting heterogeneous kinetics on angiomap (**m**). The central nonenhancing tissue represents mucin within the tumor. Axial 70 s slice at the level of the nipple (**n**) shows part of the index lesion and unexpected segmental linear NME. Sagittal and coronal reconstructed images (**o, p**) are shown. Ultrafast 14 s thin slab axial image (**q**, *arrow*) and sagittal image (**r**, *arrow*) show to advantage the additional finding of NME in the anterior breast. Histology: IDC grade 2 with mucinous features and low-grade solid DCIS, ER/PR (+), HER-2/neu (–). Two axillary nodes were positive for malignancy (2/17).

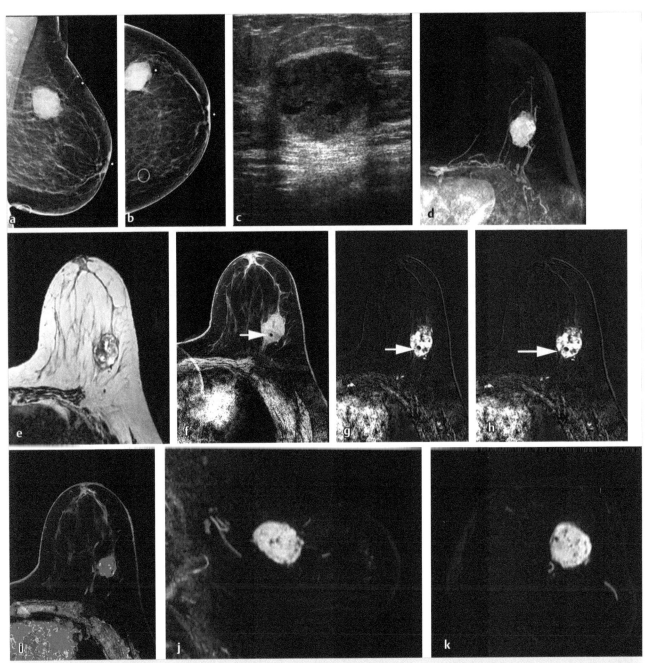

Fig. 8.49 IDC. Mucinous subtype. Age 82: a palpable mass, marked with a skin BB, is seen in the posterior left breast at 2:00 on MG-MLO/CC views of the right breast (**a, b**). This high-density oval mass is also visible, demonstrating mixed echogenicity, on ultrasound image (**c**). A unifocal 2.5-cm mass with heterogeneous internal enhancement is seen on MIP image (**d**). The T2w image (**e**) shows high internal signal intensity, a hallmark finding in mucinous cancer. T1w precontrast image (**f**) is isointense, heterogeneous internal enhancement seen on postcontrast source and subtraction images (**g, h**). A marker clip from prior transcutaneous biopsy is seen within the mass (**f, g, h,** *arrows*) which exhibits persistent kinetics on angiomap (**i**). Sagittal and coronal reconstructed images (**j, k**) are shown. Histology: IDC grade 2 with mucinous features. The patient was treated only with aromatase inhibitors. Follow-up imaging 5 years later showed the mass to be smaller, measuring 12 mm at mammography. Histology: IDC mucinous subtype grade 2: ER/PR (+), HER-2/neu (−).

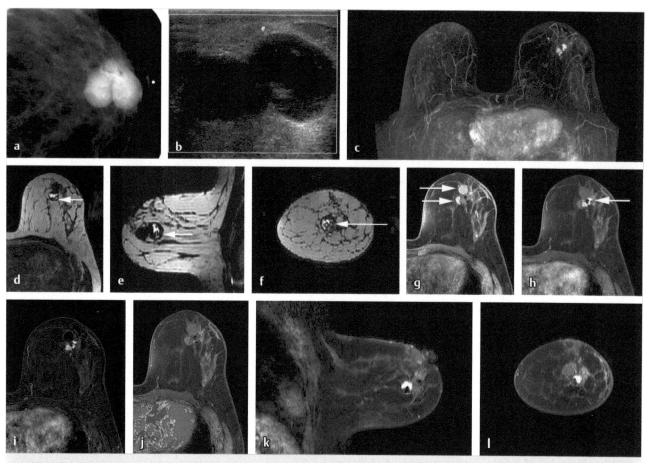

Fig. 8.50 IDC. Mucinous subtype. Age 41: a palpable high-density mass, marked with a skin BB is seen on subareolar spot CC-MG view (**a**) and the bilobed cystic component of the mass is seen on ultrasound image (**b**). MIP subtraction image (**c**) shows an irregular enhancing mass, immediately lateral and inferior to the unenhancing cystic component of the mass. The T2w axial image (**d**) and sagittal and coronal reformatted images (**e, f**) show high internal signal intensity within the mass (*arrows*), immediately posterior to the round enhancing low signal mass representing proteinaceous material within a cyst. T1w precontrast image (**g**) demonstrates the cyst with high internal signal (*short arrow*) and adjacent high signal representing the mucin within component of the cancer (*long arrow*). Postcontrast source, subtraction, and angiomap images (**h-j**) show an irregular mass with predominantly persistent enhancement and an internal marker clip from prior biopsy. Sagittal and coronal reconstructed images (**k, l**) are shown. Histology: IDC mucinous subtype grade 2, ER/PR (+), HER-2/neu (–).

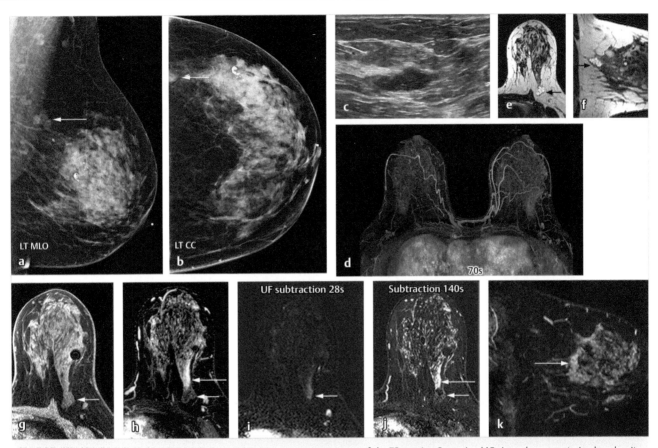

Fig. 8.51 IDC. Mucinous subtype. Example of a nonenhancing cancer. Importance of the T2w series. Screening MG views show a posterior, low-density lobulated mass at 1:00 (**a**, **b**, *arrows*) in the left breast, with an ultrasound correlate (**c**). MIP image at 70 s postcontrast (**d**) exhibits marked BPE. T2w images (**e**, **f**) show a lobulated high-signal mass, correlating in size and location with the mammographic findings. Pre- and postcontrast source and subtraction T1w images (**g-j**) show no discernable enhancement within the identified mass (*short arrows*). Focal increased BPE is seen laterally (*long arrows*) also visible on sagittal view (**k**, *arrow*). Histology: IDC mucinous subtype, 1.5 cm, grade 1 with associated cribriform DCIS, ER/PR (+), HER-2/neu (−), Ki-67: 5%. Axillary nodes were negative for malignancy (0/3).

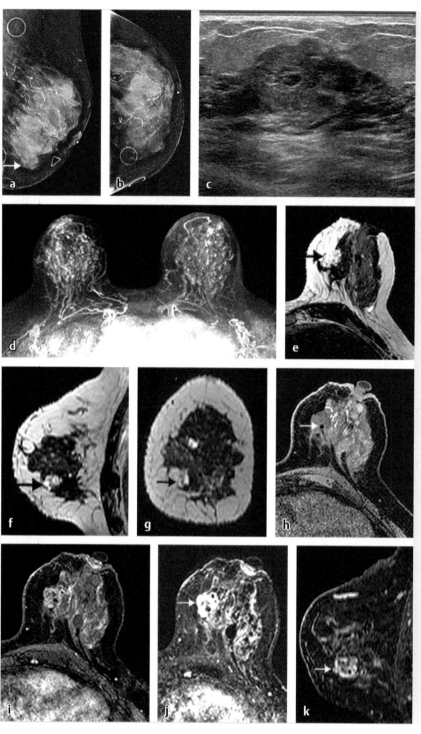

Fig. 8.52 IDC. Mucinous subtype. Screening MG views of the left breast (**a**, **b**) show dense breast tissue and a partially obscured palpable mass is seen in the inferior breast (*arrow*) identified by a triangular skin marker. Multiple round sebaceous markers denote skin lesions and ultrasound image (**c**) identifies a lobulated mass with mixed echogenicity. MIP image (**d**) exhibits marked BPE. Multiplanar T2w images (**e-g**) show a lobulated high-signal mass, correlating in size and location with the palpable lesion (*arrows*). Precontrast T1w image (**h**) exhibits benign high-signal in medial ducts and a postbiopsy marker clip in the mass (*arrow*). Source and subtraction T1w images (**i**, **j**) show rim and internal heterogeneous enhancement within the mass (*short arrows*), also visible on sagittal view (**k**, *arrow*). Histology: IDC mucinous subtype, grade1, size 1.8 cm with associated low-grade DCIS, ER/PR (+), HER-2/neu (−), Ki-67: 5%. Sentinel nodes negative for malignancy (0/4).

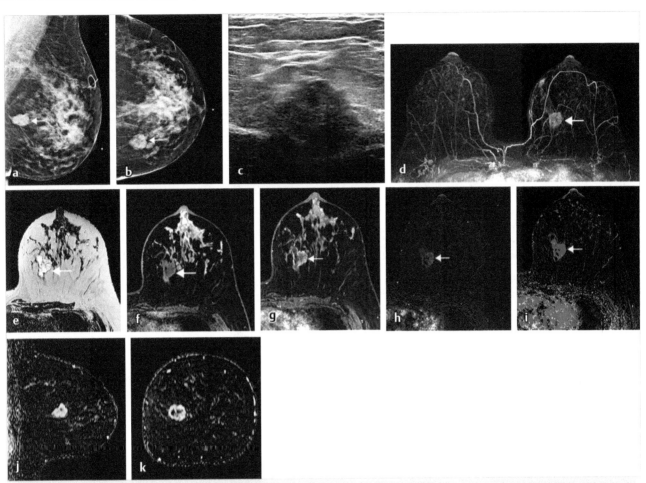

Fig. 8.53 IDC. Mucinous subtype (1.5 T). Screening MG views of the left breast (**a, b**) show a lobulated circumscribed mass at 9:00, posterior depth (*arrows*). Incidental note is made of round and linear skin markers, representing a skin lesion and a surgical scar (benign lesion), respectively. Ultrasound image (**c**) identifies a hypoechoic microbulated mass, seen on MIP image (**d**, *arrow*) as a round enhancing mass. T2w image (**e**) exhibits high signal intensity within the mass, representing mucin within the tumor (*arrows*). The mass is also seen, containing a biopsy clip, on precontrast T1w image (**f**, *arrow*). Postcontrast source and subtracted images (**g-i**) exhibit heterogeneous persistent mass enhancement (*arrows*). Reformatted sagittal and coronal images (**j, k**) are shown. Histology: IDC mucinous subtype grade 1, ER/PR (+), HER-2/neu (–), Ki-67: 5–9%. Sentinel nodes were negative for malignancy (0/2).

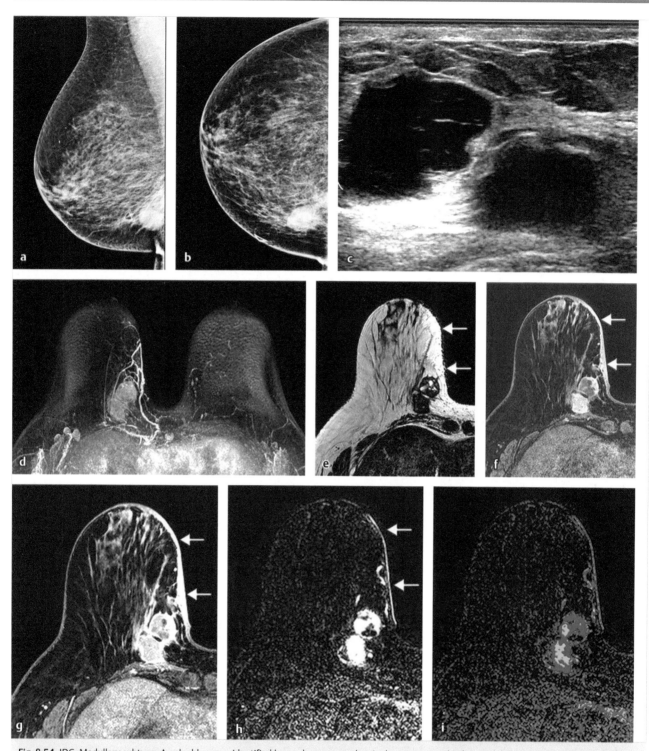

Fig. 8.54 IDC. Medullary subtype. A palpable mass, identified by a sebaceous marker, is shown as a partly obscured, bilobed, high-density mass in the posterior inferomedial right breast on MG–MLO/CC views (**a**, **b**). Ultrasound image (**c**) identifies two adjacent hypoechoic masses, visible on MIP image (**d**). Medial subcutaneous edema (*arrows*), and high signal intensity within the two masses is noted on T2w image (**e**). Both masses exhibit isointensity on precontrast image (**f**) and medial skin thickening is identified (*arrows*). Postcontrast source and subtracted images (**g**, **h**) exhibit heterogeneous enhancement and skin enhancement indicates extension to the dermis (*arrows*). Angiomap (**i**) exhibits heterogeneous enhancement. Histology: IDC medullary subtype, grade 2, ER (+), PR (–), HER-2/neu (–). The sentinel node was negative for malignancy (0/1).

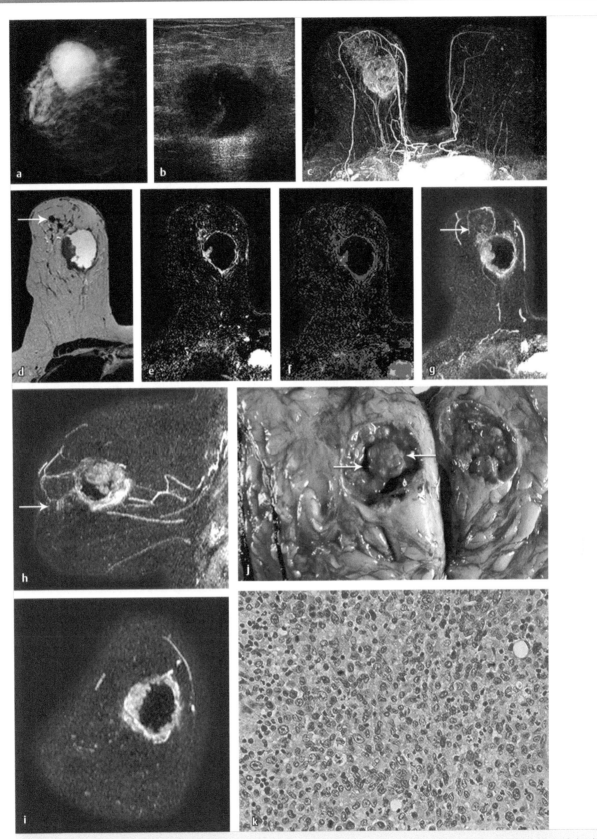

Fig. 8.55 IDC. Cystic medullary subtype. A large palpable mass is shown as a high-density, round, circumscribed mass in the medial right breast on MG-ML view (**a**). Ultrasound image (**b**) shows a thick-wall, largely anechoic, cystic mass with a thick internal septum. MIP image (1.5 T) exhibits heterogeneous mass enhancement with NME extending to the nipple (**c**). T2w image (**d**) shows a cystic mass with a thick wall, mural nodule, peritumoral edema and dilated subareolar ducts (*arrow*). Postcontrast T1w subtraction image (**e**) exhibits enhancement of the cyst wall, with angiomap (**f**) demonstrating persistent kinetics. Reformatted axial, sagittal, and coronal partial MIP images (**g–i**) show to advantage the cystic lesion and anterior NME (*arrows*). A slice through the excised breast specimen shows the medullary cancer located within the cyst (**j**, *arrows*), and tumor cells are seen in the cyst wall on histologic specimen (**k**). Histology: IDC cystic medullary subtype with internal necrosis, grade 3, size 6.5 cm, with associated DCIS, solid and high grade, ER (–), PR (+), HER-2/neu (–). Sentinel nodes were negative for malignancy (0/5).

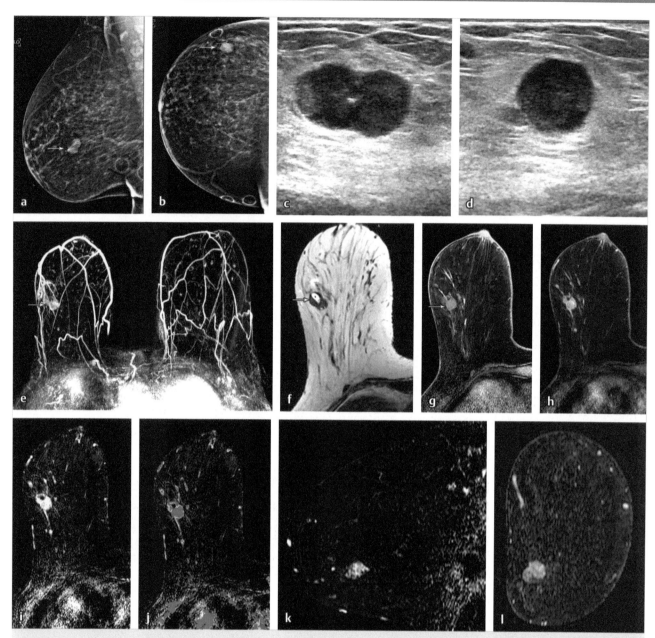

Fig. 8.56 Encysted papillary subtype (noninvasive). Age 68: screening MG views of the right breast identify an oval lobulated mass at 9:00 mid-depth (**a, b,** *arrows*) (multiple, ring sebaceous markers are present) and correlative ultrasound images are shown (**c, d**). The mass enhances robustly on MIP image (**e**). T2w image (**f**) shows a mass (*arrow*) with central clip artifact, also visible on precontrast image (**g,** *arrow*). Rapid enhancement is noted on postcontrast images (**h, i**) with homogeneous washout kinetics seen on angiomap (**j**). Reformatted sagittal and coronal images (**k, l**) are shown. Histology: 1.9 cm encapsulated (intracystic) papillary cancer, intermediate grade, ER (+), PR (−), HER-2/neu (−).

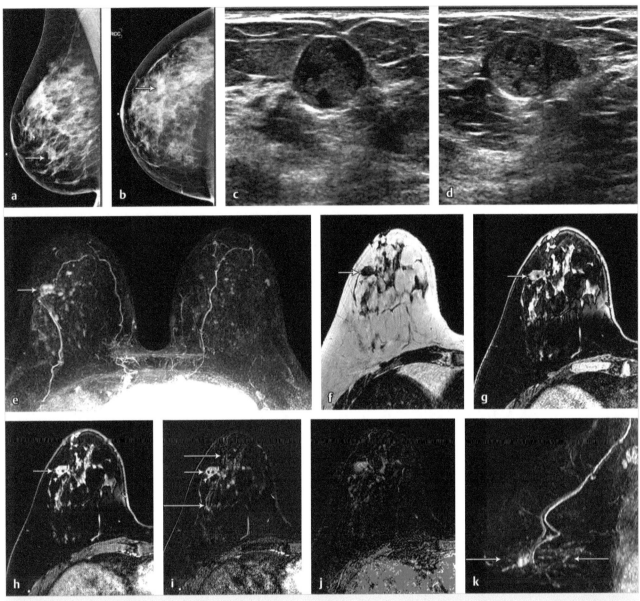

Fig. 8.57 Encysted papillary subtype (noninvasive) (1.5 T). Screening MG views of the right breast identify an obscured oval mass at 8:00, anterior depth (**a, b,** *arrows*), correlative ultrasound images showing a lobulated isoechoic mass (**c, d**). MIP image (**e**) demonstrates an enhancing circumscribed mass (*arrow*), which is seen as a low-signal mass on T2w image (**f,** *arrow*), and as an isointense mass with central clip artifact on precontrast image (**g,** *arrow*). Postcontrast images (**h, i**) show homogeneous mass enhancement (*short arrows*), NME extending beyond the index mass (*long arrows*), washout kinetics shown on angiomap (**j**). Reformatted sagittal image (**k**) shows linear NME extending from the index cancer (*arrows*). Histology: 1.2 cm encapsulated (intracystic) papillary cancer, intermediate grade, with DCIS, papillary type, extending from the index mass. Total extent of disease area is 5.5 cm. ER (+), PR (+), HER-2/neu (–). Sentinel nodes were negative for malignancy 0/4.

8.6 Molecular Signatures of Breast Cancer

Breast cancer is diagnosed with varying clinical presentations, histologic subtypes, and a classification based on the similarities between tumors at the genetic level. These distinct differences in tumor genetics are unevenly distributed among women with various patterns of disease expression, response to therapy, and patient survival outcomes. DNA microarray technology is a method involving isolation of genetic material usually messenger

RNA, from a cancer specimen. The cancer RNA is tested against certain complementary DNA microarrays, in order to determine which genes are expressed and which are lacking. Incubation of messenger RNA from the cancer to be analyzed, with many thousands of known sequences from the genes commonly expressed by breast cancers, allows determination of the unique gene expression profile of the cancer in question.

In clinical practice, a tissue sample of a patient's breast cancer is acquired at the time of diagnosis, is processed, and the isolated messenger RNA fraction is then incubated with a specific

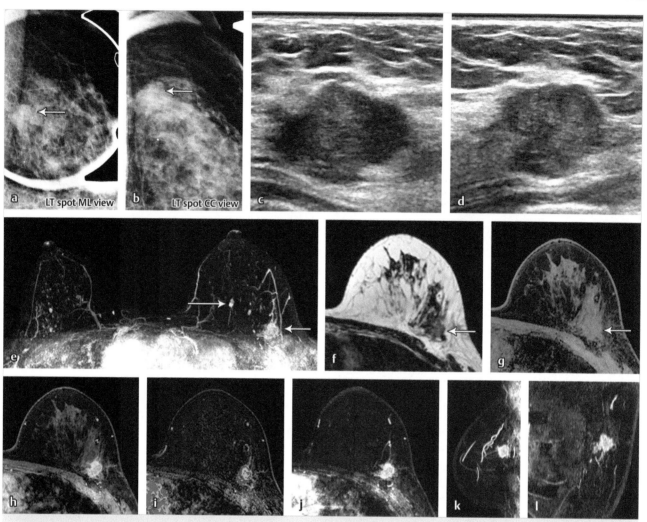

Fig. 8.58 Invasive papillary subtype. Screening MG views of the left breast identify an obscured mass at 2:00, posterior depth, adjacent to the pectoral muscle (**a, b,** *arrows*). Correlative ultrasound images show a lobulated mass with mixed echogenicity (**c, d**). MIP image (**e**) demonstrates rim enhancement in the oval index mass (*short arrow*); incidental note is made of a fibroadenoma with unenhancing internal septation (*long arrow*). The mass is partly obscured on T2w and T1w precontrast images (**f, g,** *arrows*), but enhances robustly with washout kinetics on postcontrast images, with some peritumoral NME suggesting associated DCIS (**h, i**). Reformatted slab axial, sagittal image and coronal images (**j-l**) are shown. Histology: invasive papillary cancer, intermediate grade, associated DCIS cribriform and micropapillary. ER/PR (+), HER-2/neu (–). Sentinel nodes were negative for malignancy (0/3).

microarray that contains thousands of oligonucleotides[2] commonly found in breast cancer. Computer analysis of the data is then obtained from the microarray analysis, providing a comprehensive molecular signature of the patient's breast cancer. This research has led to groupings of molecular portraits of tumors, discovered as gene expression patterns, clustered by means of growth rates, cellular composition, and specific signaling pathways that have led to the four major subtypes that are in clinical use today.

8.6.1 Luminal A Subtype

Luminal A breast cancers are the most common subtype representing more than 50% of all breast cancers. They are generally characterized by expression of both ER and PR and absence of overexpression of the gene ERBB2 (also known as the HER2/neu gene), a protooncogene that stimulates cellular growth. These tumors are usually of low grade, with a low Ki-67 proliferative index less than 15%, and are associated with an excellent prognosis and a 5-year survival rate of more than 80%.

Imaging Findings

This molecular type represents the majority of invasive luminal cancers and is usually seen on all imaging methods as a mass with irregular or spiculated margins, irregular shape, heterogeneous

---

[a] **Oligonucleotides** are short DNA or RNA molecules, oligomers, used in a wide range of applications such as in genetic testing, research, and forensics.

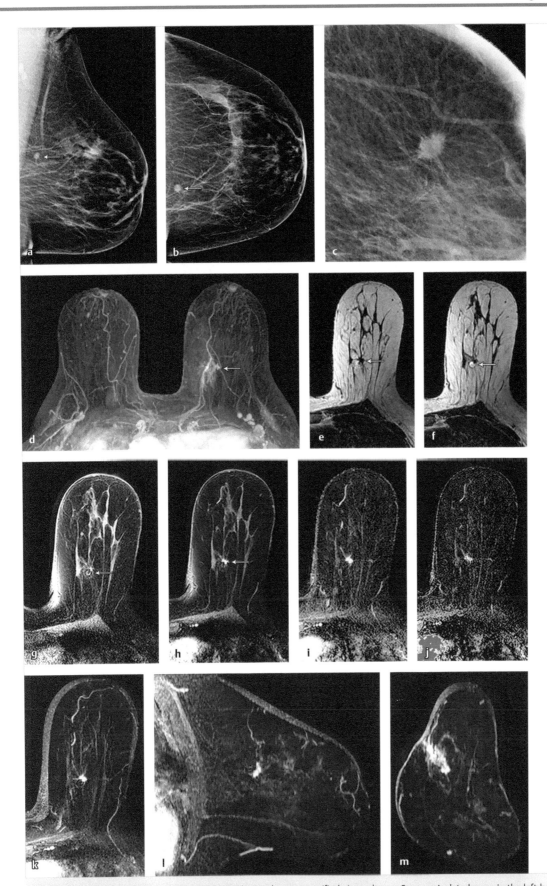

Fig. 8.59 Luminal A subtype. Screening MG–MLO/CC and spot magnified views show a 6-mm spiculated mass in the left breast at 10:00 (**a-c** *arrows*) with correlative enhancement seen on MIP image (**d**, *arrow*). Two T2w slices are shown; a spiculated mass (**e**, *arrow*), and a marker clip just posterior to the mass (**f**, *arrow*). Precontrast T1w image identifies the postbiopsy clip (**g**, *arrow*). Rapid enhancement is seen in the sunifocal mass on postcontrast source and subtraction images (**h**, *arrow* , **i**) with predominantly plateau enhancement noted on angiomap (**j**). Reformatted, slab axial, sagittal, and coronal images (**k, l, m**) are shown. Histology: IDC with lobular features, 8 mm, grades 1–2. ER (+), PR (+), HER-2/neu (–). Sentinel nodes and one nonsentinel lymph node were negative for carcinoma (0/4).

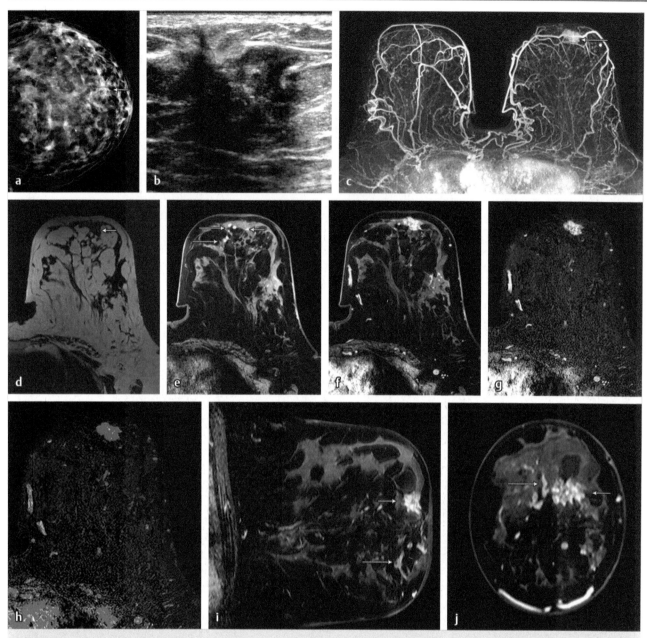

Fig. 8.60 Luminal A subtype. Age 68: patient presented with a palpable mass (triangular skin marker) in the anterior left breast, seen on MG-CC view as a subtle architectural distortion (**a**, *arrow*), and confirmed as an irregular spiculated mass on ultrasound (**b**). MIP image shows a unifocal mass with heterogeneous enhancement (**c**, *arrow*). Precontrast T2w and T1w images show subtle spiculation at the site of the mass (**d**, **e**, *arrows*), and incidental subareolar ductal fluid is noted (*long arrows*). Postcontrast source and subtraction images exhibit heterogeneous mass enhancement (**f**, **g**) with predominantly persistent kinetics seen on angiomap (**h**). Reformatted source sagittal and coronal images (**i**, **j**) show the subareolar cancer (*short arrows*) and duct fluid in the anterior breast (*long arrows*). Histology: IDC 2.2 cm, grade 2 with internal DCIS cribriform/solid. ER /PR (+), HER-2/neu (–). Sentinel nodes were negative for carcinoma (0/4).

enhancement on MRI, and with low initial enhancement and variable enhancement in the delayed phase (▶ Fig. 8.59; ▶ Fig. 8.60).

8.6.2 Luminal B Subtype

Luminal B breast cancers express both ER and PR, are usually higher grade than luminal A cancers, and have been shown to have significantly worse relapse-free survival rates than the luminal A subtype,[42] Approximately 30% of luminal B cancers are classified as HER2 enriched with overexpression of ERBB2, and exhibit higher proliferative activity, with Ki-67 levels ≥ 15%.

Imaging Findings

There is limited information regarding the specific MRI appearance of luminal B tumors. Although ER and PR status are predictors of response to tamoxifen-based therapies, unlike luminal A tumors, the luminal B subtype has been shown to be relatively insensitive to endocrine therapy. Mazurowski and colleagues have shown a large differential between the rate of enhancement of luminal B breast cancers and normal background parenchyma, implying an increase in either vascularity and/or vascular permeability due to neoangiogenesis.[43] The authors

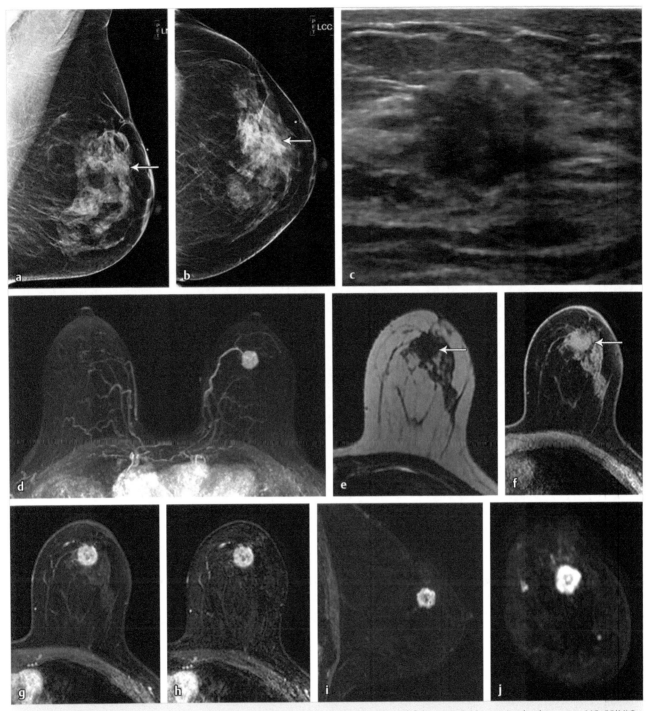

Fig. 8.61 Luminal B subtype. Patient presented with a palpable mass (BB skin marker) in the left breast at 2:00, anterior depth, seen on MG-CC/MLO views as an obscured mass (**a,b** *arrows*), and confirmed as an irregular mass on ultrasound (**c**). MIP image shows a unifocal round mass with heterogeneous enhancement (**d**). Precontrast T2w and T1w images show the partly obscured isointense mass (**e, f,** *arrows*). Postcontrast source and subtraction images exhibit heterogeneous mass enhancement (**g, h**). Reformatted sagittal and coronal images are shown (**i, j**). Histology: IDC grade 2, size 1.7 cm, with internal DCIS, cribriform/solid. ER (+), PR (−), HER-2/neu (−). The sentinel node was negative for carcinoma (0/1).

concluded that lesions with a higher ratio of lesion enhancement rate to the BPE rate were more likely to be of the luminal B subtype (▶ Fig. 8.61, ▶ Fig. 8.62). Patients with luminal A and B cancers are more likely to develop bone metastases than are those with the basal-like subtype, where lung and brain lesions are more common.[43]

8.6.3 HER2/Neu-Enriched Subtype

Patients with HER2/neu-enriched tumors often present clinically as grade 2 or 3 infiltrating cancers with high rates of multifocal disease, associated intraductal disease, lymphovascular invasion, and nodal involvement. HER2 is a member of the ErbB family of

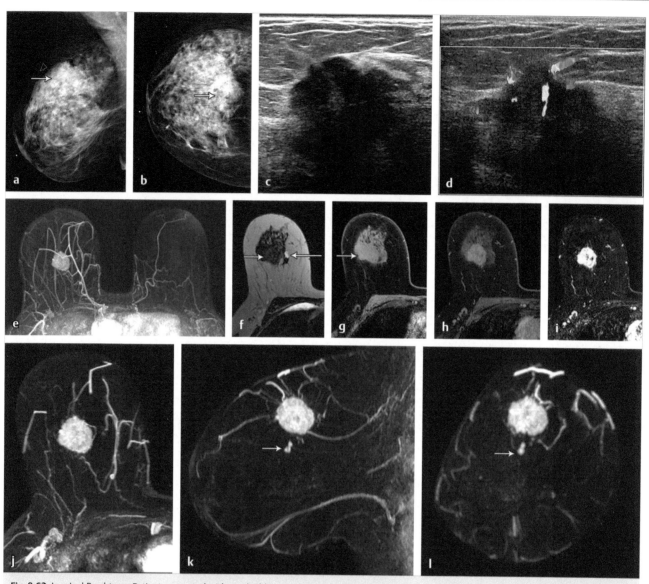

Fig. 8.62 Luminal B subtype. Patient presented with a palpable mass (triangular skin marker) in the right breast at 12:00 mid-depth, seen on MG-CC/MLO views as an obscured mass (**a, b** *arrows*), and confirmed as a microlobulated, hypoechoic mass with increased blood flow at ultrasound (**c, d**). MIP image shows a unifocal round mass with heterogeneous enhancement (**e**). Precontrast T2w and T1w images show the partly obscured isointense mass (**g, h,** *arrows*). A high signal cyst is seen on T2w image, medial to the mass (**g,** *long arrow*). Postcontrast source and subtraction images exhibit heterogeneous mass enhancement (**h, i**). Reformatted axial, sagittal, and coronal images are shown (**j-l**), revealing a satellite focus of enhancement adjacent to the index mass on sagittal and coronal images (*arrows*), proved to be malignant at subsequent MR-guided biopsy. Histology: IDC grade 2 suspicious for LVI, ER (+), PR (–), HER-2/neu (–). Sentinel nodes were negative for malignancy (0/4).

proteins and is involved in regulating cellular proliferation and apoptosis through a variety of different signaling pathways. HER2/neu-positive cancers are defined by overexpression of ERBB2, the gene that encodes the epidermal growth factor receptor type 2.[44] These tumors do not express ERs but exhibit strong HER2 overexpression: (3+) on IHC or (2+) on HER2 gene amplification, as evidenced by FISH (fluorescence in situ hybridization) or by CISH (chromogenic in situ hybridization). Because the HER2/neu gene is a protooncogene, its amplification results in increased cellular aggressiveness and faster tumor growth.

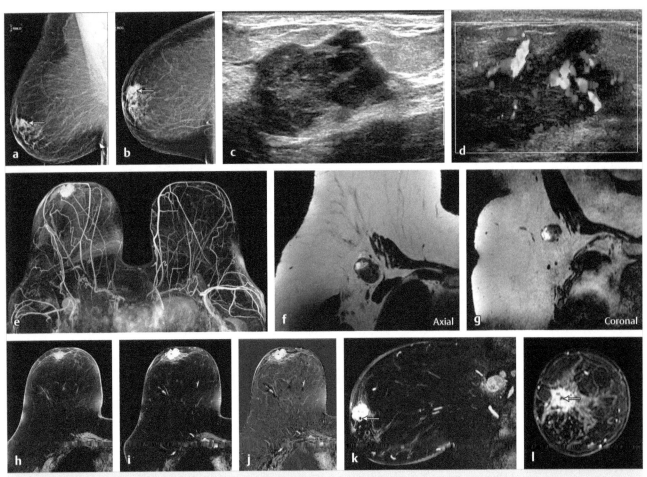

Fig. 8.63 HER2/neu-enriched subtype. Screening MG-MLO/CC of the right breast identifies a partly obscured subareolar mass (**a, b,** *arrows*), confirmed on ultrasound as an irregular mass with increased vascularity (**c, d**). MIP image shows a unifocal irregular/lobulated mass with homogeneous enhancement and a large axillary lymph node (**e**). T2w images of the axilla show to advantage the large metastatic node with internal high signal suggesting necrosis (**f, g**). Precontrast T1w image identifies the subareolar mass (**h**) with rapid mass enhancement exhibited on source and subtracted images (**i, j**). Reformatted sagittal image demonstrates an enlarged metastatic axillary lymph node, and a signal void/biopsy marker clip is found within the mass on both sagittal and coronal views (**k, l,** *arrows*). Histology: IDC grade 3, ER/PR (+), HER-2/neu (+), Ki-67: 15%, One, axillary lymph node confirmed to be malignant, patient underwent neoadjuvant therapy.

Imaging Findings

The imaging findings of HER2/neu-positive lesions on mammography are variable, the tumors most often presenting as an irregular mass, with or without malignant-appearing calcifications representing associated DCIS. MRI shows that HER2/neu-positive cancers are more likely to exhibit non–mass enhancement as the primary imaging finding than other types of invasive cancer, where mass findings predominate (▶ Fig. 8.63; ▶ Fig. 8.64; ▶ Fig. 8.65). A 30% prevalence of NME was found in one report on triple-negative cancer.[45] Findings reflecting tumor aggressiveness on T2w series, such as high intratumoral signal, peritumoral edema, prepectoral edema, and dilated posterior lymphatics, are more frequently found in high-grade lesions than in luminal cancers (▶ Fig. 8.66).[46,47] Additional examples of these T2w findings, given their importance as an imaging prognostic marker, are shown (▶ Fig. 8.67; ▶ Fig. 8.68; ▶ Fig. 8.69). HER2-positive tumors have also been shown to demonstrate rapid early contrast uptake to a greater extent than other molecular subtypes, another sign of tumor aggressiveness.[48]

The development of targeted therapy for HER2/neu-positive cancers with the introduction of trastuzumab therapy has significantly improved patient outcome, resulting in a 52% reduction in disease recurrence and a 33% reduction in the death rate.[49] In addition to the molecular markers discussed earlier, research in this field has identified additional markers of cell proliferation and invasion. These markers include the p53 gene, TP53, a tumor-suppressor gene; the Bcl-2 gene, BCL2, a proto-oncogene involved in the regulation of cell death or apoptosis; Claudin, a protein involved in the formation of epithelium; and UPA/PAI1 (urokinase plasminogen activator/plasminogen activator inhibitor 1), which is involved in tumor spread.

8.6.4 Triple-Negative and Basal-Like Subtype

Basal-like tumors are high-grade, rapidly growing, biologically aggressive tumors with a high mitotic index.[50] Compared with other breast cancer subtypes, these tumors are often larger at

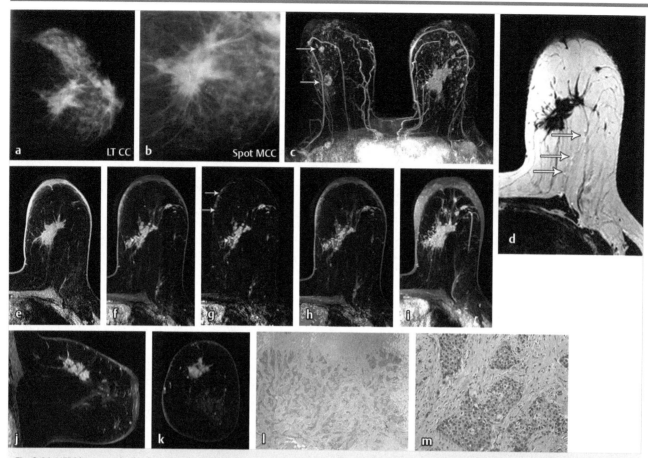

Fig. 8.64 HER2/neu-enriched subtype. Patient presented with a palpable mass in the left midbreast at 10:00, seen on MLO and MCC spot views as a 2.5-cm spiculated mass with associated microcalcifications (**a, b**). MIP image shows a large irregular mass in the central left breast with satellite lesions and two stable circumscribed benign masses in the right breast (**c**, *arrows*). T2w image shows an irregular hypointense mass, with linear hyperintense signal extending from the posterior aspect of the mass to the pectoral muscle (**d**, *arrows*). Precontrast T1w image shows anterior skin thickening (**e**), and postcontrast source, subtraction, and angiomap images (**f-h**) show enhancement extending to the medial-anterior breast with heterogeneous washout kinetics. Focal medial skin enhancement likely reflects biopsy change (*arrows*). Slab axial image demonstrates the extent of disease (**i, j**). Reformatted sagittal and coronal images are shown (**j, k**). Histology: IDC grade 3, multifocal with DCIS high grade, solid, no skin involvement. ER/PR (−), HER-2/neu (+) Ki-67: 25%. (**l, m**) Two axillary lymph nodes were confirmed to be malignant (2/14).

the time of diagnosis and lymph node metastases are more frequently found. Lymph node involvement, however, is probably less important in triple-negative tumors than other subtypes, because these tumors display a propensity toward node-negative progression and early systemic involvement.[51] Cancers are grouped into the basal category if the cancer cells display characteristics that are similar to the myoepithelial cells (basal cells) that line the inner surface of the basement membrane. The most common basal-type gene signature is that of the triple-negative subtype. This subtype is defined as a tumor that does not express ER or PR, and does not overexpress or amplify the HER2/neu gene. As this definition is one of exclusion, it would be reasonable to expect that triple-negative cancers likely represent a heterogeneous population of malignancies. A P53-gene mutation is seen in most of these tumors, and numerous other genomic changes with loss of chromosome segments are often found. There is no universally accepted definition of basal-like breast cancer, and the majority of triple-negative cancers (80%) are also basal-like, the two terms often being used interchangeably.[51] Medullary and metaplastic breast cancer subtypes are strongly associated with the triple-negative subtype. Triple-ne-

gative cancer comprises 12 to 17% of all breast malignancies and is commonly found in BRCA1 mutation carriers and also in premenopausal African American women. On the other hand, BRCA2-related cancers are less often described as ER negative and exhibit similar characteristics to nonhereditary (sporadic) breast cancer. Secretory and adenoid cystic carcinomas, both rare histologic types, share triple-negative characteristics; however, patient outcome is more favorable when compared to patients with the more common triple-negative invasive cancer subtype.[51]

Imaging Findings

Triple-negative cancers are consistent in their morphology, with a round, oval, or lobular mass shape, often with a posterior location, shown in 77 to 95% of cases.[45,51] Heterogeneous or rim enhancement on MRI is commonly found in triple-negative cancer, in addition to rapid uptake of contrast and washout kinetics.[52] Associated calcification representing DCIS is infrequently seen (► Fig. 8.70; ► Fig. 8.71; ► Fig. 8.72; ► Fig. 8.73; ► Fig. 8.74).

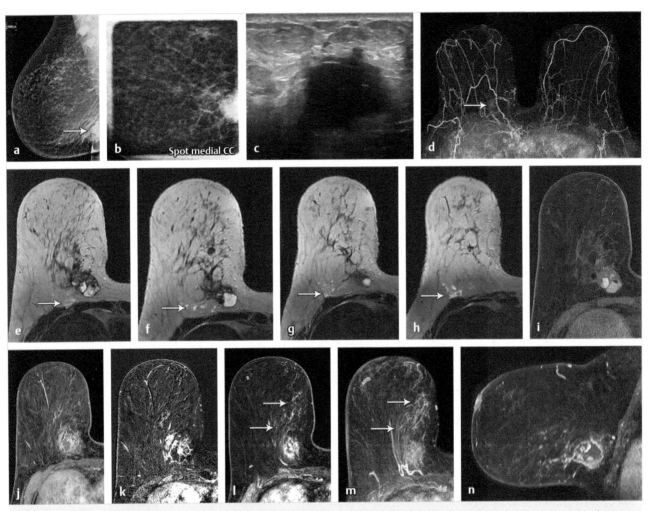

Fig. 8.65 HER2/neu-enriched subtype (1.5 T). Patient presented with a palpable mass in the inferomedial right breast as seen on MLO and CC spot views, partially visible as a high density, circumscribed mass with associated axillary lymphadenopathy (**a, b**). Ultrasound shows an irregular mass with indistinct margins and hypoechogenicity (**c**). MIP image reveals mild BPE and possible abnormal enhancement in the medial, posterior right breast (**d**, *arrow*). The mass is well seen on T2w images as a lobulated, circumscribed mass with hyperintense signal (necrosis) and associated prepectoral fluid (**e-h**, *arrows*). Mixed signal intensity is noted, including some high signal, on precontrast T1w image (**i**). Postcontrast source and subtraction images (**j, k**) show mass heterogeneous rim enhancement with a central enhancing nidus (bulls-eye). Additional slices show associated NME extending from the mass to the anterior breast (**l, m**, *arrows*). A sagittal reformatted image is shown (**n**). Histology: IDC grade 3, with DCIS high grade. ER/PR (−), HER-2/neu (+), Ki-67: 80%. Eight axillary lymph nodes were confirmed to be malignant (8/22).

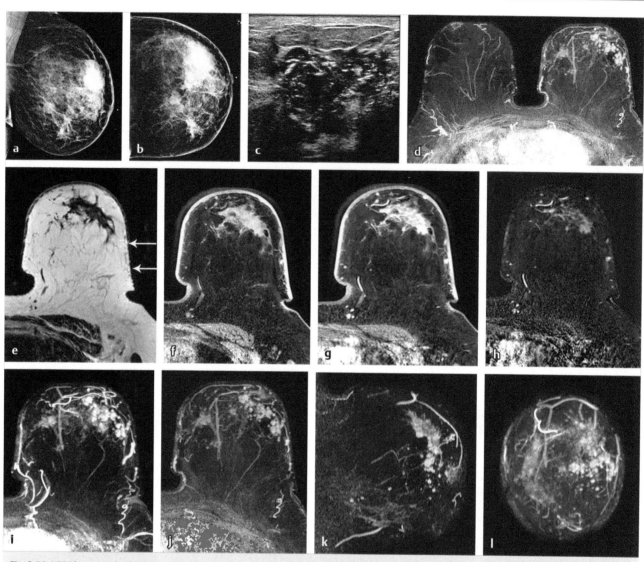

Fig. 8.66 HER2/neu-enriched subtype. Age 34: patient presented with a feeling of "heaviness" in her left breast. LT MG-MLO/CC views show skin thickening and a 15 cm × 10 cm area of pleomorphic highly suspicious calcifications, with least three spiculated masses, at 12:00, 6:00 and 9:00 (**a, b**). The mass at 12:00 is shown on ultrasound as an irregularly shaped hypoechoic mass with angular margins and multiple internal calcifications (**c**). MIP image shows mass and non–mass enhancement wrapping around the anterior and lateral left breast (**d**). The lesion is isointense on T2w image (**e**) and subtle high signal is noted laterally (*arrows*) suggesting subcutaneous edema. Skin thickening is noted on precontrast T1w image (**f**). Postcontrast T1w source and subtraction images (**g, h**) show confluent enhancement in the anterolateral breast. Axial slab image (**i**) shows to advantage the multiple enhancing masses and surrounding NME, with persistent enhancement noted on angiomap (**j**). Sagittal and coronal reformatted images are shown (**k, l**). Histology: IDC grade 2/3 with high-grade DCIS (cribriform, micropapillary, apocrine) admixed with the invasive component, constituting 50% of the tumor volume. Tumor involvement in the dermal lymphatics of the nipple: blood vessel and lymphatic invasion. ER/PR (+), HER-2/neu (+). Eight axillary lymph nodes were confirmed to be malignant (8/16).

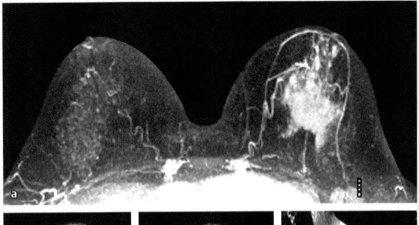

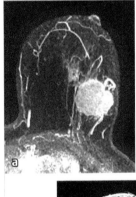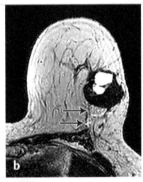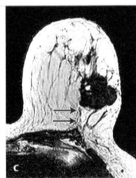

Fig. 8.67 T2w findings. A newly diagnosed breast cancer is shown on MIP image (**a**) as a large, enhancing, irregular mass in the central left breast with NME extending to the nipple. T2w images show diffuse anterolateral skin thickening, fluid posterior to the mass and prepectoral fluid, on images (**b-d**, *arrows*). Histology: IDC grade 3 with lobular features and extensive lymphovascular space invasion. Also noted is associated DCIS, high grade, solid, constituting 20% of the tumor volume. ER/PR (–), HER-2/neu (+), Ki-67: 20–30%. Eighteen axillary lymph nodes were confirmed to be malignant (18/33), with extensive extranodal extension and lymphovascular emboli in the perinodal adipose tissue.

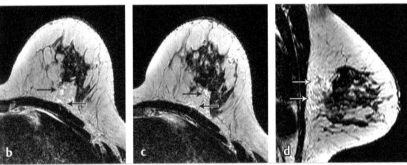

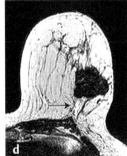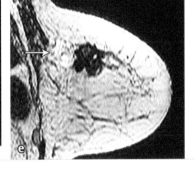

Fig. 8.68 T2w findings. A newly diagnosed breast cancer is shown on MIP image (**a**) as an enhancing mass with lobulation and an adjacent anteromedial satellite. T2w images show high signal within the hypointense mass indicating central tumor necrosis, and posterior fluid is seen between the mass and the pectoral muscle (**b-e**, *arrows*). Histology: IDC grade 3, 4 cm in size, ER (+), PR (–), HER-2/neu (–), Ki-67: 70%: Five sentinel nodes were negative for carcinoma (0/5).

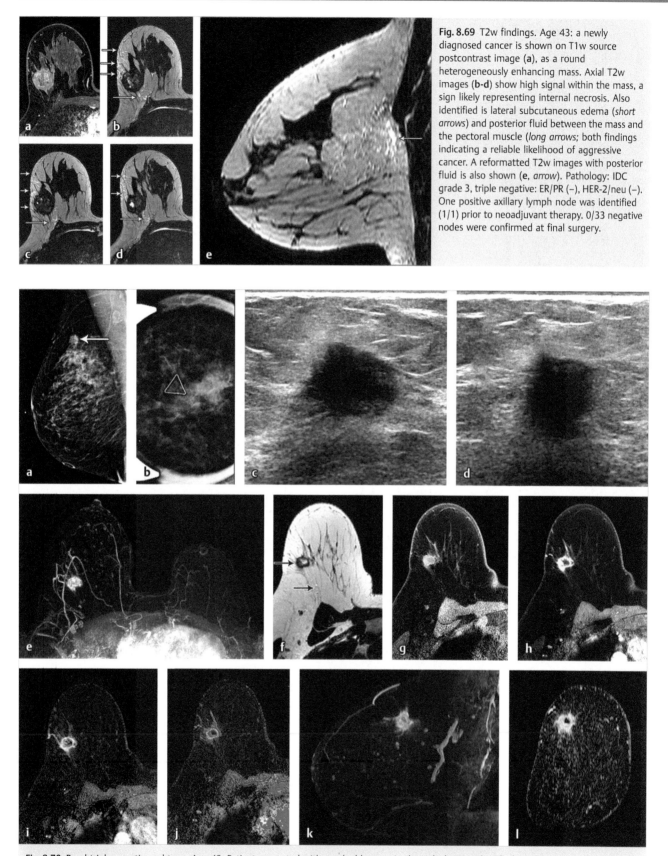

Fig. 8.69 T2w findings. Age 43: a newly diagnosed cancer is shown on T1w source postcontrast image (**a**), as a round heterogeneously enhancing mass. Axial T2w images (**b-d**) show high signal within the mass, a sign likely representing internal necrosis. Also identified is lateral subcutaneous edema (*short arrows*) and posterior fluid between the mass and the pectoral muscle (*long arrows;* both findings indicating a reliable likelihood of aggressive cancer. A reformatted T2w images with posterior fluid is also shown (**e**, *arrow*). Pathology: IDC grade 3, triple negative: ER/PR (–), HER-2/neu (–). One positive axillary lymph node was identified (1/1) prior to neoadjuvant therapy. 0/33 negative nodes were confirmed at final surgery.

Fig. 8.70 Basal-triple negative subtype. Age 49. Patient presented with a palpable mass in the right breast, identified as a round mass at 10:00, posterior depth (triangular markers) on MLO and CC spot views (**a, b**, *arrow*). Correlative ultrasound shows a round, hypoechoic mass with indistinct margins (**c, d**). MIP image shows a correlative, robustly enhancing mass with increased vascularity (**e**). The mass is well seen on T2w images as a circumscribed mass with hyperintense internal signal (necrosis) with subtle high-signal representing fluid, located between the posterior mass margin and the pectoral muscle (**f**, *arrows*). Precontrast image (**g**) shows central mass hypointensity and postcontrast images reveal classic rim enhancement (**h, i**). Heterogeneous enhancement is seen in the mass periphery (**j**). Sagittal and coronal reformatted images are shown (**k, l**). Histology: IDC grade 3, with focal necrosis. ER/PR–, HER-2/neu–, Ki67: 40%. 0/4 sentinel nodes negative for carcinoma.

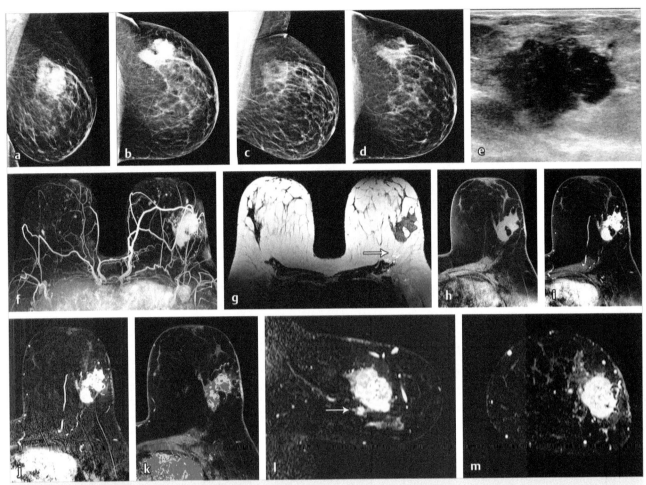

Fig. 8.71 Basal-triple negative subtype. Age 48. Patient presented with a palpable mass in the left breast identified as a developing distortion/asymmetry at 2:00 on MG-MLO/CC views (**a, b**), prior images taken at 5 months previously are shown (**c, d**). Correlative ultrasound shows an irregular, hypoechoic mass with indistinct margins (**e**). MIP image reveals a correlative, enhancing mass with increased vascularity and an enlarged axillary node (**f**). The mass is isointense on T2 and fluid between the posterior mass margin and the pectoral muscle is noted (**g**, *arrow*). Precontrast image (**h**) exhibits mass isointensity and postcontrast images reveal heterogeneous enhancement with washout kinetics (**i-k**). Sagittal and coronal reformatted images are shown (**l, m**). Histology: IDC grade 3, ER/PR–, HER-2/neu–, 2/17 axillary lymph nodes confirmed to be malignant.

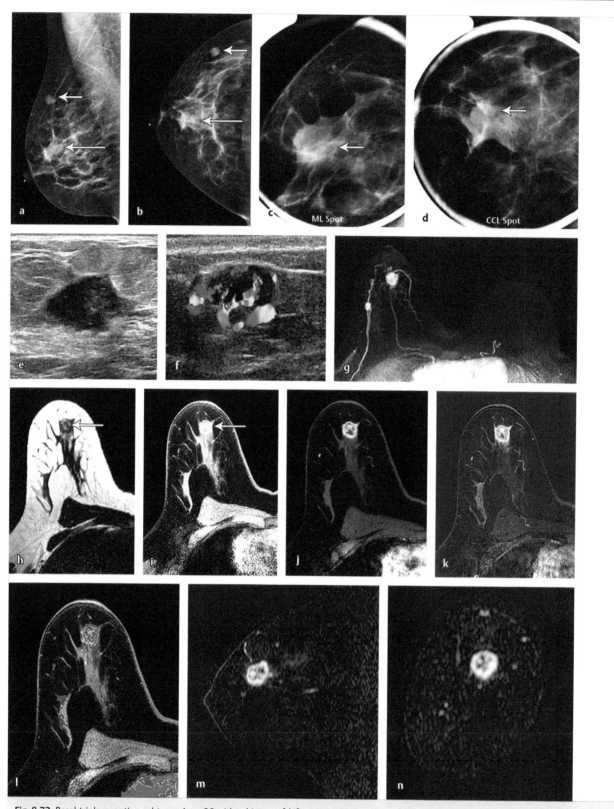

Fig. 8.72 Basal-triple negative subtype. Age: 36 with a history of left mastectomy and autologous reconstruction: Follow-up routine mammogram revealed an enlarging intramammary lymph node in the right breast (*short arrow*), in addition to an obscured mass in the subareolar region (*long arrows*) (**a, b**), better visualized on spot compression views (**c, d**). Ultrasound of the subareolar mass shows an irregular shape with mixed echogenicity (**e**), and an enlarged intramammary lymph node with marked increased blood flow (**f**). MIP image reveals a correlative enhancing mass and an enlarged node (**g**). The mass is hyperintense on T2 (**h**) and isointense on precontrast image (**i**) and exhibits rim enhancement with a central enhancing tumor nidus and washout kinetics (**j-l**). Sagittal and coronal reformatted images are shown (**m, n**). Histology: IDC grade 3, ER/PR (–), HER-2/neu (–). Six sentinel nodes negative for carcinoma (0/6).

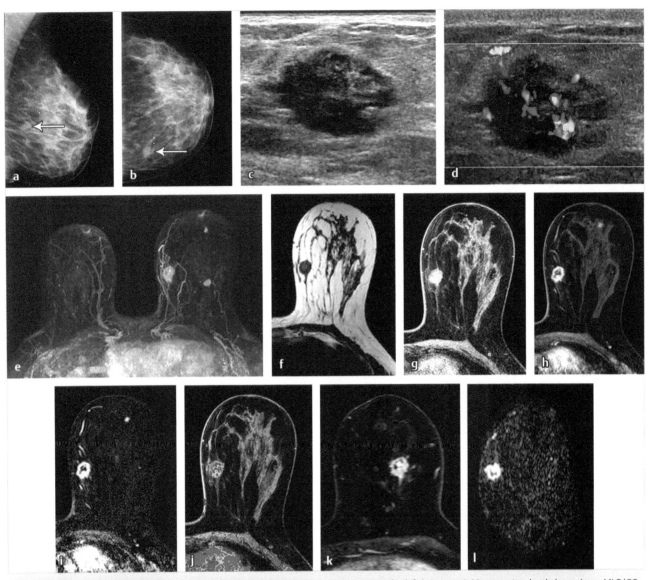

Fig. 8.73 Basal-triple negative subtype. Screening mammogram shows an oval mass in the left breast at 9:00, posterior depth (*arrow*), on MLO/CC views (**a, b**), found on ultrasound as an irregular, microlobulated mass with increased vascularity (**c, d**). MIP image reveals three masses; the largest mass at 9:00 correlates with the mammographic and ultrasound finding, a second small irregular subareolar mass and a third mass at 3:00 are identified (**e**). The mass at 9:00 is isointense on T2 (**f**), hyperintense on precontrast image (**g**), and exhibits mass rim enhancement with a central enhancing nidus on source and subtracted postcontrast series (**h, i**). The angiomap shows heterogeneous washout kinetics (**j**). Sagittal and coronal reformatted images are shown (**k, l**). Ultrasound-guided biopsy of the 3:00 mass yielded IDC grade 3. Histology 9:00 mass: IDC grade 3, size 1.5 cm. ER/PR (−), HER-2/neu (−), Ki-67: 80%. Sentinel nodes negative for carcinoma (0/4). Patient underwent NACT.

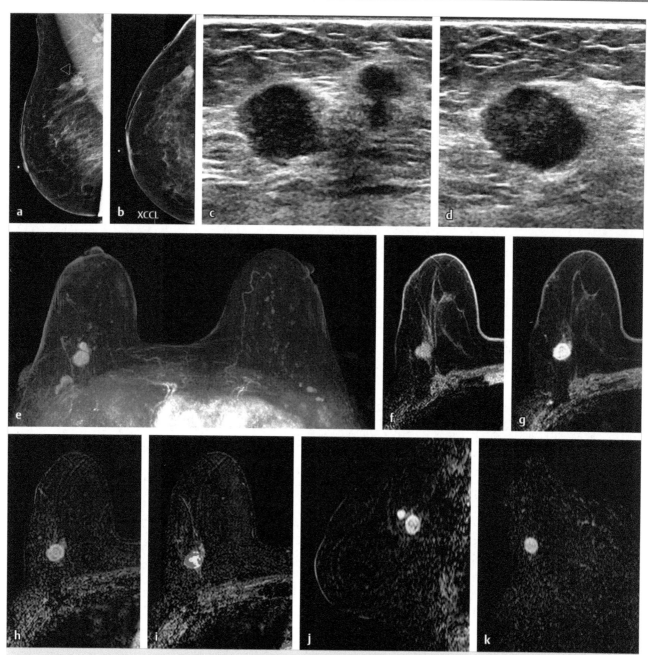

Fig. 8.74 Basal-triple negative subtype. Patient presented with a right breast palpable mass, shown on MG (triangular skin marker) as a round mass in the far posterior depth at 2:00 (**a, b**). An anterior linear skin marker denotes the site of prior benign biopsy. Ultrasound reveals a correlative hypoechoic indistinct mass with a smaller anterior satellite (**c, d**). MIP image (**e**) exhibits enhancement in both the index and satellite lesion and an enlarged axillary lymph node is noted. The mass is isointense on precontrast image (**f**), exhibits rim enhancement with a central enhancing tumor nidus "bullseye," and washout kinetics (**g-i**). Sagittal and coronal reformatted images are shown (**j, k**). Histology: IDC grade 2, 1.4 cm and 3.0 mm, ER/PR (−), HER-2/neu (−). Sentinel nodes negative for carcinoma (0/2).

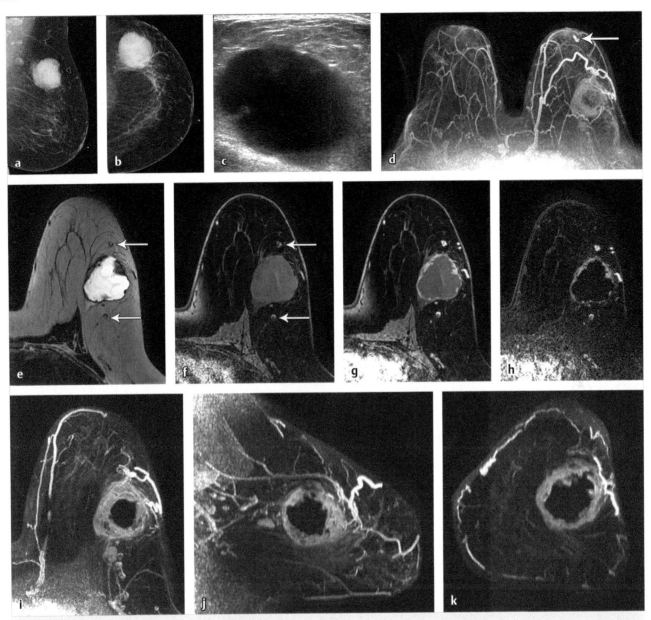

Fig. 8.75 Basal-triple negative subtype. A 58-year-old patient presented with a painful palpable mass in the left breast at 2:00, seen as a high-density mass (triangular skin marker) on MG-MLO/CC views (**a, b**). Ultrasound demonstrates a 5.5-cm anechoic mass with a thick wall, internal mural nodule and thick septum (**c**). MIP image (**d**) reveals a correlative enhancing mass with increased vascularity, and a subareolar, enhancing oval mass, representing a stable papilloma (*arrow*). The mass is fluid-filled with a thick wall on T2 (**e**) and is isointense on precontrast T1 image (**f**). IMLNs both anterior and posterior to the mass exhibit normal morphology (*arrows*). Postcontrast source and subtraction images (**g, h**) reveal rim enhancement surrounding the fluid-filled mass. Slab reformatted images, axial, sagittal, and coronal (**i-k**) are shown. Histology: IDC grade 3, with extensive necrosis and focal sarcomatoid differentiation. Histology: ER/PR (−), HER-2/neu (−). Sentinel nodes negative for carcinoma (0/2).

A salient MRI feature, commonly reported in triple-negative cancer, is that of central high signal within the index mass on T2w precontrast images. This finding likely represents tumor necrosis and is typically seen in rapidly growing lesions, which may indicate a poor prognosis. The finding of high T2 signal on precontrast images is also seen in mucinous carcinoma, a lower grade tumor, where the high signal represents mucin rather than necrosis (▸ Fig. 8.75; ▸ Fig. 8.76). It is important to note that the findings of mass margin circumscription, and uniform hypoechogenicity as seen on ultrasound, may lead to a misdiag-

nosis of benignity, resulting in a significant delay in diagnosis. MRI findings strongly indicate malignancy as shown (▸ Fig. 8.77; ▸ Fig. 8.78; ▸ Fig. 8.79).

In general, these cancers have a poor prognosis and although they remain unresponsive to standard endocrine therapy, they are chemosensitive, possibly due to their high proliferation index and/or high prevalence of the P53 gene mutation. Triple-negative cancers tend to recur early, usually within 2 to 3 years following treatment, with a relatively low risk of distant metastases after 5 years.[53] Triple-negative cancer metastases are less

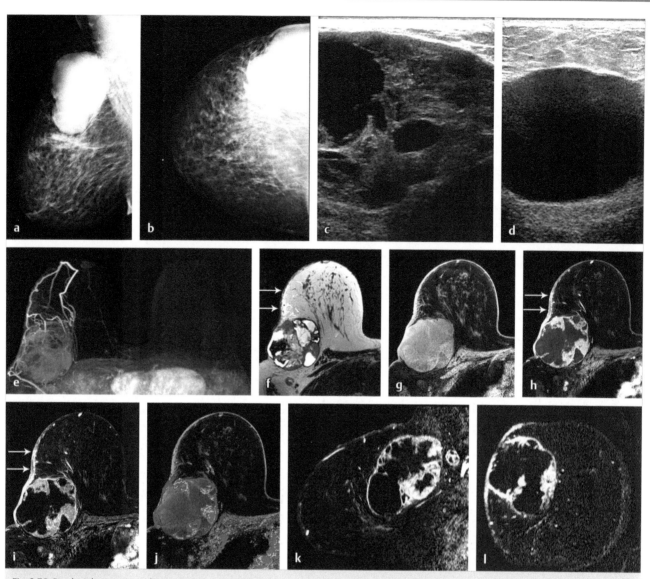

Fig. 8.76 Basal-triple negative subtype. Patient presented with a large palpable mass in the right breast at 2:00, posterior depth, seen as a high-density lobulated mass on MG-MLO/CC views (**a, b**). Ultrasound demonstrates a 9.5-cm mass with internal fluid (necrosis) and solid components (**c, d**). MIP image (**e**) reveals a correlative enhancing mass with increased vascularity, seen on T2 as a complex mass with fluid and solid components and lateral subcutaneous edema (**f**, *arrows*). The mass is isointense on precontrast T1 image and lateral skin thickening is present (**g**). Postcontrast source and subtraction images (**h-j**) reveal rim and internal tumor enhancement, with washout kinetics, and skin enhancement in the lateral breast (*arrows*). Sagittal and coronal reformatted images are shown (**k, l**). Histology: IDC grade 3, with extensive necrosis, associated internal DCIS, and direct extension of tumor into the skin with ulceration. ER/PR (−), HER-2/neu (−). Twelve axillary lymph nodes confirmed to be malignant (12/20).

likely to involve bony structures and are more likely to involve the viscera, particularly the lungs and brain. A summary of the main imaging findings, categorized by molecular subtypes, is shown (▶ Table 8.5).

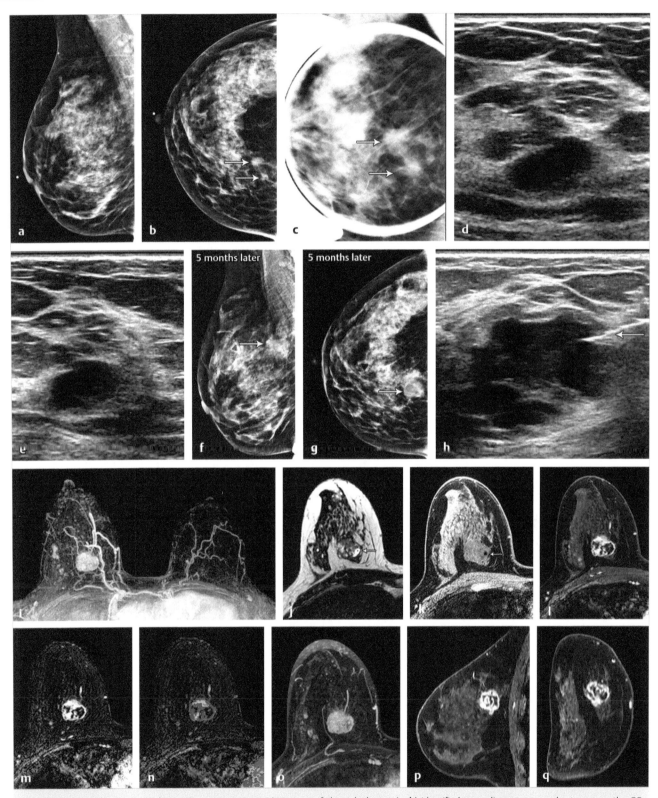

Fig. 8.77 Basal-triple negative subtype. Screening MG-MLO/CC views of the right breast (**a, b**) identified two adjacent masses, best seen on the CC view (*arrows*) and further evaluated with spot compression view (**c**) and ultrasound (**d, e**). Although the lesions appear anechoic, the margins are not circumscribed. An erroneous diagnosis of "cysts" was made. The patient presented 5 months later with a right breast palpable mass, seen on MLO and CC views as a larger, partly obscured mass (**f, g**) and identified on ultrasound as an irregular hypoechoic mass. The mass was biopsied under ultrasound guidance and the biopsy needle is shown (**h,** *arrow*). MIP image (**i**) reveals a correlative enhancing mass with increased vascularity, seen on T2 as a hyperintense mass with signal void representing a biopsy marker clip (**J,** *arrow*). The mass is isointense on precontrast T1 image and the marker clip is identified (**k,** *arrow*). Postcontrast source and subtraction images (**l-n**) reveal rim and heterogeneous internal tumor enhancement suggesting central necrosis. Slab axial, sagittal, and coronal reformatted images are shown (**o-q**). Histology: IDC grade 3, with extensive metaplastic (chondrosarcomatous) differentiation. ER/PR (−), HER-2/neu (−), Ki67: 60%. Sentinel nodes negative for carcinoma (0/3).

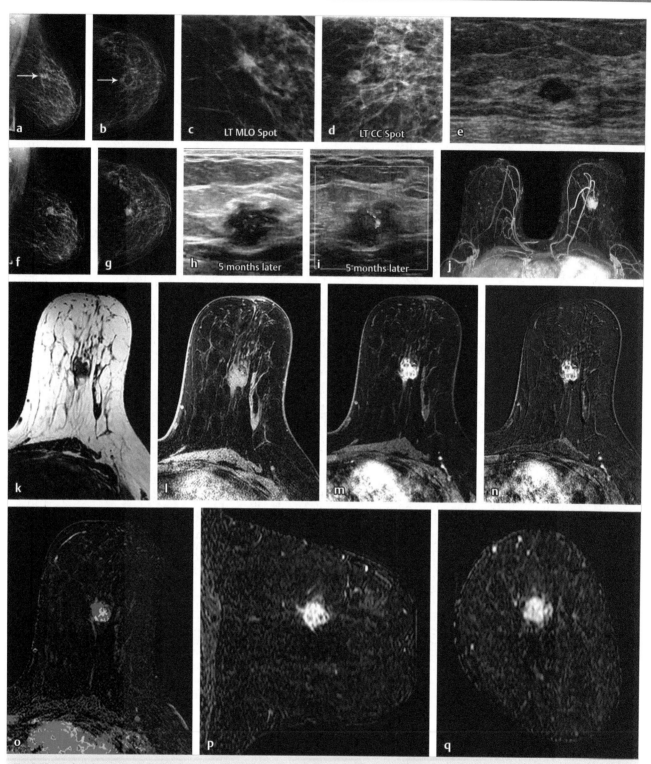

Fig. 8.78 Basal-triple negative subtype. Screening MG-MLO/CC views of the left breast (**a, b**) identified a mass at 12:00 (*arrows*) and further evaluation was recommended with spot compression view (**c, d**) and ultrasound (**e**). The lesion was diagnosed as "probable fibroadenoma" and a 6-month follow-up MG was recommended. The patient presented 5 months later with a palpable mass, marked with a skin BB, and seen on MLO and CC views as an irregular mass, increased in size since the previous MG examination (**f, g**). Correlative ultrasound shows an irregular hypoechoic mass with increased blood flow (**h, i**), subsequently biopsied under ultrasound guidance. MIP image (**j**) reveals a correlative enhancing mass with increased vascularity, seen on both T2 and precontrast T1 images as an isointense mass (**k, l**). Postcontrast source and subtraction images (**m, n**) reveal heterogeneous internal tumor enhancement and predominantly persistent and plateau enhancement as seen on angiomap (**o**). Reformatted sagittal and coronal images are shown (**p, q**). Histology: IDC grade 3, ER/PR (–), HER-2/neu (–). Sentinel nodes negative for carcinoma (0/4).

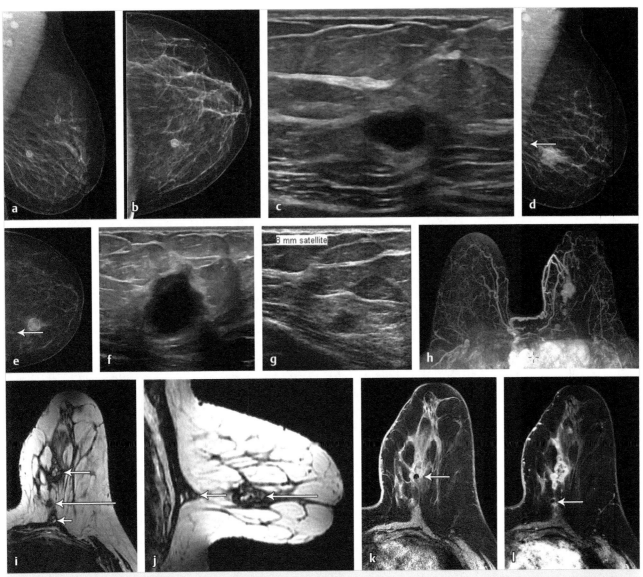

Fig. 8.79 Basal-triple negative subtype. Screening MG-MLO/CC views of the left breast (**a, b**) identify a potential mass at 9:00, seen on CAD (a false-positive mark is present in the superior left breast). Further diagnostic evaluation with ultrasound (**c**) show an oval anechoic mass incorrectly diagnosed as a "cyst." The patient presented 7 months later with a palpable mass seen on MLO and CC views as a mass with indistinct margins, increased in size since the previous MG examination, and a new small mass identified posterior to the index lesion (**d, e** *arrows*). Correlative ultrasound shows an irregular anechoic mass with a thick wall and through transmission (**f**), and a posterior microlobulated satellite lesion (**g**), both subsequently biopsied under ultrasound guidance. The enhancing index mass is seen on MIP image (**h**) in addition to the enhancing satellite. T2w axial and sagittal images (**i, j**) demonstrate the index mass with internal high signal indicating necrosis (*arrows*) in the isointense satellite lesion (*long arrow*) and posterior fluid adjacent to the pectoral muscle (*short arrows*). Precontrast isointense T1w image (**k**) shows a marker clip in the posterior aspect of the index lesion (*arrow*) and a second clip is seen in the satellite lesion on postcontrast source image (**l**). (*Continued*)

8.6.5 Inflammatory Breast Cancer

Inflammatory breast cancer (IBC) presents clinically with findings of rapid-onset breast enlargement, erythema, tenderness, and typical thickening of the skin described as "peau d'orange" or "orange peel-like." IBC has no specific histological characteristics and is not a recognized morphological subtype of invasive cancer. Axillary adenopathy is often evident at diagnosis. The hallmark signature of IBC is the presence of tumor embolization in dermal lymphatics at histology, accounting for the clinical skin changes. The underlying invasive breast cancer is usually a high-grade IBC-NST with highly angiogenic, lymphangiogenic, and vasculogenic features. This aggressive cancer is rare, comprising 2.5% of all breast cancer patients in the United States[54] and may or may not be associated with a palpable finding in the affected breast. A tissue diagnosis is essential for accurate diagnosis because acute mastitis and other rare tumors such as lymphoma and sarcoma may mimic the presentation of IBC.

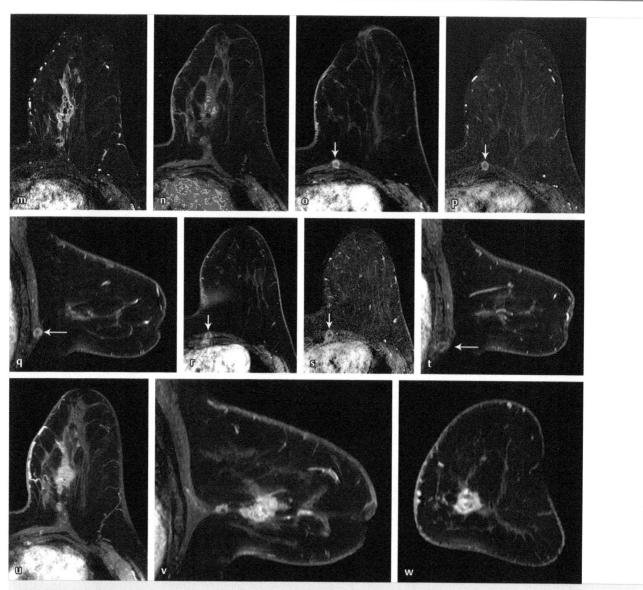

Fig. 8.79 (*continued*) Subtraction and angiomap images (**m,n**) reveal heterogeneous internal tumor enhancement with washout kinetics and anterior and posterior extension of enhancing tumor. Two areas of pectoral muscle invasion are shown (**o–t,** *arrows*). Slab reformatted images are shown (**u-w**). Histology: IDC grade 3, ER/PR (–), HER-2/neu (–), Ki67: 80%. Sentinel nodes negative for carcinoma (0/3).

Table 8.5 Molecular subtypes of breast cancer

Molecular subtype	MG (typical findings)	US (typical findings)	MRI (typical findings)	IHC (surrogate marker)	Grade (proliferative index)
Luminal A	Irregular/Spiculated mass ± calcifications Architectural distortion	Irregular mass Angulation/Echogenic halo Indistinct margins	Irregular mass Heterogeneous/Variable Enhancement	Commonly ER (+) PR (+)	Low grade Low Ki67
Luminal B	Irregular/Round mass Spiculated/Indistinct margins	Irregular/Round mass Angulation Indistinct margins	Irregular/Round mass Spiculated margins Heterogeneous Washout kinetics	Commonly ER (+) PR (+)/(–)	Intermediate/High grade High Ki67
HER2 enriched	Irregular, spiculated mass ± calcifications Pleomorphic/Fine-linear	Irregular mass, Indistinct, microlobulated/spiculated margins ± calcification	Irregular mass and/or NME ± High T2 signal Washout kinetics	Commonly HER2 + ER (–)	High grade High Ki67
Basal-like (triple negative)	Round/Oval/Lobular mass Irregular margins (Ca + + infrequent)	Circumscribed mass Marked hypoechogenicity	Round/Oval mass T2 hyperintense Rim enhancement	Commonly ER– PR– HER2–	High grade High Ki-67

Abbreviations: ER, estrogen receptor; HER2, human epidermal growth factor receptor 2; IHC, immunohistochemical; NME, nonmass enhancement; PR, progesterone receptor; US, ultrasound.

Punch biopsy of the skin in order to identify tumor emboli in dermal lymphatics is generally required to confirm a malignant diagnosis. Malignant growth often exhibits a diffuse infiltrative pattern, with or without an additional tumor mass or masses.[55]

Imaging Findings

Mammography is usually limited for patients with IBC. Breast tenderness generally precludes optimal breast compression often resulting in suboptimal image quality, some women being unable to tolerate the examination. Diffuse trabecular thickening, breast edema, and skin thickening all produce increased breast density, further hindering diagnostic efficacy at mammography. Despite these limitations,[56] evidence of an underlying tumor mass, architectural distortion, calcifications, and axillary adenopathy may be apparent.[55] Ultrasound is useful for identifying the primary malignancy and for evaluating lymph nodes in the axilla, supraclavicular and infraclavicular regions. High-resolution ultrasound provides a localized target in over 90% of cases, thus facilitating percutaneous biopsy.[57] MRI is a superior method of detection, not only for identification of the primary breast malignancy and extent of disease but also for evaluation of the contralateral breast. Typical findings include skin thickening (greater than normal skin thickness measurements of 0.5–2 mm), and subcutaneous, peritumoral, prepectoral, or diffuse edema on T2w precontrast series.[57,58,59] Skin enhancement and diffuse NME, a common finding reflecting infiltrating malignancy, is often seen on the T1w dynamic sequence.[60] Multiple, irregular, confluent, heterogeneously enhancing masses in a diffuse distribution are seen in many cases. Rapid enhancement with washout or plateau intensity curves are seen in 85 to 100% of IBC lesions (▶ Fig. 8.80; ▶ Fig. 8.81).[58,59] Skin enhancement is not unique to IBC, and may be seen in mastitis, locally advanced skin cancer with skin involvement, in addition to postradiation and postsurgical changes. The prognosis for inflammatory carcinoma patients is poor; 20% of patients initially present with distant metastases and 55 to 85% of patients have metastatic involvement of axillary or supraclavicular nodes.[60] The survival time averages 12 to 36 months and treatment generally includes neoadjuvant chemotherapy, followed by mastectomy and chest wall irradiation.[61]

8.7 Uncommon Tumor Subtypes

8.7.1 Phyllodes Tumor

Phyllodes tumor is rare in the United States (< 1% all breast tumors), typically presenting in women at 40 to 52 years of age, but is more common in Asian women (7% all breast tumors) with earlier age onset (mean: 25–30 years). The tumor arises from periductal stroma and is characterized as a biphasic fibroepithelial neoplasm with double-layered epithelium. Papillary growths of epithelial-lined stroma forming "leaf-like" projections, interspersed with clefts "cystic" spaces, are found. Unlike fibroadenoma, also a fibroepithelial lesion, these tumors have greater stromal cellularity and are locally aggressive. Histology varies within any given mass and differentiation of phyllodes tumors between benign (75%), borderline (16%), and malignant (9%) may be challenging.[62] This classification is based on a number of factors, the mitotic index, stromal cellularity and overgrowth, tumor margin characteristics, and the presence of heterologous components and necrosis. Prediction of biologic behavior in phyllodes tumors is uncertain; however, in general, benign tumors do not metastasize and have a (20%) likelihood of local recurrence after wide excision, whereas borderline tumors have a small (< 5%) likelihood of metastasis and are more likely to recur locally. A malignant phyllodes tumor has about a 22% likelihood of metastasis and is prone to local recurrence (27%).

The classic clinical presentation of a phyllodes tumor is that of a woman aged 40 to 60 years, with a rapidly enlarging, firm, painless breast mass.

Imaging Findings

Typically seen on mammography and ultrasound is a noncalcified mass, with a round, oval, or lobulated shape and circumscribed margins. When small, this lesion cannot be differentiated from a fibroadenoma. It has been reported that increasing size and a tumor diameter of 3 cm or more is associated with a higher likelihood of malignancy.[62] There are scant reports in the literature on the MRI features of phyllodes tumors and the existing descriptions are variable. Reported features include a round, oval, or lobulated mass with a circumscribed margin and mixed signal intensity on T2w and T1w series. Septations, cystic spaces, slit-like pattern, and hemorrhage are often seen within the index mass and kinetic patterns may vary between slow persistent, rapid plateau, and rapid washout.[63] Features suggesting malignancy include large size, irregular shape, hypointense/isointense signal on T2w images, hyperintense signal on T1w images (hemorrhage), cystic change (tumor necrosis), and low ADC on DWI (stromal hypercellularity).[64,65,66] Examples of a benign and a malignant phyllodes tumor are shown (▶ Fig. 8.82; ▶ Fig. 8.83).

8.7.2 Metaplastic Breast Cancer

This neoplasm is rare (< 1% of all breast cancers) and is of either epithelial or myoepithelial cell origin. The lesion comprises a heterogeneous group of tumors with mixed epithelial and mesenchymal differentiation and consists in whole or in part of either squamous or spindle cell, matrix-producing and true malignant mesenchymal component (carcinosarcoma). The molecular signature is similar to but distinct from basal-like cancer and resembles claudin-low cancers. These are mostly intermediate or high-grade triple negative, p63 (+) tumors, with generally a worse patient outcome than triple-negative lesions.

Imaging Findings

A large dense circumscribed mass with round or oval shape is typically seen on mammography, rarely with osteoid-like calcifications and segmental linear pleomorphic calcifications and microlobulation and mixed echogenicity seen on ultrasound. MRI usually exhibits a large hyperintense mass on T2w images with rapid enhancement often showing central necrosis and rim enhancement on T1w series. MRI is the most accurate imaging method for determining disease extent. Most breast "sarcomas" are actually metaplastic cancers and the diagnosis

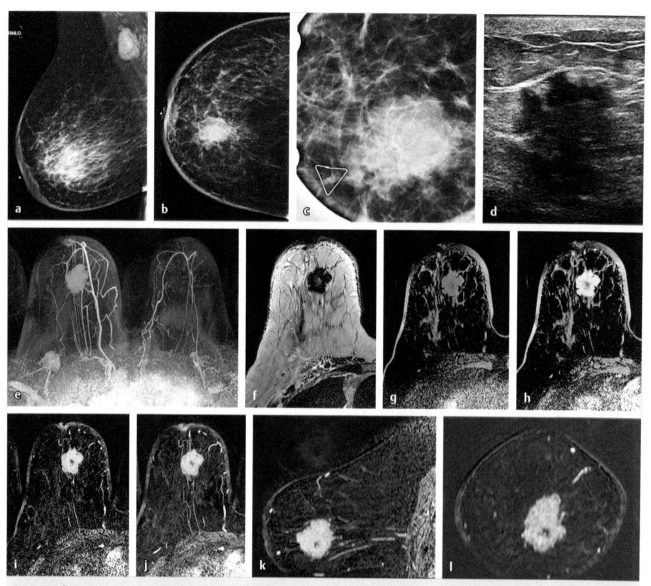

Fig. 8.80 Inflammatory cancer. Patient presented with a swollen, painful right breast with periareolar erythema. MG-MLO/CC views of the right breast (**a, b**) reveal a 2.5-cm, partly obscured mass in the anterior breast, with diffuse skin thickening and axillary lymphadenopathy. MG spot compression view (**c**) reveals an oval palpable mass (*triangular skin marker*), seen well on ultrasound (**d**) as a hypoechoic irregular mass with microlobulation. MIP image (**e**) shows homogeneous mass enhancement and a large abnormal axillary lymph node. The index lesion is shown as a hypointense mass with extensive skin thickening and subcutaneous/prepectoral edema on T2w image (**f**). Precontrast T1w image (**g**) identifies the isointense mass with extensive skin thickening and postcontrast images (**h, i**) exhibit robust mass enhancement. Reformatted slab images (**j-l**) are shown. Histology: IDC grade 3, ER/PR (–), HER-2/neu (+). Axillary nodes positive for metastatic disease. Patient was treated with neoadjuvant chemotherapy.

can be confidently made only after excision of the entire lesion.[67] Metastases are generally hematogenous to lung and liver. An example of metaplastic cancer is shown (▶ Fig. 8.84).

8.7.3 Spindle Cell Tumor

This rare neoplasm (< 1% of all breast cancers) is also known as pleomorphic spindle cell sarcoma and falls under the umbrella of breast sarcomas, including not only pleomorphic spindle cell tumor but also angiosarcoma, osteosarcoma, liposarcoma, leiomyosarcoma, rhabdomyosarcoma, and malignant fibrous histiocytoma. Breast sarcomas may arise de novo or in a field of prior radiation therapy, usually angiosarcomas, 5 to 7 years

from prior breast cancer treatment. These tumors grow rapidly, are high grade, cytokeratin negative, and exhibit malignant spindle cell proliferation in a storiform or herringbone pattern.

Imaging Findings

Typical mammographic findings include a large noncalcified round or oval mass with circumscribed or indistinct margins and findings of a solid hypoechoic mass with indistinct margins, posterior acoustic enhancement, and internal hypervascularity predominate on ultrasound.[68] The task to distinguish phyllodes tumors from primary breast sarcomas and benign fibroepithelial lesions is difficult on mammography and ultra-

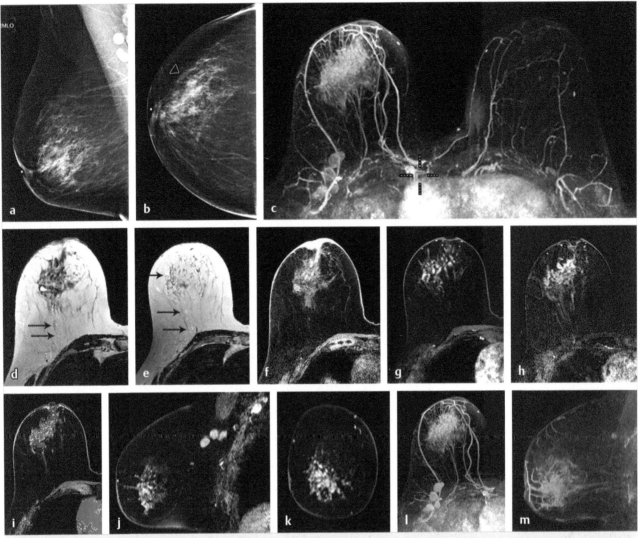

Fig. 8.81 Inflammatory cancer. Patient presented with a swollen, erythematous right breast and a palpable "thickening." MG-MLO/CC views (**a, b**) reveal an anterior global asymmetry (*triangular skin marker*), with anterior skin thickening and axillary lymphadenopathy. MIP image (**c**) shows an extensive anterior NME and several enlarged axillary lymph nodes. T2w images show peritumoral fluid and posterior breast fluid, indicating an aggressive lesion (**d, e**, *arrows*). Precontrast T1w image (**f**) exhibits anterior, periareolar skin thickening and postcontrast images (**g-i**) exhibit diffuse anterior NME with washout kinetics. Reformatted sagittal and coronal images (**j, k**) and slab axial and sagittal images (**l, m**) are shown. Histology: IBC, 6.7 cm, grade 3, with mixed ductal and lobular features, and extensive lymphovascular space invasion, involvement of dermal lymphatics and blood vessel and lymphatic invasion. ER/PR (+). Six axillary lymph nodes confirmed to be malignant (6/21).

sound. MRI findings may show mass hyperintensity or isointensity on T2w images with rapid uptake of contrast on T1w images, central necrosis, and a persistent enhancement pattern (▶ Fig. 8.85). A report on a multicenter study of primary breast sarcomas ($n = 42$) found no pathognomonic imaging features; however, overall, MR findings exhibited irregular mass shape (81.8% [9/11]) with irregular or spiculated margins and inter-mediate or heterogeneous enhancement. T2w images showed hyperintense or isointense signal (66.7% [6/9]). Kinetic analysis indicated a rapid initial signal increase with delayed washout.[69] Treatment usually includes a wide local excision or mastectomy. Axillary node sampling is not routine because nodal metastases are rare. Hematogenous metastases to lungs, bone marrow, and liver are most common. The role of chemotherapy is unclear.

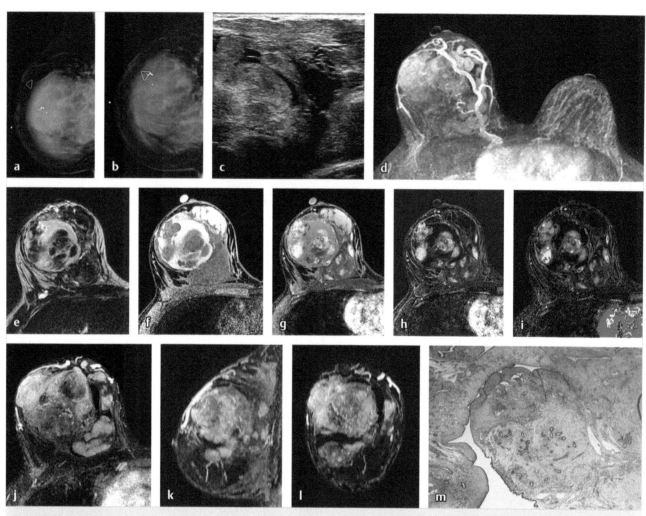

Fig. 8.82 Phyllodes tumor (benign). A 30-year-old patient presented with an 8-cm enlarging mass in the right breast. MG-MLO/CC views (**a, b**) reveal a circumscribed mass occupying most of the right breast, (*triangular skin marker*) with internal benign calcification. Ultrasound exhibits a mass with mixed echogenicity and internal vascularity with multiple hypoechoic regions (**c**). A large circumscribed enhancing mass with increased vascularity is seen on MIP image (**d**). Precontrast T2w (**e**) and postcontrast images T1w (**f**) reveal mixed signal intensity regions within the mass. Postcontrast images (**g-i**) show slit-like and cystic spaces, heterogeneous enhancement within some internal areas of the lesion, and washout noted. Slab reformatted axial, sagittal, and coronal images (**j-l**) are shown. Histology: benign phyllodes tumor. A fibroepithelial lesion with prominent leaf-like architecture is demonstrated (**m**), 9.8 cm in greatest dimension, surgical resection margins widely free. One IMLN confirmed negative for malignancy (0/1) and one axillary node confirmed negative for malignancy (0/1).

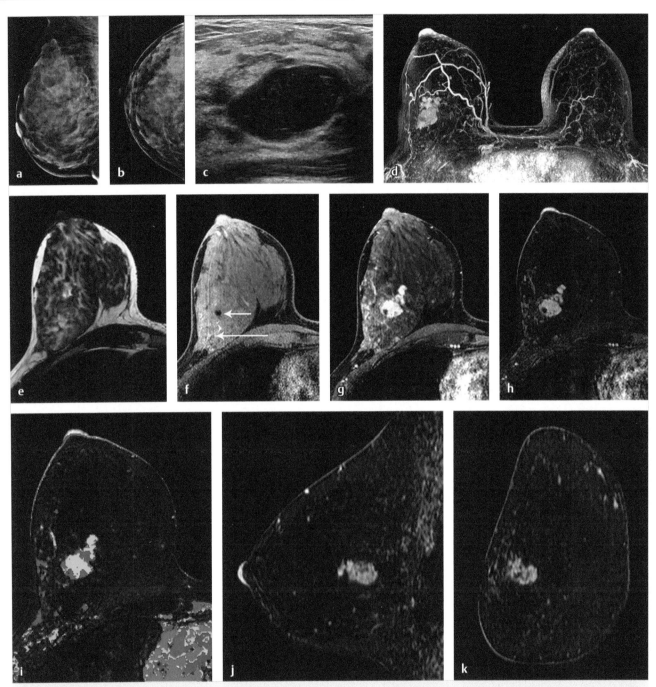

Fig. 8.83 Phyllodes tumor (malignant). A 41-year-old patient presented with a palpable mass in the right breast at 9:00. MG-MLO/CC views (**a, b**) reveal extremely dense breast tissue but no abnormal findings. An oval hypoechoic mass is identified on ultrasound (**c**) correlating with the palpable lesion, and an irregular mass with anterior adjacent satellites is noted on MIP Image (**d**). No significant findings are found on T2 (**e**) but precontrast T1w image (**f**) shows a marker clip from prior biopsy (*short arrow*), and a focal high signal region in the lateral posterior breast representing fluid (*long arrow*). BPE is shown in this region on subsequent series. Postcontrast images (**g-i**) show homogeneous enhancement with predominantly persistent kinetics and adjacent anteromedial tumor extension away from the index mass. Reformatted sagittal and coronal images, (**j, k**) are shown. Histology: malignant phyllodes tumor, 2.5 cm in greatest dimension, surgical margins negative. Prominent leaf-like architecture is demonstrated and there is marked cytologic atypia and focally high mitotic activity. Wide local excision revealed margins free of tumor.

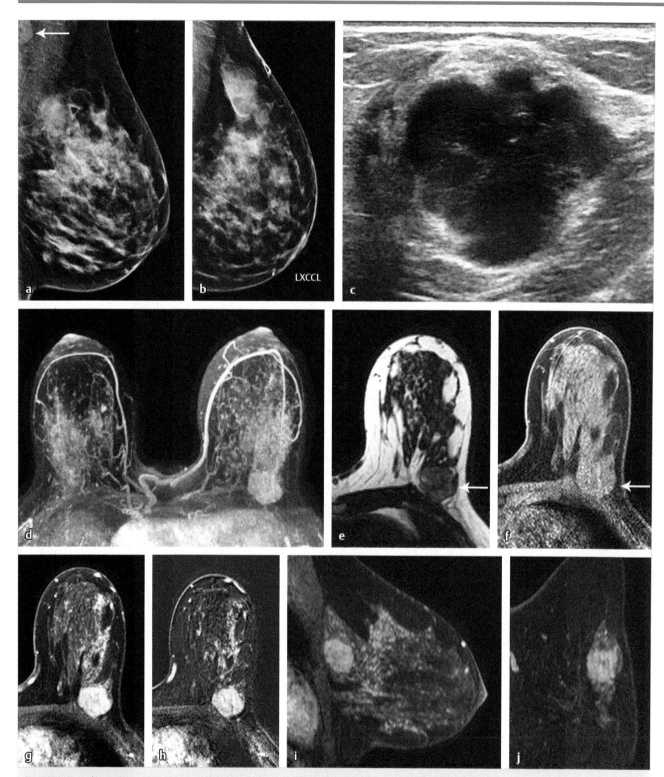

Fig. 8.84 Metaplastic cancer. Patient presented with a palpable mass in the posterior left breast at 1:00, a correlative round mass is identified on MG-MLO/XCCL views (**a, b**) and an enlarged left axillary lymph node is also noted (**a**, *arrow*). The mass is seen as a complex hypoechoic, microlobulated mass on ultrasound (**c**). MIP image, obtained at the first postcontrast time point, reveals the enhancing mass and marked BPE (**d**). The mass is hyperintense on T2 (**e**, *arrow*) and isointense on precontrast T1w image (**f**, *arrow*). Postcontrast images (**g, h**) show homogeneous enhancement. Reformatted sagittal and coronal images (**i, j**) are shown. Histology: IDC grade 3, size 3.4 cm, ER/PR (faint+), HER-2/neu (–), Ki-67: 30%. Associated DCIS low to high nuclear grades with solid and cribriform patterns. Two axillary nodes confirmed positive for carcinoma (2/12).

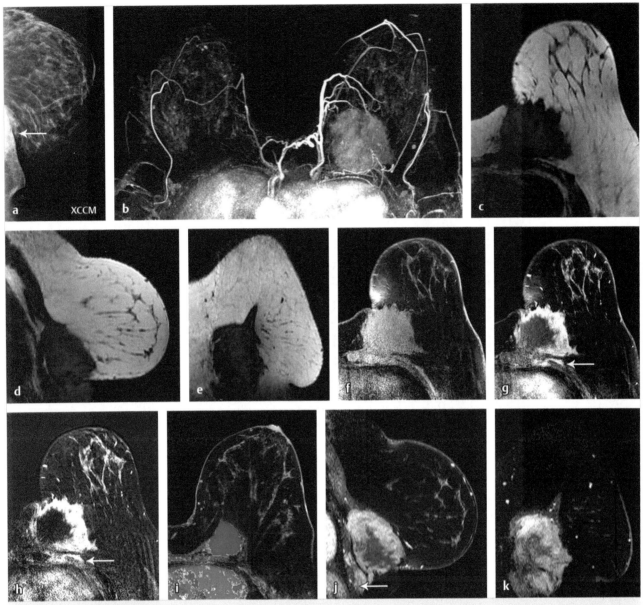

Fig. 8.85 Spindle cell lesion. Patient presented with a palpable mass partly seen on the far posteromedial left breast on MG-XCCM view (**a**). MIP image obtained at the first postcontrast time point reveals the 8.0-cm enhancing mass with increased vascularity (**b**). MPR T2w (**c-e**) images show an irregular mass abutting the pectoral muscle. The mass is isointense on precontrast T1w image and obliteration of the fat plane between the mass and the pectoral muscle is noted (**f**). Postcontrast source and subtraction images (**g-i**) show rim enhancement, central necrosis, and persistent kinetics, with pectoral muscle enhancement indicating invasion (*arrows*). Reformatted sagittal image (**j**) shows pectoral muscle invasion (*arrow*) and coronal image (**k**) is shown. Histology: spindle cell lesion consistent with fibromatosis. B-catenin shows nuclear staining.

8.7.4 Fibromatosis

Fibromatosis, also known as extra-abdominal desmoid tumor, desmoid tumor, and desmoid fibromatosis, is a locally aggressive proliferation of fibroblasts and myofibroblasts without metastatic potential, and usually arises from the pectoralis fascia. This tumor is distinct from stromal fibrosis (also known as focal fibrous disease, fibrous tumor, focal fibrosis, and fibrous mastopathy) and is a benign finding characterized by proliferation of fibrous stroma with obliteration and atrophy of mammary ducts and lobules.[70] Patients usually present with a palpable, firm painless mass in the posterior breast, which may be fixed to the pectoralis muscle.

Imaging Findings

A dense mass in the posterior breast, adjacent or attached to the pectoralis muscle, is typically seen at mammography with varying shapes and marginal characteristics, ultrasound showing a hypoechogenic mass with circumscribed, irregular, or angular margins and an echogenic rim. MRI findings include variable T2 mass intensity, with both slow persistent enhance-

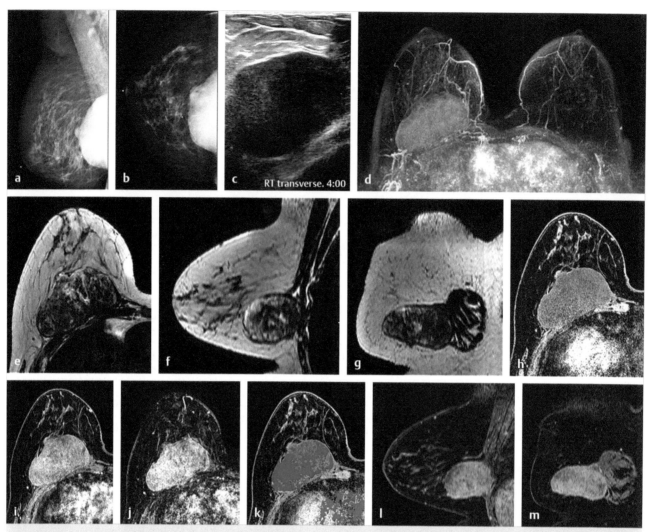

Fig. 8.86 Desmoid-type fibromatosis. Patient presented with a palpable mass in the inferior right breast on MG-MLO/CC views (**a, b**), ultrasound yielding a 5.8 × 8.7 cm circumscribed, mixed echogenicity mass (**c**). MIP image shows some homogeneous enhancement within the mass, which abuts the pectoral muscle (**d**). MPR T2w images (**e-g**) show mixed signal intensity within the mass, which appears to arise from the pectoral muscle, but does not involve the costochondral cartilage of the adjacent ribs, nor the intercostal muscles. The mass is isointense on precontrast T1w image (**h**), postcontrast source and subtraction images (**i-k**) showing homogeneous enhancement with persistent kinetics. Reformatted sagittal and coronal images (**l, m**) are shown. Histology: wide-excision. Desmoid-type fibromatosis, 10.5 cm.

ment and rapid plateau/washout enhancement reported on T1w series.[71] An example of desmoid-type fibromatosis is shown (▶ Fig. 8.86).

8.8 Summary

In this chapter, we have reviewed the imaging characteristics of invasive breast cancer, focusing primarily on their various morphologic and kinetic findings on MRI. Additionally, we have discussed the heterogeneous nature of not only imaging findings but also the clinical, histologic, and molecular characteristics of breast cancer as they apply to patient outcome. As future research unfolds, it is possible that the imaging phenotype of invasive breast cancer, particularly as applied to DCE-MRI with advanced computer analysis, may well provide even more inde-

pendent prognostic and predictive markers, complementing existing biomarkers, and thus improving patient care.

References

[1] Lakhani SR, Ellis IO, Schnitt SJ, et al. WHO Classification of Tumors of the Breast. 4th ed. Lyon: International Agency for Research on Cancer; 2012

[2] AJCC Cancer Staging Manual, Eighth Edition. The American College of Surgeons (ACS), Chicago, Illinois.

[3] Weigelt B, Geyer FC, Reis-Filho JS. Histological types of breast cancer: how special are they? Mol Oncol. 2010; 4(3):192–208

[4] Simpson PT, Reis-Filho JS, Lakhani SR. Breast pathology: beyond morphology. Semin Diagn Pathol. 2010; 27(1):91–96

[5] Guiu S, Michiels S, André F, et al. Molecular subclasses of breast cancer: how do we define them? The IMPAKT 2012 Working Group Statement. Ann Oncol. 2012; 23(12):2997–3006

[6] Perou CM, Sorlie T, Eisen MB, et al. Molecular portraits of human breast tumours. Nature. 2000; 406:747–752

[7] Sørlie T, Perou CM, Tibshirani R, et al. Gene expression patterns of breast carcinomas distinguish tumor subclasses with clinical implications. Proc Natl Acad Sci U S A. 2001; 98(19):10869–10874

[8] American College of Radiology ACR BI-RADS. Magnetic resonance imaging. In: ACR Breast Imaging Reporting and Data System, Breast Imaging Atlas. Reston, VA: American College of Radiology; 2013:1–178

[9] Shimauchi A, Abe H, Schacht DV, et al. Evaluation of kinetic entropy of breast masses initially found on MRI using whole-lesion curve distribution data: comparison with the standard kinetic analysis. Eur Radiol. 2015; 25(8):2470–2478

[10] Mahoney MC, Gatsonis C, Hanna L, DeMartini WB, Lehman C. Positive predictive value of BI-RADS MR imaging. Radiology. 2012; 264(1):51–58

[11] Michael M, Garzoli E, Reiner CS. Mammography, sonography and MRI for detection and characterization of invasive lobular carcinoma of the breast. Breast Dis. 2008–2009; 30:21–30, 20080

[12] Qayyum A, Birdwell RL, Daniel BL, et al. MR imaging features of infiltrating lobular carcinoma of the breast: histopathologic correlation. AJR Am J Roentgenol. 2002; 178(5):1227–1232

[13] Stivalet A, Luciani A, Pigneur F, et al. Invasive lobular carcinoma of the breast: MRI pathological correlation following bilateral total mastectomy. Acta Radiol. 2012; 53(4):367–375

[14] Lopez JK, Bassett LW. Invasive lobular carcinoma of the breast: spectrum of mammographic, US, and MR imaging findings. Radiographics. 2009; 29(1):165–176

[15] Dixon JM, Anderson TJ, Page DL, Lee D, Duffy SW. Infiltrating lobular carcinoma of the breast. Histopathology. 1982; 6(2):149–161

[16] Iorfida M, Maiorano E, Orvieto E, et al. Invasive lobular breast cancer: subtypes and outcome. Breast Cancer Res Treat. 2012; 133(2):713–723

[17] Tabár L, Dean PB, Chen SL, et al. Invasive lobular carcinoma of the breast: the use of radiological appearance to classify tumor subtypes for better prediction of long-term outcome. J Clin Exp Pathol. 2014; 4:1000179

[18] Mendelson EB, Harris KM, Doshi N, Tobon H. Infiltrating lobular carcinoma: mammographic patterns with pathologic correlation. AJR Am J Roentgenol. 1989; 153(2):265–271

[19] Mann RM, Hoogeveen YL, Blickman JG, Boetes C. MRI compared to conventional diagnostic work-up in the detection and evaluation of invasive lobular carcinoma of the breast: a review of existing literature. Breast Cancer Res Treat. 2008; 107(1):1–14

[20] Levrini G, Mori CA, Vacondio R, Borasi G, Nicoli F. MRI patterns of invasive lobular cancer: T1 and T2 features. Radiol Med (Torino). 2008; 113(8):1110–1125

[21] Kim SH, Cha ES, Park CS, et al. Imaging features of invasive lobular carcinoma: comparison with invasive ductal carcinoma. Jpn J Radiol. 2011; 29(7):475–482

[22] Schelfout K, Van Goethem M, Kersschot E, et al. Preoperative breast MRI in patients with invasive lobular breast cancer. Eur Radiol. 2004; 14(7):1209–1216

[23] Mann RM, Veltman J, Huisman H, Boetes C. Comparison of enhancement characteristics between invasive lobular carcinoma and invasive ductal carcinoma. J Magn Reson Imaging. 2011; 34(2):293–300

[24] Caramella T, Chapellier C, Ettore F, Raoust I, Chamorey E, Balu-Maestro C. Value of MRI in the surgical planning of invasive lobular breast carcinoma: a prospective and a retrospective study of 57 cases: comparison with physical examination, conventional imaging, and histology. Clin Imaging. 2007; 31(3):155–161

[25] Mann RM, Loo CE, Wobbes T, et al. The impact of preoperative breast MRI on the re-excision rate in invasive lobular carcinoma of the breast. Breast Cancer Res Treat. 2010; 119(2):415–422

[26] Hansen CJ, Kenny L, Lakhani SR, et al. Tubular breast carcinoma: an argument against treatment de-escalation. J Med Imaging Radiat Oncol. 2012; 56(1):116–122

[27] Rakha EA, Lee AH, Evans AJ, et al. Tubular carcinoma of the breast: further evidence to support its excellent prognosis. J Clin Oncol. 2010; 28(1):99–104

[28] Monzawa S, Yokokawa M, Sakuma T, et al. Mucinous carcinoma of the breast: MRI features of pure and mixed forms with histopathologic correlation. AJR Am J Roentgenol. 2009; 192(3):W125–W131

[29] Yuen S, Uematsu T, Kasami M, et al. Breast carcinomas with strong high-signal intensity on T2-weighted MR images: pathological characteristics and differential diagnosis. J Magn Reson Imaging. 2007; 25(3):502–510

[30] Okafuji T, Yabuuchi H, Sakai S, et al. MR imaging features of pure mucinous carcinoma of the breast. Eur J Radiol. 2006; 60(3):405–413

[31] Woodhams R, Kakita S, Hata H, et al. Diffusion-weighted imaging of mucinous carcinoma of the breast: evaluation of apparent diffusion coefficient and sig-

nal intensity in correlation with histologic findings. AJR Am J Roentgenol. 2009; 193(1):260–266

[32] Hatakenaka M, Soeda H, Yabuuchi H, et al. Apparent diffusion coefficients of breast tumors: clinical application. Magn Reson Med Sci. 2008; 7(1):23–29

[33] Liberman L, LaTrenta LR, Samli B, Morris EA, Abramson AF, Dershaw DD. Overdiagnosis of medullary carcinoma: a mammographic-pathologic correlative study. Radiology. 1996; 201(2):443–446

[34] Linda A, Zuiani C, Girometti R, et al. Unusual malignant tumors of the breast: MRI features and pathologic correlation. Eur J Radiol. 2010; 75(2):178–184

[35] Jeong SJ, Lim HS, Lee JS, et al. Medullary carcinoma of the breast: MRI findings. AJR Am J Roentgenol. 2012; 198(5):W482–W487

[36] Rakha EA, Gandhi N, Climent F, et al. Encapsulated papillary carcinoma of the breast: an invasive tumor with excellent prognosis. Am J Surg Pathol. 2011; 35(8):1093–1103

[37] Pal SK, Lau SK, Kruper L, et al. Papillary carcinoma of the breast: an overview. Breast Cancer Res Treat. 2010; 122(3):637–645

[38] Liberman L, Feng TL, Susnik B. Case 35: intracystic papillary carcinoma with invasion. Radiology. 2001; 219(3):781–784

[39] Lam WWM, Chu WCW, Tang APY, Tse G, Ma TK. Role of radiologic features in the management of papillary lesions of the breast. AJR Am J Roentgenol. 2006; 186(5):1322–1327

[40] Linda A, Londero V, Mazzarella F, Zuiani C, Bazzocchi M. Rare breast neoplasms: is there any peculiar feature on magnetic resonance mammography? Radiol Med (Torino). 2007; 112(6):850–862

[41] Harvey JA. Unusual breast cancers: useful clues to expanding the differential diagnosis. Radiology. 2007; 242(3):683–694

[42] Tran B, Bedard PL. Luminal-B breast cancer and novel therapeutic targets. Breast Cancer Res. 2011; 13(6):221

[43] Mazurowski MA, Zhang J, Grimm LJ, Yoon SC, Silber JI. Radiogenomic analysis of breast cancer: luminal B molecular subtype is associated with enhancement dynamics at MR imaging. Radiology. 2014; 273(2):365–372

[44] Elias SG, Adams A, Wisner DJ, et al. Imaging features of HER2 overexpression in breast cancer: a systematic review and meta-analysis. Cancer Epidemiol Biomarkers Prev. 2014; 23(8):1464–1483

[45] Uematsu T, Kasami M, Yuen S. Triple-negative breast cancer: correlation between MR imaging and pathologic findings. Radiology. 2009; 250(3):638–647

[46] Uematsu T. Focal breast edema associated with malignancy on T2-weighted images of breast MRI: peritumoral edema, prepectoral edema, and subcutaneous edema. Breast Cancer. 2015; 22(1):66–70

[47] Kaiser CG, Herold M, Baltzer PA, et al. Is "prepectoral edema" a morphologic sign for malignant breast tumors? Acad Radiol. 2015; 22(6):684–689

[48] Blaschke E, Abe H. MRI phenotype of breast cancer: kinetic assessment for molecular subtypes. J Magn Reson Imaging. 2015; 42(4):920–924

[49] Romond EH, Perez EA, Bryant J, et al. Trastuzumab plus adjuvant chemotherapy for operable HER2-positive breast cancer. N Engl J Med. 2005; 353(16):1673–1684

[50] Chen JH, Agrawal G, Feig B, et al. Triple-negative breast cancer: MRI features in 29 patients. Ann Oncol. 2007; 18(12):2042–2043

[51] Youk JH, Son EJ, Chung J, Kim JA, Kim EK. Triple-negative invasive breast cancer on dynamic contrast-enhanced and diffusion-weighted MR imaging: comparison with other breast cancer subtypes. Eur Radiol. 2012; 22(8):1724–1734

[52] Sung JS, Jochelson MS, Brennan S, et al. MR imaging features of triple-negative breast cancers. Breast J. 2013; 19(6):643–649

[53] Eiermann W, Bergh J, Cardoso F, et al. Triple negative breast cancer: proposals for a pragmatic definition and implications for patient management and trial design. Breast. 2012; 21(1):20–26

[54] Rea D, Francis A, Hanby AM, et al. UK Inflammatory Breast Cancer Working group. Inflammatory breast cancer: time to standardise diagnosis assessment and management, and for the joining of forces to facilitate effective research. Br J Cancer. 2015; 112(9):1613–1615

[55] Robertson FM, Bondy M, Yang W, et al. Inflammatory breast cancer: the disease, the biology, the treatment. CA Cancer J Clin. 2010; 60(6):351–375

[56] Lee KW, Chung SY, Yang I, et al. Inflammatory breast cancer: imaging findings. Clin Imaging. 2005; 29(1):22–25

[57] Alunni JP. Imaging inflammatory breast cancer. Diagn Interv Imaging. 2012; 93(2):95–103

[58] Le-Petross HT, Cristofanilli M, Carkaci S, et al. MRI features of inflammatory breast cancer. AJR Am J Roentgenol. 2011; 197(4):W769–W776

[59] Uematsu T. MRI findings of inflammatory breast cancer, locally advanced breast cancer, and acute mastitis: T2-weighted images can increase the specificity of inflammatory breast cancer. Breast Cancer. 2012; 19(4):289–294

[60] Girardi V, Carbognin G, Camera L, et al. Inflammatory breast carcinoma and locally advanced breast carcinoma: characterisation with MR imaging. Radiol Med (Torino). 2011; 116(1):71–83

[61] Yang WT, Le-Petross HT, Macapinlac H, et al. Inflammatory breast cancer: PET/CT, MRI, mammography, and sonography findings. Breast Cancer Res Treat. 2008; 109(3):417–426

[62] Liberman L, Bonaccio E, Hamele-Bena D, Abramson AF, Cohen MA, Dershaw DD. Benign and malignant phyllodes tumors: mammographic and sonographic findings. Radiology. 1996; 198(1):121–124

[63] Wurdinger S, Herzog AB, Fischer DR, et al. Differentiation of phyllodes breast tumors from fibroadenomas on MRI. AJR Am J Roentgenol. 2005; 185(5):1317–1321

[64] Tan H, Zhang S, Liu H, et al. Imaging findings in phyllodes tumors of the breast. Eur J Radiol. 2012; 81(1):e62–e69

[65] Yabuuchi H, Soeda H, Matsuo Y, et al. Phyllodes tumor of the breast: correlation between MR findings and histologic grade. Radiology. 2006; 241(3): 702–709

[66] Plaza MJ, Swintelski C, Yaziji H, Torres-Salichs M, Esserman LE. Phyllodes tumor: review of key imaging characteristics. Breast Dis. 2015; 35(2):79–86

[67] Choi BB, Shu KS. Metaplastic carcinoma of the breast: multimodality imaging and histopathologic assessment. Acta Radiol. 2012; 53(1):5–11

[68] Smith TB, Gilcrease MZ, Santiago L, Hunt KK, Yang WT. Imaging features of primary breast sarcoma. AJR Am J Roentgenol. 2012; 198(4):W386–W393

[69] Wienbeck S, Meyer HJ, Herzog A, et al. Imaging findings of primary breast sarcoma: results of a first multicenter study. Eur J Radiol. 2017; 88:1–7

[70] Lee SJ, Mahoney MC, Khan S. MRI features of stromal fibrosis of the breast with histopathologic correlation. AJR Am J Roentgenol. 2011; 197(3):755–762

[71] Linda A, Londero V, Bazzocchi M, Zuiani C. Desmoid tumor of the breast: radiologic appearance with a focus on its magnetic resonance features. Breast J. 2008; 14(1):106–107

9 Management of Findings Initially Detected at MRI

Hiroyuki Abe

Abstract

When abnormal findings are detected on breast MRI studies, the next step is to differentiate between probably benign lesions that do not need tissue sampling and suspicious lesions that need to be biopsied. The morphologic characteristics, kinetic assessment, patient risk factors, and the indications for MRI studies are taken into account in deciding whether tissue sampling is needed. Probably benign lesions can be followed in short term. For suspicious lesions, the next step is to determine a method of percutaneous biopsy. Although the mainstay of the biopsy method is MRI-guided biopsy, an ultrasound-guided biopsy or a stereotactic biopsy may be performed depending on the lesion type. Selection of a biopsy method must be made with careful observation of relevant images. Any suspicious lesions that are not visualized on any imaging modalities other than MRI should be biopsied under MRI guidance. The technical difficulty of MRI-guided biopsy is variable depending on the lesion location. Once a biopsy is performed, the physician who performed the biopsy should determine whether the pathologic result is concordant or discordant with imaging findings. The decision-making process in this series of studies requires considerable breast imaging experience.

Keywords: MRI-guided biopsy, MR-directed ultrasound, second look ultrasound, short-term follow-up, introducer, obturator, trocar

9.1 Introduction

Magnetic resonance imaging (MRI) is more sensitive in detecting breast lesions than conventional imaging by far, and is very useful for screening purposes. It is also true that MRI can be used for regional staging of a patient with known breast cancer, to look for satellites and determine the extent of a known malignancy. Due to its high sensitivity, however, MRI detects not only malignant lesions but also benign lesions. The challenge for MRI is to differentiate clearly between benign lesions that do not need tissue sampling and those suspicious lesions that need to be biopsied.

▶ Table 9.1 shows a summary of negative, benign, and probably benign lesions. In general, large mass lesions (> 15 mm)

with irregular shape, irregular or spiculated margins, heterogeneous or thick rim enhancement, and rapid enhancement tend to be malignant. Masses with homogeneous enhancement or dark internal septations and persistent kinetics tend to be benign. When evaluating any given lesion, it is important not only to evaluate the morphologic and kinetic characteristics, but also to take into account the patient's risk factors, such as the presence of a genetic mutation or a strong family or personal history of breast cancer, before deciding whether tissue sampling is needed.

Patient indications for MRI studies may also influence management. For example, an enhancing lesion initially seen on MRI tends to be malignant in patients who have metastatic axillary lymph nodes of unknown origin (CUP [carcinoma unknown primary] syndrome). Similarly, a finding on MRI in a patient referred with positive or close surgical margins following breast cancer surgery or with newly diagnosed breast cancer is more likely to require further investigation. A lesion identified in the same quadrant as that of a known cancer is likely to be a satellite lesion, and should be evaluated further. Availability of prior MRI examinations is very helpful for diagnosis, and when available, a search for interval change and new and developing lesions will aid in cancer detection.

See related cases (▶ Fig. 9.1; ▶ Fig. 9.2; ▶ Fig. 9.3; ▶ Fig. 9.4; ▶ Fig. 9.5; ▶ Fig. 9.6; ▶ Fig. 9.7; ▶ Fig. 9.8; ▶ Fig. 9.9; ▶ Fig. 9.10; ▶ Fig. 9.11; ▶ Fig. 9.12; ▶ Fig. 9.13).

Table 9.1 MRI features of normal, benign, and probable benign lesions

1. Normal	Edge enhancement
	Nodular parenchymal enhancement
	Lymph node
2. Benign lesions	Multiple similar-shaped and similar-sized lesions
	Thin, regular rim enhancement
	Nonenhancing lesions
	Skin lesion
3. Probable benign lesions	Enhancing mass with dark internal septations
	Slowly enhancing, circumscribed mass
	Fat-containing lesion
	Small linear NME (nonbranching)

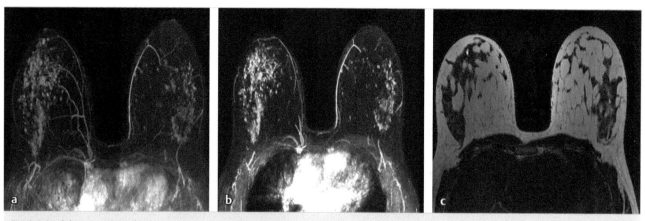

Fig. 9.1 Nodular parenchymal enhancement. Multiple enhancing foci are distributed in both breasts on MIP image **(a)** and on postcontrast axial T1-weighted subtraction image **(b)**. The distribution appears asymmetric between the breasts, but the enhancing foci are distributed within the parenchyma, as is confirmed by comparison to axial T2-weighted image **(c)**.

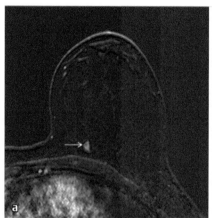
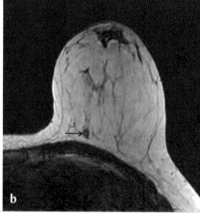

Fig. 9.2 Intramammary lymph node. An enhancing focus associated with a suggestion of small area of nonenhancing area (*arrow*) is present in the left posterior inner breast on postcontrast axial T1-weighted subtraction image **(a)**. On the same slice of axial T2-weighted image **(b)**, the nonenhancing area (*arrow*) shows fat signal, consistent with fatty hilum of intramammary lymph node.

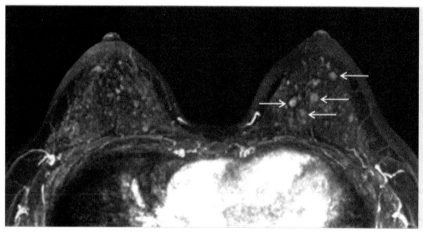

Fig. 9.3 Multiple similar-shaped and similar-sized lesions. There are multiple similar-shaped and similar-sized masses (*arrows*) in the left breast in postcontrast axial T1-weighted subtraction image (partial MIP image). These masses were stable for 3 years.

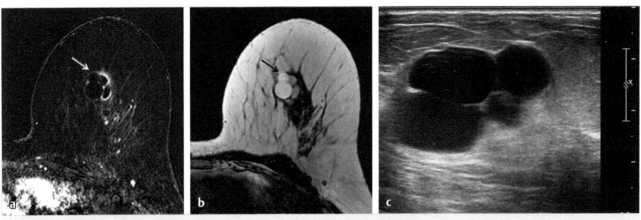

Fig. 9.4 Thin, regular rim enhancement. A rim enhancing lesion (*white arrow*) is present in the left breast on postcontrast axial T1-weighted subtraction image (**a**). The rim enhancement is smooth and thin. On the axial T2-weighted image (**b**), the lesion (*arrow*) shows homogenous water signal. Focused ultrasound (**c**) confirms it to be a simple cyst.

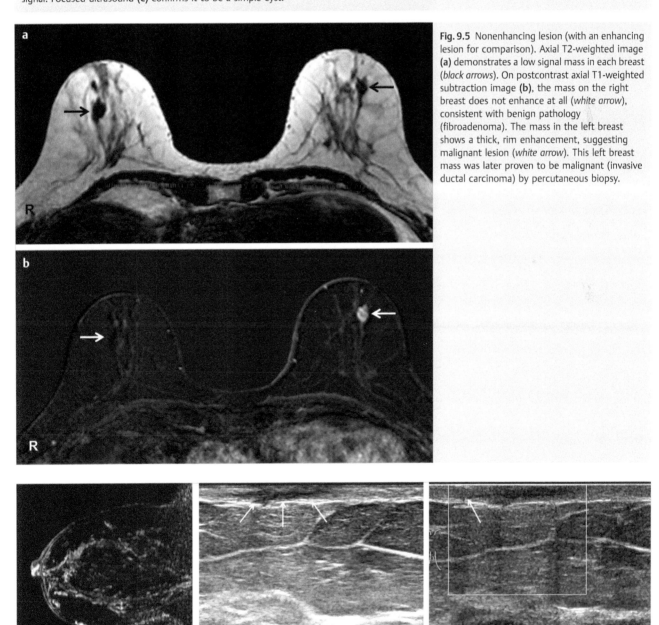

Fig. 9.5 Nonenhancing lesion (with an enhancing lesion for comparison). Axial T2-weighted image (**a**) demonstrates a low signal mass in each breast (*black arrows*). On postcontrast axial T1-weighted subtraction image (**b**), the mass on the right breast does not enhance at all (*white arrow*), consistent with benign pathology (fibroadenoma). The mass in the left breast shows a thick, rim enhancement, suggesting malignant lesion (*white arrow*). This left breast mass was later proven to be malignant (invasive ductal carcinoma) by percutaneous biopsy.

Fig. 9.6 Skin lesion; an enhancing lesion is usually benign. There is an enhancing lesion (*arrow*) in the lower portion of the breast on postcontrast sagittal T1-weighted subtraction image (**a**). Ultrasound (**b**) confirms that the lesion has the typical appearance of sebaceous cyst, located within the skin layer (*white arrows*). Mild blood flow (*white arrow*) on color Doppler image (**c**) suggests that there is mild inflammation.

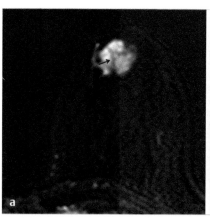
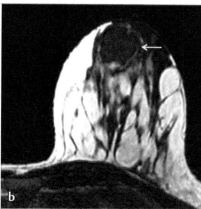

Fig. 9.7 Enhancing mass with dark internal septations. An oval enhancing mass with dark internal septations (*small black arrow*) is present in the left anterior breast on postcontrast axial T1-weighted subtraction image (**a**). Axial T2-weighted image shows a circumscribed low signal mass (**b**, *white arrow*). Ultrasound of this lesions shows a circumscribed homogeneously hypoechoic mass, suggesting fibroadenoma, which was confirmed by ultrasound-guided biopsy.

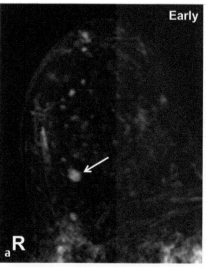
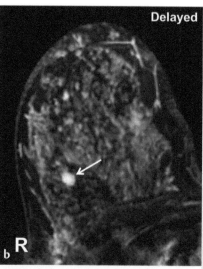

Fig. 9.8 Slowly enhancing, circumscribed mass. A circumscribed, oval mass (*white arrow*) is enhancing slowly in the right breast on postcontrast axial T1-weighted subtraction image (**a, b**). Magnitude of enhancement is obviously higher on the delayed phase (**b**) than on the early phase (**a**). Kinetic curve (**c**) shows slow initial uptake and persistent pattern. The mass was stable for 2 years with ultrasound follow-up.

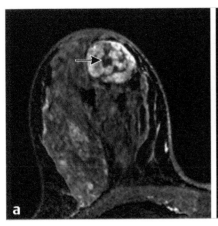
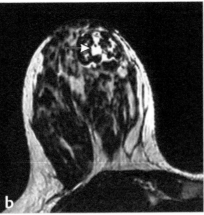

Fig. 9.9 Fat-containing lesion. A circumscribed, round mass showing heterogeneous internal enhancement is present in the right breast on postcontrast axial T1-weighted fat-suppression image (**a**). Nonenhancing components on T1-weighted image (**a**, *black arrow*) correspond to areas of fat signal (*white arrow*) on axial T2-weighted image (**b**). This lesion is consistent with a benign fibroadenolipoma.

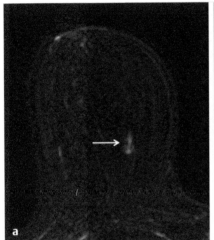
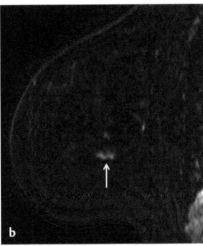

Fig. 9.10 Small linear NME (nonbranching). A linear nonmass enhancement (9 mm) was newly detected in a high-risk woman (strong family history of breast cancer) on postcontrast axial and sagittal T1-weighted subtraction image (**a, b**, *white arrow*). This nonmass enhancement is less than 1 cm and nonbranching type. The lesion was proven to be benign with subsequent MRI-guided biopsy.

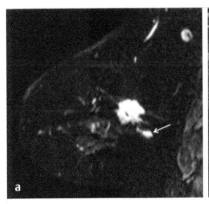
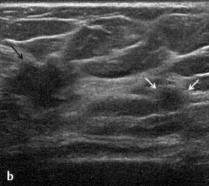

Fig. 9.11 Staging MRI for known cancer, with unexpected satellite lesion. A 47-year-old woman with biopsy-proven cancer (invasive lobular carcinoma) in the right breast. Staging MRI shows a satellite lesion (*white arrow*) posterior and inferior to the known cancer on postcontrast sagittal T1-weighted subtraction image (**a**). MR-directed ultrasound shows a correlating mass (**b**, *white arrows*) posterior to the index malignancy (*black arrow*). This satellite lesion was proven to be malignant (invasive lobular carcinoma) upon a surgical excision. Being a lesion in the same quadrant as that of a known cancer, the lesion should be treated as malignant until proven otherwise, unless there are definite signs of benignity.

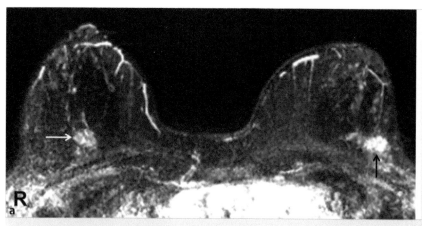
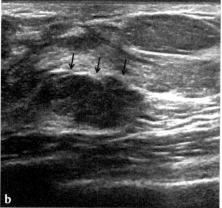

Fig. 9.12 Staging MRI for known cancer, with unexpected contralateral lesion. A 47-year-old woman with biopsy-proven cancer (invasive ductal carcinoma, grade 1) in the left breast (*black arrow*). An unexpected enhancing mass (*white arrow*) is present on postcontrast axial T1-weighted subtraction MIP image **(a)**. MR-directed ultrasound shows a correlated mass (*black arrows*) in the right breast **(b)**. Ultrasound-guided biopsy of this right breast mass revealed DCIS, grade 1.

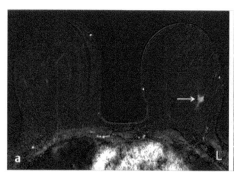
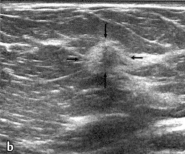

Fig. 9.13 Typical malignant lesion detected on high-risk screening. The patient was a 61-year-old BRCA 1 mutation carrier. A new, irregular-shaped, speculated enhancing mass (*white arrow*) is present on postcontrast axial T1-weighted subtraction image **(a)**. MR-directed ultrasound shows a correlated irregular hypoechoic mass with thick echogenic rim **(b**, *black arrows*).

9.2 Follow-up for Probably Benign Lesions

There are no systematic methods for differentiating probably benign lesions from suspicious lesions. Published articles generally report that a BI-RADS 3 assessment made by experienced radiologists may result in a malignancy rate of 2 to 3%. Follow-up MRI is usually performed after 6 months when a BI-RADS 3 assessment is made, with short-term follow-up usually continuing at 6, 12, and 24 months, as long as the lesion does not change in appearance. Two-year stability of the lesion is usually considered to be sufficient for a benign diagnosis. If the lesion appears smaller or less enhancing, or if it disappears during the follow-up period, it can be downgraded as benign. A decision to downgrade a lesion must be made prudently, as the change in appearance of a lesion can be easily influenced by various factors: the injection rate/volume of contrast, differences in magnetic field strength, or even the patient's positioning. On the other hand, if a lesion shows an increase in size or a change in its kinetic pattern from a benign to a suspicious pattern, a biopsy should be performed.

See related cases (▶ Fig. 9.14; ▶ Fig. 9.15).

9.3 How to Work Up Suspicious Lesions Initially Detected on MRI

A percutaneous biopsy should be performed for any suspicious lesion. The work-up process and the biopsy method may vary, according to the lesion type (focus, mass or nonmass enhancement [NME]). The mainstay biopsy method for such lesions is MRI-guided biopsy. Conventional imaging can be used in some cases in order to avoid an MRI-guided biopsy, which is expensive, time-consuming, and uncomfortable for some patients.

First of all, one should review the most recent mammogram to search for any lesion that might correlate with the MR findings (subtle calcification or asymmetry). If there is a finding seen that is amenable for biopsy, then a stereotactic biopsy should be considered. If the mammogram does not reveal a possible correlate, then MR-directed (second-look) ultrasound is the next option. There is variability in the rate of detection of MR-detected findings on ultrasound, depending on the MR lesion type (focus, mass, NME). In general, masses are most likely to be correlated with MRI, but a focus and NME are not. One study reports that the correlation rates of mass, focus, and NME are 67, 46, and 12%, respectively. The overall correlation rate was 57.5% (1,266/2,201) in one review series.

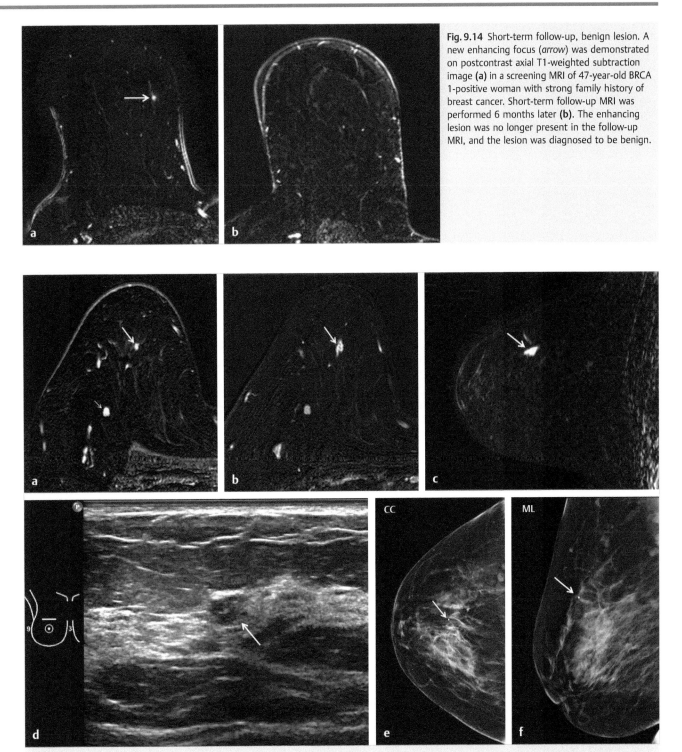

Fig. 9.14 Short-term follow-up, benign lesion. A new enhancing focus (*arrow*) was demonstrated on postcontrast axial T1-weighted subtraction image (**a**) in a screening MRI of 47-year-old BRCA 1-positive woman with strong family history of breast cancer. Short-term follow-up MRI was performed 6 months later (**b**). The enhancing lesion was no longer present in the follow-up MRI, and the lesion was diagnosed to be benign.

Fig. 9.15 Short-term follow-up, malignant lesion. A new enhancing focus (*white arrow*) was demonstrated on postcontrast axial T1-weighted subtraction image (**a**) in a screening MRI of 49-year-old woman with personal history of left breast cancer. There was a stable intramammary lymph node in the same breast (*small white arrow*). Short-term follow-up MRI was performed 6 months later. The lesion shows interval enlargement, associated with rim enhancement (*white arrow*), on follow-up postcontrast axial and sagittal T1-weighted subtraction images (**b, c**). MR-directed ultrasound found a correlating 5-mm mass (**d**, *white arrow*). Two views of postbiopsy mammogram (**e, f**) demonstrate a marker clip (*arrow*) to be placed in approximately the same location as the target tumor on MRI (**b, c**). Ultrasound-guided biopsy revealed invasive ductal carcinoma grade 3 with high-grade DCIS. The final pathology of the surgical specimen revealed the lesion had 3-mm invasive component, and there was no lymph node metastasis.

9.3.1 Focus

MRI-guided biopsy is the first choice for work-up, because it is not easy to correlate a focus with MR-directed ultrasound. There are, however, some exceptions. It is worth attempting an MR-directed ultrasound if a focus is in close proximity to a visible anatomic landmark lesion or structure. A landmark, for example, could be a known mass, a cyst, a surgical seroma, the nipple, etc. If there are such landmarks near the target, an ultrasound study could be performed, focused on a specific region for detection and biopsy.

9.3.2 Mass

It is worth trying to perform an MR-directed ultrasound for any kind of mass.

9.3.3 NME

One should look at the most recent mammogram to see if there are any correlative findings, such as calcifications or focal asymmetry. If recent mammography has not been performed, it should be obtained. MR-directed ultrasound for small NME lesions has a remote chance of identifying a correlate on ultrasound; however, a sizable NME may be identified. This is especially true if the pathology of such a sizable NME represents ductal carcinoma in situ (DCIS), which may contain invasive components that can be detected with ultrasound.

9.4 MR-Directed Ultrasound (Second-Look Ultrasound)

An ultrasound study performed for identification of a lesion initially detected on MRI is often called "a second-look ultrasound." However, the term "second-look" is a misnomer, because ultrasound used for this indication is usually a first examination, and no prior ultrasound study targeted to the new lesion has been performed. "MR-directed ultrasound" therefore is a preferred term for this procedure.

When performing MR-directed ultrasound, the operator should have adequate knowledge of the location of the lesion as well as its shape and size. One needs to consider the lesion position given that the patient is imaged in the prone position on MRI and in the supine position on ultrasound. The patient's breast size and shape should also be taken into account. Lesion location (quadrants, o'clock position, and distance from the nipple), lesion characteristics, and, if possible, landmarks near the lesion are useful indicators for identification of an MR correlate. Often, a lesion initially detected on MRI is subtle on ultrasound, and lowering one's threshold for detection may help identify the correlate lesion. Use of Doppler is also very useful, because increased vascularity may be present in the target lesion reinforcing the likelihood of successful correlation with MRI. When a correlate lesion is identified, ultrasound-guided biopsy should be performed unless the lesion appears to be definitely benign. A review paper on MR-directed ultrasound found that malignant lesions tend to be detected more often (75.8%; 380/501) than benign lesions (52.4%; 829/1581).

See related cases (▶ Fig. 9.7; ▶ Fig. 9.9; ▶ Fig. 9.11; ▶ Fig. 9.12; ▶ Fig. 9.13; ▶ Fig. 9.15).

Placement of a marker clip at the site of ultrasound biopsy is mandatory. Ideally, a marker clip that is visible on both mammography and MRI should be used. With such a marker clip, the lesion's location can be checked on postprocedure mammography and on the follow-up MRI. The purpose of a post-biopsy mammogram is to assess an approximate correlation between the clip location (biopsy site) and the location of the lesion on MRI (▶ Fig. 9.15). If the ultrasound-placed clip location on the mammogram is obviously in a different position from the lesion localized on MRI, an MRI-guided biopsy should be performed, because it is likely that an incorrect lesion was biopsied on ultrasound. An MRI with a T1 nonenhanced scan may be performed for confirmation of the clip location after the biopsy.

Pathology results should be reviewed for concordance with imaging findings. If the results are discordant with MRI/ultrasound findings, then MRI-guided biopsy or surgical excision should be considered. When the pathology results are malignant and concordant, a surgical consultation should follow. If the pathology is benign and concordant, follow-up MRI may be performed in 6 to 12 months, to exclude a false-negative biopsy result. On follow-up MRI, interval changes in the lesion can be assessed in addition to checking the relationship of the marker clip to the lesion.

9.5 MR-Guided Biopsy

9.5.1 Lesion and Patient Selection

Any suspicious MR lesion that is not detected on any other imaging modality should be biopsied with MRI guidance. Patients have already undergone a prior contrast-enhanced MRI of breast; therefore, there is little safety concern regarding MR-guided biopsy for these patients. The difficulty of lesion accessibility for biopsy can be variable, depending on its location. Challenging cases (multiple lesions, posterior lesions, thin breasts, medial lesions, superficial lesions, breasts with implants) and the issue of lesion nonvisualization on the day of biopsy will be discussed later in this section.

9.5.2 Informed Consent

In obtaining informed consent for an MR-guided biopsy, a detailed explanation of the procedure is needed in order to reassure the patient and gain her cooperation. In addition to explaining the course of action, it is important that she should be informed about the possibility of cancellation of the procedure due to nonvisualization of the target. Possible patient complications to be discussed include hematoma, skin bruising, and the rare occurrence of an abscess.

9.5.3 Patient Positioning and MR Technique

The patient is positioned on the MR table in the prone position in the same manner as for a diagnostic MRI. The target breast is compressed for immobilization and also for gaining a grid impression on the breast (the grid itself is not visible, but the skin impression is visible on MR images) (▶ Fig. 9.16). The

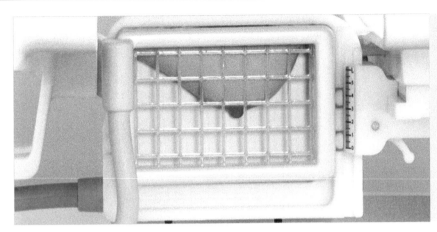

Fig. 9.16 Patient in a breast coil with biopsy grid (courtesy of Hologic, Inc Marlborough, Massachusetts).

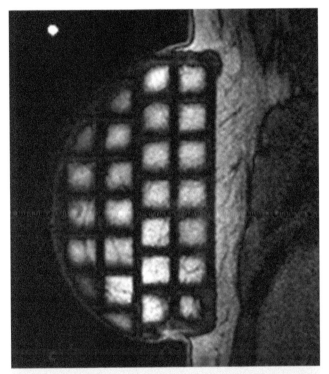

Fig. 9.17 Grid impression on sagittal T1-weighted image. Location of a target lesion relative to the coverage by the grid should be assessed. The target lesion must be within a range of the grid impression on x–y axes.

breast compression should not be excessively strong, as hard compression can compromise blood circulation and prevent contrast enhancement of the target lesion.

The breast coil used for biopsy may or may not be the same coil that was used for the diagnostic study, depending on the practice setting. If the coil is different, the target lesion might not be similarly visualized; therefore, identification of neighboring structures, such as the shape of neighboring fat lobules and the outline of glandular tissue, is helpful for finding the exact location of the lesion. Therefore, it is important to position the breast as on the prior study. In order to move the lesion to the optimal location for biopsy once the patient is placed in the coil, one can utilize the same techniques for positioning as used in stereotactic biopsy, such as rolling of the breast tissue; however, this technique should be used only when it is

absolutely necessary because the features of the neighboring structure are also modified.

After localizing images, sagittal non-fat-suppression T1-weighted images are obtained (sagittal reformatted images are also good for this purpose if a slice is reasonably thin) (▶ Fig. 9.17). With these images, the grid position relative to the target lesion should be evaluated. The target lesion must be within the coverage area of the grid. Contrast injection can be performed only once; therefore, the patient's position must be appropriately confirmed before the contrast is injected. Pre- and postcontrast T1-weighted images are then acquired. Imaging sequence and volume/rate of contrast injection should be the same as those used for diagnostic MRI. The number of post-contrast scans can be reduced (three rather than five or six) because the delayed images are not important for the detection of the target lesion. Additional images are obtained after placement of an introducer with an obturator for confirmation of the proper lesion depth and location. Additional images are also obtained after biopsy so that the biopsy changes at the target site can be seen.

9.5.4 Guidance Equipment

Basically, there are two types of guidance equipment, a grid device and a pillar-and-post device. In a grid device, the needle goes in horizontally using a lateral or a medial approach. With a pillar-and-post device, an angular approach is possible. The technique using a grid device is now described.

The grid of the biopsy system is placed on the lateral or medial surface of the breast, depending on the approach. For localization of a target lesion, the grid has to provide a fiducial marker, which is visible on T1-weighted images. Some grids have built-in markers for a CAD (computer-aided detection) system to assist in targeting, whereas manual placement of a fiducial marker is needed for the other types of grid. A vitamin E capsule is often used as a fiducial marker and is placed in one of the grid openings, but not in the vicinity of the target lesion.

9.5.5 Targeting

Although there are commercially available CAD systems that can provide localizing information by identifying the needle insertion location and depth, one needs to know how to use a manual technique because not every practice may have access to such a system, or the CAD device may fail on the day of

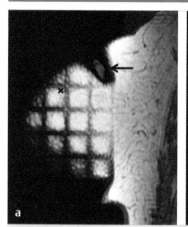 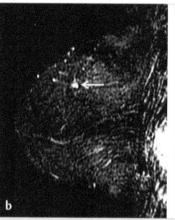 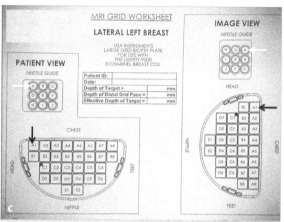

Fig. 9.18 Targeting by a grid diagram. A T1-weighted sagittal non-fat-suppression image **(a)** shows a grid impression with a fiducial marker (*black arrow*). The target lesion is a small enhancing mass (*white arrow*) on postcontrast T1-weighted sagittal subtraction image **(b)**, and an x marker points to the target position on x–y axes over the grid impression image **(a)**. A diagram has two grid maps: a grid on monitor (image view) on the right, and an actual grid view (patient view) on the left. In addition, a grid guide with nine holes is shown superior to each grid map. Initially, the position of a fiducial marker (*black arrow*) and the target lesion (x) are marked on the image view correlated to the actual image on the monitor. A hole "a" of the grid guide (*white arrow*) is selected by the target position **(c)**. Finally, markings on the image view are translated on the patient view.

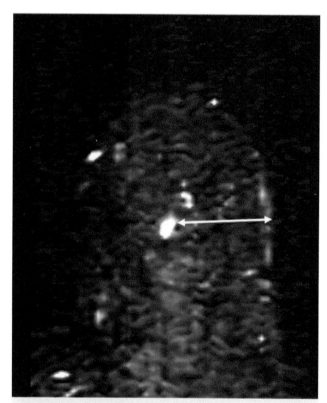

Fig. 9.19 Distance from skin surface to the target lesion (*arrow*) is measured on T1-weighted axial subtraction image.

biopsy due to problems with a picture archiving and commutation system (PACS) or with the workstation.

The orientation of the grid as seen on the monitor and its actual orientation on the patient are different. Diagrams of the localization grid are commonly used, and the settings provided (right or left breast, and lateral or medial approach) are useful for avoiding mistakes and for identification of the correct aper-

ture for needle insertion (▶ Fig. 9.18). Once the target lesion is identified, the grid aperture to be used for biopsy can be determined on the postcontrast sagittal images (or subtraction images) by placing a cursor on the lesion and viewing of the grid impression slice. The location of the specific apertures on the grid for biopsy can be determined by counting the number of apertures from the fiducial marker. The position of the needle guide can be determined by checking of the location of the cursor in the designated opening; the x, y coordinates on the grid are thus determined. The depth of the lesion is best determined by measuring the distance from the skin on the reformatted axial or coronal postcontrast images. Lesion depth can also be measured by counting the number of slices from the skin to the target on sagittal images, then by multiplying of the number of slices by the known slice thickness. Measuring the distance on the reformatted axial or coronal images is much simpler (▶ Fig. 9.19).

9.5.6 Local Anesthesia and Sampling

Local anesthesia should be given before the needle guide is placed in the grid opening. After the skin at the appropriate opening is cleaned, 1 to 2% lidocaine is placed for superficial anesthesia, and 1% lidocaine with 1:100 epinephrine is placed for deep anesthesia. Because the skin is usually most sensitive, a skin wheal should be made with lidocaine for superficial anesthesia and epinephrine is useful for deeper anesthesia to reduce bleeding from the procedure, unless there is a contraindication for epinephrine use. Epinephrine should be avoided for superficial anesthesia as tissue necrosis may occur. In some biopsy devices, anesthesia can be placed simultaneously with tissue sampling during the biopsy.

After placement of the local anesthesia, the needle guide is positioned at the grid opening. A skin nick can be made before placement of the needle guide. Some biopsy devices use a sharp trocar, thus placing the introducer within the breast without a skin nick. The introducer with the trocar should be advanced into the tissue with a twisting motion in order for the tissue to

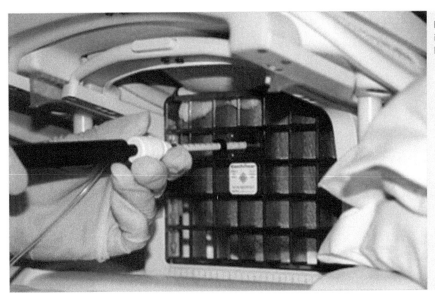

Fig. 9.20 An introducer with trocar is advanced in the tissue (courtesy of Hologic, Inc Marlborough, Massachusetts).

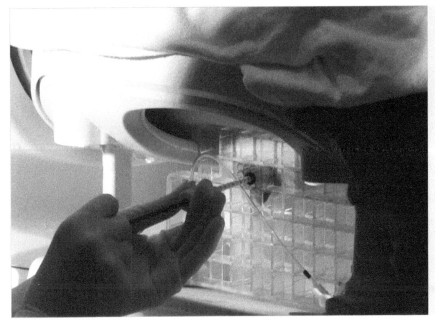

Fig. 9.21 A trocar is replaced by a plastic obturator.

be cut efficiently (▶ Fig. 9.20). When the introducer is placed at an appropriate depth, the skin entry site is checked to see whether the introducer causes "skin tenting," which is a depression of the skin entry by the device. Skin tenting indicates that the introducer is placed at an inappropriate depth. To avoid skin tenting, the introducer could be placed a little deeper than the predetermined depth and pulled back to the appropriate depth. Once the introducer is appropriately placed, the trocar will be removed and replaced by a plastic obturator (▶ Fig. 9.21). The obturator is seen as a signal void within the introducer, on the subsequent confirmation scan, so that the location of the introducer can be positioned at the target lesion (▶ Fig. 9.22). After confirmation of the positioning of the obturator, sampling is performed (▶ Fig. 9.23). The obturator is then removed and replaced by a hand-held sampling device and 6 to 12 samples are usually obtained. Unlike stereotactic biopsy, the biopsy needle is held manually by the radiologist, allowing the needle to be moved relatively freely. Care must be taken to

avoid an accidental "push-in" or "pull-back" of the biopsy needle at the time of sampling. Because MRI-guided biopsy is not a real-time image-guided procedure such as ultrasound-guided biopsy, the targeting is not as accurate as ultrasound or stereotactic biopsy. A large-core needle, such as a 9-gauge needle, is thus preferred to avoid undersampling and mistargeting. After sampling, the biopsy needle is removed from the introducer and replaced by the obturator. A postbiopsy scan is then obtained to confirm appropriate sampling and to check for biopsy changes such as hematoma (▶ Fig. 9.24). Subsequently, a marker clip is placed through the introducer (▶ Fig. 9.25). When a sizable hematoma is present, suction can be used and a marker clip is subsequently placed at the appropriate location. The breast is then released from the grid and pressure is held over the biopsy site. Once hemostasis is established, the skin is cleaned, the skin incision is closed with sterile surgical strips, and a pressure dressing is positioned over the biopsy site.

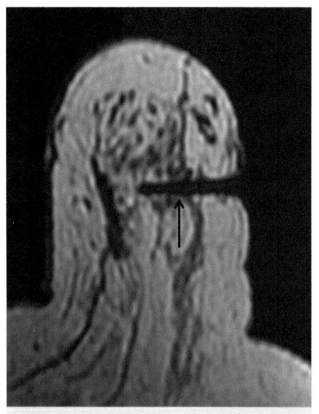

Fig. 9.22 A linear signal void (*arrow*) by the plastic obturator within the introducer at the confirmation scan on T1-weighted axial non-fat-suppression image.

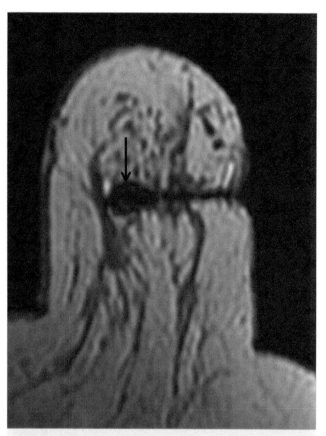

Fig. 9.24 A postbiopsy image (T1-weighted axial non-fat-suppression image) shows a biopsy cavity (*arrow*) with a linear signal void by the obturator.

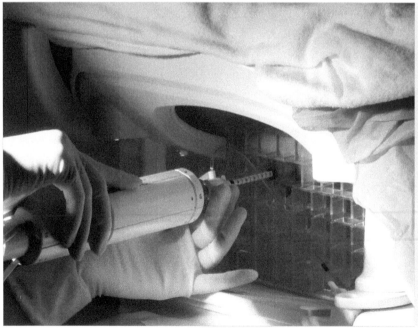

Fig. 9.23 A sampling is performed with a hand-held device.

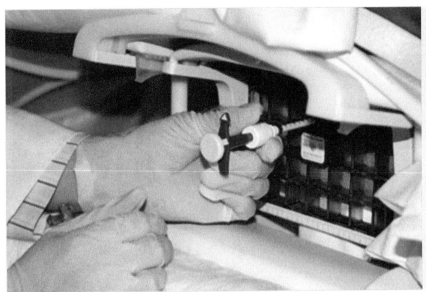

Fig. 9.25 A marker clip is placed through the introducer (courtesy of Hologic, Inc Marlborough, Massachusetts).

Following the biopsy procedure, a two-view mammogram is obtained to document marker clip placement. Displacement of the marker clip does not occur often because mild breast compression is used during the procedure unlike stereotactic biopsy, where moderate compression is used and the "accordion effect" may facilitate clip movement. Postbiopsy written instructions include no strenuous activity within 24 hours and placement of an ice pack over the biopsy site as needed, and are reviewed with the patient before she leaves the MRI suite.

9.6 Challenging Cases

9.6.1 Multiple Lesions

Multiple targets can be sampled in one session. If all targets are located in one breast, multiple sampling can be performed by using either the same approach or two different approaches, a lateral and a medial approach, for example. Sampling of the contralateral breast is also possible, as long as all of the lesions can be accessed by a lateral approach. A medial approach cannot be used when sampling both breasts in one session because the medial approach requires the contralateral breast to be displaced. When a target lesion is visible on noncontrast images, however, biopsy can be performed in two continuous sessions, because one or both sessions do not require contrast injection. In this case, the patient can be repositioned, and a medial approach could be used for either breast. Separate vacuum devices must be used for each tissue sampling procedure, and different types of marker clips should be placed, if possible, when multiple biopsies are performed in the same breast.

9.6.2 Posterior Lesions

Posterior lesions are sometimes difficult to access because the posterior part of the breast may not be placed deep enough in the breast coil to be covered by the grid. In such cases, the solution can be as follows: removal of table padding to minimize the dead space between the chest wall and breast, pulling of

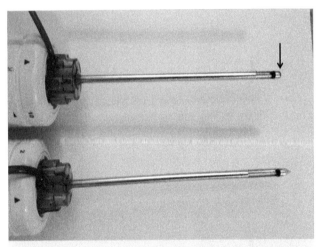

Fig. 9.26 Two types of biopsy needle. The one at the top is a "petite" needle with a short trough (1.2 cm) and a blunt tip (*arrow*), and the other is a regular needle that has a 2-cm trough with a sharp tip (courtesy of Hologic, Inc Marlborough, Massachusetts).

the breast into the coil and immobilizing with the grid, or angling the patient to position the breast deeper into the coil. If the target is partially accessible, the target lesion can be sampled at least partially. If all efforts fail, MR-guided wire localization and excisional biopsy should be considered. In this situation, successful needle localization for a far posterior lesion can be accomplished by an angled approach. The needle guide can be removed and an angled approach of the needle to the target can be achieved.

9.6.3 Thin Breasts

Vacuum-assisted needles usually provide a 2-cm-long trough with an approximately 0.8-cm sharp tip. In order for MR-guided biopsy to be performed, the breast thickness should be at least 2.8 cm when the breast is placed in the grid with mild compression applied. For a thinner breast, needles with a shorter trough (1.2 cm) and a blunt and shorter tip (▸ Fig. 9.26) can be used, but a thickness of at least a 1.7 cm is required. To accommodate this situation, measures using less compression of the breast or rolling of the breast to maximize thickness can be used.

When biopsying a thin breast, an accidental skin biopsy should be avoided. Because the trough length is about the same as the breast thickness, the trough might be partially outside the breast when the needle is placed exactly at the target. If vacuum biopsy is performed in such a setting, a large amount of skin may be removed by the vacuum system, and this could result in a skin defect. In order to avoid such a complication, the whole trough should be placed within the breast, even if the needle is placed deeper than the target location. As long as the target is somewhere within the trough length, the target lesion can be sampled. A visual assessment should be made to confirm that the trough is completely within the tissue before actual sampling is performed. It may be difficult, however, to ascertain that the trough is completely placed within the tissue because of the presence of the needle guide. To avoid an accidental skin biopsy, a precise measurement of the breast thickness on the monitor and appropriate planning of the needle placement are needed.

9.6.4 Medial Lesions

Some biopsy coil designs only allow a medial approach for anterior lesions. When a medial approach for central or posterior lesions is required, the patient may be angled in the coil or the table padding can be removed. If these techniques fail, a lateral access may be necessary. If the lesion is extremely medially located, the risk of piercing the breast is high with a lateral approach. In such a case, a needle with a blunt tip should be used.

9.6.5 Superficial Lesions

As in the case of patients with thin breasts, an accidental skin biopsy should be avoided when the target lesion is located superficially. The key to avoiding skin suction at biopsy is to keep the entire suction trough within the breast, as previously noted. The biopsy system is designed so that the target position is at the center of the trough and it is necessary for the lesion depth to be positioned at more than half the length of the trough in order to avoid an accidental skin biopsy. When the distance between the target and skin, as measured on the monitor, is shorter than half the length of the trough, the needle should be advanced further than the target position to avoid skin injury. On the other hand, when a superficial lesion is at the far side from the skin entry, skin piercing is a risk. To avoid this, a needle with a blunt tip should be used.

9.6.6 Implants

The presence of an implant is not a contraindication for MRI-guided biopsy if the lesion can be localized with the implant positioned outside the needle trajectory. If the implant cannot be avoided during the localizing technique, however, an MRI-guided biopsy cannot be performed. If the lesion is located very close to the implant, an MRI-guided wire localization is the procedure of choice, but care must be taken not to perforate the implant. Another option would be to place an MRI-guided skin marker over the lesion for surgical localization. In this situation, close communication between the radiologist and the breast surgeon is imperative.

9.6.7 Lesion Nonvisualization on the Day of Biopsy

Lesion nonvisualization at the time of biopsy may occur either because the lesion is falsely positive (BPE) or because the lesion is actually present, but not visualized for technical reasons. The first thing to do is to examine all current MR images and compare them with the prior images to make sure that the lesion is not visible. If the lesion is visible on precontrast images, targeting is possible by use of precontrast images. The next thing to do is to obtain delayed-phase MR images to see whether there is any sign of the lesion. If the breast is compressed too tightly, it should be loosened, and another scan should be obtained. Even though the lesion is not visualized, a biopsy can be performed with use of the neighboring landmarks, when the lesion is sufficiently suspicious on the prior MR images. If the radiologist is not comfortable with this approach, the biopsy should be canceled. Usually, nonvisualized lesions are followed up with MRI in 6 months. The follow-up protocol is the same as that for BI-RADS 3 lesions.

9.6.8 Follow-up for Lesions Proven Benign

When the pathology of an MRI-guided biopsy is benign and concordant, follow-up MRI is encouraged because there are possible false-negative cases (▶ Table 9.2). Li et al reported that 4 malignant lesions were confirmed among 177 lesions with benign concordant results, and Hayward et al reported 2 false-negative cases among 84 lesions. The follow-up interval may be 6 to 12 months. If the lesions are stable or disappear, a benign result will be confirmed. On the other hand, if the lesions become larger, another biopsy may be needed at the radiologist's discretion.

Table 9.2 Follow-up results of benign concordant MRI-guided biopsy

	No. of lesions	Biopsy equipment	Follow-up period, mo (mean [range])	Smaller or Resolved	Stable	Increased	No. of rebiopsy	No. of malignancy in rebiopsy	Mean interval from initial biopsy	FN rate %
Li et al	117	9G, vacuum	24 (7–53)	155	14	8	17	4	6 (2–12)	3.4
Hayward et al	84	9G, vacuum	33.1 (0.4–100.8)	62	21	1	4	2	15 (6–24)	2.4
Shaylor et al	113	9G, vacuum	27 (5–63)	69	42	2	3	1	24	0.5

Table 9.3 High risk lesions initially detected on MRI

	High risk lesions	Rate of high risk lesion	Upgrade rate	Size of upgraded lesion, mm (mean [range])	Biopsy equipment
Liberman	ADH	6.3% (15/237)	38.5% (5/13)	10 (7–28)	MR Bx:9G
Han	ADH, LCIS, ALH, RS, PL	14% (21/150)	25% (4/16)	NA	MR Bx:9,10G
Norrozian	ADH, LCIS, ALH	9.3% (7/75)	16.7% 1/6)	NA	MR Bx:9G
Malhaire	ADH, LCIS, ALH, RS, PL, OA	13.8% (10/72)	12.5% (1/8)	NA	MR Bx:10G
Strigel	ADH	10.6% (51/482)	32.4% (11/34)	10 (4–70)	MR Bx:9, 14G, US Bx: 14G, stereo Bx:9, 11G
Pavel	ADH, LCIS, ALH, RS, PL, FEA	19.3% (31/161)	50% (13/26)	24.3 (2.8–45.8)	MR Bx: 9G

Abbreviations: ADH, atypical ductal hyperplasia; ALH, atypical lobular hyperplasia; FEA, flat epithelial atypia; LCIS, lobular carcinoma in situ; OA, other atypia; PL, papillary lesion; RS, radial scar.

9.6.9 Proven High-Risk Lesions

When pathology confirms the presence of a high-risk lesion, such as atypical ductal hyperplasia, lobular carcinoma in situ, atypical lobular hyperplasia, and complex sclerosing lesions, within a biopsy specimen, the lesion may be upgraded to malignancy at surgical excision. The rate of upgrade for lesions initially detected on MRI has ranged from 12.5 to 50% (▶ Table 9.3). Therefore, all cases with high-risk lesions proven by MRI-guided biopsy need surgical consultation.

9.7 Summary

A multimodal approach is essential for the management of findings initially detected on MRI. A decision to perform a biopsy or follow-up imaging must be made with careful observation of the relevant images. If a detected lesion needs further evaluation, a less invasive examination should be conducted initially. At the same time, each examination at work-up must be meaningful. Unnecessary examinations (e.g., MR-directed ultrasound for a small NME) will be a waste of time. Once a biopsy is performed, the physician who performs the biopsy should decide if the imaging findings are concordant or discordant with the pathologic result. The decision-making process after detection of a lesion on MRI is complex, necessitating considerable physician experience with all imaging methods.

Suggested Readings

Abe H, Schmidt RA, Shah RN, et al. MR-directed ("Second-Look") ultrasound examination for breast lesions detected initially on MRI: MR and sonographic findings. AJR Am J Roentgenol. 2010; 194(2):370–377

Eby PR, Demartini WB, Peacock S, Rosen EL, Lauro B, Lehman CD. Cancer yield of probably benign breast MR examinations. J Magn Reson Imaging. 2007; 26(4): 950–955

Hayward JH, Ray KM, Wisner DJ, Joe BN. Follow-up outcomes after benign concordant MRI-guided breast biopsy. Clin Imaging. 2016; 40(5):1034–1039

Li J, Dershaw DD, Lee CH, Kaplan J, Morris EA. MRI follow-up after concordant, histologically benign diagnosis of breast lesions sampled by MRI-guided biopsy. AJR Am J Roentgenol. 2009; 193(3):850–855

Machida Y, Tozaki M, Shimauchi A, Yoshida T. Two distinct types of linear distribution in nonmass enhancement at breast MR imaging: difference in positive predictive value between linear and branching patterns. Radiology. 2015; 276(3): 686–694

Schrading S, Strobel K, Keulers A, Dirrichs T, Kuhl CK. Safety and efficacy of magnetic resonance-guided vacuum-assisted large-volume breast biopsy (MR-guided VALB). Invest Radiol. 2017; 52(3):186–193

Shaylor SD, Heller SL, Melsaether AN, et al. Short interval follow-up after a benign concordant MR-guided vacuum assisted breast biopsy–is it worthwhile? Eur Radiol. 2014; 24(6):1176–1185

Spick C, Baltzer PA. Diagnostic utility of second-look US for breast lesions identified at MR imaging: systematic review and meta-analysis. Radiology. 2014; 273(2): 401–409

Yamaguchi K, Schacht D, Sennett CA, et al. Decision making for breast lesions initially detected at contrast-enhanced breast MRI. AJR Am J Roentgenol. 2013; 201(6): 1376–1385

10 Diagnostic MRI: Breast Cancer Applications

Gillian M. Newstead

Abstract

The goal of MRI is to establish the size and extent of the known index malignancy in women with a newly diagnosed breast cancer, to identify additional sites of malignancy and to improve surgical treatment planning. Identification of multifocal, multicentric, diffuse and contralateral tumors helps to guide treatment planning. In this chapter we discuss the literature that relates to the use of breast MRI for assessment of disease in the preoperative setting, and the increasing evidence of the efficacy of preoperative MRI in decreasing re-operation rates.

Many practices now rely on MRI for monitoring of assessment response during neoadjuvant systemic chemotherapy (NACT; chemotherapy prior to surgery for invasive cancer) and is widely used to provide improved surgical outcomes, recurrence free survival and overall survival in certain subtypes of breast cancer, with the additional potential benefit that reduced tumor volume during treatment may allow for more conservative surgery. MRI also allows superior assessment of tumor size, volume and surface area measurements reflecting a more accurate characterization of overall tumor burden especially during NACT monitoring of tumor response. Diagnostic MRI is also used for management of residual disease following cancer excision and evaluation of suspected recurrent disease following breast conserving surgery.

Keywords: MR imaging of known cancer, tumor measurements, management of additional disease, breast conserving therapy (BCS) diagnosis of residual disease, reoperation rates, MRI for reducing rates of re-excision, neoadjuvant chemotherapy monitoring (NACT), recurrent tumor

10.1 Introduction

The increased numbers of small cancers detected at mammography screening allow breast-conserving surgery (BCS) for many women, underscoring the importance of accurate assessment of tumor extent. Traditional breast cancer treatment is determined by two major factors: tumor histology, assessed by classifications based on grade and morphology, and the TNM staging method, based on cancer size, nodal status, and presence or absence of distant metastases. Breast cancer therapy relies primarily on surgical treatment when cancers are nonpalpable and detected at screening. Complete imaging evaluation for each individual cancer patient should guide the surgical approach. In the pre–magnetic resonance imaging (MRI) era, surgical and oncologic treatment planning methods were judged primarily by clinical examination, mammography, and ultrasound imaging. Precise assessment of tumor size at mammography was often difficult to achieve, particularly for the patient with dense breast tissue, resulting in the large variation in postsurgical positive margins reported in the literature (5–70%).[1] Breast MRI provides superior sensitivity and accuracy in determining the tumor burden in patients with newly diagnosed breast cancer. MRI allows precise identification not only of the index lesion, be it invasive or noninvasive, but also of the presence and extent of additional previously undetected cancer. It has been well documented that presence of multifocal and diffuse (multicentric) breast cancer provides an independent negative prognostic factor, affecting therapeutic decision-making.[2,3] MRI allows identification of 15% (12–27%) additional occult malignancies in the ipsilateral breast and 4% (3–6%) in the contralateral breast.[4,5,6,7,8,9,10,11,12] Accurate MRI depiction of disease extent may serve patients well by selecting those patients with a large tumor burden at initial diagnosis, thus avoiding immediate lumpectomy and allowing change in therapy to mastectomy or neoadjuvant chemotherapy. MRI also plays an important role in the assessment of tumor burden when margins are positive at lumpectomy, when recurrent tumor is suspected, and when monitoring tumor response for the patient undergoing neoadjuvant chemotherapy.

10.2 Imaging of the Patient with Known Cancer

Breast cancer is known to be a heterogeneous disease with characteristic molecular and genetic subtypes, and although the traditional histologic classification of breast cancer offers limited prognostic value, molecular characterization, cellular markers, and imaging phenotypes of breast tumors, especially MRI, have changed the treatment landscape. Most breast cancers are multifocal at histology, with MRI identifying a substantial number of additional lesions, both invasive and noninvasive, in the ipsilateral and contralateral breast. A report on 500 consecutive breast cancer cases, retrospectively analyzed and documented by large-format histologic sectioning, determined the distribution of both in situ and invasive components of breast tumors. The large-section histology method has proven to be the most accurate way of achieving precise estimation of malignancy extent. The distribution of cancer found in this study was follows: unifocal 34%, multifocal 36%, diffuse 28%, and mixed 2%. It is not surprising therefore that the exquisite sensitivity of MRI allows detection of additional disease not identified by other imaging methods (▶ Fig. 10.1; ▶ Fig. 10.2).[13]

Preoperative MRI can assess disease extent more accurately than other imaging techniques, and over time may also provide improved prognostication and prediction. Quantitative analyses of image-based phenotypes have opened the door to provision of MR image–based predictive and prognostic biomarkers. A biomarker is defined as a characteristic that is objectively measured and evaluated as an indicator of normal biologic

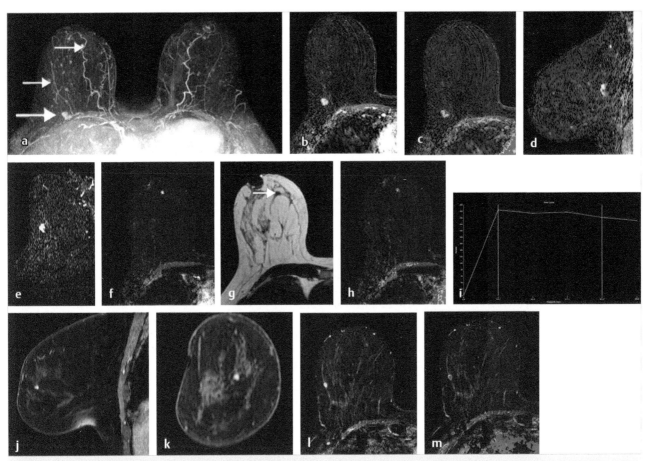

Fig. 10.1 Multicentric disease; age 51, newly diagnosed right breast IDC grade 1, MRI for disease extent assessment. MIP image **(a)** shows the index cancer in the far posterolateral right breast (*long arrow*). Two additional small masses are shown in the anterior and lateral breast (*short arrows*). The index cancer is shown as an irregular mass **(b)**, with heterogeneous washout kinetics **(c)** and sagittal and coronal images **(d, e)**. The additional unsuspected anterior mass is shown on subtraction imaging to enhance robustly **(f)** and an isointense correlate is seen on T2w image **(g,** *arrow***)**. Plateau kinetic mass enhancement is shown **(h, i)**. The additional lateral mass exhibits benign findings with circumscribed margins and homogeneous kinetics **(j–m)**. MR-guided biopsy of the anterior mass yielded IDC grade 2 ER/PR (+), HER2 (–). Patient management was changed from lumpectomy to mastectomy. Histologic confirmation of additional findings before patient management is changed is shown in this case.

or pathogenic processes, or a pharmacological response to a therapeutic intervention that could aid in therapeutic decision-making. MRI tumor characteristics have been shown to correlate with both histologic and molecular subgroups, as shown in Chapter 8. Although gene expression profiling is increasingly used for treatment planning, immunohistochemical (IHC) markers are commonly used as substitute measures of tumor biology. These markers include the presence of estrogen and progesterone receptors (ER, PR), overexpression of the oncogene HER-2/neu, and proliferation rate, as measured by Ki-67. Imaging biomarkers need confirmation of accuracy and efficacy to be appropriately validated as surrogate end points. Their measurements should be accurate and reproducible and closely connected to the target lesion or treatment effect. Quantitative radiomics, a discipline that has developed quantitative image-based techniques with clinical applications such as cancer risk assessment and risk recurrence, are discussed further in Chapter 13.

Diagnostic accuracy is improved when preoperative MRI is performed, prompting changes in patient management. However, both overestimation and underestimation of disease can

occur and confirmative biopsy, of suspicious lesions found only at MRI, is necessary before changes in therapeutic management are put into effect. The decision to change the surgical approach from lumpectomy to mastectomy based on MRI findings, for example, should only be made after biopsy proof of additional cancer (▸ Fig. 10.3; ▸ Fig. 10.4). Cancer patients will benefit if treatment planning is made after careful review of all clinical, imaging, and histologic findings in a multidisciplinary setting. Individualized therapeutic regimens can aid in determining optimal patient outcome.

10.2.1 Tumor Measurements

Accurate tumor measurements are necessary for surgical and oncologic treatment planning, not only at initial diagnosis, but also when monitoring chemotherapeutic treatment. It is evident that tumor multifocality identified at MRI cannot be accurately assessed in most cases by a single maximum diameter measurement of the index cancer and satellites.[14] Complete assessment of the tumor burden requires measurement of not only the size of the individual tumor component(s) but also the

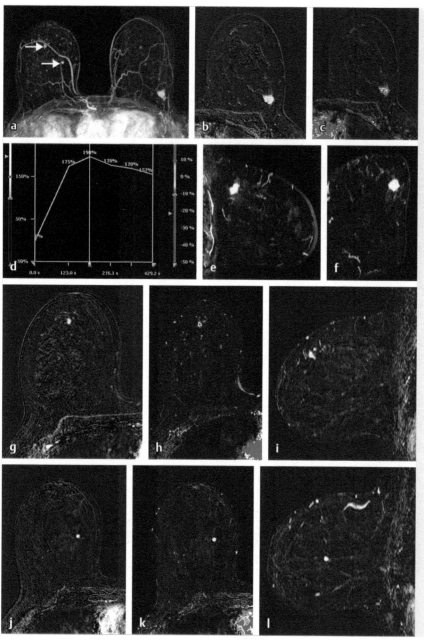

Fig. 10.2 Contralateral disease. Age 56: high-risk woman with newly diagnosed left breast IDC grade 3 with associated DCIS, MRI was recommended for disease extent assessment. MIP image (**a**) shows the index cancer in the far posterolateral left breast, and two additional small masses are shown in the anterior and lateral right breast (*arrows*). The index cancer is seen as an irregular mass on subtraction image (**b**), with heterogeneous washout kinetics (**c, d**). Sagittal and coronal images reformatted images are shown (**e, f**). Subtraction images of the right breast reveal an irregular anterior 5-mm mass with heterogeneous washout kinetics (**g, h**) also shown on sagittal image (**i**), and an additional circumscribed mass medial mass with plateau kinetics is shown on subtracted images (**j–l**). MR-guided biopsy of both small masses in the right breast yielded LCIS, classic, and pleomorphic subtypes. The patient requested bilateral mastectomy and right breast histology yielded LCIS, 7 cm in size, classic and pleomorphic types.

full volume of the extent of disease, both invasive and in situ. Multifocal disease may present as in situ cancer only, multiple invasive cancers with intervening normal tissue, or multiple invasive cancers associated with an in situ component, necessitating carefully imaging and histologic correlation. It is logical therefore that breast cancer patients might benefit from the accurate MRI identification of multifocal and diffuse disease that would otherwise go undetected. It has been shown in many studies that the use of multimodal imaging, and the additional use of percutaneous biopsy techniques, can provide precise maps of the extent and localization of breast disease. Computer-generated volume and surface area calculations reflect a more accurate estimate of tumor burden and can be automatically generated using newer advanced analytic software.

In rare circumstances, a patient may present with enlarged axillary lymph nodes, biopsy indicating metastatic disease likely of breast origin; however, clinical breast examination, mammography, and ultrasound studies are normal. MRI is usually able to identify the primary lesion if it indeed originates in the ipsilateral breast (▶ Fig. 10.5; ▶ Fig. 10.6).

MRI frequently detects ductal carcinoma in situ (DCIS) and associated invasive components not seen on mammography. Holland et al reported that mammographically occult DCIS was present histologically in 16% of higher-grade DCIS lesions larger than 20 mm, with necrosis, whereas occult disease was found in 47% cases with predominantly micropapillary-cribriform growth patterns.[15] Women undergoing surgical excision of DCIS diagnosed only at mammography may experience an inadequate surgical resection resulting in positive margins and the

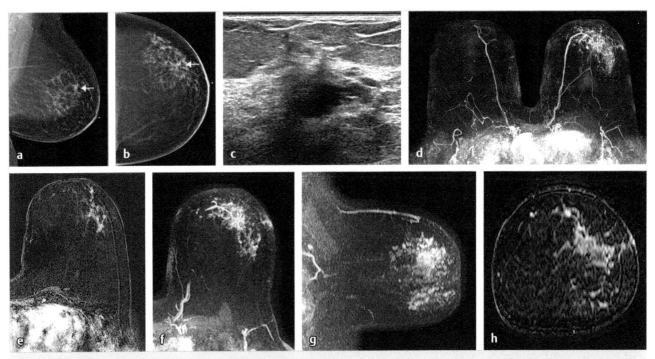

Fig. 10.3 Extent of disease assessment. Age 71, mammographic screening detected a focal asymmetry as shown on MLO and CC views (**a, b,** *arrows*). An ill-defined irregular mass is shown on ultrasound image (**c**). MIP image (**d**) reveals correlative anterior regional NME, more extensive than found at mammography, as shown on additional subtracted images (**e–h**). Histology yielded left breast IDC grade 2 with lobular features ER (+), PR (–), HER2/neu (–), Ki-67: 10%. Axillary nodes were negative for malignancy (0/6).

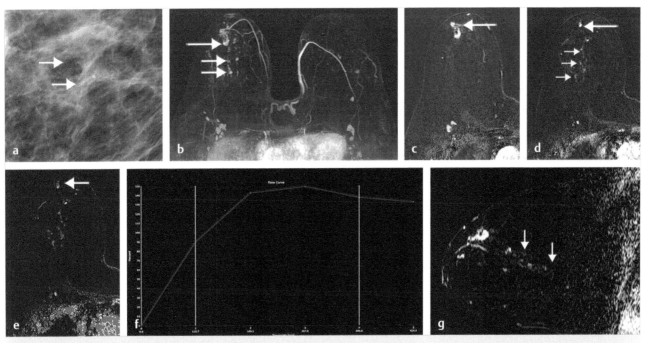

Fig. 10.4 Extent of disease assessment. Age 63, screen-detected new faint punctate calcifications are seen in the anterior right breast on mammographic CC magnification view (**a,** *arrows*). Stereotaxic biopsy yielded DCIS. MIP image (**b**) reveals the biopsy site (*long arrow*) and surrounding extensive NME (*short arrows*). Subtraction images (**c, d**) show a small enhancing mass anterior to the site of prior biopsy (*long arrows*) and extensive NME is also seen on image (**d,** *short arrows*). Angiomap and TIC (**e, f**) show plateau kinetics, and posterior NME is seen on sagittal image (**g,** *arrows*). MR-guided biopsy of the posterior extent of NME yielded DCIS intermediate grade. Histology at mastectomy yielded a 9 mm IDC grade 1 with 8 cm low and intermediate grade DCIS, cribriform, micropapillary and papillary, ER/PR (+).

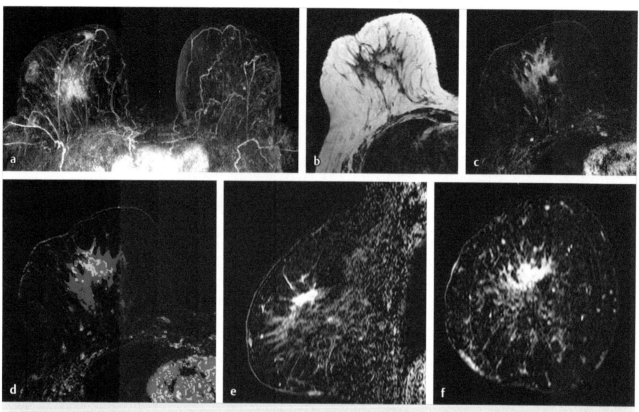

Fig. 10.5 Cancer of unknown primary (CUP syndrome). Age 85, with plaque-like sebaceous lesions diagnosed as cancer likely of breast origin. Physical examination of the right and left breasts, mammography, and ultrasound were normal. MIP image **(a)** reveals extensive NME in the central right breast and slight retraction of the anterior breast tissue. T2w image **(b)** reveals flattening of the anterior tissue and diffuse anterior and central NME is seen on subtraction image **(c)**. Angiomap **(d)** exhibits heterogeneous washout enhancement. Sagittal and coronal images are shown **(e, f)**. Histology yielded IDC grade 2. ER (+), PR (−), HER2/Neu (−).

need for re-excision surgery. Moreover, axillary nodal metastases may be found in 5 to 15% of patients with DCIS diagnosed at mammography; sentinel node (SLN) biopsy is justified in women with DCIS who have a high risk of invasive carcinoma, such as those with large tumors, a mass, or high-grade lesions.[16] MRI is able to detect the extent of DCIS and identify foci of invasion not present on mammography and ultrasound (▶ Fig. 10.7; ▶ Fig. 10.8).

10.3 Breast-Conserving Therapy (BCS)

BCS is used as an alternative to mastectomy for patients with diagnosis of early-stage breast cancer and is the most commonly performed breast surgical procedure. Partial mastectomy, or lumpectomy, consists of surgical removal of the tumor and the immediate surrounding normal breast tissue. Lumpectomy followed by radiation therapy (RT) has been shown in randomized clinical trials to be as effective as mastectomy when disease-free and overall survival rates are calculated.[17,18,19,20,21] The goal for successful BCS requires that the entire malignant lesion be removed with margins negative for tumor; therefore, knowledge of the true extent of the cancer is an important requisite for successful surgery. The literature is varied, however, as to whether MR identification of additional ipsi-lateral or contralateral occult malignancy is beneficial, given current therapeutic regimens.

Factors influencing treatment options among patients considered suitable for BCS include tumor size, location, nipple involvement, and presence or absence of tumor multifocality or multicentricity/diffuse disease. Additional considerations include tumor size as related to breast volume, cosmetic options, and patient preference. Identification of additional cancers can lead to a more extensive lumpectomy than originally planned, or even a mastectomy. In clinical practice, most patients have received a percutaneous biopsy prior to the MR examination and a postbiopsy seroma may be visible (▶ Fig. 10.9). MRI may detect an occult invasive component in a region of previously diagnosed DCIS, for example, or demonstrate axillary and internal mammary lymphadenopathy, all of which can impact surgical management. Preoperative MRI planning is especially useful for detection of mammographically occult DCIS. In some cases, DCIS may be found to be much more extensive on MR than on mammography and findings may even extend to the large subareolar ducts. Careful discussion of preoperative MR findings between the radiologist and the surgeon is necessary for favorable outcome. Two recent papers investigated the efficacy of preoperative breast MR imaging, MR-guided surgery and surgical outcome, showing improved depiction of disease extent and resulting change in therapeutic management (▶ Fig. 10.10; ▶ Fig. 10.11).[22,23]

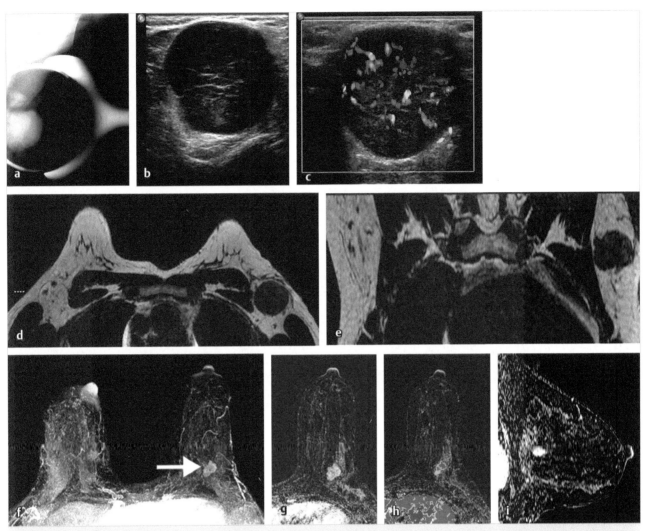

Fig. 10.6 Cancer of unknown primary (CUP syndrome). Age 37: newly enlarged left axillary lymph node, physical examination of the left breast, mammography, and ultrasound and were normal. Mammographic spot compression view of the left axilla reveals an enlarged axillary lymph node (a), shown to advantage on ultrasound image (b) with increased vascular flow shown on ultrasound color Doppler image (c). The enlarged lymph node is seen on axial and coronal T2w images (d, e). MIP image (f) shows marked BPE and an enhancing mass in the posterior left breast (*arrow*). The mass exhibits robust enhancement on subtracted image (g), and washout kinetics are noted on angiomap (h). Sagittal image (i) is shown. Histology yielded IDC, grade 3, with squamous features, triple-negative, Ki-67: 80%.

MRI is also very useful for identification of the associated features of malignancy, identified in ▶ Table 10.1.

Important benefits of preoperative MRI include identification of tumor invasion extending deep to fascia and determination of the relationship of tumor to fascia and its extension into the pectoralis major, serratus anterior, and/or intercostal muscles. MRI can detect muscle involvement, which impacts tumor staging, surgical planning, and the overall therapeutic approach—an extremely difficult, if not impossible, task to diagnose on clinical examination, mammography, or ultrasound.[24,25] Careful MR assessment is needed for diagnosis of pectoral muscle invasion. Enhancement that approaches or violates the prepectoral fat plane is not sufficient. Enhancement within the muscle itself is necessary for detection of invasion, superficial muscle enhancement allowing partial muscle excision, whereas radical mastectomy may be needed if the full thickness of the muscle is involved with tumor (▶ Fig. 10.12; ▶ Fig. 10.13).

Table 10.1 Associated features of malignancy

Nipple retraction	Axillary adenopathy
Nipple invasion	Pectoralis muscle invasion
Skin retraction	Chest wall invasion
Skin thickening	Architectural distortion
Skin invasion: direct invasion, inflammatory cancer	

Source: Morris EA, Comstock CE, Lee CH, et al. ACR BI-RADS® Magnetic Resonance Imaging. In: ACR BI-RADS® Atlas, Breast Imaging Reporting and Data System. Reston, VA, American College of Radiology; 2013.

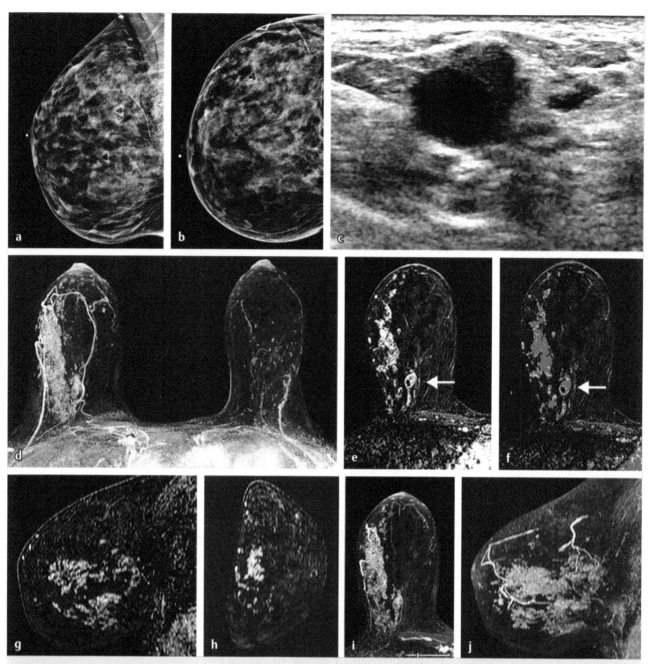

Fig. 10.7 Extent of disease assessment: DCIS. Age 47: patient with a history of prior right benign breast excisional biopsy, presented with a right breast "*thickening*." MLO and CC mammographic views (**a, b**) show no abnormal findings; a linear scar marker indicates prior biopsy site and triangular markers denote the site of palpable concern. Ultrasound (**c**) detected an indistinct complex mass, biopsy yielding DCIS. MIP image (**d**) exhibits mild BPE and segmental NME in the lateral right breast extending from the pectoral muscle to the subareolar region. Subtracted images (**e, f**) reveal NME, the site of prior ultrasound biopsy is indicated (*arrows*) and persistent kinetics are noted on angiomap (**f**). Reformatted sagittal and coronal images (**g, h**) show NME and sagittal and axial slab images (**i, j**) reveal the disease extent. Histology at mastectomy yielded DCIS, grade 3, with necrosis, ER/PR (–).

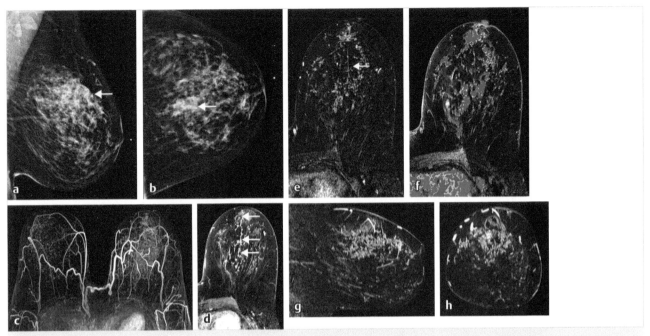

Fig. 10.8 Extent of disease assessment: DCIS. Age 59, presents with a palpable lump in the left breast: MLO and CC mammographic views **(a, b)** reveal a focal asymmetry (*arrows*), ultrasound did not indicate an abnormal finding. MIP image **(c)** shows diffuse NME in the central left breast. T1w source and subtraction images reveal duct enhancement **(d, e** *arrows*). Source angiomap image **(f)** shows persistent enhancement. Sagittal and coronal reformatted images **(g, h)** are shown. Histology yielded DCIS, high grade, solid, and cribriform types with associated central necrosis, ER/PR (−).

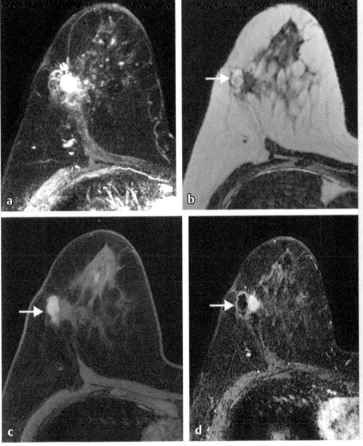

Fig. 10.9 Postbiopsy seroma. Age 65 with a newly diagnosed right breast IDC at 9 o'clock position: T1w source postcontrast image **(a)** shows the irregular enhancing index mass with surrounding NME. T2w image **(b)** reveals a hyperintense round mass representing a seroma following percutaneous core biopsy (*arrow*), located just lateral to the isointense malignant mass. Precontrast source T1w image **(c)** shows a hyperintense seroma (*arrow*), and subtraction image **(d)** shows a rim-enhancing seroma located lateral to the enhancing cancer (*arrow*).

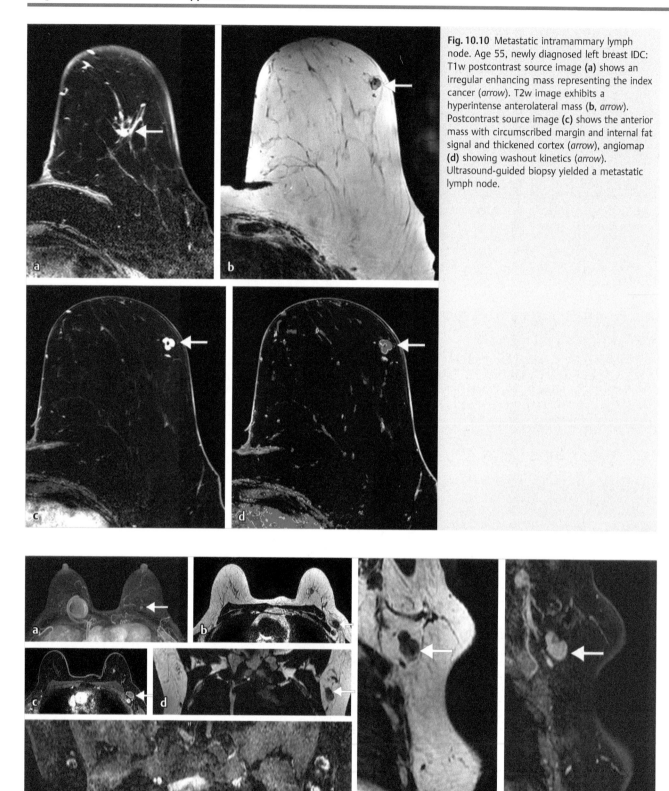

Fig. 10.10 Metastatic intramammary lymph node. Age 55, newly diagnosed left breast IDC: T1w postcontrast source image (**a**) shows an irregular enhancing mass representing the index cancer (*arrow*). T2w image exhibits a hyperintense anterolateral mass (**b**, *arrow*). Postcontrast source image (**c**) shows the anterior mass with circumscribed margin and internal fat signal and thickened cortex (*arrow*), angiomap (**d**) showing washout kinetics (*arrow*). Ultrasound-guided biopsy yielded a metastatic lymph node.

Fig. 10.11 Metastatic axillary lymph nodes. Age 48, newly diagnosed triple-negative IDC in the left breast: the index cancer is shown on MIP image (**a**) in the posterior left breast (*arrow*). A chemo-port artifact overlies the medial right breast. An enlarged left axillary metastatic node is seen on both T2w and postcontrast T1w source images; in the axial plane (**b, c**, *arrows*), the coronal plane (**d, e**, *arrows*) and the sagittal plane (**f, g**, *arrows*).

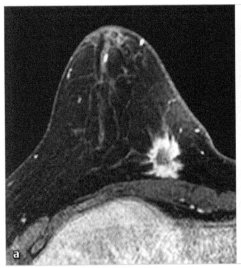

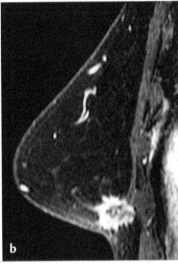

Fig. 10.12 IDC located close to the pectoral muscle. Newly diagnosed IDC grade 3, ER/PR (+), Her2/Neu (−): a spiculated enhancing mass is seen on postcontrast T1w postcontrast axial and sagittal images **(a, b)**. The mass is located posteriorly, adjacent to, but not invading the pectoral muscle. The sagittal reformatted plane is very helpful for diagnosis in this situation, and enhancement of the pectoral muscle is the key for diagnosis of invasion, which is not seen in this case.

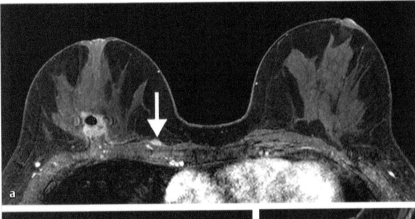

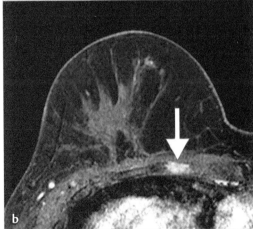

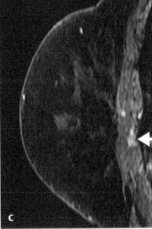

Fig. 10.13 IDC with pectoral muscle invasion. Newly diagnosed IDC grade 3, ER/PR (−), Her2/Neu (+): an irregular enhancing mass containing a signal void at the site of a marker clip is seen on postcontrast T1w postcontrast axial image **(a)**. The mass abuts the pectoral muscle and enhancement is noted within the muscle (*arrow*) indicating invasion. Additional muscle enhancement is shown on T1w postcontrast axial image **(b**, *arrow)* and sagittal image **(c**, *arrow)*.

Nipple and subareolar duct involvement can be seen either by direct involvement from an anterior invasive cancer or by linear enhancing extension of a DCIS lesion.[26,27] Surgeons will usually resect the nipple–areola complex if tumor is documented. MRI can identify DCIS lesions that exhibit linear enhancement extending into the subareolar region close to the nipple, which are occult at mammography (▶ Fig. 10.14). Skin enhancement suggests skin involvement with malignancy. Skin edema and skin thickening may be due to lymphatic obstruction with or without malignant involvement. Direct skin infiltration from an underlying malignant lesion is generally evident clinically and is well seen on MRI (▶ Fig. 10.15; ▶ Fig. 10.16).[28,29]

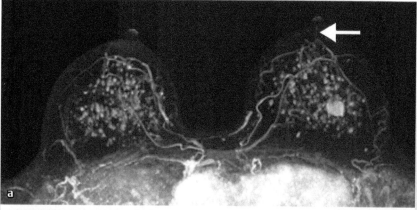
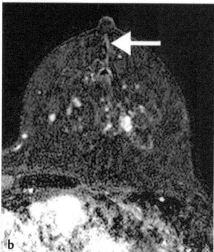
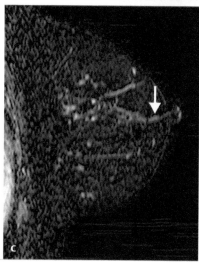

Fig. 10.14 Nipple involvement. Age 56: newly diagnosed IDC grade 2, triple-negative, Ki-67: 15%. MIP image **(a)** exhibits a round, irregular, posterior, left breast mass, representing the index cancer, in the setting of marked BPE. Linear enhancement of a single large duct in the left subareolar region is shown (*arrow*). T1w postcontrast axial and sagittal subtraction images **(b, c)** demonstrate extensive segmental NME extending from the known invasive cancer to the nipple (*arrows*). MR biopsy of anterior NME yielded high-grade DCIS, solid type with necrosis. Patient management was changed, and mastectomy was performed rather than lumpectomy as originally planned.

10.4 Management of Additional Disease

Identification of additional invasive cancer or DCIS at preoperative MRI has changed surgical management, by allowing a more accurate assessment of disease extent. When additional suspicious occult foci or masses are identified, image-guided percutaneous biopsy of the MR findings is usually required if the presence of cancer will alter surgical management. Identification of unsuspected invasive lesion(s) associated with a DCIS diagnosis will often change surgical management of the axilla. BI-RADS 3 assessments in this setting are generally not warranted as a specific diagnosis is needed.

Mapping of MRI-only visible DCIS in the preoperative setting often requires MR-guided biopsy (or biopsies) and clip placement(s) to document lesion extent. Multiple-wire placement is often needed to bracket imaging findings, resulting in complex surgical excisions. Successful outcome requires close collaboration between the surgeon, radiologist, and pathologist on the day of the surgical procedure. Despite improved DCIS mapping with MRI, some reports suggest that this capability does not always result in a decrease in the number of patients with positive margins at surgical excision.[15] Translation of imaging data from the magnet to the surgical environment is challenging. One explanation might relate to the position of the patient, who is supine in the operating room and prone in the magnet. Correlation of lesion(s) location using prone MR images for

guidance may prove to be difficult for the surgeon, particularly when attempting to resect multifocal disease. Contributing to this problem is the surgical approach, which may be oriented orthogonally to the length of the target DCIS lesion, thus increasing the difficulty of complete resection, even when the lesions are appropriately bracketed. Examples of the difference between the location of breast tissue in the prone and supine positions are shown (▶ Fig. 10.17; ▶ Fig. 10.18).

10.5 Reoperation Rates

A review of the literature indicates that the frequency of tumor in second surgical excision specimens ranges from 32 to 63%, with microscopic residual disease being found in about 50% of patients overall.[30,31] Findings of residual tumor have been shown to be associated with an increasing risk of recurrent cancer in the ipsilateral breast, for both invasive and noninvasive cancer, with some investigators showing increased local recurrence rates.[32,33] Other reports have indicated no increase in recurrence rates.[34,35,36] A retrospective observational trial conducted in four large institutions in the United States between 2003 and 2008 evaluated 2,206 women with 2,220 invasive breast cancers undergoing partial mastectomy.[1] The aim was to assess hospital- and surgeon-specific variation in reoperation rates following initial surgery. Overall, 22.9% patients underwent additional surgery on the affected breast. Among these patients, 89.2% underwent a single operative procedure, 9.4%

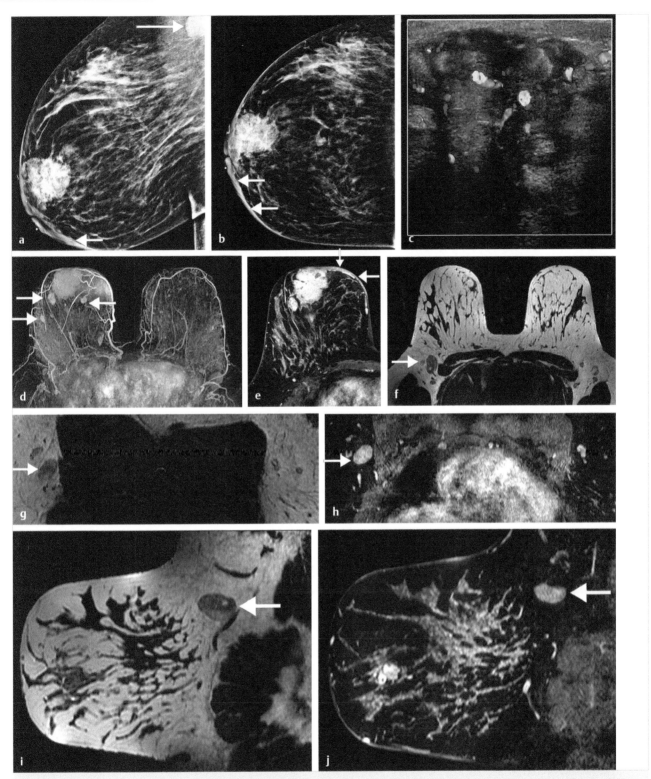

Fig. 10.15 Direct skin involvement and axillary adenopathy. Age 47, newly diagnosed right breast IDC with lobular features and high-grade DCIS with necrosis, ER/PR (+), Her2/Neu (−), Ki-67: 30%. MLO and CC mammographic views (**a, b**) demonstrate a round irregular mass in the subareolar region with adjacent skin thickening (*short arrows*) and a partly visible axillary lymph node (**a**, *long arrow*). Ultrasound image (**c**) shows an irregular mass with marked increased vascularity. MIP image (**d**) reveals marked BPE with a large subareolar enhancing mass and satellite lesions (*arrows*). T1w source postcontrast image (**e**) exhibits the irregular subareolar mass with adjacent skin enhancement (*arrows*). Punch biopsy of the skin revealed direct malignant perivascular and lymphocytic infiltration. Axial T2w image exhibits right axillary adenopathy (**f**, *arrow*). T2w and postcontrast source T1w images demonstrate right axillary adenopathy in the coronal and sagittal planes (**g–j**, *arrows*).

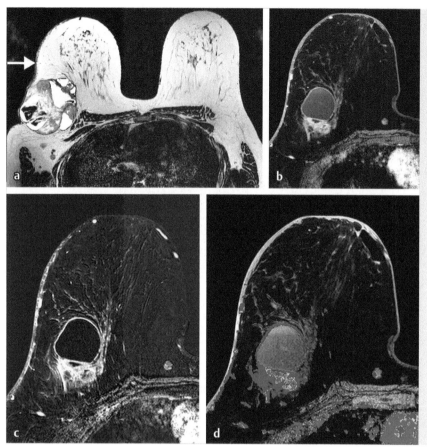

Fig. 10.16 Direct dermal extension. Age 45, newly diagnosed triple-negative right breast IDC grade 3, 12.0 cm, with extensive central necrosis and direct dermal extension and ulceration. 12/20 axillary lymph nodes are involved with malignancy. T2w axial image **(a)** shows a mixed signal mass with necrotic fluid, overlying skin thickening, and subcutaneous edema (*arrow*) representing skin involvement. Postcontrast T1w source and subtraction images **(b, c)** reveal the necrotic mass and diffuse lateral skin enhancement. Angiomap **(d)** shows washout kinetics in the solid component of the necrotic mass.

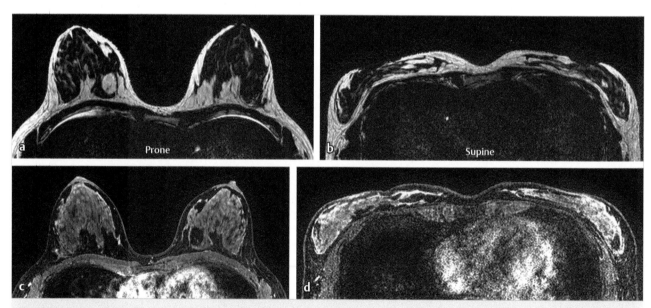

Fig. 10.17 Prone supine positioning. Breast MRI is performed in the prone position and the patient is supine in the operating room. We imaged a patient with normal findings in both the supine and the routine prone position, in order to demonstrate the differences in breast appearance. T2w images **(a, b)** and postcontrast T1w image **(c, d)** are shown.

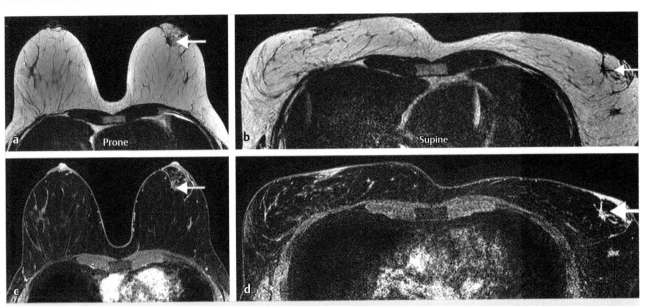

Fig. 10.18 Prone and supine positioning. Breast MRI is performed in the prone position and the patient is supine in the operating room. We imaged a patient with a postoperative scar in the left subareolar region (*arrows*) in both the supine and the routine prone position, in order to demonstrate the differences in breast appearance. T2w images (**a, b**) and postcontrast T1w image (**c, d**) are shown.

underwent two re-excisions, and 4% underwent three re-excisions. Subsequent mastectomy was required in 8.4%. The authors concluded that substantial surgeon and institutional variation existed; however, re-excision rates were somewhat lower than previously reported rates of 36 to 50%.[37,38] Morrow et al reported a 37.9% re-excision rate following initial BCS in a similarly large series of 1,459 patients in 2009, with 26.0% patients undergoing local repeat surgery and 11.9% ultimately undergoing mastectomy.[37]

Another study published in 2016 showed that nearly one in four women who underwent BCS in New York State between 2011 and 2013 required a reoperation within 90 days.[39] The reoperation rate averaged 30%, decreasing from a 38.5% rate during 2003 to 2005, to a 23.1% rate during 2011 to 2013. It is important to note that surgeons with higher volume of procedures were independently associated with lower reoperation rates, whereas procedures performed by low-volume surgeons were associated with a 50% higher risk for reoperation, the difference persisting in multivariable analyses.

A modified surgical technique known as "cavity shaving" involves re-excision of the entire surgical cavity by removing additional tissue from each face of the cavity at time of initial cancer resection. This surgical method has proved successful as reported in a recent randomized trial, by significantly reducing the rate of positive margins from 34 to 19% and the rate of re-excision from 21 to 10%, in the "shaved" versus the standard surgical approach.[40]

10.5.1 Role of MRI for Reducing Rates of Re-excision

Can preoperative breast MRI help reduce reoperation rates by providing careful mapping of disease extent? Questions remain as to whether the improved sensitivity of preoperative breast MRI improves patient outcomes and the use of MRI for staging of newly diagnosed breast cancer has been controversial. The clinical outcome literature on the benefits of preoperative MRI shows conflicting results regarding rates of re-excision and local recurrence.

A randomized controlled trial conducted in the United Kingdom known as the COMICE trial, published in 2010, compared two patient groups: one group received preoperative MRI and the other group received standard care. Re-excision rates were identical (19%) for both the MRI and non-MRI groups.[41] This trial was widely criticized, partly because older MRI technology was used across the imaging sites, and partly because radiological and surgical experience was varied. Another problem with this trial involved the lack of MR-guided biopsy procedures, which were not generally available at the trial sites. This deficiency resulted in management changes to mastectomy in 28% of the MRI group, who went to surgery without presurgical confirmation of malignancy. The MONET trial found an increase in re-excision rates in patients with MRI (34%) versus for patients without MRI (12%). This paradoxical higher rate of positive margins and re-excision rates in the MRI group was partly attributed to surgical bias; critics of this study noted that, overall, the volume of the excised tissue in the MRI group (69.1 cm^3) was much smaller than the volume in the non-MRI group (90.2 cm^3). Additional variability was noted in surgical resection volumes, which were even smaller in patients with DCIS and negative MRI examinations (40.3 cm^3).[42] A later study in 2012, where biopsy confirmation of malignancy was made prior to management change, found a significant improvement in reoperation rates using preoperative breast MRI. Patients in the MRI group in this study had a reoperation rate of only 11% compared to 25% in the non-MRI group, without an increase in the mastectomy rates,[43] and recently published studies have shown decreased rates of re-excision when preoperative MRI was used.[44,45] The data on the efficacy of use of preoperative MRI for patients with invasive lobular carcinoma (ILC) lesions are particularly convincing.[46,47,48]

It is important to note that use of reoperation rates as a metric for clinical efficacy of preoperative MRI is confounded by the wide variation in surgical practice, which may override any impact that MRI findings might make.[1] There is considerable inconsistency in recommendations for preoperative MRI in the United States. Some surgeons and oncologists request MRI before surgery or neoadjuvant chemotherapy routinely, while others may select preoperative MRI for younger women only or for those with ILC histology, and others do not recommend preoperative MRI. Several studies have documented the critical role of preoperative MRI for women selected for partial breast irradiation.[49,50] No survival benefit has been demonstrated until now. A prospective randomized controlled trial is currently under development by the American College of Radiology Imaging Network (ACRIN) on the short- and long-term benefits and cost analysis of preoperative MRI staging.[51]

10.6 Diagnosis of Residual Disease

Diagnosis of positive margins at the tumor resection site is best achieved with MRI. Early reports have shown that a delay in MRI of 28 days or more is preferable to imaging immediately after surgery.[52] Today, however, the patient is usually scanned as soon as is feasible, between 2 and 3 weeks after surgery when the pathology report is available for review and the patient has discussed further treatment options with her surgeon.

10.6.1 Imaging Findings

Normal postsurgical MRI findings typically include the presence of a seroma at the surgical site, seen as a thin smoothly enhancing < 3-mm rim, often with findings of focal skin thickening and edema (▶ Fig. 10.19). Most of these benign changes diminish completely over time, but some seromata may persist for many years. Identification of the precise location of residual tumor has the potential to lead to more appropriate selection of re-resection procedures. Suspicious findings include irregular thickening of the seroma wall, ≥ 5 mm, with adjacent mass or nonmass enhancement (▶ Fig. 10.20). Unsuspected findings may be detected in the ipsilateral or contralateral breast remote from the surgical site, especially if MRI was not performed prior to initial surgery (▶ Fig. 10.21; ▶ Fig. 10.22).[53] When this occurs, MR-guided biopsy with clip placement can be employed to confirm and document the additional site(s) of tumor, prior to needle localization and re-excision surgery. When residual disease is identified close to the resection site, a needle localization procedure alone, without a prior MR-guided biopsy, can be used to guide the surgeon to the site of possible residual tumor.

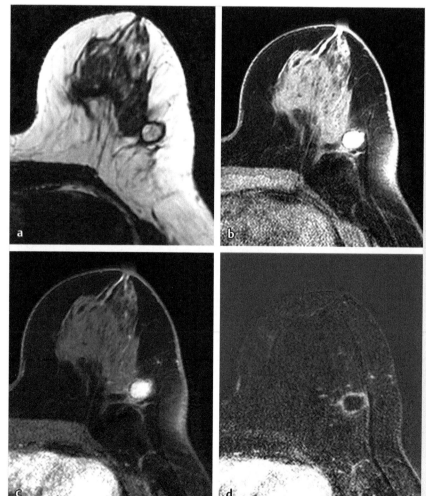

Fig. 10.19 Postoperative seroma: no residual tumor. A seroma cavity at 21 days following surgery for IDC with close margins is shown. T2w image (a) reveals an oval seroma with high internal signal in the lateral left breast, also shown on T1w precontrast image (b). Postcontrast source image (c) reveals high signal within the seroma and benign high ductal signal in the subareolar region. Subtraction image (d) shows an enhancing seroma rim < 5 mm, with several scattered foci. Re-excision surgery did not identify any residual tumor.

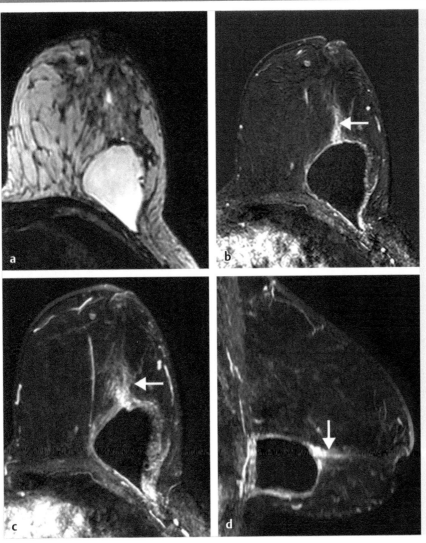

Fig. 10.20 Postoperative seroma: fat necrosis. A seroma cavity at 19 days following surgery for IDC with close margins is shown. T2w image (a) reveals a large seroma with fluid signal in the lateral left breast. T1w postcontrast axial source image (b) shows linear enhancement extending from the anterior aspect of the normal enhancing seroma rim (*arrow*) also seen on axial slab (c) and sagittal (d) images (*arrows*). MR-guided biopsy of the anterior enhancement yielded fat necrosis and granulomatous change.

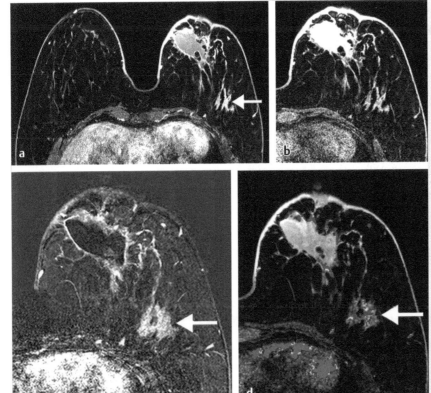

Fig. 10.21 Postoperative seroma: residual tumor. Age 60, screening mammogram detected a 7-mm cluster of microcalcifications in the anterior left breast, histology yielding DCIS, solid and cribriform with necrosis, ER/PR +, SLNB negative for nodal metastases. No preoperative MRI was obtained. Patient subsequently underwent three surgical excisions for positive margins and was then referred for MRI. Axial source postcontrast image (a) shows volume loss, with diffuse skin thickening, distortion and a large anteromedial seroma cavity and NME in the lateral left breast, remote from the resection seroma (*arrow*). Precontrast T1w image (b) shows high signal within the seroma cavity, and subtraction image (c) shows irregular peri-seromal enhancement and regional NME in the posterolateral quadrant (*arrow*). Angiomap (d) reveals NME with heterogeneous washout kinetics (*arrow*). Mastectomy found 7.0 cm of residual DCIS, intermediate and high grade, solid and cribriform type with a 3 mm associated IDC grade1.

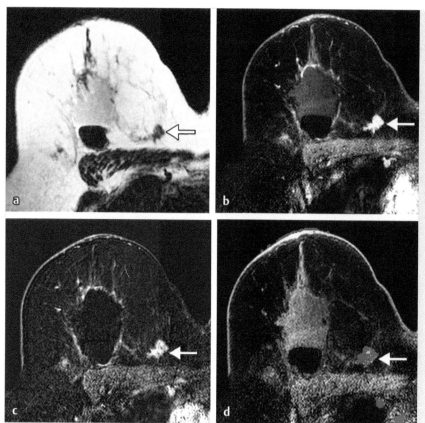

Fig. 10.22 Postoperative seroma: residual tumor. Age 51, patient underwent three excisions for removal of a 2.1 cm IDC in the central posterior aspect of the right breast: no prior MRI was obtained. Axial T2w image (**a**) shows a large mixed signal posterior seroma cavity and a hypointense irregular mass in the medial breast (*arrow*), also seen as a robustly enhancing mass on source postcontrast T1w image (**b**, *arrow*). Subtraction image (**c**) also shows the enhancing mass (*arrow*) and associated periseromal enhancement. The mass exhibits heterogeneous washout kinetics as shown on angiomap (**d**, *arrow*). Mastectomy yielded IDC grade 2 with foci of DCIS, solid and cribriform, and 1/16 nodes positive for malignancy.

Differentiation of residual and recurrent tumor from fat necrosis is often the most challenging differential diagnosis.[54] Fat necrosis is thought to result from a localized response to the hematoma that develops after surgical trauma. The histologic appearance of fat necrosis depends on the temporal stage of the lesion. Blood and tissue lipase in the early stages cause sterile saponification of fat, which results in the formation of vacuoles surrounded by fat-filled macrophages, foreign body giant cells, and plasma cells, exhibiting irregular enhancement on MRI. During the healing phase, fibrosis develops along the periphery of the necrotic debris and may replace the entire lesion. Areas of fat necrosis may form a fluid-filled cavity and eventually calcify, with no residual enhancement, but in some instances, enhancement may remain for many years. The enhancement of fat necrosis may mimic malignancy, and even though fat signal may be evident on imaging, biopsy may be necessary for proof of benignity in some cases. Delayed periareolar fat necrosis may be found in some women who underwent a periareolar injection of radionuclide prior to SLN biopsy. Two examples are shown (▶ Fig. 10.23; ▶ Fig. 10.24).

10.7 Neoadjuvant Chemotherapy Monitoring (NACT)

Neoadjuvant systemic chemotherapy (chemotherapy prior to surgery for invasive cancer) is widely used to provide improved surgical outcomes, recurrent-free survival, and overall survival in certain subtypes of breast cancer, with the additional potential benefit that reduced tumor volume during treatment may allow for more conservative surgery.[55] The opportunity to monitor treatment response in vivo as early in the treatment as possible and to be able to identify nonresponders, by using MRI monitoring, is a critical patient benefit. Change in tumor size has been shown to be a clinically useful measure of tumor response and is predictive of patient survival. MRI is the most accurate imaging method for monitoring treatment response during therapy and for assessment of the extent of residual disease, before surgery, when chemotherapy is completed (▶ Fig. 10.25; ▶ Fig. 10.26).

The NACT protocol generally requires a preoperative MRI and two subsequent MRI examinations—a second after initial treatment and a third after final treatment before surgery. MRI documentation of treatment response is traditionally recorded as follows. Absence of any enhancement at the site of the prior index lesion(s) is recorded as a complete response (CR). Reduction in the index cancer size by > 30% is recorded as a partial response (PR). Decrease in the size of the index cancer by < 30% is recorded as no response (NR). MR studies performed after the first cycle of chemotherapy often provide the best opportunity for the radiologist to assess early response. In the event that a tumor shows no response or even progression of disease on imaging after the first treatment, modifications to the treatment protocol can be considered, thus sparing the patient from prolonged and ineffective chemotherapy. Assessment of tumor volumes and surface areas using computerized analytical software can provide more accurate comparison measures than traditional linear measure of maximum tumor diameter.[14,56]

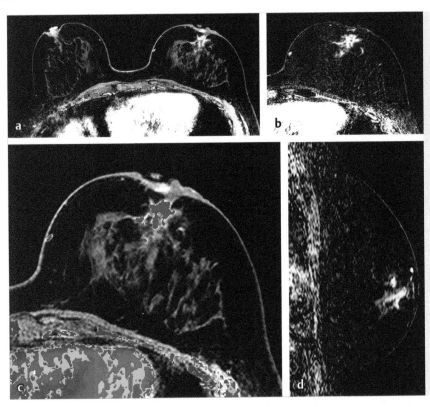

Fig. 10.23 Subareolar fat necrosis following radionuclide injection. Age 50, patient was treated with BCS for a triple-negative IDC in the posterior medial left breast: routine MRI surveillance at I year shows volume loss irregular left subareolar enhancement on axial postcontrast source image (a) and on subtracted image (b). The enhancing finding exhibits persistent kinetics on angiomap (c) and subtraction sagittal view (d) is shown. Ultrasound-guided biopsy yielded fat necrosis, and subsequent MRI at 3 years showed resolution of the findings. The patient received a periareolar injection of radionuclide prior to sentinel node surgery and this is thought to be the cause of the fat necrosis remotely located from the surgical site.

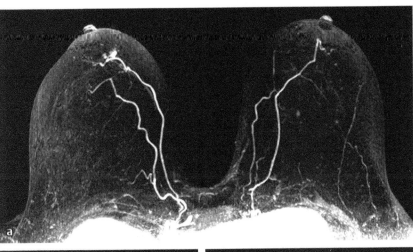
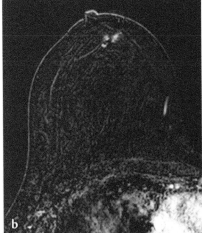
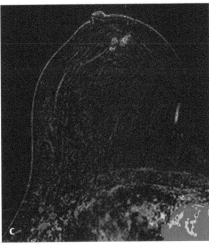

Fig. 10.24 Subareolar fat necrosis following radionuclide injection. Age 50, patient was treated with BCS for IDC grade 3, ER/PR (+), in the posterior lateral right breast: routine MRI surveillance at 2 years shows slight volume loss and irregular right subareolar enhancement on MIP image (a) also seen on subtracted image (b). The enhancing finding exhibits washout kinetics on angiomap (c). Ultrasound-guided biopsy yielded fat necrosis, and subsequent MRI at 2 years showed resolution of the findings. The patient received a periareolar injection of radionuclide prior to sentinel node surgery and this is thought to be the cause of the fat necrosis remotely located from the surgical site.

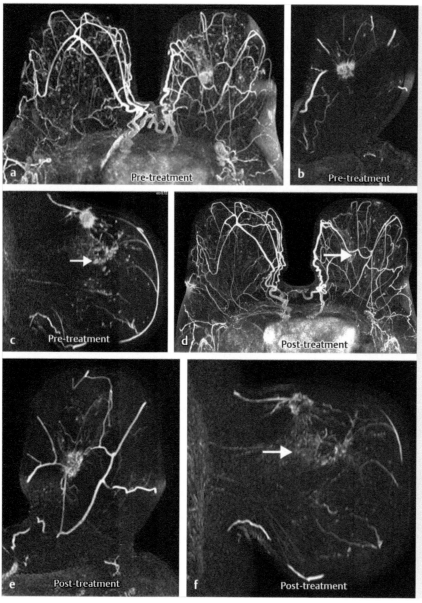

Fig. 10.25 Monitoring of NACT response. Age 57, new diagnosis of IDC grade 3 triple-negative, Ki-67: 15%, presenting as a 2.1 cm mass in the superior left breast with associated DCIS spanning 6.0 cm. Pretreatment MIP image (a) reveals an enhancing mass, superficially located at 11 o'clock position, with associated anterior NME. Axial slab image (b) shows mass marginal spiculation and sagittal image (c) reveals regional NME located anterior and inferior to the mass (arrow). Posttreatment MIP image (d) reveals diminished mass enhancement and subtracted axial and sagittal slab images (e, f) reveal a partial response to NACT (>30%), with diminished but persistent mass enhancement and persistent NME as shown on image (f, arrow). Histology at mastectomy yielded a partial response with IDC grade 3, 2.1 cm remaining with extensive treatment changes and <5% tumor cellularity. 7/11 axillary nodes were positive for malignancy.

Cancers undergoing treatment generally exhibit two different patterns of response. Masses often exhibit concentric shrinkage, are easier to measure, and accord good histologic and imaging concordance after therapy. Diffuse or multifocal lesions and those initially presenting as NME may exhibit an overall volume decrease with heterogeneous tumor regression following therapy, but without a significant change in maximum tumor diameter.[57,58,59,60] Prediction of in-breast residual cancer burden in the ACRIN 6657 trial showed that MRI measurements of tumor volume and longest tumor diameter were superior to clinical examination, and changes in tumor volume showed the greatest predictive value for response after the first cycle of NACT.[61] A more recent study from the ACRIN 6657 Trial sought to investigate the accuracy of preoperative measurements for detecting pathologic complete response (CR) and assessing residual disease after neoadjuvant chemotherapy (NACT) in patients with locally advanced breast cancer. These results indicated that measurement of longest diameter by MRI is more accurate than

by mammography and clinical examination for preoperative assessment of tumor residua after NACT and may improve surgical planning. Care must be taken not to overlook subtle signs of residual cancer. Underestimation of residual disease has been reported with both ILC and DCIS lesions likely because a low degree of angiogenesis is often seen with these tumors. Careful inspection of the last postcontrast subtracted series may exhibit faint enhancement and may be the only indication of residual disease. Other acquisitions such as diffusion-weighted imaging (DWI) can be added to the DCE series and may improve diagnostic accuracy in the neoadjuvant setting.[62] It is important to remember that MRI-compatible localization tissue markers should always be placed in the tumor prior to the first chemotherapy dose. The marker may prove to be essential at time of surgery, when no imaging evidence of disease is found. Further investigation is needed to assess the potential benefit of tumor response to NAC among all molecular subtypes of breast cancers.

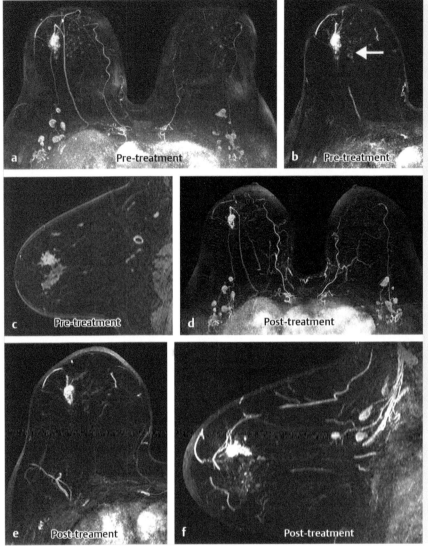

Fig. 10.26 Monitoring of NACT response. Age 61, newly diagnosed grade 3 IDC, HER2/neu enriched subtype and high-grade DCIS, presenting as a 1.7 cm enhancing irregular mass in the superior right breast with associated NME spanning 5.0 cm medially, as seen on pretreatment MIP image (a). Axial slab image (b) shows the irregular mass and medial focal NME (*arrow*). Sagittal Image (c) is shown. Posttreatment MIP image (d) reveals minimal diminution in mass size and subtracted axial and sagittal slab images (e, f) show no change in the extent of NME (<30%). Histology at mastectomy yielded IDC gross measurement 2.1 cm, indicating IDC grade 3, size 2.1 cm, Ki-67: 23%, with 70% residual cellularity. Axillary nodes were negative for malignancy (0/7).

10.8 Recurrent Tumor

It is well known that whole breast RT reduces overall local recurrence by about 50% in DCIS cases and treatment of ER (+) cases with tamoxifen reduces this risk by an additional 50%.[63] The absolute benefit of RT in low-risk DCIS is uncertain and there is no widespread agreement as to the effect on survival. The management of low-risk DCIS with BCS and no subsequent RT has been studied retrospectively, with evidence that ipsilateral breast tumor recurrence is low.[64] Low-risk cases with negative margins achieved at BCS result in a recurrence rate of 22.5% when treated without RT. The recurrence rate increases if close or positive margins are present at surgical resection. There is inconsistent evidence that DCIS with human epidermal growth factor receptor HER-2/neu-positive tumors and ER-negative tumors has a worse prognosis. It is important to consider that regardless of the therapeutic protocol (mastectomy, lumpectomy with RT, or wide surgical excision alone), half of the DCIS lesions are invasive when they recur, and 20% of cases present with distant metastases at 10 years.[65] MR readily identifies recurrent tumor (▶ Fig. 10.27), the differential diagnosis being

generally that of tumor versus fat necrosis. Any new enhancement should be carefully evaluated given that background parenchymal enhancement in the normal postirradiated breast is usually diminished. Tumor characteristics associated with recurrence following BCS include young patient age, large lesion size, high nuclear grade, necrosis with or without microinvasion, and adequacy of the surgical resection. Recurrent cancers, those that present clinically, generally have a poorer prognosis than subclinical recurrent cancers. Reports have shown that a greater number of small second cancers are detected on posttreatment MRI surveillance than on mammography. MRI is often added to the surveillance regimen when the patient's age, imaging features, cancer histology, and genetic profiles are taken into account. A report published by Houssami and colleagues in 2009 showed the prognostic benefit of early diagnosis of a second tumor (invasive or in situ) in a study of 1,044 cancer survivors. Improved relative survival, between 27 and 47%, was found in asymptomatic women whose recurrent cancers were diagnosed at an early stage.[65] Tumor recurrence rates after breast conservation therapy are relatively low, 1 to 2% per year, and these rates continue to

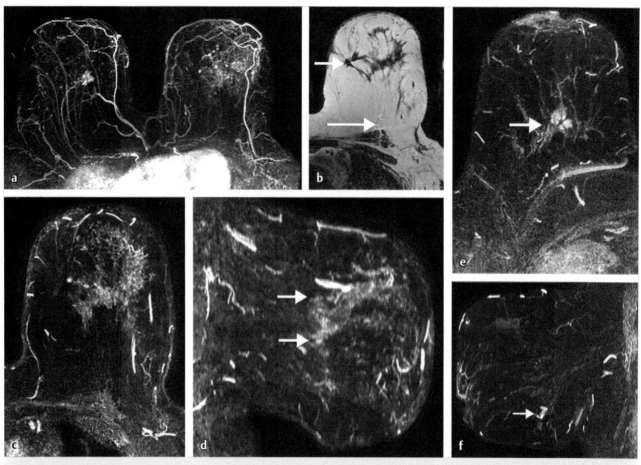

Fig. 10.27 Recurrent tumor; patient age 45 with a diagnosis of low-grade DCIS in the left breast upper inner quadrant treated 10 years ago with BCS and radiation therapy, presented with new calcifications near the resection site at mammography. Stereotactic biopsy yielded IDC, grade 2, with micropapillary features and DCIS, intermediate and high-grade, solid type, ER/PR +. MIP image (a) reveals extensive NME in the central and lateral anterior left breast, and an unsuspected irregular enhancing mass in the central right breast. T2w image (b) reveals scarring at the left breast lumpectomy site (*short arrow*), and prepectoral fluid, a sign of aggressive disease (*long arrow*). Extensive NME is seen in the anterior left breast on subtracted axial slab image (c) and skin thickening, and enhancement is also present. Sagittal image (d) shows extensive NME (*arrows*). Histology at left mastectomy yielded IDC grade 2, with micropapillary features and DCIS intermediate to high nuclear grade, solid type. MRI of the right breast detected an ILC lesion occult at mammography, as shown on axial and sagittal slab images (e, f, *arrows*).

decrease due to ongoing improvement in chemotherapy and hormonal treatment.[66]

10.9 Summary

Breast MRI demonstrates superior accuracy for assessment of tumor size, location, and extent of malignant disease. Identification of multifocal, multicentric, diffuse, and contralateral tumors not only helps to guide treatment planning but also provides an independent negative prognostic indicator. Most practices now rely on MRI for monitoring of assessment response during NACT. While there is no consensus as yet as to the routine use of MRI for assessing extent of disease, further evidence has shown preoperative MRI to be beneficial in certain subsets of patients. There is increasing evidence of the efficacy of preoperative MRI in decreasing reoperation rates.

References

[1] McCahill LE, Single RM, Aiello Bowles EJ, et al. Variability in reexcision following breast conservation surgery. JAMA. 2012; 307(5):467–475

[2] Tot T, Gere M, Pekár G, et al. Breast cancer multifocality, disease extent, and survival. Hum Pathol. 2011; 42(11):1761–1769

[3] Iacconi C, Galman L, Zheng J, et al. Multicentric cancer detected at breast MR imaging and not at mammography: important or not? Radiology. 2016; 279 (2):378–384

[4] Lehman CD, Gatsonis C, Kuhl CK, et al. ACRIN Trial 6667 Investigators Group. MRI evaluation of the contralateral breast in women with recently diagnosed breast cancer. N Engl J Med. 2007; 356(13):1295–1303

[5] Fischer U, Kopka L, Grabbe E. Breast carcinoma: effect of preoperative contrast-enhanced MR imaging on the therapeutic approach. Radiology. 1999; 213(3):881–888

[6] Hollingsworth AB, Stough RG, O'Dell CA, Brekke CE. Breast magnetic resonance imaging for preoperative locoregional staging. Am J Surg. 2008; 196 (3):389–397

[7] Liberman L, Morris EA, Kim CM, et al. MR imaging findings in the contralateral breast of women with recently diagnosed breast cancer. AJR Am J Roentgenol. 2003; 180(2):333–341

[8] Berg WA, Gutierrez L, NessAiver MS, et al. Diagnostic accuracy of mammography, clinical examination, US, and MR imaging in preoperative assessment of breast cancer. Radiology. 2004; 233(3):830–849

[9] Gutierrez RL, DeMartini WB, Silbergeld JJ, et al. High cancer yield and positive predictive value: outcomes at a center routinely using preoperative breast MRI for staging. AJR Am J Roentgenol. 2011; 196(1):W93–9

[10] Lehman CD, DeMartini W, Anderson BO, Edge SB. Indications for breast MRI in the patient with newly diagnosed breast cancer. J Natl Compr Canc Netw. 2009; 7(2):193–201

[11] Schnall MD, Blume J, Bluemke DA, et al. MRI detection of distinct incidental cancer in women with primary breast cancer studied in IBMC 6883. J Surg Oncol. 2005; 92(1):32–38

[12] Barco I, Chabrera C, García-Fernández A, et al. Magnetic resonance imaging in the preoperative setting for breast cancer patients with undetected additional disease. Eur J Radiol. 2016; 85(10):1786–1793

[13] Tot T. Clinical relevance of the distribution of the lesions in 500 consecutive breast cancer cases documented in large-format histologic sections. Cancer. 2007; 110(11):2551–2560

[14] Eisenhauer EA, Therasse P, Bogaerts J, et al. New response evaluation criteria in solid tumours: revised RECIST guideline (version 1.1). Eur J Cancer. 2009; 45(2):228–247

[15] Holland R, Hendriks JH, Vebeek AL, Mravunac M, Schuurmans Stekhoven JH. Extent, distribution, and mammographic/histological correlations of breast ductal carcinoma in situ. Lancet. 1990; 335(8688):519–522

[16] Amersi F, Hansen NM. The benefits and limitations of sentinel lymph node biopsy. Curr Treat Options Oncol. 2006; 7(2):141–151

[17] Bleicher RJ, Ciocca RM, Egleston BL, et al. Association of routine pretreatment magnetic resonance imaging with time to surgery, mastectomy rate, and margin status. J Am Coll Surg. 2009; 209(2):180–187, quiz 294–295

[18] Veronesi U, Saccozzi R, Del Vecchio M, et al. Comparing radical mastectomy with quadrantectomy, axillary dissection, and radiotherapy in patients with small cancers of the breast. N Engl J Med. 1981; 305(1):6–11

[19] Fisher B, Anderson S, National Surgical Adjuvant Breast and Bowel Project. Conservative surgery for the management of invasive and noninvasive carcinoma of the breast: NSABP trials. World J Surg. 1994; 18(1):63–69

[20] Fisher B, Anderson S, Bryant J, et al. Twenty-year follow-up of a randomized trial comparing total mastectomy, lumpectomy, and lumpectomy plus irradiation for the treatment of invasive breast cancer. N Engl J Med. 2002; 347 (16):1233–1241

[21] Veronesi U, Cascinelli N, Mariani L, et al. Twenty-year follow-up of a randomized study comparing breast-conserving surgery with radical mastectomy for early breast cancer. N Engl J Med. 2002; 347(16):1227–1232

[22] Benveniste AP, Ortiz-Perez T, Ebuoma LO, et al. Is breast magnetic resonance imaging (MRI) useful for diagnosis of additional sites of disease in patients recently diagnosed with pure ductal carcinoma in situ (DCIS)? Eur J Radiol. 2017; 96: 7479

[23] Kuhl CK, Strobel K, Bieling H, et al. Impact of Preoperative breast MR imaging and MR-guided surgery on diagnosis and surgical outcome of women with invasive breast cancer with and without DCIS component. Radiology. 2017; 284(3): 645–655

[24] Morris EA, Schwartz LH, Drotman MB, et al. Evaluation of pectoralis major muscle in patients with posterior breast tumors on breast MR images: early experience. Radiology. 2000; 214(1):67–72

[25] Kazama T, Nakamura S, Doi O, Suzuki K, Hirose M, Ito H. Prospective evaluation of pectoralis muscle invasion of breast cancer by MR imaging. Breast Cancer. 2005; 12(4):312–316

[26] Sakamoto N, Tozaki M, Hoshi K, Fukuma E. Is MRI useful for the prediction of nipple involvement? Breast Cancer. 2013; 20(4):316–322

[27] Steen ST, Chung AP, Han SH, Vinstein AL, Yoon JL, Giuliano AE. Predicting nipple-areolar involvement using preoperative breast MRI and primary tumor characteristics. Ann Surg Oncol. 2013; 20(2):633–639

[28] Renz DM, Baltzer PA, Böttcher J, et al. Inflammatory breast carcinoma in magnetic resonance imaging: a comparison with locally advanced breast cancer. Acad Radiol. 2008; 15(2):209–221

[29] Girardi V, Carbognin G, Camera L, et al. Inflammatory breast carcinoma and locally advanced breast carcinoma: characterisation with MR imaging. Radiol Med (Torino). 2011; 116(1):71–83

[30] Schnitt SJ, Connolly JL, Khettry U, et al. Pathologic findings on re-excision of the primary site in breast cancer patients considered for treatment by primary radiation therapy. Cancer. 1987; 59(4).675–681

[31] Beron PJ, Horwitz EM, Martinez AA, et al. Pathologic and mammographic findings predicting the adequacy of tumor excision before breast-conserving therapy. AJR Am J Roentgenol. 1996; 167(6):1409–1414

[32] Freedman G, Fowble B, Hanlon A, et al. Patients with early stage invasive cancer with close or positive margins treated with conservative surgery and radiation have an increased risk of breast recurrence that is delayed by adjuvant systemic therapy. Int J Radiat Oncol Biol Phys. 1999; 44(5):1005–1015

[33] Smitt MC, Nowels KW, Zdeblick MJ, et al. The importance of the lumpectomy surgical margin status in long-term results of breast conservation. Cancer. 1995; 76(2):259–267

[34] Cowen D, Houvenaeghel G, Bardou V, et al. Local and distant failures after limited surgery with positive margins and radiotherapy for node-negative breast cancer. Int J Radiat Oncol Biol Phys. 2000; 47(2):305–312

[35] Gage I, Schnitt SJ, Nixon AJ, et al. Pathologic margin involvement and the risk of recurrence in patients treated with breast-conserving therapy. Cancer. 1996; 78(9):1921–1928

[36] Solin LJ, Fourquet A, Vicini FA, et al. Mammographically detected ductal carcinoma in situ of the breast treated with breast-conserving surgery and definitive breast irradiation: long-term outcome and prognostic significance of patient age and margin status. Int J Radiat Oncol Biol Phys. 2001; 50(4):991–1002

[37] Morrow M, Jagsi R, Alderman AK, et al. Surgeon recommendations and receipt of mastectomy for treatment of breast cancer. JAMA. 2009; 302(14):1551–1556

[38] Waljee JF, Hu ES, Newman LA, Alderman AK. Predictors of re-excision among women undergoing breast-conserving surgery for cancer. Ann Surg Oncol. 2008; 15(5):1297–1303

[39] Isaacs AJ, Gemignani ML, Pusic A, Sedrakyan A. Association of breast conservation surgery for cancer with 90-day reoperation rates in New York State. JAMA Surg. 2016; 151(7):648–655

[40] Chagpar AB, Killelea BK, Tsangaris TN, et al. A randomized, controlled trial of cavity shave margins in breast cancer. N Engl J Med. 2015; 373(6):503–510

[41] Turnbull L, Brown S, Harvey I, et al. Comparative effectiveness of MRI in breast cancer (COMICE) trial: a randomised controlled trial. Lancet. 2010; 375(9714):563–571

[42] Peters NH, van Esser S, van den Bosch MA, et al. Preoperative MRI and surgical management in patients with nonpalpable breast cancer: the MONET - randomised controlled trial. Eur J Cancer. 2011; 47(6):879–886

[43] Grady I, Gorsuch-Rafferty H, Hadley P, Preoperative staging with magnetic resonance imaging, with confirmatory biopsy, improves surgical outcomes in women with breast cancer without increasing rates of mastectomy. Breast J. 2012; 18(3):214–218

[44] Sung JS, Li J, Da Costa G, et al. Preoperative breast MRI for early-stage breast cancer: effect on surgical and long-term outcomes. AJR Am J Roentgenol. 2014; 202(6):1376–1382

[45] Gonzalez V, Sandelin K, Karlsson A, et al. Preoperative MRI of the breast (POMB) influences primary treatment in breast cancer: a prospective, randomized, multicenter study. World J Surg. 2014; 38(7):1685–1693

[46] Fortune-Greeley AK, Wheeler SB, Meyer AM, et al. Preoperative breast MRI and surgical outcomes in elderly women with invasive ductal and lobular carcinoma: a population-based study. Breast Cancer Res Treat. 2014; 143(1):203–212

[47] Mann RM, Loo CE, Wobbes T, et al. The impact of preoperative breast MRI on the re-excision rate in invasive lobular carcinoma of the breast. Breast Cancer Res Treat. 2010; 119(2):415–422

[48] McGhan LJ, Wasif N, Gray RJ, et al. Use of preoperative magnetic resonance imaging for invasive lobular cancer: good, better, but maybe not the best? Ann Surg Oncol. 2010; 17 Suppl 3:255–262

[49] Al-Hallaq HA, Mell LK, Bradley JA, et al. Magnetic resonance imaging identifies multifocal and multicentric disease in breast cancer patients who are eligible for partial breast irradiation. Cancer. 2008; 113(9):2408–2414

[50] Godinez J, Gombos EC, Chikarmane SA, Griffin GK, Birdwell RL. Breast MRI in the evaluation of eligibility for accelerated partial breast irradiation. AJR Am J Roentgenol. 2008; 191(1):272–277

[51] ACRIN American College of Radiology Imaging Network website. Protocol 6694: effect of preoperative breast MRI on surgical outcomes, costs and quality of life in women with breast cancer (Alliance A011104/ACRIN 6694). Available at: www.acrin.org/protocolsummarytable/protocol6694.aspx. Accessed July 25, 2017

[52] Frei KA, Kinkel K, Bonel HM, Lu Y, Esserman LJ, Hylton NM. MR imaging of the breast in patients with positive margins after lumpectomy: influence of the time interval between lumpectomy and MR imaging. AJR Am J Roentgenol. 2000; 175(6):1577–1584

[53] Krammer J, Price ER, Jochelson MS, et al. Breast MR imaging for the assessment of residual disease following initial surgery for breast cancer with positive margins. Eur Radiol. 2017; 27(11):4812–4818

[54] Kinoshita T, Yashiro N, Yoshigi J, Ihara N, Narita M. Fat necrosis of breast: a potential pitfall in breast MRI. Clin Imaging. 2002; 26(4):250–253

[55] Jochelson MS, Lampen-Sachar K, Gibbons G, et al. Do MRI and mammography reliably identify candidates for breast conservation after neoadjuvant chemotherapy? Ann Surg Oncol. 2015; 22(5):1490–1495

[56] Kaufmann M, von Minckwitz G, Bear HD, et al. Recommendations from an international expert panel on the use of neoadjuvant (primary) systemic treatment of operable breast cancer: new perspectives 2006. Ann Oncol. 2007; 18(12):1927–1934

[57] Chen JH, Feig B, Agrawal G, et al. MRI evaluation of pathologically complete response and residual tumors in breast cancer after neoadjuvant chemotherapy. Cancer. 2008; 112(1):17–26

[58] Woodhams R, Kakita S, Hata H, et al. Identification of residual breast carcinoma following neoadjuvant chemotherapy: diffusion-weighted imaging–comparison with contrast-enhanced MR imaging and pathologic findings. Radiology. 2010; 254(2):357–366

[59] Yeh E, Slanetz P, Kopans DB, et al. Prospective comparison of mammography, sonography, and MRI in patients undergoing neoadjuvant chemotherapy for palpable breast cancer. AJR Am J Roentgenol. 2005; 184(3):868–877

[60] Kim TH, Kang DK, Yim H, Jung YS, Kim KS, Kang SY. Magnetic resonance imaging patterns of tumor regression after neoadjuvant chemotherapy in breast cancer patients: correlation with pathological response grading system based on tumor cellularity. J Comput Assist Tomogr. 2012; 36(2):200–206

[61] Scheel JR, Kim E, Partridge SC, et al. ACRIN 6657 trial team and I-SPY investigators network. MRI, clinical examination, and mammography for preoperative assessment of residual disease and pathologic complete response after neoadjuvant chemotherapy for breast cancer: ACRIN 6657 trial. AJR Am J Roentgenol. 2018; 210(6): 1376-1385

[62] Wu LM, Hu JN, Gu HY, Hua J, Chen J, Xu JR. Can diffusion-weighted MR imaging and contrast-enhanced MR imaging precisely evaluate and predict pathological response to neoadjuvant chemotherapy in patients with breast cancer? Breast Cancer Res Treat. 2012; 135(1):17–28

[63] Wapnir IL, Anderson SJ, Mamounas EP, et al. Prognosis after ipsilateral breast tumor recurrence and locoregional recurrences in five National Surgical Adjuvant Breast and Bowel Project node-positive adjuvant breast cancer trials. J Clin Oncol. 2006; 24(13):2028–2037

[64] Anderson SJ, Wapnir I, Dignam JJ, et al. Prognosis after ipsilateral breast tumor recurrence and locoregional recurrences in patients treated by breast-conserving therapy in five National Surgical Adjuvant Breast and Bowel Project protocols of node-negative breast cancer. J Clin Oncol. 2009; 27(15): 2466–2473

[65] Houssami N, Ciatto S, Martinelli F, Bonardi R, Duffy SW. Early detection of second breast cancers improves prognosis in breast cancer survivors. Ann Oncol. 2009; 20(9):1505–1510

[66] Wapnir IL, Dignam JJ, Fisher B, et al. Long-term outcomes of invasive ipsilateral breast tumor recurrences after lumpectomy in NSABP B-17 and B-24 randomized clinical trials for DCIS. J Natl Cancer Inst. 2011; 103(6):478–488

11 Advanced Breast MRI Techniques

Milica Medved

Abstract

In women at high risk for development or recurrence of breast cancer, annual MRI screening is recommended. The current screening protocol relies heavily on information obtained from dynamic contrast-enhanced MRI, utilizing gadolinium-based contrast media (GBCM) which carry some risk. Currently, screening participation in the high-risk population can be as low as 50%, and a significant percentage of women quote use of intravenous GBCM as the main concern. Thus, development of a non-contrast enhanced breast cancer screening MRI protocol would be a significant advancement in breast cancer prevention. We discuss four non-contrast enhanced MRI techniques which hold potential for forming the basis of a screening breast MRI protocol: diffusion weighted imaging (DWI) which provides information on movement of water molecules within tissue; high spectral and spatial resolution (HiSS) MRI which provides information on the spectral structure of the water resonance in small voxels; arterial spin labeling (ASL) which can be used to quantify perfusion; and electrical properties tomography (EPT) which provides information on conductivity and permittivity of tissue. These techniques have been studied in the context of breast lesion characterization, with promising results. They provide lesion information that can be complementary to that obtained from contrast enhanced screening MRI examinations, often improving accuracy, and further technical development may also increase their utility in breast lesion detection. An effective non-contrast screening MRI protocol could be offered in a non-hospital setting, lowering the barriers of cost, risk, and inconvenience.

Keywords: non-contrast magnetic resonance imaging (MRI) breast cancer screening, gadolinium-based contrast media, diffusion-weighted imaging (DWI), high spectral and spatial resolution (HiSS) MRI, arterial spin labeling (ASL), electrical properties tomography (EPT)

11.1 Non–Contrast-Enhanced Breast MRI

In this chapter, we discuss four non–contrast-enhanced breast magnetic resonance imaging (MRI) techniques: diffusion-weighted imaging (DWI), high spectral and spatial resolution (HiSS) MRI, arterial spin labeling (ASL), and electrical properties tomography (EPT). Although none are currently included in the Breast Imaging Reporting and Data System (BIRADS), these techniques have been studied as auxiliary tools for breast lesion characterization, with promising results. They have the potential to provide complementary information on lesions identified on contrast-enhanced screening MRI examinations, which can be used to rule out malignancy and thus increase the accuracy of the examinations. There are additional challenges in breast imaging that these sequences could potentially address. A major advancement would be the development of a non–contrast-enhanced breast cancer screening MRI protocol. Thus, the

techniques discussed here should also be evaluated in the context of lesion detection. The current breast cancer screening MRI protocols are based on dynamic contrast-enhanced MRI (DCE-MRI), which requires the use of gadolinium-based contrast media (GBCM). The use of GBCM comes with established clinical risks and introduces barriers to uptake of MRI screening examinations in the high-risk population. These will be discussed briefly here.

11.2 Risks Inherent to Use of Gadolinium-Based Contrast Media

The rates of immediate adverse reactions to GBCM have been shown to be low, but non-negligible.[1] The adverse reaction rate is variable depending on the contrast agent used, and is generally below 1%.[2] However, it was observed to be as high as 2.4% for gadopentetate dimeglumine (Magnevist®, Bayer Healthcare).[3] The most frequent adverse reactions were nausea and headaches at the time of injection.[2,4,5,6] Less frequently, extravasation of intravenous (IV) contrast can occur during power injection of contrast media, with a reported incidence of 0.1 to 0.9%,[7,8,9] and can cause severe tissue damage, such as compartment syndrome, skin necrosis and ulceration. In addition, serious allergic reactions sometimes occur as a consequence of GBCM administration, including anaphylactic shock[10,11,12,13,14,15,16,17,18] which can result in death.[17] The occurrence of such allergic reactions to GBCM is unpredictable. However, it is known that individuals with a history of allergies, such as food or other medication allergies, and those with features of atopy, such as asthma, dermatitis, and urticaria, are at higher risk.[15,19]

Nephrogenic systemic fibrosis (NSF) is a rare but serious adverse reaction to GBCM that typically occurs within days to months following administration.[20,21] Early symptoms and signs include skin discoloration, swelling, and pain. Later, skin and subcutaneous sclerosis, induration, inflexibility, hair loss, shiny skin surface, brownish discoloration, and skin thickening can occur. The skin thickening can lead to reduced joint movement and flexion contractures of the limbs, resulting in significant disability.[21] Although initially introduced to clinical practice as a safer alternative to iodine-based contrast agents for patients with compromised kidney function, in 2006 GBCMs were recognized as a trigger for NSF in this population.[20,21] Consequently, guidelines for administration of GBCM were introduced by the Food and Drug Administration (FDA), the European Society of Urogenital Radiology, and the American College of Radiology, with all three organizations recommending patient screening for chronic kidney disease and acute renal failure, as well as transition to low-risk GBCM.[22] Published studies from several academic medical centers indicated that no new NSF cases have been reported following the implementation of these guidelines.[20] However, as the risk cannot be absolutely excluded, NSF is still a deterrent to some women who would otherwise have considered a screening breast MRI.[23]

Beginning in 2014, anecdotal evidence of long-term gadolinium (Gd) accumulation in the dentate nucleus (DN) and globus

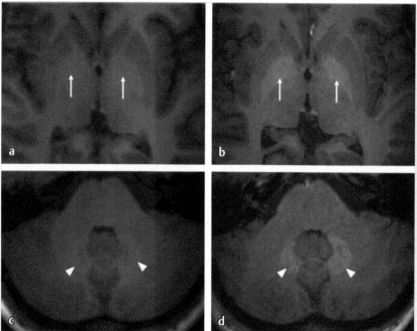

Fig. 11.1 Gadolinium deposition in deep brain structures is illustrated. Axial non-enhanced T1-weighted MR images of the basal ganglia (**a,b**) and cerebellum (**c,d**) from a patient with numerous prior MRIs performed with GBCM demonstrate bilateral intrinsic T1 hyperintensity of the globus pallidus (**b**, *arrows*) and the dentate nucleus (**d**, *arrowheads*). On a brain MRI exam from several years earlier (**a, c**), these same structures were not intrinsically T1 hyperintense. Overall, these findings are consistent with Gd deposition from repeated GBCM exposure. The globus pallidus and dentate nucleus are two of the most common sites in the brain to be affected by gadolinium deposition. (Reproduced with permission from Fraum et al.[22])

pallidus (GP) in patients with normal renal function began to be reported in literature.[24,25] Retrospective studies conducted since continued to demonstrate this effect,[26,27,28] and have included histological confirmation.[29] The Gd deposition can be evidenced as hyperintensity of the DN or GP on unenhanced T1-weighted MRI images (▶ Fig. 11.1).[22] The dependence of Gd deposition on the type of GBCM is established and consistent with known data on GBCM stability.[26,27,28] An in vitro study established that after a 15-day incubation period, the release rate of linear nonionic GBCMs was 20 to 21%, in contrast to 1.1 to 1.9% for linear ionic GBCMs, and under 0.1% for macrocyclic GBCMs.[30] To put these findings in perspective, there have been no unequivocal reports of clinical symptomatology due to Gd deposition in the brain or elsewhere in the body. However, caution is warranted. The U.S. FDA currently recommends that the need for GBCM be assessed and the minimum effective dose be used, and that use of a macrocyclic GBCM, rather than a linear agent be considered.[31] As of May 2018, the FDA additionally requires that all MRI centers provide a Medication Guide the first time an outpatient is administered any GBCM.[32] The European Medicines Agency has restricted the use or suspended the authorization of most linear GBCM since July 2017.[33]

11.3 Underutilization of Screening Breast MRI in High-Risk Women

The American Cancer Society currently recommends that women who are at high risk for breast cancer (20–25% lifetime risk or higher) undergo annual breast MRI exams in addition to annual screening mammograms.[34] While the use of breast MRI has increased approximately 18-fold between 2000 and 2011—to 105 per 10,000 women[35]—in a sample of women enrolled in two non-profit health insurance plans, several studies have found that utilization among women at high risk is low.[35,36,37] In a study by Stout et al that quantified this utilization, it was

Table 11.1 The distribution of self-reported primary reasons for declining a screening MRI examination in the cohort of women accrued to the ACRIN 6666 study[23] (data from study)

Primary reason for screening MRI refusal	
Claustrophobia	25.4%
Time constraints and/or other priorities	18.2%
Physician would not provide referral or did not believe MR was indicated	9.2%
Patient not interested or did not want to participate	7.8%
Patient had contraindications for MRI examinations	7.6%
Patient did not want to undergo IV injection	5.7%
Patient concerned about additional biopsies and testing that MRI may indicate	5.3%
MRI scheduling constraints	4.1%
Travel-related concerns	2.2%
Gadolinium intolerance or fear of reaction, including nephrogenic systemic fibrosis	1.4%
Unknown	1.2%

found to be as low as 50%,[35] and in a study by Berg et al, only 58% of high-risk women who were offered an MRI screening examination agreed to participate.[23] Berg et al examined the data acquired as part of the MRI sub-study of the ACRIN 6666 trial on screening breast ultrasound in women with high breast cancer risk, and compiled a list of primary reasons why these women declined to undergo screening MRI examinations (▶ Table 11.1).[23] While the most frequent reason for screening MRI refusal was claustrophobia, a significant percentage of women (7.1%) quoted use of intra-venous (IV) GBCM as the main concern. In addition, the 7.6% of women who had contraindications for an MRI exam included women who were contraindicated for GBCM use because of lack of IV access and/or impaired kidney function. A further 24.5% cited time, scheduling, and travel constraints—basically, inconvenience—as the primary reason. Other issues, such as concern about unnecessary follow-up procedures for lesions that will ultimately be found to be benign and inaccurate perception of risk[38] were also recorded.

If the low MRI screening participation rate in the high-risk group increased, this group would reap great benefits via reduction in mortality and morbidity. Obviously, women who cited GBCM use as their primary concern would benefit immediately from a non–contrast-enhanced screening MRI protocol. In addition, such a protocol would also reduce the barriers of cost and inconvenience. By forgoing the use of a contrast agent, several current components of the breast MRI examinations would be eliminated: establishing IV access, administration of GBCM, kidney function screening and testing, need for medical supervision, and need for access to emergency procedures in case of a serious reaction. These changes would significantly lower the cost and allow screening breast MRI examinations to be offered in a nonmedical setting. Today, screening X-ray mammography is often offered in shopping malls. By utilizing noncontrast protocol and teleradiology, a similar approach could be applied to screening breast MRIs. This would go a long way toward overcoming the inconvenience barrier to access by reducing travel times and allowing easier scheduling. The lower cost would also figure in more general cost-benefit analyses, possibly enlarging the pool of women who would be offered and could benefit from MRI screening.

11.4 Diffusion-Weighted Imaging

11.4.1 Introduction to Diffusion-Weighted Imaging

The first applications of diffusion-weighted imaging (DWI) came in the 1990s, in the differential diagnosis of ischemic versus hemorrhagic acute stroke. It has since been used for a variety of brain disorders, primarily white matter disorders, as well as for monitoring therapy response in brain tumors. The first applications in cancer imaging outside the brain came in the early 2000s,[39,40,41,42] and included early breast cancer imaging.[43,44,45,46,47,48] Today, DWI is well established as a breast MR imaging technique, particularly as a lesion diagnostic tool, but also for cancer imaging in general.[49]

Diffusion is displacement due to random brownian motion of a particle within a volume, such as a water molecule within an imaging voxel. In tissue, diffusion occurs within and across various water compartments, such as intra- and extracellular compartments. In the intracellular compartment, diffusion is restricted, as water molecules diffuse across cell membranes into the extracellular compartment relatively slowly and are thus effectively trapped within cells on the timescales relevant to DWI. In the extracellular compartment, diffusion is hindered —not restricted, but still slower than free diffusion—as water molecules navigate proteins and other macromolecules present in this compartment, as well as boundaries of cells that reduce the available volume and give it an irregular shape. Thus, DWI can yield information on properties and relative volume of different water compartments.

Although there is no undisputed consensus on the appropriate biophysical interpretation of in vivo quantitative measures

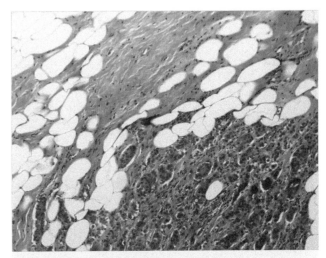

Fig. 11.2 This pathology slide section shows an invasive ductal carcinoma (grade II/III, *bottom right*), adjacent to normal stroma (*top left*). Dark purple spots represent cell nuclei, which are sparse in normal stroma (*pink*). In carcinoma, stroma is invaded by invasive cancer with high cellularity, which is evident from the higher concentration of nuclei and thus darker overall staining.

of water diffusion, an intuitive model describing restricted intracellular diffusion coupled with hindered extracellular diffusion is often accepted.[49] Because the restricted-diffusion intracellular signal contributes little to the overall diffusion-induced signal loss, DWI is primarily sensitive to extracellular diffusion. A reduced rate of extracellular diffusion is generally interpreted as a sign of a reduced extracellular volume, which may be due to higher cellularity—a hallmark of cancerous lesions, as illustrated in ▶ Fig. 11.2. The diffusion rate has an inverse relationship with cellularity, and thus with tumor grade, and DWI has emerged as a useful tool for cancer detection or lesion characterization.

DWI Pulse Sequence

Today, DWI is most frequently implemented as a spin-echo echo-planar imaging (SE-EPI) sequence. We will review here the elements of the SE sequence, the adaptation of the SE sequence for diffusion weighting, and finally the inclusion of the EPI component for acceleration of imaging. The SE sequence (▶ Fig. 11.3, *top*) excites spins into the transverse plane using a 90° pulse and, after spins have dephased due to local gradients over time TE/2, an 180° pulse is applied. The 180° pulse causes spins to regain phase coherence under unchanged local gradients, until an echo is formed at TE. In DWI, an additional strong linear diffusion-encoding gradient G_{diff} is used to additionally dephase the spins during the time to TE/2 (▶ Fig. 11.3, *middle*). After the 180° RF pulse, a second diffusion gradient pulse G_{diff} is applied, matched in intensity and polarity to the first. The net phase change due to application of the two diffusion-encoding gradients is zero for spins that have not changed position along the diffusion-encoding direction. For spins that have drifted over time Δ, the net phase change is non-zero and is dependent on the displacement along the diffusion-encoding direction. This results in a residual dephasing due to the

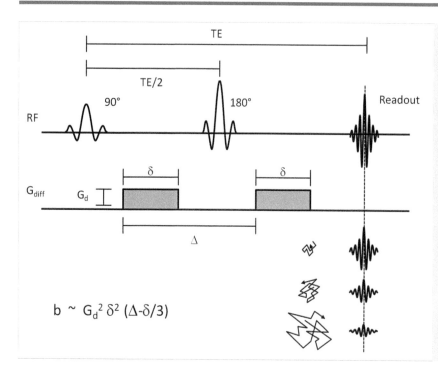

$$b \sim G_d^2\, \delta^2\, (\Delta\text{-}\delta/3)$$

Fig. 11.3 A basic diagram of a spin-echo diffusion-weighted pulse sequence is shown. The two diffusion encoding gradients (G_{diff}) are matched and with same polarity. Diffusion-induced displacement of water molecules causes residual dephasing at TE and loss of MRI signal. In clinical applications, the spin-echo echo-planar imaging (SE-EPI) sequence is used to implement DWI.

random diffusive motion of the water molecules and a reduction in the measured signal (▶ Fig. 11.3, *bottom*). The amount of diffusion encoding is quantified via parameter b, which is proportional to $G_d^2\delta^2(\Delta - \delta/3)$ and expressed in s/mm². Stronger diffusion encoding b and higher diffusion rate (D) lead to higher residual dephasing at TE and thus lower DWI signal. In the simplest model, DWI signal decays exponentially with b, with a decay constant D:

$$S_{DWI} = S_{SE}e^{-Db} \sim (1 - e^{-TR/T1})e^{-TE/T2}e^{-Db} \qquad (11.1)$$

where S_{DWI} is the MRI signal of the diffusion-weighted sequence, S_{SE} is the signal of the spin-echo sequence on which the diffusion-weighted sequence is based, T1 and T2 are the longitudinal and transverse relaxation constants in the given voxel, and TR and TE are the sequence repetition and echo times. As evidenced in equation (11.1), in addition to the exponential decay with b, S_{DWI} also decays exponentially with TE. In clinical DWI, the shortest possible TE is typically selected to maximize signal-to-noise ratio (SNR). However, there is evidence that the observed diffusion decay constant can vary with TE, with longer TE values yielding better diagnostic performance.[50]

To allow fast DWI, the SE sequence is modified so that an EPI echo train, centered around TE, is acquired. The use of the SE-EPI sequence makes DWI susceptible to artifacts generally associated with EPI, such as blurring and spatial distortion. Decreasing effective interecho spacing by increasing bandwidth results in less chemical shift artifact and less image distortion.[51] Parallel imaging can achieve a similar effect and shorten the echo train to reduce artifacts and spatial distortion, but there is an increase in noise that is nonlinear and spatially inhomogeneous.[51,52] Partial Fourier imaging is commonly applied to shorten the EPI echo train, though with an SNR penalty. Shortening the echo train using alternative

k-space filling trajectories, such as in segmented EPI, results in lower artifact level but increased acquisition times.[52] Thus, imaging parameters should be optimized to achieve balance between artifact levels, SNR, and imaging times. Partridge and McDonald provide an excellent review of protocol optimization considerations.[53] ▶ Table 11.2 shows DWI sequence parameters currently used for breast MRI at the University of Chicago Medical Center, at 1.5 and 3 T.

Table 11.2 DWI sequence parameters currently used at the University of Chicago Medical Center.

	1.5T	3.0T
Pulse sequence	SE-EPI	SE-EPI
orientation	Axial	Axial
Field of view	300 × 300 × 200 mm³	300 × 300 × 200 mm³
Spatial resolution	2.5 × 2.5 × 2.5 mm³	2 × 2 × 2.5 mm³
Rest slab	No	Over heart
TR / TE	15000 / 63 ms	13000 / 64 ms
EPI echo train length	43, single shot	53, single shot
Fat suppression / inversion delay	SPAIR / 90 ms	SPAIR / 70 ms
Fat-water separation / Bandwidth	6.4 pix / 34.1 Hz	15.8 pix / 27 Hz
Partial Fourier factor	0.62	0.62
b values (number of acquisitions)	0 (1), 50 (1), 800 (2)	0 (1), 50 (1), 800 (2)
Number of averages	2	2
Coil	16 channel dedicated breast coil	16 channel dedicated breast coil
SENSE	3 in RL direction	3 in RL direction
Acquisition Time	5'14"	4'33"

Technical Considerations

The diagnostic value of high b-value images ($b > \sim 500\,\text{s/mm}^2$) is derived from the fact that cancer lesions appear very bright due to hindered diffusion in the tissue. However, voxels with high T2 values have intrinsically high signal compared to the background, which propagates to the high b-value DW image and mimics the appearance of cancer (► Fig. 11.4). This effect is called "T2 shine-through" and can lower the diagnostic value of the DW images. In order to differentiate high T2 tissue from cancer, DW signal dependence on b is modeled quantitatively to eliminate T2 contrast—i.e., D is calculated (see equation 11.1). As "D" is commonly used to represent free water diffusivity, in tissue this constant is instead termed "apparent diffusion coefficient", or ADC. ADC is a quantitative measure of overall diffusive motion in the tissue and is lower in regions with higher cellularity, such as cancer.[54] In principle, ADC can be calculated from signal intensity acquired at $b = 0\,\text{s/mm}^2$ and one higher b value, typically in the 800 to 1,500 s/mm² range:

$$ADC = -\frac{1}{b(>0)}\ln\left(\frac{S_{b(>0)}}{S_{b(=0)}}\right) \qquad (11.2)$$

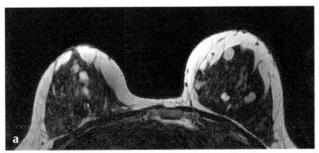
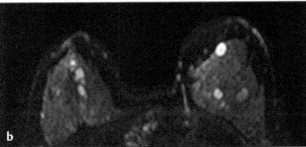
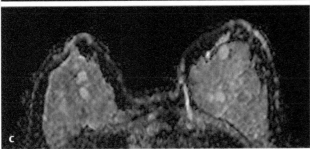

Fig. 11.4 T2-weighted image (**a**), DW image at $b = 800\,\text{s/mm}^2$ (**b**), and the ADC map (**c**), acquired at 3 T, are shown for a 38-year-old patient with benign findings and multiple cysts (isointense with fat on T2-weighted image). Due to the "T2 shine-through" effect, the cysts are strongly hyperintense relative to parenchyma in the $b = 800\,\text{s/mm}^2$ image, mimicking appearance of cancer. The ADC map shows that their ADC values are higher, rather than lower, than those of the surrounding parenchyma, excluding cancer and providing an image with a higher diagnostic utility.

where $S_{b=0}$ and $S_{b>0}$ represent DWI signal measured at $b = 0\,\text{s/mm}^2$ and at some higher b value, respectively.

With equation (11.2), the question of choosing the optimum $b > 0\,\text{s/mm}^2$ value is introduced. When a single high b value DW image is acquired, there is an obvious tradeoff between SNR of the image, and accuracy of the ADC calculation—higher b values improve estimation of ADC, but the resulting SNR penalty degrades it. Additionally, there is a tradeoff between SNR (higher at low b values) and contrast-to-noise ratio (CNR, higher at high b values) in $b > 0\,\text{s/mm}^2$ images, because accurate outlining of the lesion is necessary for accurate measurement of ADC. To improve SNR, manufacturers often provide options to acquire high b value images with a higher number of averages than those at $b = 0\,\text{s/mm}^2$.

Additionally, the decay of the DWI signal with b is often not mono-exponential, and thus ADC, as calculated from equation (11.2), can be dependent on the choice of the high b value (► Fig. 11.5). Microperfusion is well accepted as a source of incoherent motion and hence of signal loss at very low b values (up to $\sim 100\,\text{s/mm}^2$). In fact, the fast decay of DWI signal at low b values has been studied as a method for noncontrast quantification of tissue perfusion via intra-voxel incoherent motion (IVIM) modeling.[55,56,57] Microperfusion is thought to be negligible in breast parenchyma[58,59] but is obviously of significance in tumors.[60] To exclude perfusion effects and eliminate the dependence of ADC on the single high b value selection, DWI is now commonly acquired with multiple b values, and only b values larger than about 50 to 100 s/mm² are used to calculate ADC via an exponential fit.

Uniform fat suppression is crucial for reduction of artifacts, and modern scanners with dual and multiple transmit coils can achieve high-quality fat suppression. Fat suppression implementation in DWI varies by manufacturer, but generally relies on a spectrally selective fat suppression (90°) or inversion (180°) RF pulse. Spectrally selective excitation performs better at 3 T, due to the better spectral separation of water and fat peaks, and thus better fat suppression can be achieved at 3 T. Proper positioning of breast MRI patients to avoid tissue folds can minimize local susceptibility differences and B0 gradients that degrade fat suppression and is thus very important.

Gd-based contrast agents act to shorten the T2 to some extent in the extracellular space, but not in the intracellular space, potentially compromising ADC measurements. Currently, DWI is typically acquired after the DCE-MRI sequence, to avoid patient fatigue and resulting motion artifacts in the DCE-MRI sequence. However, the differences in dose and timing of the contrast relative to the DWI acquisition introduce variability that is difficult to control or predict. To achieve standardization and improve quantitative interpretation of DWI, precontrast imaging is preferable.

A recent study introduced the concept of synthetic DWI, which uses ADC and T2 maps to eliminate T2 shine-through and extrapolate signal from a lower b (e.g., $b \leq 800\,\text{s/mm}^2$) DW image to generate a higher b (e.g., $b = 1,000\,\text{s/mm}^2$) DW image.[61] This approach seems intuitively beneficial: it uses high SNR images to generate high CNR images with presumably higher diagnostic utility. However, image contrast at very high b values can be intrinsically different from that at lower b values. Even after perfusion effects are taken into account, the pure diffusion signal decay is itself not monoexponential, due to the presence

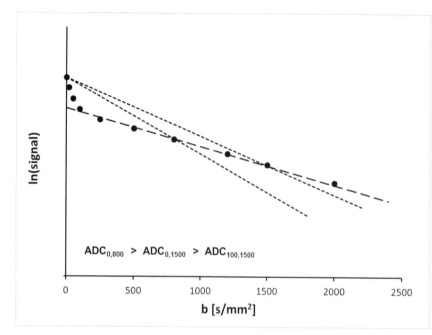

Fig. 11.5 DWI signal as a function of *b* value for a hypothetical voxel with measurable microperfusion is shown on a logarithmic scale (*solid circles*). Exponential fits using two different high *b* values are shown (*dotted lines*), demonstrating the ADC dependence on the b value used to acquire DWI data. A lower ADC value (negative slope on the logarithmic scale) is calculated for a DW dataset acquired using $b = 0$, 1,500 s/mm², as compared to that using $b = 0$, 800 s/mm². An exponential fit could also be performed using only $b \geq 100$ s/mm² values (*dashed line*). The ADC value thus calculated is lower still, as it excludes perfusion effects and more closely represents the true rate of diffusion in the tissue.

$$ADC_{0,800} > ADC_{0,1500} > ADC_{100,1500}$$

In(signal)

b [s/mm²]

of multiple water compartments in the tissue. Thus, synthetic DW images obtained via extrapolation from lower *b* values should be clearly identified and distinguished from DW images that were truly acquired at a very high *b* value. The authors of the study do stress this point in the discussion and use short extrapolation ranges where contrast is unlikely to change significantly. However, as this technique gains acceptance and surely becomes used for ever farther extrapolation, it is important to keep this distinction in mind.

Currently, the main limitation of DWI is the low resolution necessary to achieve clinically realistic imaging times. This is relevant when non-mass lesions suffer from partial volume ADC dilution, and higher resolution DWI would allow their better characterization. In addition, calculating an ADC map from a fixed optimal TE value and fixed optimal $b \geq 100$ s/mm² values, as well as precontrast acquisition of DW images, would allow for standardization of ADC measurement and a more confident use of ADC values for lesion diagnostics. This would aid ongoing work on DWI standardization in acquisition and postprocessing methods.[62,63,64,65] As of today, BIRADS mainly relies on the description of T1-weighted, contrast-enhanced MR images. Standardization would allow future inclusion of DWI characteristics in BIRADS description of breast lesions.

Characteristics of Normal Fibroglandular Tissue

▶ Fig. 11.6 shows DWI images and ADC maps of two patients with negative findings, acquired at 1.5 and 3.0 T. Several studies have attempted to describe the range of ADC values of normal parenchymal tissue and the variations due to physiological factors.[66,67,68,69,70,71] Of most importance is the variation during the menstrual cycle, though variation due to lactation and menopausal status were also examined. There is a nonsignificant trend toward lower values and thus presumably lower contrast with cancerous lesions during week 2 of the menstrual cycle,[71] but these changes are likely too small to affect the

utility of DWI.[69,72] Although large variations are observed with age or menopausal status,[68,73] and lactation,[74] where DWI may improve clinical utility over DCE-MRI alone, overall, the range of ADC values in normal parenchyma remains above that of cancerous lesions. Therefore, DWI can be expected to be diagnostically useful at any age or time during the menstrual cycle.[72] Reported mean ADC values in normal breast parenchyma range from 1.51 to 2.09×10^{-3} mm²/s.[53]

Characterization of Breast Lesions

The clinical utility of DWI is derived from the fact that ADC values in cancerous lesions are lower than those in benign lesions and normal fibroglandular tissue. ▶ Fig. 11.7 and ▶ Fig. 11.8 show examples of a benign (fibroadenoma) and a cancerous (IDC grade III) lesion, in DW images and ADC maps. Similarly, ▶ Fig. 11.9 illustrates DWI of multiple metastatic axillary lymph nodes. A 2010 meta-analysis, which included 13 studies and 964 total lesions, demonstrated pooled sensitivity of 84% (95% confidence interval [CI] 0.82, 0.87) and specificity of 79% (95% CI 0.75, 0.82) for DWI.[75] In reports included in this study, the mean ADC of malignant lesions ranged from 0.87 to 1.36 10^3 mm²/s, with the recommended cutoffs ranging from 0.90 to 1.76×10^3 mm²/s.[75] A different meta-analysis study, which included 12 publications, recommended a threshold for malignancy of 1.23×10^{-3} mm²/s.[76] While the diagnostic utility of DWI is high in each individual study, the wide ranges of cancer ADC and recommended cutoff values illustrate the significant variability of ADC measurements with sequence parameters and physiologic changes. This variability underscores the need for standardization of breast DWI, including prescribing fixed optimal *b* values to acquire DW images. For greater reproducibility, care must be taken to ensure that areas of necrosis or hemorrhage are avoided. Normalization of lesion ADC to that of ipsilateral normal parenchyma can be helpful.[77]

While the ADC of cancer is in general lower than that of benign lesions, there are numerous exceptions to this rule. For

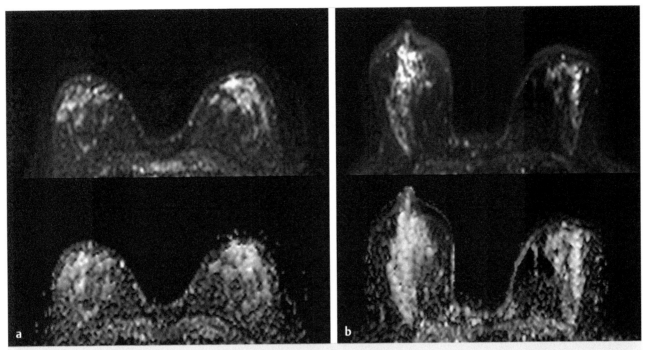

Fig. 11.6 Normal breast parenchyma from two subjects with negative findings is shown in $b = 800$ s/mm^2 DW images top, and ADC maps bottom. The images on the left (a) were acquired at 1.5 T and the images on the right (b) at 3.0 T. The $b = 800$ s/mm^2 images show a wide range of signal intensity in the parenchyma, while the signal in the ADC maps, calculated to eliminate T2 contrast, is more uniform.

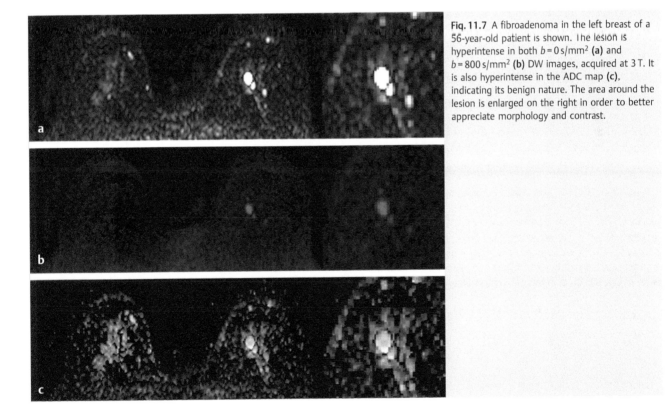

Fig. 11.7 A fibroadenoma in the left breast of a 56-year-old patient is shown. The lesion is hyperintense in both $b = 0$ s/mm^2 (a) and $b = 800$ s/mm^2 (b) DW images, acquired at 3 T. It is also hyperintense in the ADC map (c), indicating its benign nature. The area around the lesion is enlarged on the right in order to better appreciate morphology and contrast.

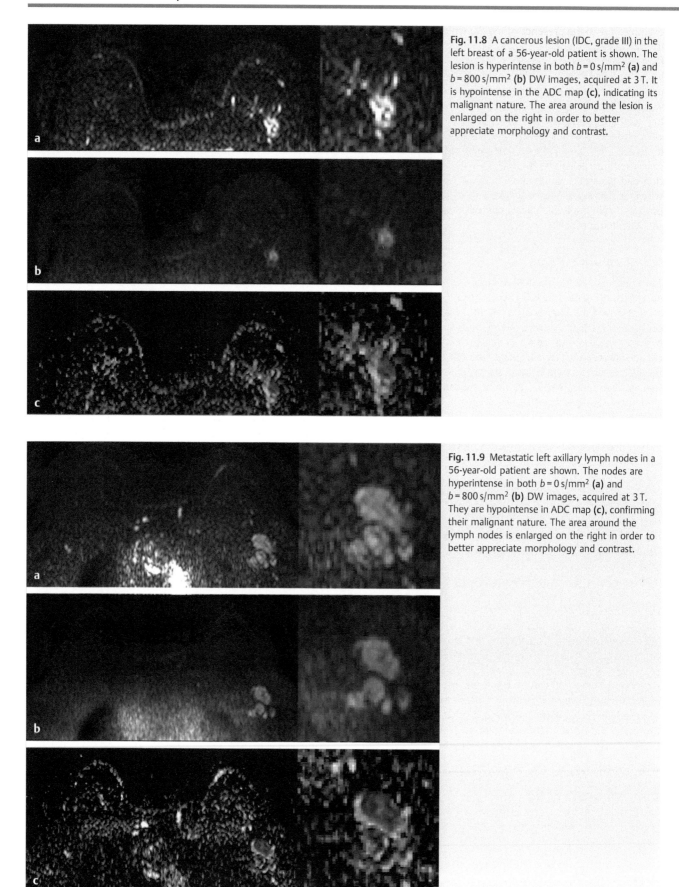

Fig. 11.8 A cancerous lesion (IDC, grade III) in the left breast of a 56-year-old patient is shown. The lesion is hyperintense in both $b = 0\,s/mm^2$ **(a)** and $b = 800\,s/mm^2$ **(b)** DW images, acquired at 3 T. It is hypointense in the ADC map **(c)**, indicating its malignant nature. The area around the lesion is enlarged on the right in order to better appreciate morphology and contrast.

Fig. 11.9 Metastatic left axillary lymph nodes in a 56-year-old patient are shown. The nodes are hyperintense in both $b = 0\,s/mm^2$ **(a)** and $b = 800\,s/mm^2$ **(b)** DW images, acquired at 3 T. They are hypointense in ADC map **(c)**, confirming their malignant nature. The area around the lymph nodes is enlarged on the right in order to better appreciate morphology and contrast.

example, due to the presence of mucin, which has low cellularity, mucinous carcinoma displays ADC values that can be higher than those of benign lesions.[78] On the other hand, benign papillomas[79] as well as high risk lesions[80] can present with ADC values as low or lower than those found in cancer. In addition, ADC values of ductal carcinoma in situ (DCIS) are intermediate and have significant overlap with both benign and malignant ADC value ranges.[79,81] Thus, despite generally high diagnostic performance, DWI does suffer to a degree from low specificity for cancer and low sensitivity to DCIS. Other MRI-derived information and physical examination findings should be considered when diagnosing a breast lesion. For an excellent review of practices and pitfalls in clinical application of DWI of the breast, see Woodhams et al.[51]

Other Applications

The cytotoxic effects of chemotherapeutic agents include cell apoptosis, necrosis, and cell lysis. As cell membranes deteriorate and become increasingly more permeable during the course of the treatment, the rate of exchange across cell membranes increases and hence water mobility increases. These changes precede tumor shrinkage and are directly observable by DWI, leading to the hypothesis that DWI can be used as a tool for evaluating early treatment response to neoadjuvant chemotherapy. Specifically, several studies have explored the hypothesis that an early increase in ADC value will predict favorable treatment response, with promising results.[82,83,84,85] In addition, low ADC values were explored as a pretreatment predictive marker of positive response, also with promising results.[84,86,87,88]

A study that included 70 excised cancerous lesions assessed breast DWI as a tool for detection of residual tumors and found that it demonstrated the same accuracy as DCE-MRI.[89] As DWI detected residual cancers that DCE-MRI did not, DWI could potentially be used to increase diagnostic accuracy of MRI for residual tumor evaluation.

Given the recent concerns about Gd deposition in tissues and its unclear clinical consequences,[26,27,28] there is an increasing interest in effective noncontrast breast cancer screening protocols. Multiple studies have assessed DWI as a noncontrast MR screening tool, usually in combination with a T2-weighted sequence.[90,91,92,93,94,95] Compared to mammography, such protocols perform better, though not as well as DCE-MRI-based protocols.[95] However, in combination with mammography, excellent cancer detection rates can be achieved, with receiver operating characteristic area under the curve (ROC AUC) values as high as 0.96.[92]

11.5 High Spectral and Spatial Resolution MRI

11.5.1 Introduction to High Spectral and Spatial Resolution MRI

A number of MR spectroscopic imaging methods were originally used for measurement of low concentrations of metabolites,[96,97,98,99,100,101,102] but in the early 1990s these methods were adapted for high spectral and spatial resolution (HiSS)

anatomic and functional imaging,[103] and new methods for analyzing and interpreting water and fat spectra were developed.[104,105,106,107,108] Initially tested for neuroimaging,[109] it was first applied to breast in the early 2000s, and has since advanced to producing images of high diagnostic utility.[110,111, 112,113] In conventional spectroscopic imaging, spectral peaks of metabolites are of primary interest and voxel sizes on the order of 1 cm^3 are used to achieve practical SNRs. In HiSS MRI, on the other hand, the water proton resonance and its structure are of primary interest, and fat resonance can be characterized as well. Voxel size in HiSS MRI of the human breast is generally on the order of ~1 mm^3, although higher spatial resolution has been demonstrated.

Even in small tissue voxels (~1 mm^3), where macroscopic B0 gradients can be assumed to be weak and linear, the water resonance can present as non-Lorentzian. This can be a result of the presence of multiple water compartments within the voxel, as well as of line broadening due to susceptibility gradients caused by the presence of deoxyhemoglobin or hemosiderin, microcalcifications, local microanatomy, or tissue boundaries. As cancerous lesions show greater inhomogeneity than normal breast tissue, it can be hypothesized that non-Lorentzian line shapes will be more pronounced there, and this has been observed.[111,112,114,115,116] Often, multiple spectral components can be clearly and reproducibly resolved, yielding information on subvoxel compartments.[114] Signals from these compartments were demonstrated to respond differently to injected contrast agents[104,108,117] (▶ Fig. 11.10) or changes in blood oxygenation levels.[117] Such sub-voxel information cannot be obtained via conventional imaging, and thus HiSS can be considered a form of functional MR imaging. The spectral information in HiSS datasets can be used to provide a wide array of images carrying different physiological information,[104,108,114, 115,118,119] and postprocessing methods are an ongoing area of research.

11.5.2 Acquisition and Postprocessing

HiSS imaging is usually implemented as a high spatial resolution 2D multislice echo-planar spectroscopic imaging (EPSI)[96,97] sequence, though a multiple gradient echo sequence can also be used. In either case, slices are acquired sequentially, and for each slice a series of MR images are acquired over a number of distinct time points, or echo times. This means that for a given slice, each k-space line is acquired at all echo times in a single RF excitation. A variable phase-encoding gradient determines the k-space line to be acquired at each RF excitation. At the end of a single-slice acquisition, a 3D k-space matrix is populated as a time series of 2D k-space matrices, each corresponding to a specific echo time. Although multiecho gradient echo and sometimes EPSI sequences are commercially available, at this time they are not implemented adequately for HiSS imaging. Instead, HiSS MRI has been implemented as a patch on Philips, GE, and Siemens scanner consoles. It is reasonable to expect that in the future clinically available sequences may be adequate for HiSS MRI applications.

Performing a Fourier transform in 2D k-spaces corresponding to each echo time, time-dependent MR images of a slice are reconstructed, and the evolution over time of the MR signal in each voxel can be observed. This initial 2D reconstruction can

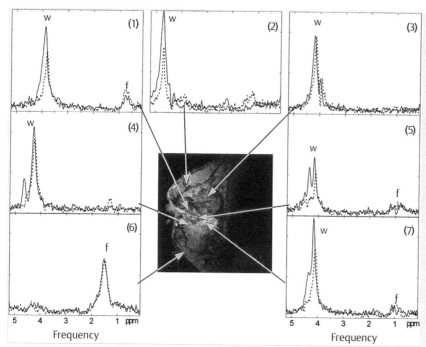

Fig. 11.10 Representative spectra from selected voxels before (*dotted lines*) and after (*solid lines*) contrast medium injection illustrate its selective effect on different water resonance components. The reference image shows a sagittal section through a breast with ductal carcinoma (sampled with spectra 1, 4, 5, and 7). All spectra are on the same scale and referenced to the same carrier frequency and the water (w) and fat (f) peaks are labeled. Spectra in some voxels (3 and 6) show minimal changes after contrast media injection, indicating that effects of inter-image motion have been minimized. (Reproduced with permission from Du et al.[105])

be combined with accelerated imaging (e.g., sensitivity encoding, or SENSE)[120] and is handled by the imaging console at the time of the scan. In MR imaging, both the k-space and the reconstructed images are matrices of complex values, but conventionally only magnitude MR images are shown and stored. When full complex information is retained, a further Fourier transform in the temporal direction can be applied, with some corrections, to yield the proton spectrum in each voxel. This and subsequent postprocessing described below are not currently performed on the scanner console, though research options allow installation of custom postprocessing algorithms on consoles.

Further postprocessing steps that are used to extract information from the proton spectra and produce a varied array of HiSS-derived images are detailed in multiple publications.[104, 105,108,114,115,119,121] In the first step, water and fat peaks are identified based on their spectral location and separation[119] and modeled as Lorentzian peaks (i.e., fit with modulus Lorentzian functions). This allows removal of the baseline and fat signal and isolation of the water resonance signal. From such "pure" water signal, the structure of the water resonance can be explored, and a large variety of HiSS-derived images can be generated. Most frequently used is the HiSS water peak height image, for anatomical imaging. Other types used for morphological imaging include water peak integral and fat peak height and integral images. ▶ Fig. 11.11 displays axial water peak height and integral images showing a cancerous lesion and compares them on SNR and internal contrast within the lesion. Additional HiSS-derived images can be generated to capture a variety of functional information. These include T2* and B0,[118] as well as water peak asymmetry,[122] Fourier component (FC) images (maps of water resonance amplitude at multiple frequency bins),[114,115] main off-peak component (OPC) frequency offset and amplitude,[111,112] and other measures of water

resonance broadening, such as those derived from dispersion/absorption analysis.[116]

Advantages

In HiSS MRI, almost complete removal of the fat signal can be achieved in postprocessing, without use of additional RF pulses. This produces effective fat suppression that is often superior to that of conventional imaging (▶ Fig. 11.12),[119,123] as well as images that can be interpreted more quantitatively, e.g., for breast density measurement. The advantage of HiSS MRI over conventional fat suppression methods is two-fold. First, additional RF fat saturation or inversion pulses can partially suppress the water resonance, and magnetization transfer effects can further reduce the water signal. Such effects are variable and difficult to model, which presents challenges for quantitative image analysis, but are avoided in HiSS MRI. Second, spectrally selective RF pulses used for fat suppression are sensitive to B0 inhomogeneities, leading to variation in the degree of fat suppression across the breast, whereas HiSS spectral postprocessing takes B0 variation into account. Finally, current advanced methods such as Dixon,[124,125] and therefrom derived IDEAL,[126] use spectral modeling of one or multiple lipid peaks with fixed T2* values, which can produce inaccuracies in fat and water separation. This can potentially pose problems for quantitative imaging. In HiSS imaging, full spectral information is used, and T2* of both water and fat are taken into account, while neither is treated as a fixed parameter. In addition, HiSS MR imaging retains the full fat signal with spectroscopic information, whose distribution and spectral characteristics can be analyzed and potentially augment the diagnostic information or breast cancer risk assessment.[127,128]

In conventional imaging, the integral of the broadened water resonance is used to generate images, which can cause the

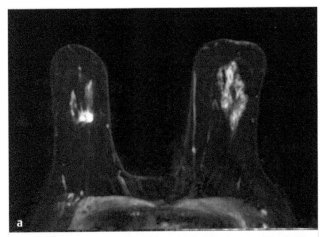

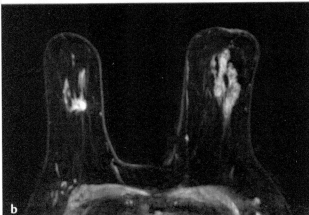

Fig. 11.11 HiSS water peak height (a) and HiSS water peak integral (b) images of an axial slice through the breasts of a 73-year-old woman are shown. While the water peak integral image shows higher signal-to-noise ratio and lower artifact level water peak height image shows better contrast and internal structure definition in the parenchyma and in the IDC lesion in central right breast.

signal to partially bleed into neighboring pixels and cause blurring. Thus the ability to resolve individual FCs (frequencies) within the water resonance results in sharper images. For example, when the amplitude of the water peak frequency is resolved and selectively displayed, there is less blurring at tissue boundaries and image quality is improved.[119] Further, the high spectral resolution allows description of new types of MRI contrast based on the water resonance structure, which constitute forms of functional imaging. B0,[118] peak asymmetry,[122] FC amplitudes,[114,115] frequency offset and amplitude of the strongest off-peak (different from main) component,[111,112] and measures of water resonance broadening derived from dispersion/absorption analysis[116] have been explored for enhancing diagnostic performance. Additionally, spectral information allows advanced lesion and parenchymal texture analysis, resulting in lesion discrimination performance that is comparable or higher than that of DCE-MRI, even in non–contrast-enhanced HiSS MRI.[113] HiSS images are also very sensitive to the local magnetic field and allow accurate B0 mapping, which can accentuate morphology of the lesion margin, as illustrated in ▶ Fig. 11.13.[118] Even when the structure of the water resonance is not directly examined, e.g., for lack of sufficient SNR or spectral resolution, there are benefits to using spectroscopic imaging to reduce blurring at tissue boundaries and improve image quality.

In general, non–contrast-enhanced imaging methods do not exhibit artifacts intrinsic to contrast-enhanced images, such as blurring due to contrast diffusion and/or convection,[110,129] or blurring due to the changing contrast concentration during data acquisition. ▶ Fig. 11.14 shows an example of image degradation due to the use of contrast agent. Contrast agents can also introduce susceptibility gradients, further degrading image quality. Because of the recently discovered problems with Gd deposition[22,24,25] in a variety of tissues, noncontrast imaging is preferred when diagnostic performance can be preserved. HiSS MRI could be useful in achieving this goal.

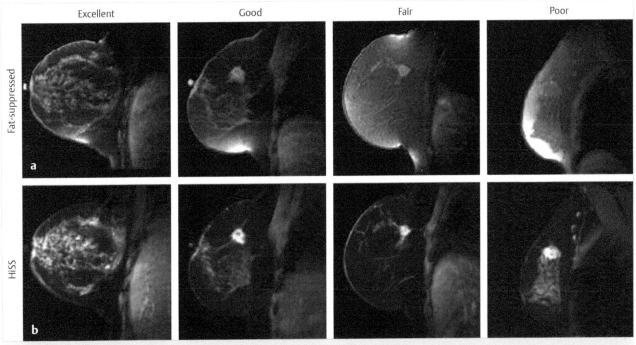

Fig. 11.12 Conventional T1-weighted MR images obtained using a spectrally selective inversion method show variable effectiveness of fat suppression (a). These are compared to the corresponding HiSS water peak height images showing higher and more consistent quality of fat suppression (b). (Reproduced with permission from Fan et al.[123])

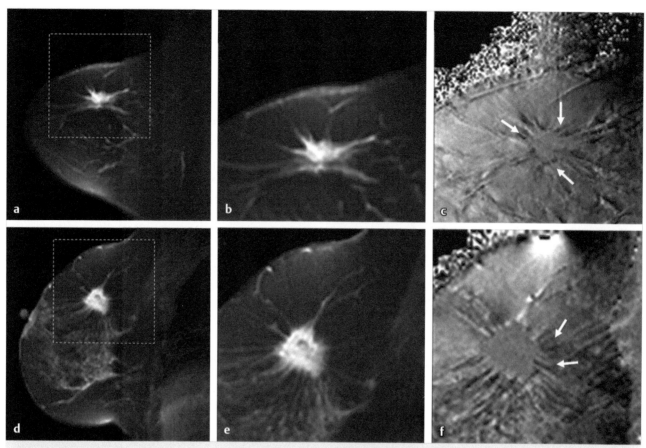

Fig. 11.13 Postcontrast T1-weighted fat-suppressed images of two malignancies are shown, an infiltrating ductal carcinoma (**a**, Patient 1) and an infiltrating ductal carcinoma with ductal carcinoma in situ (**d**, Patient 2). In (**b**) and (**e**), a small region around the lesion (square in **a**, **d**) is shown. Images proportional to B0, calculated from HiSS data, (**c** and **f**) are shown in the same region. B0 maps highly accentuate spiculations at the lesion boundary, which could facilitate lesion assessment. Some spiculations were only observed in the B0 maps (*arrows*). (Reproduced with permission from Medved et al.[118])

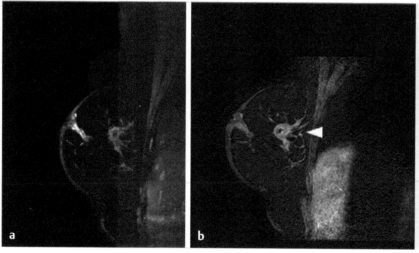

Fig. 11.14 A 69-year-old woman with an invasive ductal carcinoma was imaged using HiSS MRI (**a**) and conventional T1-weighted fat-suppressed postcontrast DCE-MRI (**b**). The lesion is indicated with the arrowhead. Spiculations surrounding the lesion are better visualized in the HiSS water peak height image, likely because contrast agent diffusion blurs the lesion edges in the postcontrast image. (Reproduced with permission from Medved et al.[110])

Applications

Lesion Diagnostics

To date, the primary application of HiSS MRI is to produce images with intensity proportional to the peak amplitude of the isolated water resonance, which provide the best CNR in morphological HiSS images. These images are heavily T2*-weighted, and thus provide very high contrast, but without the distortion and loss of SNR generally associated with T2*-weighted gradient echo imaging. Multiple studies have compared non–contrast-enhanced HiSS water peak height images to conventional postcontrast T1-weighted MRI, which is traditionally used for lesion diagnostics, and have demonstrated improved image quality[119,121,130] and comparable diagnostic performance.[110,113]

Of particular interest is the study by Bhooshan et al that used computer-aided diagnostics (CADx) with neural networks to analyze and compare 2D (single-slice, single time point) nonenhanced HiSS water peak height images to 4D (multislice, multiple time points) DCE-MRI T1-weighted images in the task of classification of benign and malignant breast lesions.[113] Thirty-four malignant and seven benign lesions were scanned and automatically segmented on both types of images using a fuzzy c-means method (▶ Fig. 11.15). For HiSS images, morphological features were generated, while for T1-weighted DCE-MRI, both morphological and kinetic features were generated. Area under the ROC curve (ROC AUC) was used as the performance metric, and ROC AUC values of 0.92 ± 0.06 (HiSS) and 0.90 ± 0.05 (DCE-MRI) were obtained, satisfying a non-inferiority condition for HiSS performance (▶ Fig. 11.16). Such high diagnostic performance of non-enhanced HiSS MRI could result from reduced blurring at edges—a benefit of spectroscopic and non-

contrast imaging. Another reason could be that heavy T2* weighting produces internal contrast in the lesion that differs from that found in contrast-enhanced T1-weighted images. For DCE-MRI data, full 3D signal and its temporal dependence were included in the analysis; yet, the diagnostic performance of HiSS MRI was comparable or better than that of DCE-MRI. As new information on Gd deposition in tissues and the resulting risks becomes available,[22,123] this is an increasingly important result.

Additional studies have sought to further improve the diagnostic performance of noncontrast HiSS MRI by analyzing the full water resonance spectral information. The methods have ranged from assessing spatial variation in the water resonance structure,[114,115] to analyzing properties of the strongest water signal component other than the main peak,[111,112] to describing the overall deviation of the water resonance shape from a Lorentzian function.[116] The non-Lorentzian structure of the water resonances in cancerous lesions likely arises from local magnetic susceptibility gradients caused by deoxygenated tumor blood vessels and calcifications, and thus contains diagnostically useful information concerning local tissue physiology. This information cannot be obtained using conventional MRI and is likely to complement other available metrics to increase diagnostic performance.

In FC imaging, maps of spectral intensity at given frequencies within the water resonance (FC images) are generated and analyzed for presence of clusters of voxels with marked irregularities in the water resonance shape.[114,115] Cluster analysis takes spatial correlation into account and is illustrated in ▶ Fig. 11.17 for five IDC lesions. In a study including 33 malignant and 9 benign lesions, when the number of cluster voxels with marked irregularities was used as a classifier of benign versus cancerous

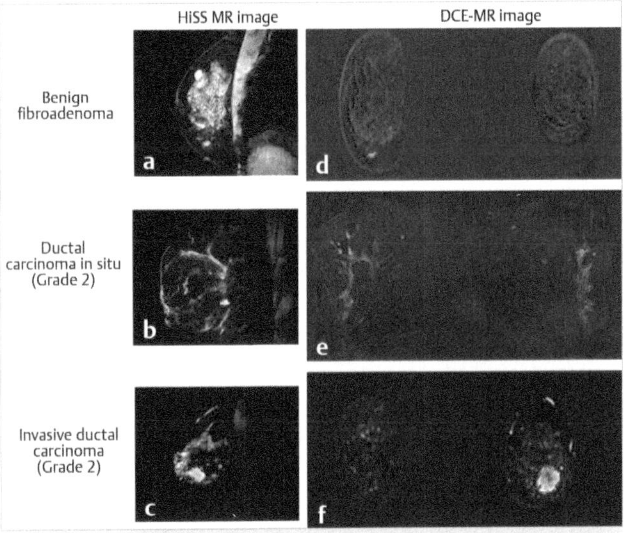

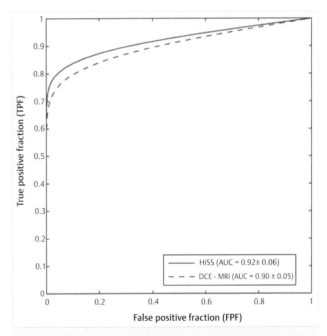

Fig. 11.15 Sagittal precontrast HiSS water peak height MR images **(a-c)** and coronal DCE-MRI images acquired at the first minute postinjection **(d-f)** are shown for three patients with breast lesions (top to bottom: benign fibroadenoma, ductal carcinoma in situ [grade 2], and invasive ductal carcinoma [grade 2]). Computerized segmentations of lesions are shown in red. (Reproduced with permission from Bhooshan et al.[113])

Fig. 11.16 ROC curves illustrating the performance of precontrast HiSS and postcontrast DCE-MRI images in the task of malignant versus benign breast lesion differentiation are shown. (Reproduced with permission from Bhooshan et al.[113])

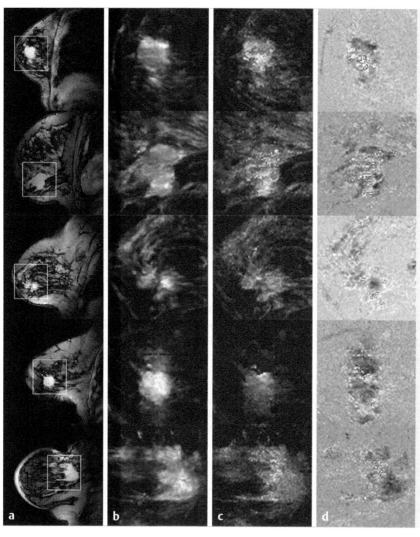

Fig. 11.17 T1-weighted **(a)** images are shown for five patients with IDC lesions confirmed on biopsy, and a 5 × 5 cm region surrounding the lesion is outlined by the white square. Fourier component images generated at peak frequency **(b)** and Fourier component images generated at 10 Hz offset from the water resonance peak **(c)** are shown for the outlined region. The subtractions of **(c)** and **(b)**, normalized to same average intensity, are shown in **(d)**. Clusters of voxels with irregularities in the spectral shape, evidenced by differences in contrast in **(b)** and **(c)** are highlighted in yellow. (Reproduced with permission from Medved et al.[115])

lesions, ROC AUC of 0.83 was obtained.[115] Further, non-spatially correlated, voxel-by-voxel analysis of OPCs of the water resonance has also proven useful.[111,112] When the voxels with the top 10% main off-peak component (OPC) amplitude values were selected and the mean of the OPC amplitudes over this set was used as a classifier, the ROC AUC value in the task of separating benign ($N = 8$) from malignant ($N = 15$) lesions reached 0.86.[112] Analysis of the overall resonance shape (dispersion versus absorption analysis), yielded an ROC AUC value of 0.90 on the same dataset.[116] Similar analysis of the main OPC frequency offset yielded an ROC AUC of 0.83.[111] While the sample sizes of these studies are limited, they do clearly demonstrate the potential for high diagnostic utility of non–contrast-enhanced HiSS MRI.

Lesion Detection and Other Applications

Recently, it was shown that full bilateral HiSS MRI of the breast can be achieved in 6 to 7 minutes with some reduction of the spectral resolution.[121] The ability to perform full bilateral breast examinations opens HiSS MRI to new applications such as

lesion detection and breast density measurement. Several examples of maximum intensity projections of HiSS water peak height images are shown in ▶ Fig. 11.18. The use of HiSS MRI as a screening tool is of great interest due to its ability to visualize and reliably characterize breast lesions without the administration of contrast agent. After recent reports of Gd deposition in tissue, including deep brain structures, with repeated exposure to GBCM,[22,131] any population-wide breast screening programs will almost certainly require imaging without contrast media injection. DWI has been studied for this purpose,[90,91,92,93,94,95] and HiSS MRI could provide complementary information that could improve diagnostic performance.

Such screening MRI examinations could also be used to stratify women according to breast density and thus allow individualized breast cancer risk management. Currently, mammography is used to stratify women into four BIRADS-defined breast density groups, but this method is reader-dependent and often results in significant overlap between the categories.[132,133] Most importantly, the stratifying is coarse and thus provides little quantitative information. Breast MRI can provide quantitative 3D measurements of breast density and glandular

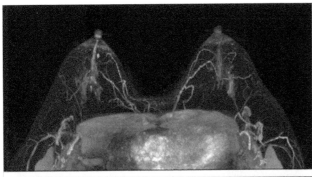
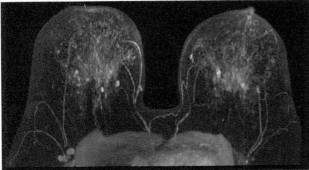
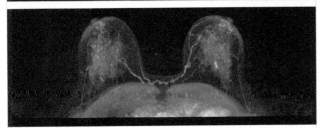
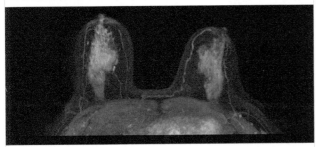
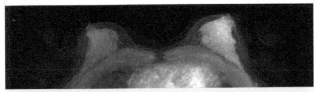

Fig. 11.18 Maximum intensity projections of unenhanced HiSS water peak height images through breasts of five healthy women are shown. The breast density increases from top to bottom. All images are shown within the same field of view.

11.6 Arterial Spin Labeling

ASL is a contrast-free method for quantitative mapping of tissue perfusion, in absolute units.[134] It was pioneered in neuroimaging,[135,136] e.g., in MR angiography and in functional MRI, where it allowed direct activation visualization via tracking of arterial inflow, rather than in a derivative way via the change in tissue oxygenation state. In ASL MRI, water protons in arterial blood are tagged—or "labeled"—using inversion pulses over a limited tagging zone proximal to the area of interest. The inverted water proton spins act as an endogenous contrast medium, exchanging magnetization with local water molecules in the imaged area and thus reducing signal. ASL images are subtracted from images obtained without labeling, and under proper conditions, the difference is directly proportional to local blood flow and can be used to quantify tissue perfusion.[134]

ASL has been implemented with a variety of MRI sequences, including EPI, single-shot fast spin echo (FSE), single-shot gradient-and-spin-echo (GRASE), true-steady state free precession (true-FISP), and other sequences.[137,138,139] Further, there are four main methods for velocity encoding that is read out using the above sequences: continuous ASL (CASL) which was the first method to be introduced, pseudocontinuous ASL (PCASL), which reduces SAR and magnetization transfer effects relative to CASL, pulsed ASL (PASL), including flow-sensitive alternating inversion recovery (FAIR), and velocity-sensitive ASL (VS-ASL).[134,137,140] The most frequently used method is PCASL, which does not pose any special hardware requirements and has been implemented on unmodified clinical scanner hardware from all of the major MR systems manufacturers.[134] In PCASL, a large gradient is applied along the direction of flow and a train of slice-selective RF pulse is used to invert spins within a well-defined region proximal to the imaged volume.[137] As the time spent within the excited plane is inversely proportional to blood velocity, the degree of inversion and thus signal loss is proportional to blood velocity.[134]

As the perfusion-induced signal decrease is only ~1–2% of the initial signal, ASL images are typically averaged over several acquisitions, significantly increasing imaging times and restricting body applications to limited volumes.[134,135,137] In neuroimaging, arterial blood in the carotid arteries is labeled, and the effect is observed in axial slices through the brain. In breast imaging, the area behind the chest wall, including the heart, is labeled, and the effect is observed in coronal slices through the breasts.[141] Other body applications include perfusion imaging of kidney, spleen, lung, muscle, and multiple glands.[142]

In breast, ASL has been used to assess the likelihood of malignancy for a detected lesion, based on the higher perfusion detected in malignant lesions as compared to benign lesions or normal tissue.[139,141,143] In breast, perfusion shows excellent diagnostic performance, but is typically assessed using Gd-based contrast agents, which carry risks. Thus, a reliable non–contrast-enhanced method for perfusion evaluation of breast lesions would be highly valuable. Two small studies have investigated the feasibility of perfusion imaging of breast lesions using an ASL technique.[139,141] Kawashima et al were able to demonstrate successful measurement of perfusion in 13 of 14 breast tumors using PASL EPI, and established significant correlation between ASL-based and CT-based perfusion values in breast cancer.[141] Buchbender et al used FAIR true-FISP

tissue volume, which would be of greater value in cancer risk management. HiSS MRI is well suited for this purpose, as it is sensitive in voxels with low water content, and able to selectively visualize the parenchymal tissue without the use of fat-suppressing RF pulses that may affect water signal as well.

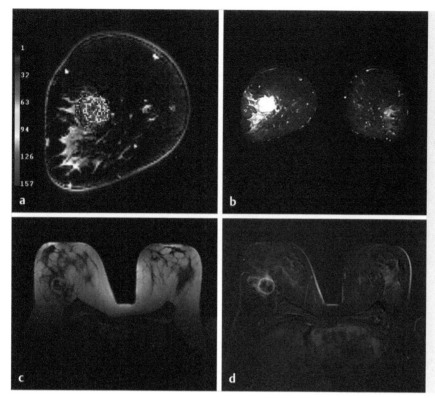

Fig. 11.19 An invasive ductal carcinoma in the right breast is depicted. The color map of the ASL perfusion measurement within the lesion is shown in (**a**), demonstrating higher perfusion at the rim of the tumor. Coronal and axial views obtained using STIR (**b**), native T1-weighted FLASH 3D (**c**), and contrast-enhanced subtracted T1-weighted (**d**) sequences are also shown. (Reproduced with permission from Buchbender et al.[139])

perfusion imaging to demonstrate that breast cancers show higher perfusion than benign lesions or normal tissue (▶ Fig. 11.19).[139]

11.7 Electrical Properties Tomography

The dielectric properties of human tissue correlate well with their sodium and water content,[144] and thus differences can be expected between cancerous and normal tissue. Specifically, the conductivity and permittivity of the tissue is expected to be higher in cancer, due to higher water content, and this premise has been tested in multiple studies. At frequencies relevant for MRI, it was found that permittivity and conductivity were 30% higher in glioma than in surrounding brain tissue[145] and around 15% higher in malignant colorectal versus normal tissue samples.[146] In breast, permittivity and conductivity were found to be 233% and 577%, respectively, higher in mammary malignancies than in normal mammary tissue.[147]

Thus, visualizing electrical properties of the tissue could potentially be useful for detection of malignancies.[148] EPT relies on accurate mapping of the transmit B1 field, which describes the spatial sensitivity of the transmit coil. Both magnitude and phase B1 information are important for conductivity and permittivity calculations, and current implementations have used a variety of sequences, though most frequently a T2-weighted FSE sequence[49,150,151,152] or a steady-state-free-precession (SSFP) sequence.[153] Systematic work on EPT theory and implementation has been ongoing since 2009.[154] EPT has initially been tested in the brain,[155,156,157,158,159] and is now finding

applications in body imaging. In breast tissue, conductivity and permittivity could in principle be used for lesion detection, but as smaller lesions could be obscured, EPT is better suited to the task of lesion characterization. Better distinction of malignant from benign breast lesions is arguably the most pressing issue in breast MRI today, and new sources of MRI contrast could potentially increase specificity and reduce the number of biopsies performed on indeterminate lesions. Monitoring of breast cancer therapy response and outcome prediction are other possible applications of breast EPT.

The first applications in breast date only from 2012 on,[160,161] and are largely still at the stage of technical development.[152,162] However, a clinical study from 2016 by Kim et al examined the correlation between conductivity and prognostic factors of invasive breast cancer (▶ Fig. 11.20).[151] In tumors larger than 2 cm, higher conductivity was associated with higher mitosis grades and high Ki-67 values, which are markers of cell proliferation and correlate strongly with poor prognosis. In addition, tumors with HER-2 overexpression showed lower mean conductivity values. This finding may be related to microcalcifications often found in DCIS, which in turn is often associated with HER-2-positive cancers.[151]

In a rat model study published in 2015, Hancu et al have compared the utility of diffusive and electrical properties of tissue as cancer markers. Although the authors found that conductivity is moderately correlated with ADC ($r = -0.65$), it contributed little benefit to lesion discrimination performance, while permittivity showed independent discriminating power that was comparable to that of ADC.[163] These findings are likely relevant to future work on human in vivo EPT development.

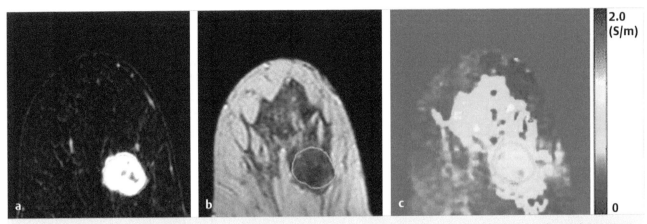

Fig. 11.20 An axial cross-section through a breast of a 67-year-old woman with a 2.2 cm invasive ductal carcinoma with lymphovascular invasion in the right upper medial breast is shown. **(a)** T1-weighted fat-suppressed contrast-enhanced image demonstrates an irregular enhancing mass. **(b)** T2-weighted fast spin echo image demonstrates iso-to-hypointense mass with respect to breast parenchyma. **(c)** Conductivity map shows a lower mean conductivity value within the tumor region, as compared with uninvolved parenchyma. (Reproduced with permission from Kim et al.[151])

References

[1] Rose TA , Jr, Choi JW. Intravenous Imaging Contrast Media Complications: The Basics That Every Clinician Needs to Know. Am J Med. 2015; 128(9): 943–949

[2] Li A, Wong CS, Wong MK, Lee CM, Au Yeung MC. Acute adverse reactions to magnetic resonance contrast media–gadolinium chelates. Br J Radiol. 2006; 79(941):368–371

[3] Nelson KL, Gifford LM, Lauber-Huber C, Gross CA, Lasser TA. Clinical safety of gadopentetate dimeglumine. Radiology. 1995; 196(2):439–443

[4] Hunt CH, Hartman RP, Hesley GK. Frequency and severity of adverse effects of iodinated and gadolinium contrast materials: retrospective review of 456,930 doses. AJR Am J Roentgenol. 2009; 193(4):1124–1127

[5] Canga A, Kislikova M, Martínez-Gálvez M, et al. Renal function, nephrogenic systemic fibrosis and other adverse reactions associated with gadolinium-based contrast media. Nefrologia. 2014; 34(4):428–438

[6] ACR Committee on Drugs and Contrast Media. ACR Manual on Contrast Media v10.2. https://www.acr.org/quality-safety/resources/contrast-manual: American College of Radiology;2016. ISBN 978–1–55903–012–0

[7] Bellin MF, Jakobsen JA, Tomassin I, et al. Contrast Media Safety Committee of the European Society of Urogenital Radiology. Contrast medium extravasation injury: guidelines for prevention and management. Eur Radiol. 2002; 12(11):2807–2812

[8] Hardie AD, Kereshi B. Incidence of intravenous contrast extravasation: increased risk for patients with deep brachial catheter placement from the emergency department. Emerg Radiol. 2014; 21(3):235–238

[9] Wang CL, Cohan RH, Ellis JH, Adusumilli S, Dunnick NR. Frequency, management, and outcome of extravasation of nonionic iodinated contrast medium in 69,657 intravenous injections. Radiology. 2007; 243(1):80–87

[10] Beaudouin E, Kanny G, Blanloeil Y, Guilloux L, Renaudin JM, Moneret-Vautrin DA. Anaphylactic shock induced by gadoterate meglumine (DOTAREM). Eur Ann Allergy Clin Immunol. 2003; 35(10):382–385

[11] Bertherat J, Hoeffel C, Pariente-Khayat A, et al. [Anaphylactic reactions after intravenous injection of gadolinium for pituitary or cerebral magnetic resonance imaging]. Presse Med (Paris, France: 1983). 1996; 25(40):2050

[12] Monmeneu Menadas JV, Lopez-Lereu MP, Estornell Erill J, Garcia Gonzalez P, Igual Muñoz B, Maceira Gonzalez A. Pharmacological stress cardiovascular magnetic resonance: feasibility and safety in a large multicentre prospective registry. Eur Heart J Cardiovasc Imaging. 2016; 17(3):308–315

[13] Nomura M, Takeshita G, Katada K, et al. [A case of anaphylactic shock following the administration of Gd-DTPA]. Nippon Igaku Hoshasen Gakkai Zasshi. 1993; 53(12):1387–1391

[14] Singer BD, Woodrick RS, Pedicano JB. Severe adverse drug reaction to gadobenate dimeglumine. ScientificWorldJournal. 2009; 9:363–365

[15] Jung JW, Kang HR, Kim MH, et al. Immediate hypersensitivity reaction to gadolinium-based MR contrast media. Radiology. 2012; 264(2):414–422

[16] Prince MR, Zhang H, Zou Z, Staron RB, Brill PW. Incidence of immediate gadolinium contrast media reactions. AJR Am J Roentgenol. 2011; 196(2): W138–43

[17] Takahashi S, Takada A, Saito K, Hara M, Yoneyama K, Nakanishi H. Fatal Anaphylaxis Associated With the Gadolinium-Based Contrast Agent Gadoteridol (ProHance). J Investig Allergol Clin Immunol. 2015; 25(5):366–367

[18] Rahman SL, Harbinson MT, Mohiaddin R, Pennell DJ. Acute allergic reaction upon first exposure to gadolinium-DTPA: a case report. J Cardiovasc Magn Reson. 2005; 7(5):849–851

[19] Beckett KR, Moriarity AK, Langer JM. Safe Use of Contrast Media: What the Radiologist Needs to Know. Radiographics. 2015; 35(6):1738–1750

[20] Daftari Besheli L, Aran S, Shaqdan K, Kay J, Abujudeh H. Current status of nephrogenic systemic fibrosis. Clin Radiol. 2014; 69(7):661–668

[21] Thomsen HS, Morcos SK, Almén T, et al. ESUR Contrast Medium Safety Committee. Nephrogenic systemic fibrosis and gadolinium-based contrast media: updated ESUR Contrast Medium Safety Committee guidelines. Eur Radiol. 2013; 23(2):307–318

[22] Fraum TJ, Ludwig DR, Bashir MR, Fowler KJ. Gadolinium-based contrast agents: A comprehensive risk assessment. J Magn Reson Imaging. 2017; 46(2):338–353

[23] Berg WA, Blume JD, Adams AM, et al. Reasons women at elevated risk of breast cancer refuse breast MR imaging screening: ACRIN 6666. Radiology. 2010; 254(1):79–87

[24] Errante Y, Cirimele V, Mallio CA, Di Lazzaro V, Zobel BB, Quattrocchi CC. Progressive increase of T1 signal intensity of the dentate nucleus on unenhanced magnetic resonance images is associated with cumulative doses of intravenously administered gadodiamide in patients with normal renal function, suggesting dechelation. Invest Radiol. 2014; 49(10):685–690

[25] Kanda T, Ishii K, Kawaguchi H, Kitajima K, Takenaka D. High signal intensity in the dentate nucleus and globus pallidus on unenhanced T1-weighted MR images: relationship with increasing cumulative dose of a gadolinium-based contrast material. Radiology. 2014; 270(3):834–841

[26] Beomonte Zobel B, Quattrocchi CC, Errante Y, Grasso RF. Gadolinium-based contrast agents: did we miss something in the last 25 years? Radiol Med (Torino). 2016; 121(6):478–481

[27] Runge VM. Safety of the Gadolinium-Based Contrast Agents for Magnetic Resonance Imaging, Focusing in Part on Their Accumulation in the Brain and Especially the Dentate Nucleus. Invest Radiol. 2016; 51(5):273–279

[28] Stojanov D, Aracki-Trenkic A, Benedeto-Stojanov D. Gadolinium deposition within the dentate nucleus and globus pallidus after repeated administrations of gadolinium-based contrast agents-current status. Neuroradiology. 2016; 58(5):433–441

[29] McDonald RJ, McDonald JS, Kallmes DF, et al. Intracranial Gadolinium Deposition after Contrast-enhanced MR Imaging. Radiology. 2015; 275 (3):772–782

[30] Frenzel T, Lengsfeld P, Schirmer H, Hütter J, Weinmann HJ. Stability of gadolinium-based magnetic resonance imaging contrast agents in human serum at 37 degrees C. Invest Radiol. 2008; 43(12):817–828

[31] Malayeri AA, Brooks KM, Bryant LH, et al. National Institutes of Health Perspective on Reports of Gadolinium Deposition in the Brain. J Am Coll Radiol. 2016; 13(3):237–241

[32] US Food and Drug Administration. FDA Drug Safety Communication: FDA warns that gadolinium-based contrast agents (GBCAs) are retained in the body; requires new class warnings. 2018; https://www.fda.gov/Drugs/DrugSafety/ucm589213.htm. Accessed 06/10/2018

[33] European Medicines Agency. Gadolinium-containing contrast agents. 2017; http://www.ema.europa.eu/ema/index.jsp?curl=pages/medicines/human/referrals/Gadolinium-containing_contrast_agents/human_referral_prac_000056.jsp&mid=WC0b01ac05805c516f. Accessed 06/10/2018

[34] Saslow D, Boetes C, Burke W, et al. American Cancer Society Breast Cancer Advisory Group. American Cancer Society guidelines for breast screening with MRI as an adjunct to mammography. CA Cancer J Clin. 2007; 57(2):75–89

[35] Stout NK, Nekhlyudov L, Li L, et al. Rapid increase in breast magnetic resonance imaging use: trends from 2000 to 2011. JAMA Intern Med. 2014; 174(1):114–121

[36] Miller JW, Sabatino SA, Thompson TD, et al. Breast MRI use uncommon among U.S. women. Cancer Epidemiol Biomarkers Prev. 2013; 22(1):159–166

[37] Wernli KJ, DeMartini WB, Ichikawa L, et al. Breast Cancer Surveillance Consortium. Patterns of breast magnetic resonance imaging use in community practice. JAMA Intern Med. 2014; 174(1):125–132

[38] Haas JS, Hill DA, Wellman RD, et al. Disparities in the use of screening magnetic resonance imaging of the breast in community practice by race, ethnicity, and socioeconomic status. Cancer. 2016; 122(4):611–617

[39] Chan I, Wells W, III, Mulkern RV, et al. Detection of prostate cancer by integration of line-scan diffusion, T2-mapping and T2-weighted magnetic resonance imaging; a multichannel statistical classifier. Med Phys. 2003; 30(9):2390–2398

[40] Sumi M, Sakihama N, Sumi T, et al. Discrimination of metastatic cervical lymph nodes with diffusion-weighted MR imaging in patients with head and neck cancer. AJNR Am J Neuroradiol. 2003; 24(8):1627–1634

[41] Squillaci E, Manenti G, Di Stefano F, Miano R, Strigari L, Simonetti G. Diffusion-weighted MR imaging in the evaluation of renal tumours. J Exp Clin Cancer Res. CR (East Lansing Mich). 2004; 23(1):39–45

[42] Charles-Edwards EM, deSouza NM. Diffusion-weighted magnetic resonance imaging and its application to cancer. Cancer Imaging. 2006; 6:135–143

[43] Sinha S, Lucas-Quesada FA, Sinha U, DeBruhl N, Bassett LW. In vivo diffusion-weighted MRI of the breast: potential for lesion characterization. J Magn Reson Imaging. 2002; 15(6):693–704

[44] Guo Y, Cai YQ, Cai ZL, et al. Differentiation of clinically benign and malignant breast lesions using diffusion-weighted imaging. J Magn Reson Imaging. 2002; 16(2):172–178

[45] Kinoshita T, Yashiro N, Ihara N, Funatu H, Fukuma E, Narita M. Diffusion-weighted half-Fourier single-shot turbo spin echo imaging in breast tumors: differentiation of invasive ductal carcinoma from fibroadenoma. J Comput Assist Tomogr. 2002; 26(6):1042–1046

[46] Kuroki Y, Nasu K, Kuroki S, et al. Diffusion-weighted imaging of breast cancer with the sensitivity encoding technique: analysis of the apparent diffusion coefficient value. Magn Reson Med Sci. 2004; 3(2):79–85

[47] Woodhams R, Matsunaga K, Iwabuchi K, et al. Diffusion-weighted imaging of malignant breast tumors: the usefulness of apparent diffusion coefficient (ADC) value and ADC map for the detection of malignant breast tumors and evaluation of cancer extension. J Comput Assist Tomogr. 2005; 29(5):644–649

[48] Woodhams R, Matsunaga K, Kan S, et al. ADC mapping of benign and malignant breast tumors. Magn Reson Med Sci. 2005; 4(1):35–42

[49] Padhani AR, Liu G, Koh DM, et al. Diffusion-weighted magnetic resonance imaging as a cancer biomarker: consensus and recommendations. Neoplasia. 2009; 11(2):102–125

[50] Wang S, Peng Y, Medved M, et al. Hybrid multidimensional T(2) and diffusion-weighted MRI for prostate cancer detection. J Magn Reson Imaging. 2014; 39(4):781–788

[51] Woodhams R, Ramadan S, Stanwell P, et al. Diffusion-weighted imaging of the breast: principles and clinical applications. Radiographics. 2011; 31(4):1059–1084

[52] Huang SY, Seethamraju RT, Patel P, Hahn PF, Kirsch JE, Guimaraes AR. Imaging: Artifacts, k-Space, and Solutions. Radiographics. 2015; 35(5):1439–1460

[53] Partridge SC, McDonald ES. Diffusion weighted magnetic resonance imaging of the breast: protocol optimization, interpretation, and clinical applications. Magn Reson Imaging Clin N Am. 2013; 21(3):601–624

[54] White NS, McDonald C, Farid N, et al. Diffusion-weighted imaging in cancer: physical foundations and applications of restriction spectrum imaging. Cancer Res. 2014; 74(17):4638–4652

[55] Chen W, Zhang J, Long D, Wang Z, Zhu JM. Optimization of intra-voxel incoherent motion measurement in diffusion-weighted imaging of breast cancer. J Appl Clin Med Phys/American College of Medical Physics. 2017; 18(3):191–199

[56] Liu C, Liang C, Liu Z, Zhang S, Huang B. Intravoxel incoherent motion (IVIM) in evaluation of breast lesions: comparison with conventional DWI. Eur J Radiol. 2013; 82(12):e782–e789

[57] Turner R, Le Bihan D, Maier J, Vavrek R, Hedges LK, Pekar J. Echo-planar imaging of intravoxel incoherent motion. Radiology. 1990; 177(2):407–414

[58] Delille JP, Slanetz PJ, Yeh ED, Kopans DB, Garrido L. Breast cancer: regional blood flow and blood volume measured with magnetic susceptibility-based MR imaging–initial results. Radiology. 2002; 223(2):558–565

[59] Baron P, Dorrius MD, Kappert P, Oudkerk M, Sijens PE. Diffusion-weighted imaging of normal fibroglandular breast tissue: influence of microperfusion and fat suppression technique on the apparent diffusion coefficient. NMR Biomed. 2010; 23(4):399–405

[60] Jin G, An N, Jacobs MA, Li K. The role of parallel diffusion-weighted imaging and apparent diffusion coefficient (ADC) map values for evaluating breast lesions: preliminary results. Acad Radiol. 2010; 17(4):456–463

[61] Cheng L, Blackledge MD, Collins DJ, et al. T2-adjusted computed diffusion-weighted imaging: A novel method to enhance tumour visualisation. Comput Biol Med. 2016; 79:92–98

[62] Gatidis S, Schmidt H, Martirosian P, Schwenzer NF. Development of an MRI phantom for diffusion-weighted imaging with independent adjustment of apparent diffusion coefficient values and T2 relaxation times. Magn Reson Med. 2014; 72(2):459–463

[63] Malyarenko D, Galbán CJ, Londy FJ, et al. Multi-system repeatability and reproducibility of apparent diffusion coefficient measurement using an ice-water phantom. J Magn Reson Imaging. 2013; 37(5):1238–1246

[64] Newitt DC, Tan ET, Wilmes LJ, et al. Gradient nonlinearity correction to improve apparent diffusion coefficient accuracy and standardization in the american college of radiology imaging network 6698 breast cancer trial. J Magn Reson Imaging. 2015; 42(4):908–919

[65] Zeilinger MG, Lell M, Baltzer PA, Dörfler A, Uder M, Dietzel M. Impact of post-processing methods on apparent diffusion coefficient values. Eur Radiol. 2017; 27(3):946–955

[66] Delille JP, Slanetz PJ, Yeh ED, Kopans DB, Garrido L. Physiologic changes in breast magnetic resonance imaging during the menstrual cycle: perfusion imaging, signal enhancement, and influence of the T1 relaxation time of breast tissue. Breast J. 2005; 11(4):236–241

[67] Kim JY, Suh HB, Kang HJ, et al. Apparent diffusion coefficient of breast cancer and normal fibroglandular tissue in diffusion-weighted imaging: the effects of menstrual cycle and menopausal status. Breast Cancer Res Treat. 2016; 157(1):31–40

[68] O'Flynn EA, Morgan VA, Giles SL, deSouza NM. Diffusion weighted imaging of the normal breast: reproducibility of apparent diffusion coefficient measurements and variation with menstrual cycle and menopausal status. Eur Radiol. 2012; 22(7):1512–1518

[69] Partridge SC, McKinnon GC, Henry RG, Hylton NM. Menstrual cycle variation of apparent diffusion coefficients measured in the normal breast using MRI. J Magn Reson Imaging. 2001; 14(4):433–438

[70] Shin S, Ko ES, Kim RB, et al. Effect of menstrual cycle and menopausal status on apparent diffusion coefficient values and detectability of invasive ductal carcinoma on diffusion-weighted MRI. Breast Cancer Res Treat. 2015; 149(3):751–759

[71] Clendenen TV, Kim S, Moy L, et al. Magnetic resonance imaging (MRI) of hormone-induced breast changes in young premenopausal women. Magn Reson Imaging. 2013; 31(1):1–9

[72] Partridge SC, Nissan N, Rahbar H, Kitsch AE, Sigmund EE. Diffusion-weighted breast MRI: Clinical applications and emerging techniques. J Magn Reson Imaging. 2017; 45(2):337–355

[73] Zhang L, Tang M, Min Z, Lu J, Lei X, Zhang X. Accuracy of combined dynamic contrast-enhanced magnetic resonance imaging and diffusion-weighted imaging for breast cancer detection: a meta-analysis. Acta Radiol (Stockholm, Sweden: 1987). 2016; 57(6):651–660

[74] Nissan N, Furman-Haran E, Shapiro-Feinberg M, Grobgeld D, Degani H. Diffusion-tensor MR imaging of the breast: hormonal regulation. Radiology. 2014; 271(3):672–680

[75] Chen X, Li WL, Zhang YL, Wu Q, Guo YM, Bai ZL. Meta-analysis of quantitative diffusion-weighted MR imaging in the differential diagnosis of breast lesions. BMC Cancer. 2010; 10:693

[76] Tsushima Y, Takahashi-Taketomi A, Endo K. Magnetic resonance (MR) differential diagnosis of breast tumors using apparent diffusion coefficient (ADC) on 1.5-T. J Magn Reson Imaging. 2009; 30(2):249–255

[77] Ei Khouli RH, Jacobs MA, Mezban SD, et al. Diffusion-weighted imaging improves the diagnostic accuracy of conventional 3.0-T breast MR imaging. Radiology. 2010; 256(1):64–73

[78] Woodhams R, Kakita S, Hata H, et al. Diffusion-weighted imaging of mucinous carcinoma of the breast: evaluation of apparent diffusion coefficient and signal intensity in correlation with histologic findings. AJR Am J Roentgenol. 2009; 193(1):260–266

[79] Marini C, Iacconi C, Giannelli M, Cilotti A, Moretti M, Bartolozzi C. Quantitative diffusion-weighted MR imaging in the differential diagnosis of breast lesion. Eur Radiol. 2007; 17(10):2646–2655

[80] Parsian S, Rahbar H, Allison KH, et al. Nonmalignant breast lesions: ADCs of benign and high-risk subtypes assessed as false-positive at dynamic enhanced MR imaging. Radiology. 2012; 265(3):696–706

[81] Rahbar H, Partridge SC, Eby PR, et al. Characterization of ductal carcinoma in situ on diffusion weighted breast MRI. Eur Radiol. 2011; 21(9):2011–2019

[82] Pickles MD, Gibbs P, Lowry M, Turnbull LW. Diffusion changes precede size reduction in neoadjuvant treatment of breast cancer. Magn Reson Imaging. 2006; 24(7):843–847

[83] Sharma U, Danishad KK, Seenu V, Jagannathan NR. Longitudinal study of the assessment by MRI and diffusion-weighted imaging of tumor response in patients with locally advanced breast cancer undergoing neoadjuvant chemotherapy. NMR Biomed. 2009; 22(1):104–113

[84] Li XR, Cheng LQ, Liu M, et al. DW-MRI ADC values can predict treatment response in patients with locally advanced breast cancer undergoing neoadjuvant chemotherapy. Med Oncol. 2012; 29(2):425–431

[85] Iwasa H, Kubota K, Hamada N, Nogami M, Nishioka A. Early prediction of response to neoadjuvant chemotherapy in patients with breast cancer using diffusion-weighted imaging and gray-scale ultrasonography. Oncol Rep. 2014; 31(4):1555–1560

[86] Iacconi C, Giannelli M, Marini C, et al. The role of mean diffusivity (MD) as a predictive index of the response to chemotherapy in locally advanced breast cancer: a preliminary study. Eur Radiol. 2010; 20(2):303–308

[87] Park SH, Moon WK, Cho N, et al. Diffusion-weighted MR imaging: pretreatment prediction of response to neoadjuvant chemotherapy in patients with breast cancer. Radiology. 2010; 257(1):56–63

[88] Richard R, Thomassin I, Chapellier M, et al. Diffusion-weighted MRI in pretreatment prediction of response to neoadjuvant chemotherapy in patients with breast cancer. Eur Radiol. 2013; 23(9):2420–2431

[89] Woodhams R, Kakita S, Hata H, et al. Identification of residual breast carcinoma following neoadjuvant chemotherapy: diffusion-weighted imaging-comparison with contrast-enhanced MR imaging and pathologic findings. Radiology. 2010; 254(2):357–366

[90] McDonald ES, Hammersley JA, Chou SH, et al. Performance of DWI as a Rapid Unenhanced Technique for Detecting Mammographically Occult Breast Cancer in Elevated-Risk Women With Dense Breasts. AJR Am J Roentgenol. 2016; 207(1):205–216

[91] Trimboli RM, Verardi N, Cartia F, Carbonaro LA, Sardanelli F. Breast cancer detection using double reading of unenhanced MRI including T1-weighted, T2-weighted STIR, and diffusion-weighted imaging: a proof of concept study. AJR Am J Roentgenol. 2014; 203(3):674–681

[92] Kazama T, Kuroki Y, Kikuchi M, et al. Diffusion-weighted MRI as an adjunct to mammography in women under 50 years of age: an initial study. J Magn Reson Imaging. 2012; 36(1):139–144

[93] Kuroki-Suzuki S, Kuroki Y, Nasu K, Nawano S, Moriyama N, Okazaki M. Detecting breast cancer with non-contrast MR imaging: combining diffusion-weighted and STIR imaging. Magn Reson Med Sci. 2007; 6(1):21–27

[94] Baltzer PA, Benndorf M, Dietzel M, Gajda M, Camara O, Kaiser WA. Sensitivity and specificity of unenhanced MR mammography (DWI combined with T2-weighted TSE imaging, ueMRM) for the differentiation of mass lesions. Eur Radiol. 2010; 20(5):1101–1110

[95] Yabuuchi H, Matsuo Y, Sunami S, et al. Detection of non-palpable breast cancer in asymptomatic women by using unenhanced diffusion-weighted and T2-weighted MR imaging: comparison with mammography and dynamic contrast-enhanced MR imaging. Eur Radiol. 2011; 21(1):11–17

[96] Guilfoyle DN, Mansfield P. Chemical-shift imaging. Magn Reson Med. 1985; 2(5):479–489

[97] Mansfield P. Spatial mapping of the chemical shift in NMR. Magn Reson Med. 1984; 1(3):370–386

[98] Duijn JH, Matson GB, Maudsley AA, Weiner MW. 3D phase encoding 1H spectroscopic imaging of human brain. Magn Reson Imaging. 1992; 10(2):315–319

[99] Fernandez EJ, Maudsley AA, Higuchi T, Weiner MW. Three-dimensional 1H spectroscopic imaging of cerebral metabolites in the rat using surface coils. Magn Reson Imaging. 1992; 10(6):965–974

[100] Maudsley AA, Lin E, Weiner MW. Spectroscopic imaging display and analysis. Magn Reson Imaging. 1992; 10(3):471–485

[101] Spielman D, Meyer C, Macovski A, Enzmann D. 1H spectroscopic imaging using a spectral-spatial excitation pulse. Magn Reson Med. 1991; 18(2):269–279

[102] Spielman D, Pauly J, Macovski A, Enzmann D. Spectroscopic imaging with multidimensional pulses for excitation: SIMPLE. Magn Reson Med. 1991; 19(1):67–84

[103] Kovar DA, Al-Hallaq HA, Zamora MA, River JN, Karczmar GS. Fast spectroscopic imaging of water and fat resonances to improve the quality of MR images. Acad Radiol. 1998; 5(4):269–275

[104] Du W, Du YP, Bick U, et al. Breast MR imaging with high spectral and spatial resolutions: preliminary experience. Radiology. 2002; 224(2):577–585

[105] Du W, Du YP, Fan X, Zamora MA, Karczmar GS. Reduction of spectral ghost artifacts in high-resolution echo-planar spectroscopic imaging of water and fat resonances. Magn Reson Med. 2003; 49(6):1113–1120

[106] Fan X, Du W, MacEneaney P, Zamora M, Karczmar G. Structure of the water resonance in small voxels in rat brain detected with high spectral and spatial resolution MRI. J Magn Reson Imaging. 2002; 16(5):547–552

[107] Karczmar GS, Du W, Medved M, et al. Spectrally inhomogeneous effects of contrast agents in breast lesion detected by high spectral and spatial resolution MRI. Acad Radiol. 2002; 9 Suppl 2:S352–S354

[108] Medved M, Du W, Zamora MA, et al. The effect of varying spectral resolution on the quality of high spectral and spatial resolution magnetic resonance images of the breast. J Magn Reson Imaging. 2003; 18(4):442–448

[109] Du W, Karczmar GS, Uftring SJ, Du YP. Anatomical and functional brain imaging using high-resolution echo-planar spectroscopic imaging at 1.5 Tesla. NMR Biomed. 2005; 18(4):235–241

[110] Medved M, Fan X, Abe H, et al. Non-contrast enhanced MRI for evaluation of breast lesions: comparison of non contrast enhanced high spectral and spatial resolution (HiSS) images versus contrast enhanced fat-suppressed images. Acad Radiol. 2011; 18(12):1467–1474

[111] Weiss WA, Medved M, Karczmar GS, Giger ML. Residual analysis of the water resonance signal in breast lesions imaged with high spectral and spatial resolution (HiSS) MRI: a pilot study. Med Phys. 2014; 41(1):012303

[112] Wood AM, Medved M, Bacchus ID, et al. Classification of breast lesions precontrast injection using water resonance lineshape analysis. NMR Biomed. 2013; 26(5):569–577

[113] Bhooshan N, Giger M, Medved M, et al. Potential of computer-aided diagnosis of high spectral and spatial resolution (HiSS) MRI in the classification of breast lesions. J Magn Reson Imaging. 2014; 39(1):59–67

[114] Medved M, Newstead GM, Fan X, et al. Fourier components of inhomogeneously broadened water resonances in breast: a new source of MRI contrast. Magn Reson Med. 2004; 52(1):193–196

[115] Medved M, Newstead GM, Fan X, et al. Fourier component imaging of water resonance in the human breast provides markers for malignancy. Phys Med Biol. 2009; 54(19):5767–5779

[116] Weiss WA, Medved M, Karczmar GS, Giger ML. Preliminary assessment of dispersion versus absorption analysis of high spectral and spatial resolution magnetic resonance images in the diagnosis of breast cancer. J Med Imaging (Bellingham). 2015; 2(2):024502

[117] Al-Hallaq HA, Fan X, Zamora M, River JN, Moulder JE, Karczmar GS. Spectrally inhomogeneous BOLD contrast changes detected in rodent tumors with high spectral and spatial resolution MRI. NMR Biomed. 2002; 15(1):28–36

[118] Medved M, Newstead GM, Abe H, Olopade OI, Karczmar GS. B0 maps highly accentuate spiculations at the tumor margin. Paper presented at: Seventeenth Scientific Meeting and Exhibition of ISMRM; 2009; Honolulu, HI

[119] Medved M, Newstead GM, Abe H, Zamora MA, Olopade OI, Karczmar GS. High spectral and spatial resolution MRI of breast lesions: preliminary clinical experience. AJR Am J Roentgenol. 2006; 186(1):30–37

[120] Medved M, Ivancevic MK, Olopade OI, Newstead GM, Karczmar GS. Echo-planar spectroscopic imaging (EPSI) of the water resonance structure in human breast using sensitivity encoding (SENSE). Magn Reson Med. 2010; 63(6):1557–1563

[121] Medved M, Li H, Abe H, et al. Fast bilateral breast coverage with high spectral and spatial resolution (HiSS) MRI at 3 T. J Magn Reson Imaging. 2017; 46(5): 1341–1348

[122] Foxley S, Fan X, Mustafi D, et al. Sensitivity to tumor microvasculature without contrast agents in high spectral and spatial resolution MR images. Magn Reson Med. 2009; 61(2):291–298

[123] Fan X, Abe H, Medved M, et al. Fat suppression with spectrally selective inversion vs. high spectral and spatial resolution MRI of breast lesions: qualitative and quantitative comparisons. J Magn Reson Imaging. 2006; 24(6):1311–1315

[124] Berglund J, Ahlström H, Johansson L, Kullberg J. Two-point dixon method with flexible echo times. Magn Reson Med. 2011; 65(4):994–1004

[125] Eggers H, Brendel B, Duijndam A, Herigault G. Dual-echo Dixon imaging with flexible choice of echo times. Magn Reson Med. 2011; 65(1):96–107

[126] Yu H, Reeder SB, Shimakawa A, McKenzie CA, Brittain JH. Robust multipoint water-fat separation using fat likelihood analysis. Magn Reson Med. 2012; 67(4):1065–1076

[127] Freed M, Storey P, Lewin AA, et al. Evaluation of Breast Lipid Composition in Patients with Benign Tissue and Cancer by Using Multiple Gradient-Echo MR Imaging. Radiology. 2016; 281(1):43–53

[128] He D, Mustafi D, Fan X, et al. MR Spectroscopy shows that high fat diet changes composition and distribution of mammary gland fat in a transgenic mouse model of breast cancer. Paper presented at: ISMRM 25th Annual Meeting and Exhibition; 2017; Honolulu, HI

[129] Fischer DR, Baltzer P, Malich A, et al. Is the "blooming sign" a promising additional tool to determine malignancy in MR mammography? Eur Radiol. 2004; 14(3):394–401

[130] Medved M, Newstead GM, Abe H, et al. Clinical implementation of a multi-slice high spectral and spatial resolution-based MRI sequence to achieve unilateral full-breast coverage. Magn Reson Imaging. 2010; 28(1):16–21

[131] Thomsen HS. Nephrogenic systemic fibrosis: A serious late adverse reaction to gadodiamide. Eur Radiol. 2006; 16(12):2619–2621

[132] Martin KE, Helvie MA, Zhou C, et al. Mammographic density measured with quantitative computer-aided method: comparison with radiologists' estimates and BI-RADS categories. Radiology. 2006; 240(3):656–665

[133] Nicholson BT, LoRusso AP, Smolkin M, Bovbjerg VE, Petroni GR, Harvey JA. Accuracy of assigned BI-RADS breast density category definitions. Acad Radiol. 2006; 13(9):1143–1149

[134] Wong EC. An introduction to ASL labeling techniques. J Magn Reson Imaging. 2014; 40(1):1–10

[135] Viallon M, Cuvinciuc V, Delattre B, et al. State-of-the-art MRI techniques in neuroradiology: principles, pitfalls, and clinical applications. Neuroradiology. 2015; 57(5):441–467

[136] Wolf RL, Detre JA. Clinical neuroimaging using arterial spin-labeled perfusion magnetic resonance imaging. Neurotherapeutics. 2007; 4(3):346–359

[137] Pollock JM, Tan H, Kraft RA, Whitlow CT, Burdette JH, Maldjian JA. Arterial spin-labeled MR perfusion imaging: clinical applications. Magn Reson Imaging Clin N Am. 2009; 17(2):315–338

[138] Vidorreta M, Wang Z, Rodríguez I, Pastor MA, Detre JA, Fernández-Seara MA. Comparison of 2D and 3D single-shot ASL perfusion fMRI sequences. Neuroimage. 2013; 66:662–671

[139] Buchbender S, Obenauer S, Mohrmann S, et al. Arterial spin labelling perfusion MRI of breast cancer using FAIR TrueFISP: initial results. Clin Radiol. 2013; 68(3):e123–e127

[140] Martirosian P, Klose U, Mader I, Schick F. FAIR true-FISP perfusion imaging of the kidneys. Magn Reson Med. 2004; 51(2):353–361

[141] Kawashima M, Katada Y, Shukuya T, Kojima M, Nozaki M. MR perfusion imaging using the arterial spin labeling technique for breast cancer. J Magn Reson Imaging. 2012; 35(2):436–440

[142] Martirosian P, Boss A, Schraml C, et al. Magnetic resonance perfusion imaging without contrast media. Eur J Nucl Med Mol Imaging. 2010; 37 Suppl 1: S52–S64

[143] Zhu DC, Buonocore MH. Breast tissue differentiation using arterial spin tagging. Magn Reson Med. 2003; 50(5):966–975

[144] Schepps JL, Foster KR. The UHF and microwave dielectric properties of normal and tumour tissues: variation in dielectric properties with tissue water content. Phys Med Biol. 1980; 25(6):1149–1159

[145] Lu Y, Li B, Xu J, Yu J. Dielectric properties of human glioma and surrounding tissue. Int J Hyperthermia. 1992; 8(6):755–760

[146] Li Z, Deng G, Li Z, et al. A large-scale measurement of dielectric properties of normal and malignant colorectal tissues obtained from cancer surgeries at Larmor frequencies. Med Phys. 2016; 43(11):5991

[147] Joines WT, Zhang Y, Li C, Jirtle RL. The measured electrical properties of normal and malignant human tissues from 50 to 900 MHz. Med Phys. 1994; 21 (4):547–550

[148] Katscher U, van den Berg CAT. Electric properties tomography: Biochemical, physical and technical background, evaluation and clinical applications. NMR Biomed. 2017; 30(8)

[149] Katscher U, Kim DH, Seo JK. Recent progress and future challenges in MR electric properties tomography. Comput Math Methods Med. 2013; 2013: 546562

[150] Kim DH, Chauhan M, Kim MO, et al. Frequency-dependent conductivity contrast for tissue characterization using a dual-frequency range conductivity mapping magnetic resonance method. IEEE Trans Med Imaging. 2015; 34 (2):507–513

[151] Kim SY, Shin J, Kim DH, et al. Correlation between conductivity and prognostic factors in invasive breast cancer using magnetic resonance electric properties tomography (MREPT). Eur Radiol. 2016; 26(7):2317–2326

[152] Shin J, Kim MJ, Lee J, et al. Initial study on in vivo conductivity mapping of breast cancer using MRI. J Magn Reson Imaging. 2015; 42(2): 371–378

[153] Stehning C, Voigt TR, Katscher U. Real-Time Conductivity Mapping using Balanced SSFP and Phase-Based Reconstruction. 19th Annual Meeting of the ISMRM; 2011; Montreal, Quebec

[154] Katscher U, Voigt T, Findeklee C, Vernickel P, Nehrke K, Dössel O. Determination of electric conductivity and local SAR via B1 mapping. IEEE Trans Med Imaging. 2009; 28(9):1365–1374

[155] Voigt T, Katscher U, Doessel O. Quantitative conductivity and permittivity imaging of the human brain using electric properties tomography. Magn Reson Med. 2011; 66(2):456–466

[156] Zhang X, Van de Moortele PF, Schmitter S, He B. Complex B1 mapping and electrical properties imaging of the human brain using a 16-channel transceiver coil at 7 T. Magn Reson Med. 2013; 69(5):1285–1296

[157] Jiaen L, Xiaotong Z, Schmitter S, Van de Moortele PF, Bin H. Gradient-based magnetic resonance electrical properties imaging of brain tissues. Conference proceedings: Annual International Conference of the IEEE Engineering in Medicine and Biology Society IEEE Engineering in Medicine and Biology Society Annual Conference.. 2014; 2014:6056–6059

[158] van Lier AL, Raaijmakers A, Voigt T, et al. Electrical properties tomography in the human brain at 1.5, 3, and 7T: a comparison study. Magn Reson Med. 2014; 71(1):354–363

[159] Tha KK, Katscher U, Yamaguchi S, et al. Noninvasive electrical conductivity measurement by MRI: a test of its validity and the electrical conductivity characteristics of glioma. Eur Radiol. 2018; 28(1):348–355

[160] Bulumulla S, Hancu I. Breast permittivity imaging. Proceedings of the 20th Scientific Meeting of the International Society of Magnetic Resonance in Medicine (ISMRM '12). 2012

[161] Katscher U, Djamshidi K, Voigt T, et al. Estimation of breast tumor conductivity using parabolic phase fitting. Proceedings of the 20th Scientific Meeting of the International Society of Magnetic Resonance in Medicine (ISMRM '12). 2012

[162] Lee J, Shin J, Kim DH. MR-based conductivity imaging using multiple receiver coils. Magn Reson Med. 2016; 76(2):530–539

[163] Hancu I, Roberts JC, Bulumulla S, Lee SK. On conductivity, permittivity, apparent diffusion coefficient, and their usefulness as cancer markers at MRI frequencies. Magn Reson Med. 2015; 73(5):2025–2029

12 Semi-Quantitative and Quantitative Analysis of Breast DCE-MRI

Gregory S. Karczmar and Federico D. Pineda

Abstract

Routine clinical interpretation of dynamic contrast-enhanced magnetic resonance imaging (DCE-MRI) by radiologists is based on subjective assessment of signal enhancement and the change in signal intensity as a function of time after the injection of contrast media. This chapter reviews semi-quantitative and quantitative methods that can help Radiologists to more accurately diagnose cancers by providing standardized MRI parameters that are markers for malignancy. Semiquantitative analysis of DCE-MRI data provides parameters such as rate of signal enhancement and the decay of enhancement during contrast media washout. Semiquantitative approaches are relatively simple to implement in routine clinical practice, as these approaches do not require specialized acquisitions or complicated calculations. Quantitative methods have potential to standardize diagnosis by correcting for variations in Radiologists' expertise, scanner, performance, and the systemic physiology of the patient (e.g. cardiac output). In addition, quantitative methods attempt to relate MRI measurements directly to intrinsic properties of tissue, such as blood flow and capillary permeability. In this chapter we discuss a number of widely used semi-quantitative and quantitative methods for DCE-MRI including the "three time point method," use of empirical mathematical models, use of compartmental models, impulse response analysis, reference tissue methods, and calibration methods required for quantitative measurements.

Keywords: dynamic contrast-enhanced MRI, quantitative MRI, two compartment model, empirical mathematical model, Brix model, Patlak model, compressed sensing, impulse response analysis, reference tissue methods

12.1 Semi-quantitative Analysis

Routine interpretation of dynamic contrast-enhanced magnetic resonance imaging (DCE-MRI) by radiologists is based on signal intensity and the change in signal intensity as a function of time after the injection of contrast media. Semi-quantitative techniques aid lesion categorization and provide excellent diagnostic accuracy in breast DCE-MRI. Semi-quantitative analysis has the advantage of being relatively simple to implement in routine practice, as approaches predominantly focus on postprocessing of standard clinical images and do not require specialized acquisitions.

The three time-point (3TP) method is a simple tool for classification of signal intensity time-course curves. The 3TP takes the first time-point in the DCE series, a "peak intensity" time-point (generally chosen roughly 2 minutes postcontrast administration), and a delayed time-point (approximately 6 minutes postcontrast).[1] Discrete thresholds are then used to classify two parts of the kinetic curve, the initial uptake and the delayed phase. An example of the types of classifications is illustrated in ▶ Fig. 12.1. The classification data can then be displayed as a

color overlay (on a voxel-by-voxel basis) on the standard images on computer-aided visualization stations.[2] For example, red, green, and blue color overlays can be placed on voxels displaying washout, plateau, and persistent delayed kinetics, respectively. The color intensity can also be adjusted to reflect the initial rise depending on whether it was slow, medium, or rapid. This provides radiologists a way of visually assessing the kinetics of lesion without the need to manually draw a region of interest (ROI). Kelcz et al evaluated the performance of observers aided by the 3TP in the detection of breast cancer, and found that this method had a sensitivity of 87% and specificity of 84%.[3]

While the discrete categorization of lesion kinetics has been shown to be diagnostically useful, previous work by Jansen et al[4] found that the BI-RADS descriptors of curve shape can vary significantly between different scanners and acquisition parameters in malignant lesions. Thus, results obtained with methods such as the 3TP may be inconsistent across different sites, as its performance will depend on the scanner used, the parameter settings, and the particular thresholds chosen.

Chen et al[5] used a robust, automated, segmentation method to find the region of a lesion with the highest initial enhancement. Four kinetic features were extracted from this region in each lesion: maximum enhancement, uptake rate, washout rate, and time to peak enhancement (TTP). TTP was defined as the time when the maximum signal enhancement was measured. Uptake and washout rates were determined from TTP and the maximum enhancement. Chen et al found that accuracy of classification was greater for automated segmentation than manual placement of ROIs. Of these features, TTP had the greatest area under the receiver operating characteristic (ROC) curve (0.85 ± 0.04); the values for uptake and washout rates were

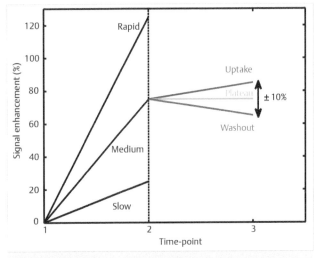

Fig. 12.1 Diagram of the three time-point (3TP) method for lesion kinetic classification.

0.71 ± 0.05 and 0.79 ± 0.05. These results suggest that these kinetic features may be diagnostically useful in the categorization of lesions.

The signal enhancement ratio (SER) was introduced by Hylton and co-workers as a way of quantifying lesion kinetic curve shape on a continuous scale.[6] The definition of SER is based on the standard interpretation of curve shape. SER is defined as:

$$SER = \frac{S_{early} - S_0}{S_{delayed} - S_0}, \tag{12.1}$$

where S_0 is the precontrast or baseline lesion signal intensity, S_{early} is the signal intensity measured at the early postcontrast phase (roughly 1–2 minutes postinjection), and $S_{delayed}$ is the signal intensity at the delayed phase (~6 minutes postinjection). SER can be thought of as a descriptor for curve shape because it indicates whether the transition from uptake to washout has occurred before, during, or after the time interval marked by S_{early} and $S_{delayed}$. SER has been shown to have diagnostic utility with a previous study reporting a sensitivity of 95%; specificity, however, was 47%.[7] SER has also been reported to be useful for evaluating tumor response to therapy, and has been shown to correlate with a parameter associated with tumor physiology (redistribution rate constant k_{ep}).[8,9,10] These results show the potential value of SER added to standard clinical practice. SER, however, is affected by the particular times at which the early and delayed phases are measured; as a result, temporal resolution will have an effect on the measured SER.

Time to enhancement (TTE) is another nonparametric semi-quantitative measure that may be of clinical utility. As its name suggests, TTE measures the time at which lesions first begin to enhance significantly. However, in order to reliably measure TTE, high temporal resolution imaging is necessary. One advantage of measuring TTE from fast acquisitions is that this allows measurement of TTE relative to the time at which the contrast bolus first reaches the breast, reducing dependence on variables such as cardiac output and leading to estimates that are more descriptive of lesion physiology. In a pilot study by Pineda et al[11] with images acquired with 6- to 10-second temporal resolution, TTE was found to be significantly different between benign and malignant lesions, with average values of 15.5 and 6.9 s after arterial enhancement in the breast, respectively. Mus et al[12] evaluated the utility of TTE (measured relative to the time of aortic enhancement) in a retrospective study with images acquired with 4.32-s temporal resolution. They found that TTE had a significantly better discriminative ability than kinetic curve type. Using a TTE threshold of 12.96 s to classify lesions (lesions below this threshold were considered malignant), the authors found an AUC as high as 0.86 using TTE alone.

12.2 Empirical Mathematical Models

As an alternative to pharmacokinetic model approaches, pure mathematical models are also common for analyzing the DCE-MRI data. These pure mathematical models make no assumptions about the underlying physiology of a tumor, but simply use functions with limited parameters to characterize the important features of contrast agent uptake and washout curves as a function of time. The mathematical models are used as a tool to smooth the signal enhancement versus time curves and interpolate the data. This approach may be advantageous because tumors are extremely heterogeneous and simple compartment models may not be consistent with the true spatio-temporal distribution of contrast agent molecules in the tumor microenvironment. For example, the two-compartment model is not consistent with initial rapid uptake of contrast media followed by a slower, more prolonged uptake phase. For noisy and/or low temporal resolution DCE-MRI data, the use of fitted curves based on empirical mathematical models (EMMs) facilitates calculation of arterial input functions (AIFs) from reference tissues,[13,14,15] improves measurements of physiological parameters, and facilitates calculation of the "area under the curve" of enhancement versus time, TTP, and initial uptake slope.

Several mathematical models have been developed for analysis of DCE-MRI data. Fan et al developed a five-parameter EMM to analyze DCE-MRI data from animal models of prostate cancer and human breast cancer.[15,16] This EMM yields five parameters descriptive of lesion kinetics. A modified three-parameter EMM was introduced by Jansen et al to describe signal enhancement of lesions in clinical breast DCE-MRI.[17,18] In the three-parameter EMM, percent signal enhancement (PSE) as a function of time is given by:

$$PSE(t) = A\left(1 - e^{-\alpha t}\right)e^{-\beta t}, \tag{12.2}$$

where A is the upper limit of enhancement, α is the uptake rate (per minute), and β is the washout rate (per minute). The EMM also allows calculation of secondary parameters such as the TTP, initial slope, and the initial area under the contrast curve. In a study that analyzed 100 patient scans with the EMM, it was shown that several of the primary and secondary parameters varied significantly between benign and malignant lesions.[17] Some of the EMM parameters also showed significant differences between tumor subtypes. The EMM was shown to have the potential of increasing the specificity of DCE-MRI with respect to BI-RADS descriptors of curve shape. The EMM has the added benefit of providing continuous variables for lesion classification; this means that thresholds can be adjusted to achieve desired sensitivity and specificity, as opposed to discrete classification of curve shape. Another class of functions that are commonly used to describe the signal increase in DCE-MRI are modified logistic functions (or sigmoid curves). Moate et al[19] [REF] proposed using a five-parameter modified logistic equation to describe signal enhancement in breast tumors, and demonstrated that parameters from this model have diagnostic value for analyzing breast DCE-MRI. Platel et al[20] used this model to fit the enhancement during an ultrafast DCE-MRI acquisition. Orth et al[21] used two modified sigmoids to fit the data from a dual tracer experiment in a preclinical model of breast cancer. While these functions have been shown to fit the shape of enhancement curves, the relationship between individual parameters and the shape of the curve is not entirely straightforward, and the inclusion of more parameters in the model means that more data along the signal time-course are required to obtain accurate fits. Gliozzi et al[22] used an

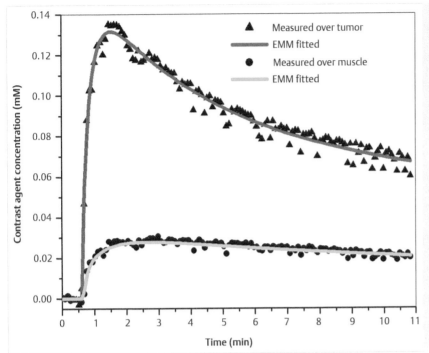

Fig. 12.2 Plots of contrast agent concentration versus time and EMM fits to the data for a rat model with prostate cancer.

"extended phenomenological universalities" (EU1) approach to analyze signal intensity versus time curves. Among these pure mathematical models, the EMM provides optimal fits to experimental DCE-MRI data and can be used to fit a range of contrast agent concentration versus time curves. ▶ Fig. 12.2 shows an example of EMM fits (red and green lines) to contrast agent concentration curves obtained from a rat model for prostate cancer (AT2.1 prostate cancer) (triangles) implanted in the hind limb and normal leg muscle (dots) acquired at 4.7 T.

12.2.1 Quantitative Analysis

Data Acquisition Methods

This section discusses acquisition techniques used to obtain information required for standardized, quantitative analysis of DCE-MRI data, specifically native T_1 measurements and maps of the transmit radiofrequency (RF) field (or B1). This information can also be used to correct semi-quantitative parameters. These measurements are not part of most routine, clinical, DCE-MRI acquisitions, because routine clinical analysis is generally based on qualitative interpretation of the images. However, quantitative methods are increasing in popularity, because they allow standardized measurements that can be compared across different scanners, sites, and patients.

T_1 Mapping

Accurate T_1 maps are essential for accurate calculation of concentration of contrast media as a function of time in each image voxel (discussed later in this chapter). Here, we summarize some of the most commonly used methods for mapping T_1. This

summary is not by any means an exhaustive list of T_1 mapping methods.

Spoiled Gradient Echo with Variable Flip Angles

This is one of the most widely used T1-mapping methods for breast MRI. Data are acquired using a series of spoiled gradient echo images with variable flip angles (VFAs).[23] The measured signal in each voxel is then fit to the gradient echo signal model as a function of flip angle, to obtain an estimate of T_1:

$$S = M_0 e^{-\frac{TE}{T_2^*}} \sin \theta \frac{1 - e^{-TR/T_1}}{1 - \cos \theta e^{-TR/T_1}}, \tag{12.3}$$

where θ is the flip angle, TE is the echo time, and T_2^* is the transverse relaxation time. Variations in the signal in equation (3) as a function of flip angle depend on TR, a known parameter, and T_1. The VFA method allows acquisitions of T_1 maps across a large volume with reasonable scan times. The accuracy of the VFA method is influenced by the accuracy of the flip angles used in equation (3), the choice and number of flip angles, and the noise present in the images.[24,25] Actual flip angles can vary spatially across the field of view (FOV), and differ significantly from the angles prescribed at the scanner console, due to an inhomogeneous transmit RF field (or B_1 field). This issue is discussed later in this chapter. Cheng and Wright showed that a bias of up to 10% in estimated T_1 can be introduced when three flip angles are used and the signal-to-noise ratio (SNR) is 150 in the VFA data (TR = 5 ms).[26] They also showed that the VFA method can be tailored to provide accurate estimates of T_1 within a narrow range when two flip angles are used. Adding more than two flip angles provides better results over a wider range of T_1 values. Interestingly, simulations by Cheng and

Wright showed that use of 10 different flip angles does not increase the performance relative to use of 3 angles, likely due to the influence of adding noisy data points (i.e., at lower flip angles). With judicious selection of flip angles,[25] and knowledge of the B_1 field, the VFA method can provide accurate T_1 maps with reasonable acquisition times, making it a suitable method for use in addition to standard clinical breast protocols.

Inversion Recovery Measurements

Inversion recovery (IR) is widely regarded as a very accurate T_1 mapping method and is commonly used to measure "gold standard" T_1 values.[27] In an IR sequence, a 180° pulse is first applied, inverting the spins and thus the net magnetization. The rate at which the spins recover to their initial alignment is determined by their T_1. This means that measurements of magnetization as a function of time after the inversion pulse leads to an estimate of T_1, derived from the IR signal model:

$$M(TI) = M_0 \left(1 - 2e^{-TI/T_1} + e^{-TR/T_1} \right),\qquad (12.4)$$

where $M(TI)$ is the magnetization measured at a given inversion time "TI," TR is the repetition time, and M_0 is the equilibrium magnetization. An additional parameter can be included in equation (4) to account for imperfect inversion pulses (i.e., not exactly 180°). The main drawback of using IR for T_1 measurements is the long acquisition times it requires. For accurate estimates of T_1, TR must be sufficiently long for magnetization to return to equilibrium following the inversion pulse (i.e., TR $\gg$ T_1).[28] A commonly used rule of thumb is that TR should at least be five times the longest T_1 being measured. The long acquisition times of IR make it ill-suited for application in routine clinical scans, especially in the case of the breast, where large FOVs are necessary for full bilateral acquisitions. To overcome this limitation of IR, sequences such as Look-Locker inversion and modified Look-Locker inversion (MOLLI) have been developed.[29,30] These sequences allow accelerated acquisition of T_1 maps in cardiac imaging, where fast acquisitions are critical. However, application of these sequences has been limited to areas of the body where small FOVs are used; thus, there is a lack of evidence about their applicability and accuracy for breast imaging.

Reference Tissue Method for T_1 Measurements

Medved et al[31] showed that, under certain conditions, the T_1 for a tissue of interest can be calculated from the signal of a reference tissue (i.e., a nearby tissue with a known T_1). The advantage of this method is that if a tissue with a homogeneous T_1 (low intra- and interpatient variability) is present in the FOV, a full T_1 measurement may not be necessary, reducing total scan time. This method relies on the fact that in a gradient echo acquisition, the product of signal × T_1 is approximately constant ($S \times T_1 \approx$ constant) if the flip angle used is greater than 30° and if the repletion time (TR) of the acquisition is much shorter than the T_1 values of the tissues being imaged, so that magnetization is highly saturated. This means that if differences in T_2^* between the reference tissue and the tissue of interest are relatively low (a realistic assumption outside the brain), and the MRI-detect-

able proton density between the two tissues is roughly the same, the following relationship can be used to obtain the T_1 for a tissue of interest with a single gradient echo acquisition:

$$\frac{S}{S_{ref}} \approx \frac{T_{1ref}}{T_1},\qquad (12.5)$$

where S is the signal measured in a given voxel and the subscript "ref" indicates the reference tissue. In the breast, fat is an ideal reference tissue, since it has a homogeneous T_1. Reported values for the T_1 of breast fat include 265 ± 2 ms[32] and 230 ± 10 ms,[33] both at 1.5 T. At 3 T, Rakow-Penner et al[34] reported a value of 367 ± 8 ms, and Pineda et al[35] measured a T_1 of 341 ± 31 ms. The relatively low standard deviation in these studies, and the similar values from different studies at the same field strength, suggests a low variability in the T_1 value of fat, both interpatient and across the breast. The reference tissue method is the simplest (and potentially fastest) method to measure T_1, but if the conditions mentioned above are not met, significant errors in the estimated T_1 values may result (e.g., if a low flip angle is used).

B_1 Mapping

Transmit RF field (B_1 or B_1^+) inhomogeneity is especially notable in breast MRI, due to the large FOVs required for bilateral breast imaging and the off-center (with respect to the center of the magnet) position of the breasts in the coil. Kuhl et al reported significant differences in the B_1 field across the FOV, with differences of nearly a factor of 2 between the left and right breasts.[36] These differences can lead to variations in image intensity across the FOV (e.g., shading), spatial variations in the signal enhancement in lesions after the administration of a contrast agent, and inaccurate T_1 values measured with a VFA sequence. Azlan et al mapped the B_1 field in several healthy volunteers at 3 T and simulated differences in enhancement due to B_1 gradients in a phantom study.[37] They found significant differences between the right and left breasts, and reductions of more than 50% relative to the nominal B_1 in some cases. They also showed that a reduction in B_1 leads to a reduction of the SER, possibly reducing the conspicuity of breast lesions. While B_1 inhomogeneity is an issue at all field strengths, the B_1 field is more inhomogeneous at larger fields.

Dual-source parallel RF excitation, combined with RF shimming methods, has been implemented by several manufacturers to reduce variations in the B_1 field.[38] Rahbar et al compared B_1 maps acquired in the breast using both single and dual-source RF excitation.[39] They found that while the use of dual-source parallel excitation reduced differences in the whole breast mean B_1 value between the right and left breasts compared to single-source excitation, significant differences between nominal and prescribed flip angles remained at many locations.

B_1 field inhomogeneity has a significant effect on the estimation of quantitative parameters in DCE-MRI.[40] Using a VFA approach, estimation of native T_1 values of tissues relies on the accurate knowledge of the flip angles used. Simulations show that for variations of up to 15% between nominal and prescribed flip angles, the relative error introduced in T_1

measurements from the VFA is twice the relative error in the flip angle (i.e., a 10% error in flip angle will lead to a 20% error in the measured T_1). Measurements of contrast agent concentration are obtained from the native and postcontrast-injection T_1 values. They are thus affected by the errors in the estimated flip angle in the ROI. In fact, when the repetition time is short and a low flip angle is used, a small error in the flip angle can lead to a large bias in concentration. In DCE-MRI of the breast, it is common to use protocols with these conditions. For this reason, accurate knowledge of the actual flip angle is essential for accurate measurements of contrast media concentration. This section outlines B_1 mapping methods that can be used in breast imaging to correct for B_1 field inhomogeneity.

Actual Flip Angle Imaging

The "actual flip angle imaging" (AFI) method, developed by Yarnykh, can be used to measure B_1 maps in vivo.[41] In this approach, the ratio of the signal of two gradient echo acquisitions at two different repetition times (TRs) is used to derive the actual flip angle in each voxel. When implementing this sequence, one must ensure that the transverse magnetization is adequately spoiled and that steady state magnetization has been achieved; otherwise, the accuracy of the AFI technique is affected.[42] Both TRs used in this sequence should be smaller than the shortest T_1 value present in the FOV. Additionally, large flip angles (40°–80°) are required for optimal implementation of this sequence; however, this leads to a reduced SNR, potential artifacts from stimulated echoes, and a distortion of slice profiles. Some vendors offer a built-in AFI option to obtain B_1 maps; otherwise, its implementation may require pulse programming knowledge.

Reference Tissue Methods for B_1 Mapping

Sung et al and Pineda et al proposed using fat as a reference tissue to obtain combined T_1 and B_1 maps, by acquiring a VFA sequence of spoiled gradient echo acquisitions.[35,43] As discussed above, fat is an ideal reference tissue in the breast because of its homogeneous T_1. A flip angle correction factor (which is proportional to B_1) can be calculated in a voxel if its true T_1 value is known (e.g., from a population average), by measuring T_1 from fitting VFA data to the gradient echo signal model (equation 3) using the nominal flip angles (those prescribed at the scanner console). This correction factor (κ) is given by:

$$\kappa = \frac{\cos^{-1}\left(e^{-TR/T_{1t}}\right)}{\cos^{-1}\left(e^{-TR/T_{1m}}\right)}, \tag{12.6}$$

where the subscript "t" and "m" denote the true and measured T_1 values for the reference tissue (fat), respectively. In these methods, the fat voxels are identified, and a value of κ is calculated for each fat voxel. The values for the rest of the FOV (i.e., all the voxels corresponding to parenchyma) are then interpolated from the surrounding fat voxels. The VFA data are then fit to the signal model again, this time using the correct flip angle for each voxel in the breast, leading to an accurate T_1 map. This method provides T_1 maps close to the "gold standard" IR T_1 maps, even in patients with dense breasts.[35] This method for obtaining T_1 and B_1 maps relies only on the assumption that the

flip angle correction factor will be constant for all angles, a reasonable assumption for the range of angles typically used in a VFA sequence.[44]

Other B_1 Mapping Methods

Other methods for in vivo B_1 mapping include the saturated double-angle method (SDAM),[45] dual refocusing echo acquisition mode (DREAM),[46] and mapping by Bloch–Siegert shift.[47] Nehrke et al compared RF shimming with DREAM, AFI, and SDAM.[48] The authors found that DREAM outperformed the other methods while significantly reducing acquisition time. Bloch–Siegert shift B_1 mapping offers the advantage of insensitivity to factors such as TR, T_1, and flip angle (DREAM has a weak dependence on T_1 and T_2), and has been shown to improve the accuracy of longitudinal T_1 measurements in the breast. In fact, there is potential to combine DREAM and Bloch–Siegert approaches to produce a new and more accurate method. One drawback of the DREAM and Bloch–Siegert B_1 mapping methods is that they require specialized sequences that are implemented through research software patches that are not currently widely available.

12.3 Calculation of Contrast Media Concentration

While the signal in a postcontrast DCE-MRI acquisition is a function of the concentration of contrast media, other factors affect the amount of signal enhancement in these images. The shortening of T_1 values in the presence of contrast media is described (in the fast-exchange regime) by the following equation:

$$\frac{1}{T_1(c)} = \frac{1}{T_{10}} + r_1 c, \tag{12.7}$$

where $T_1(c)$ is the T_1 in the presence of a concentration "c" of contrast media, T_{10} is the native T_1 of the tissue in question, and r_1 is the relaxivity of the contrast media agent, a value that is well characterized in the literature for most widely used contrast media agents. Simple inspection of equation (7) shows that a tissue with a larger native T_1 will have a larger change in T_1 for the same concentration of contrast media (and thus higher signal enhancement in a T_1-weighted image). Along with the native T_1 and the relaxivity and concentration of contrast media, the TR and flip angle of the spoiled gradient echo acquisition used for DCE-MRI (as shown in equation 3) will also affect the amount of signal enhancement seen in these images. In order to obtain images that are independent of acquisition parameters and of the native T_1 of the tissues being imaged, standard DCE-MR images are converted to images of contrast media concentration.

As mentioned above, the r_1 of each contrast agent can be found in the literature,[49,50] and the native T_1 of tissues can be measured using one of the methods described above. Once r_1 and T_{10} are known, the final step in estimating the concentration of contrast media is measurement of the postcontrast shortened T_1. Ideally, $T_1(c)$ would be measured directly by acquiring a series of T_1 maps following the administration of contrast media. However, this would require very fast T_1 mapping sequences, since contrast media concentration will be changing rapidly, especially in the time shortly after it is administered. In some areas of the body, where the volumes acquired are not large, this can be achieved.[51] Even if reasonably short T_1 mapping techniques were to be used, many of the acquired images would not be diagnostically useful, due to inadequate SNR or image contrast (i.e., at low flip angles). The alternative is to estimate postcontrast T_1 from signal changes in the routine clinical sequence and precontrast native T_1 measurements. This way, the standard clinical images are used for routine interpretation, while postprocessing is used to obtain estimates of T_1 at each time-point.

In a spoiled gradient echo sequence, the PSE as a function of time can be expressed as (from equation 3):

$$PSE(t) = \frac{S(t) - S_0}{S_0} = \frac{(E_1 - E_{10})(\cos é - 1)}{(E_{10} - 1)(E_1 \cos é - 1)}, \tag{12.8}$$

where $E_{10} = \exp(-TR/T_{10})$, $E_1 = \exp(-TR/T_1)$, T_{10} is the native T_1, T_1 is the postcontrast value, and we make the common simplifying assumption that T_2^* relaxation can be neglected. Equation (8) can be solved to obtain a nonlinear analytic solution for T_1:

$$\frac{1}{T_1(t)} = \frac{1}{TR} \log \left[\frac{PSE_t(E_{10}(1 - \cos é)}{1 + \cos é(PSE_t(E_{10} - 1) - 1)} \right]. \tag{12.9}$$

Equation (9) shows that it is possible to estimate postcontrast T_1 from the signal enhancement measured in a standard clinical sequence, the actual flip angle, and the native T_1. The value of postcontrast T_1 can then be inserted into equation (7) to obtain an estimate for the concentration of contrast media at each time point.

An alternative, and simpler approach, is to use a reference signal to estimate changes in T_1 (as described in the T_1 mapping section above).[15,31] As explained above, this method relies on the presence of a "reference tissue" with a known, and homogeneous, T_1 in the FOV and the following assumptions: $TR < T_1$, a sufficiently large flip angle (greater than 30°), and differences in T_2^* between the reference tissue and the tissue of interest are assumed to be low. Under these assumptions, the product of signal and T_1 is approximately constant ($S \times T_1 \approx$ constant). Therefore, changes in signal are directly and linearly related to changes in T_1. Under these conditions, the concentration of contrast media as a function of time can be written as:

$$C(t) \approx \frac{1}{r_1 T_{1ref} S_{ref}(t = 0)} (S(t) - S(t = 0)). \tag{12.10}$$

With the reference tissue method, concentration of contrast media can be calculated from signal changes in the DCE-MRI images and knowledge of the native T_1 of a reference tissue, either by direct measurement or by using a population average. This approach has been implemented using the liver and muscle as reference tissues,[31] and in the breast using fat as a reference.[15] Besides the conditions listed above, this method relies on the flip angle being the same at the tissue of interest and the reference tissue. Variations in the B_1 field across the relatively large FOV used in breast imaging may limit its accuracy in the breast.

12.3.1 Arterial Input Function

The AIF is the contrast media concentration ($C_A(t)$) as a function of time in the arterial blood supply following intravenous injection. The local AIF is $C_A(t)$ in local arteries feeding a suspicious lesion or a specific portion of the body, e.g., the internal mammary artery. Calculation of physiologic parameters such as K^{trans} from compartmental models (e.g., the two-compartment model) requires accurate measurement of the AIF.

The contrast media AIF can vary significantly for a single subject scanned at different times *and* between subjects. Variations in cardiac output are a major contributor to variability in the AIF. In healthy individuals, cardiac output varies from 4.0 to 8.0 L/minute,[52] and in patients who are not in good health, the range can be even larger. The local AIF near a cancer may be even more variable. Fan et al[14] showed that in tumors grown on rat hind limb, the standard deviation of the peak amplitude of the local AIF measured using a reference tissue and artery was about 40% of the mean ($n = 8$). Yang et al[53] showed large inter-patient and intrapatient variability in the AIF in bone metastases using a multiple reference tissue method. For the area under the first pass of the AIF, the within-subject coefficient of variation (relative standard deviation) was 11% (range, 0.2–20.8%) and the between-subject coefficient of variation was 24%, with values ranging from approximately 50 to 200% of the mean. Lavini and Verhoeff[54] demonstrated that the AIF measured directly in the superior sagittal sinus has a very large interpatient range, with relative standard deviation of AIF amplitude of 57% or higher (depending on protocol) and a range of a factor of 5. These data demonstrate that there are large variations in the AIF that can produce diagnostic errors as well as large errors in quantitative parameters derived from contrast media enhancement kinetics, such as K^{trans} and v_e (contrast media fractional distribution volume) if they are not properly accounted for. In some patients (especially the many who are more than one standard deviation from the mean), these errors will result in cancers missed by MRI, while in other patients benign lesions will be misdiagnosed as having high perfusion/permeability characteristic of cancers.

Several approaches are used to measure the AIF:

Population AIF

Population AIFs have been constructed from measurements of the arterial concentration of contrast media in multiple patients and producing a population average. A convenient functional form of the AIF can be used for quantitative analysis of DCE-MRI data, e.g., as part of two-compartment analysis. The most commonly used population AIF was developed by Parker et al[55] using the sum of two gaussian functions plus an exponential modulated by sigmoid function to model the AIF with both the first and second passes:

$$C_p(t) = \sum_{n=1}^{2} \frac{A_n}{ó_n \sqrt{2\eth}} \exp \left(-\frac{(t - T_n)^2}{2ó_n^2} \right)$$
$$+ \frac{áexp(-ât)}{1 + \exp(-s(t - ô))}, \tag{12.11}$$

where A_n, T_n, and σ_n are the scaling constants, centers, and widths of the nth gaussian; α and β are the amplitude and decay constant of the exponential; and s and τ are the width and center of the sigmoid, respectively. A number of other population AIFs have been published, with different functional forms. More than a quarter century ago, Tofts and Kermode[56] derived the population AIF as bi-exponential decay functions. Although the bi-exponential AIF is easy to use, it lacks an initial rising phase. A few years later, Su et al[57] added a linear growth phase between time zero and time to the peak to bi-exponential AIF, which became a piecewise function. In 1999, Simpson et al[58] introduced a rising phase to model the AIF by combining a surge function to an exponential function, which was later modified by Yankeelov et al[59] to combine the surge function with bi-exponential functions. All of these AIF models, except Parker's, could only be used to describe the first pass of contrast agent circulation, and neglected the second passes. Recently, Wang et al[60] developed a new mathematical model with eight parameters (two parameters less than Parker's 10 parameter model):

$$C_p(t) = A_1 n(1+t)\exp(-\beta t)(1 + \sum_{n=1}^{2}\frac{A_n}{\sigma_n\sqrt{2\pi}}\exp(-(t - T_n)^2/2\sigma_n^2)) \tag{12.12}$$

where A and A_n are scaling constants, T_n and σ_n are centers and widths of the nth gaussian function for first and second pass, and β is the decay constant of the exponential describing the washout of the contrast agent. Please note that for this model $C_p(t) = 0$ at $t = 0$.

Reference Region Methods

These methods were developed to infer the AIF from measurements of contrast media concentration versus time in normal tissue with known physiological properties. Reference tissue methods were originally used for analysis of PET data—to avoid the need for extensive blood sampling for measurements of plasma concentration of PET tracers.[61] They were initially adapted for MRI by Kovar et al.[62] Reference tissue methods do not require measurements of high contrast media concentration in an artery. They provide high SNR because a large volume of relatively homogeneous normal tissue can be used, and they provide a local AIF for each subject since a reference tissue close to the cancer can be selected. The original "reference tissue method" for MRI[62] relied on the literature values for the volume transfer constant (K^{trans}) and the contrast media distribution volume (v_e) in a reference tissue as a starting point. Assuming that contrast media concentration as a function of time in the reference tissue (e.g., muscle; $C_R(t)$) is well approximated by a "two-compartment model,"[63,64,65] the AIF ($C_p(t)$) can be calculated from $C_R(t)$. One can approximate that:

$$C_p(t) = \frac{1}{K^{trans}}\frac{dC_R(t)}{dt} + \frac{C_R(t)}{v_e}, \tag{12.13}$$

where K^{trans} and v_e is volume transfer constant and the fractional distribution volume of the contrast agent in muscle, respectively. Later, Yankeelov et al[59] developed a "reference region method" based on an integral form of the two-compart-

ment model without explicitly calculating $C_p(t)$. The reliance of initial reference tissue/reference region models on literature values of K^{trans} and v_e can cause problems, since these parameters may differ significantly between subjects, even in normal tissues, e.g., muscle. More recent reference tissue and reference region methods avoid reliance on literature values of K^{trans} by analyzing contrast media dynamics in multiple reference tissues to determine a consensus AIF.[53,59,66] These methods are more robust, although early versions of this approach used literature values of v_e to scale the AIF.

A recent study of patients who received both a low dose (0.015 mmol/kg) and standard dose (0.085 mmol/kg) of DCE-MRI scans showed that AIFs calculated from reference tissue following a standard dose of contrast media (to minimize T_2^* and water exchange effects) correlated strongly with AIFs measured directly from the femoral artery following a low dose of contrast media.[60] However, reference tissue methods require multiple calculations and can produce significant systematic and random errors.[67] Therefore, this approach must be used carefully and should be avoided in cases where SNR is modest (▶ Fig. 12.3).

12.4 Pharmacokinetic Analysis

12.4.1 Tofts Two-Compartment Model

The two-compartment model, originally developed by Kety[65] and adapted for MRI by Tofts et al,[65,68] is the most widely used model for analysis of DCE-MRI data. The simple Tofts model assumes that contrast agent molecules exchange between two well-mixed compartments—a blood plasma compartment, and an extravascular compartment (▶ Fig. 12.4). The rate of exchange is determined by the "forward transfer rate constant," K^{trans} (per minute). Signal enhancement in the simple Tofts model is assumed to come from contrast agent molecules in the extravascular extravascular space (EES) only; the contribution to enhancement from the blood plasma compartment is assumed to be negligible. The model assumes that the low-molecular-weight gadolinium complexes typically used for MRI do not enter cells. Some recent work suggests that there is some cellular uptake[69] but it is generally believed that intracellular contrast agent concentrations are too low to affect DCE-MRI data.[70] The extended Tofts model[64] includes a term accounting for blood plasma volume, v_p:

$$C(t) = v_p\, C_p(t) + K^{trans}\int_0^t C_p(\tau)\exp\left[\frac{-K^{trans}(t-\tau)}{v_e}\right]d\tau \tag{12.14}$$

where t is time, K^{trans} is the volume transfer constant between blood plasma and EES, v_e is the extravascular extracellular fractional volume, and $C_p(t)$ is the AIF–blood plasma contrast agent concentration. Equation (14) is based on the hypothesis that when a very sharp bolus of contrast media enters tissue (e.g., a tumor), contrast media diffuses from capillaries into the EES, and subsequently $C(t)$ decays exponentially with a time constant of "K^{trans}/v_e," as contrast media is washed out of the tissue by blood flow. Because, in practice, the AIF, $C_p(t)$, is not very sharp, $C(t)$ is given by a convolution of $C_p(t)$ with this

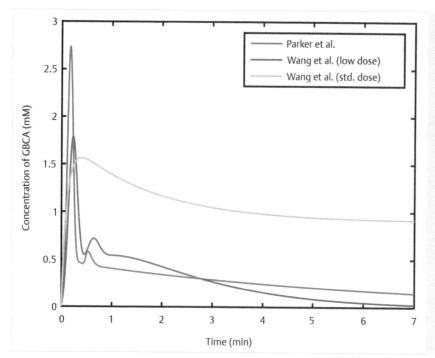

Fig. 12.3 Plots of AIF models proposed by Parker et al[56] and Wang et al.[61]

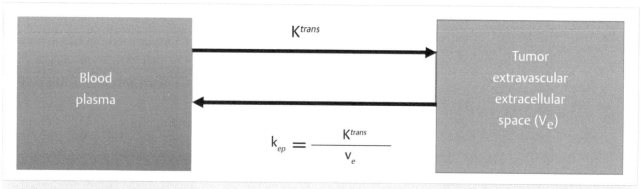

Fig. 12.4 Diagram of the two-compartment model; the transfer of contrast media from the blood plasma to the tumor EES is described by the volume transfer constant K^{trans}, and the rate of backflow of contrast media from the EES to blood plasma is given by k_{ep}.

exponential decay. $C_p(t)$ is related to the contrast agent concentration in blood vessels $C_b(t)$ through the hematocrit (Hct) as:

$$C_p(t) = C_b(t)/(1 - Hct) \tag{12.15}$$

The hematocrit in humans varies; it is normally approximately 0.45 in adults, and often lower in cancer patients. In a study by Yang et al, the hematocrit for 16 patients with prostate cancer had a mean of 0.365 (range, 0.264–0.477).[71]

12.4.2 Brix Model

The Brix model[72] was proposed for the analysis of DCE-MRI data in breast tumors. It is based on the exchange model proposed by Morales and Smith[73] (whereas the models described above are based on the Kety model); it has an independent measure for relative blood flow F/r (per minute) in addition to K^{trans} (per minute) (which in this model represents only

permeability), v_e, and v_p. The parameter "r" is a constant volume fraction between arterial, venous, and tissue concentration:

$$v_p \frac{dC_c(t)}{dt} = \frac{F}{r}\left(C_p(t) - C_c(t)\right) - K^{trans}\left(C_c(t) - C_e(t)\right) \tag{12.16}$$

$$v_e \frac{dC_e(t)}{dt} = K^{trans}\left(C_c(t) - C_e(t)\right) \tag{12.17}$$

$$C_t = v_p C_p + v_e C_e \tag{12.18}$$

Here C_C is the concentration of contrast media in the plasma in the tissue of interest. A complete derivation of this model can be found in Brix et al.[72]

12.4.3 Patlak Model

The Patlak model[74,75] was originally developed to describe the blood-to-brain transfer of contrast media. This model relies on the following assumptions[75]: (1) there is a single source of contrast media, the plasma, which may vary with time; (2) the tracer may exchange (relatively rapidly) between the plasma compartment into several exchangeable compartments; from these compartments, the tracer may move back to the plasma compartment or into another tissue compartment; (3) the tracer may enter an irreversible compartment from the plasma or exchange compartments; however, after entering this region, the tracer may not leave. The Patlak model can be seen as a special case of the Tofts-based models where there is no backflow from the EES into the blood plasma compartment. This means that the concentration in tissue can be expressed as:

$$C_t(t) = v_p C_p(t) + K^{trans} \int_0^t C_p(\hat{o}) d\hat{o} \qquad (12.19)$$

In general, the assumptions made in the Patlak model do not apply to breast tumors, specifically the assumption that there is no backflow from the tumor compartment to the plasma compartment. However, if analysis is restricted to the time immediately following the arrival of contrast media in the breast, and the data are acquired with high temporal resolution (e.g., using the ultrafast protocols described in Chapter 3), unidirectional models, such as the Patlak model, may be useful. That is, when the concentration of contrast media in plasma is much larger than in the tissue compartment, backflow into the plasma compartment may be neglected, and the Patlak model provides a relatively simple method for the estimation of K^{trans}. However, if these conditions are not met, and backflow is not negligible, the estimate of K^{trans} obtained may be biased.

12.4.4 Shutter Speed Model

Clinically approved MRI contrast agents are generally assumed to remain extracellular, with some exceptions.[76] Analysis of DCE-MRI data generally assumes that there is fast exchange across cell membranes, so that all water molecules, including intracellular water molecules, have equal access to sites on the contrast agent (usually gadolinium). As a result, the longitudinal relaxation rate for all water molecules is assumed to decrease by the same amount when contrast agents enter the tissue. This means that interactions between water protons and contrast agent molecules are approximated to be in the "fast exchange limit." However, this approximation only applies when the exchange rate of water between the intracellular and extracellular environments (the inverse of the average time that water protons spend inside of cells; $1/\tau$) is much greater than the difference between longitudinal relaxation rates of intracellular and extracellular water protons:

$$\frac{1}{\hat{o}} \ll R_{1(intracellular)} - R_{1(extracellular)}. \qquad (12.20)$$

When equation (18) does not apply, the fast exchange limit does not apply and the T_1 shortening produced by the contrast agent decreases, i.e., the effective relaxivity of the contrast agent decreases. This is particularly important when the extracellular concentration of contrast agent molecules is high (intracellular concentration is assumed to be zero), and therefore

extracellular water has a very short T_1. In this case, water exchange across cell membranes is not fast enough to maintain the longitudinal relaxation rate in the fast exchange limit. As a result, relaxation rate of intracellular water is much less effected by the contrast agent than the relaxation rate of extracellular water, and the effective relaxivity of the contrast agent is reduced. This has significant consequences for measurements of pharmacokinetic parameters. For example, in breast cancers with high blood flow and capillary permeability, high extracellular contrast media concentrations can lead to significant underestimates of K^{trans} [77] calculated from the Tofts model. Alternatively, in normal tissues with lower blood flow and capillary permeability, the fast exchange approximation applies, and K^{trans} can be measured more accurately. Work of Springer and co-workers[76,78,79] suggests that models that account for water exchange effects (referred to as "shutter speed models") can increase the diagnostic accuracy of DCE-MRI, especially in the case of breast cancer. In particular, the error in K^{trans} measurements due to water exchange is larger in cancers than in normal breast parenchyma, and the discrepancy between the "true" and measured values of K^{trans} can be a useful marker for breast cancer.[80] Shutter speed modeling of DCE-MRI data also provides an estimate of the "intracellular water lifetime"—a measure of the average intracellular residence time of water protons. A number of preclinical and clinical studies suggest that "intracellular water lifetime" reflects changes in cell physiology that occur when cells are transformed,[81,82] and therefore may be a useful biomarker for cancer.

12.4.5 Model-free Impulse Response Analysis

DCE-MRI data are frequently analyzed by using the Tofts model to extract physiological parameters. Ideally, one would like to study contrast media uptake and washout from the tumor itself, without systematic errors or bias caused by the use of inappropriate physiologic models and incorrect AIF. Therefore, it is desirable to separate the effects of the AIF from the kinetics of uptake and washout of contrast media. This can be done if the tissue is treated as a system that gives a linear, time-invariant, and causal response to the AIF. The contrast concentration curve versus time ($C_t(t)$) can be considered as the convolution between the AIF ($C_p(t)$) and the impulse response function ($C_\delta(t)$), i.e., mathematically:

$$C_t(t) = C_p(t)C_\delta(t) = \int_0^t C_p(\hat{o})C_\delta(t - \hat{o})d\hat{o}. \qquad (12.21)$$

Theoretically, the AIF can be deconvolved from the contrast concentration curve so that the impulse response function can be determined to characterize tissue contrast media uptake and washout. However, deconvolution methods are very sensitive to experimental noise. Therefore, it is difficult to accurately measure the impulse response function from experimental DCE-MRI data. In practice, numerical curve fitting is often applied to equation (19) to determine impulse response functions $C_\delta(t)$ for specific models of contrast media dynamics. For example, in Tofts model, the impulse response function is just an exponential decay:

$$C_{\tilde{a}}(t) = K^{trans} \exp\left(-\frac{K^{trans}}{ve} t\right), \qquad (12.22)$$

where K^{trans} is the volume transfer constant between blood plasma and EES, and v_e is the extravascular extracellular fractional volume. However, this simple exponential decay function from the Tofts model may not be appropriate for normal breast tissue and breast cancers. Fan and Karczmar[83] introduced a general empirical method to deconvolve the AIF from the $C(t)$. The deconvolution method is illustrated in ▶ Fig. 12.5, and can be summarized as follows: (1) the experimentally measured $C(t)$ is fitted using the EMM described above, (2) an AIF is derived from reference tissue method, and (3) the impulse response function is calculated by deconvolving the AIF from the EMM fits to $C(t)$.

Due to the complexity of the calculations, impulse response analysis has not been widely used for clinical DCE-MRI data as yet. Nevertheless, Schabel[84] demonstrated that a unified impulse response analysis (gamma capillary transit time model) is sensitive to the physiology of brain tumors and may have advantages compared to other modeling methods.

12.4.6 AATH Model

The adiabatic approximation to the tissue homogeneity (AATH) model was originally proposed by St Lawrence and Lee for the analysis of water exchange in the brain.[85] This model assumes that the tracer concentration in parenchymal tissue changes slowly relative to the change in the capillaries. This model includes a parameter (T_c) for the time it takes blood to pass from the arterial to the venous side of the capillary bed (the "transit time"). This model can be expressed as:

$$C_t(t) = F_P C_p(t) R_{AATH}(t), \qquad (12.23)$$

where F_p is the blood plasma flow (mL/(mL tissue)/ min), and R_{AATH} is the AATH impulse response function given by:

$$R_{AATH}(t) = \begin{cases} 0 & t \leq 0 \\ 1 & 0 < t \leq T_c \\ E\exp\left(\frac{-EF_p}{v_e}(t - T_c)\right) & t > T_c \end{cases} \qquad (12.24)$$

where E is the extraction fraction, the fraction of tracer extracted from the intravascular space to the EES in the first pass of the tracer through the capillary bed. For $t > T_c$, the impulse response function for the AATH model (equation 22) is identical to that in the Kety model.[86] Fusco et al[87] suggested that the AATH model may provide a better fit to clinical breast DCE-MRI data than the Tofts and Brix models when imaging with high temporal resolution, although their results were not conclusive, partly due to the relatively small sample size analyzed ($N = 4$).

12.5 Requirements for Pharmacokinetic Analysis

In order to obtain reliable and unbiased estimates of pharmacokinetic parameters, certain requirements should be met with regard to the DCE-MRI acquisition. These requirements will depend on the model being used as well as the analysis methods employed. In general, high temporal resolution is desirable to characterize the transfer of contrast media from the plasma compartment to the tissue compartment. In addition, the duration of imaging postcontrast media injection must be long enough to allow accurate measurement of parameters related to washout of contrast from the tissue compartment(s).

Knight et al[88] studied the effect of temporal resolution and total acquisition duration on estimates of pharmacokinetic parameters in an anthropomorphic prostate-mimicking flow phantom. They found large underestimation errors in wash-in parameters (up to 40%) if the temporal resolution was slower than 16 seconds per image, while washout rates did not vary across the temporal resolutions studied (from 2 to 24 seconds). Errors in the estimated values of K^{trans} were below 14% if temporal resolution was 8.1 seconds per image or greater, and acquisition durations of 360 seconds or greater. Errors in v_e were under 12% for temporal resolution of at least 16 seconds per image and scan durations of 360 seconds or larger.

Kershaw and Cheng[86] showed that to ensure minimal bias (less than 5% error) when using the AATH model, a temporal resolution of 1.5 seconds is necessary; this requirement can be relaxed to 6-second temporal resolution, if the estimated transit time need not be measured with high accuracy.

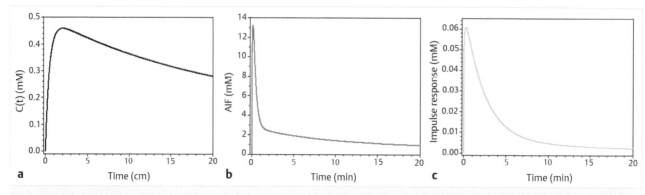

Fig. 12.5 Example plots of the concentration of GBCA in the tissue of interest **(a)**, AIF **(b)**, and the impulse response function **(c)**.

Table 12.1 Summary of representative clinical studies analyzing the utility of pharmacokinetic analysis of DCE-MRI of the breast

Study	Model	Number of patients	Findings
Radjenovic et al[90]	Brix	52	K^{trans} and k_{ep} were significantly higher in high-grade tumors (grade 3 vs. grade 1 and 2)
Furman-Haran et al[91]	Tofts	121	K^{trans} had sensitivity of 93% and specificity of 96% for distinguishing benign lesions and IDC, and increased from low-grade to high-grade DCIS
Padhani et al[92]	Tofts	25	K^{trans} after two cycles of NAC predicted clinicopathologic response—0.94 area under the ROC curve (AUC)
Vincensini et al[93]	Tofts	92	k_{ep} was significantly higher in malignant lesions with 95% sensitivity and 85% specificity
El Khouli et al[94]	Extended Tofts	95	K^{trans} (AUC = 0.76) and k_{ep} (AUC = 0.92) had significant differences between malignant and benign lesions
Schabel et al[95]	Extended Tofts	74	K^{trans} and k_{ep} performed well in classifying lesions and had AUCs of 0.88 and 0.89, respectively. When combining both parameters, sensitivity and specificity were 91 and 85% with an AUC of 0.92
Ah-See et al[96]	Tofts	28	Changes in K^{trans} and k_{ep} correlated with final clinical and pathological response to NAC. Change in K^{trans} predicted pathologic nonresponse with 94% sensitivity, 82% specificity, and a 0.93 AUC
Li et al[97]	Tofts, extended Tofts, fast exchange regime	28	k_{ep} was significantly different between pathologic complete responders and nonresponders after one cycle of NAC, with an AUC of 0.78 with the Tofts model

Abbreviations: DCIS, ductal carcinoma in situ; IDC, invasive ductal carcinoma; NAC, neoadjuvant chemotherapy.

Planey et al[89] showed that the temporal resolution requirements can be relaxed when using a reference region model for the analysis of clinical breast DCE-MRI. They showed that errors in pharmacokinetic parameters of less than 20% resulted when they analyzed data simulated to have 36-second temporal resolution, when compared to the estimates from data acquired clinically with 16-second resolution. Heisen et al[13] also showed, in a preclinical study, that a reference tissue method can be used to relax the temporal sampling requirements of pharmacokinetic analysis. For example, use of a data-derived AIF leads to significantly decreased error in K^{trans} (1–5%) when data are acquired with low temporal resolution (60 seconds) relative to using a population-based AIF (15–20% error).[13]

These results highlight the need to understand the effects of acquisition protocols on estimates of pharmacokinetic parameters. If the data are acquired with a temporal resolution that is too low, or the scan duration is not sufficient, the estimated parameters may have large biases and errors. While standard clinical acquisition protocols do not usually employ sufficiently high temporal resolution for pharmacokinetic analysis, analysis methods such as reference region approaches may be employed to reduce bias in the kinetic parameters.

12.6 Summaries of the Most Effective Diagnostic Parameters from Pharmacokinetic Analysis

Several studies have analyzed the performance of pharmacokinetic parameters in the discrimination of malignant and benign lesions, as well as in the prediction of response to neoadjuvant chemotherapy. ▶ Table 12.1 includes some examples of these studies, the number of patients imaged, the pharmacokinetic model used, and a summary of their findings.

12.7 Future of DCE-MRI

DCE-MRI is by far the most powerful tool for early detection of breast cancers. Clinical applications of DCE-MRI are likely to expand significantly in the next few years, as MRI screening is prescribed for more women with dense breasts and/or elevated breast cancer risk. However, despite the clinical importance of current DCE-MRI methods, improvements in sensitivity and specificity are needed, particularly as more women are screened with MRI. As a result, there is tremendous effort by researchers and manufacturers to improve both acquisition and analysis of DCE-MRI data. This effort from many laboratories has resulted in significant progress, and many new options are now available. The challenge in the next few years will be to develop standardized clinical protocols. While methods used at each hospital and academic center may differ, these methods must be harmonized to produce the same diagnosis regardless of the general physiology and anatomy of the patient, the scanner used, and the methods used for data acquisition and analysis. This harmonization process will require collaboration of the different labs and clinical sites to produce optimal solutions for patients.

References

[1] Furman-Haran E, Degani H. Parametric analysis of breast MRI. J Comput Assist Tomogr. 2002; 26(3):376–386

[2] Hauth EAM, Stockamp C, Maderwald S, et al. Evaluation of the three-time-point method for diagnosis of breast lesions in contrast-enhanced MR mammography. Clin Imaging. 2006; 30(3):160–165

[3] Kelcz F, Furman-Haran E, Grobgeld D, Degani H. Clinical testing of high-spatial-resolution parametric contrast-enhanced MR imaging of the breast. AJR Am J Roentgenol. 2002; 179(6):1485–1492

[4] Jansen SA, Shimauchi A, Zak L, et al. Kinetic curves of malignant lesions are not consistent across MRI systems: need for improved standardization of breast dynamic contrast-enhanced MRI acquisition. AJR Am J Roentgenol. 2009; 193(3):832–839

[5] Chen W, Giger ML, Bick U, Newstead GM. Automatic identification and classification of characteristic kinetic curves of breast lesions on DCE-MRI. Med Phys. 2006; 33(8):2878–2887

[6] Esserman L, Hylton N, George T, Weidner N. Contrast-enhanced magnetic resonance imaging to assess tumor histopathology and angiogenesis in breast carcinoma. Breast J. 1999; 5(1):13–21

[7] Lee SH, Kim JH, Cho N, et al. Multilevel analysis of spatiotemporal association features for differentiation of tumor enhancement patterns in breast DCE-MRI. Med Phys. 2010; 37(8):3940–3956

[8] Li K-L, Henry RG, Wilmes LJ, et al. Kinetic assessment of breast tumors using high spatial resolution signal enhancement ratio (SER) imaging. Magn Reson Med. 2007; 58(3):572–581

[9] Hylton N. Dynamic contrast-enhanced magnetic resonance imaging as an imaging biomarker. J Clin Oncol. 2006; 24(20):3293–3298

[10] Hylton NM, Blume JD, Bernreuter WK, et al. ACRIN 6657 Trial Team and I-SPY 1 TRIAL Investigators. Locally advanced breast cancer: MR imaging for prediction of response to neoadjuvant chemotherapy–results from ACRIN 6657/I-SPY TRIAL. Radiology. 2012; 263(3):663–672

[11] Pineda FD, Medved M, Wang S, et al. Ultrafast bilateral DCE-MRI of the breast with conventional Fourier sampling: preliminary evaluation of semi-quantitative analysis. Acad Radiol. 2016; 23(9):1137–1144

[12] Mus RD, Borelli C, Bult P, et al. Time to enhancement derived from ultrafast breast MRI as a novel parameter to discriminate benign from malignant breast lesions. Eur J Radiol. 2017; 89:90–96

[13] Heisen M, Fan X, Buurman J, van Riel NAW, Karczmar GS, ter Haar Romeny BM. The use of a reference tissue arterial input function with low-temporal-resolution DCE-MRI data. Phys Med Biol. 2010; 55(16):4871–4883

[14] Fan X, Haney CR, Mustafi D, et al. Use of a reference tissue and blood vessel to measure the arterial input function in DCEMRI. Magn Reson Med. 2010; 64 (6):1821–1826

[15] Fan X, Medved M, Karczmar GS, et al. Diagnosis of suspicious breast lesions using an empirical mathematical model for dynamic contrast-enhanced MRI. Magn Reson Imaging. 2007; 25(5):593–603

[16] Fan X, Medved M, River JN, et al. New model for analysis of dynamic contrast-enhanced MRI data distinguishes metastatic from nonmetastatic transplanted rodent prostate tumors. Magn Reson Med. 2004; 51(3):487–494

[17] Jansen SA, Fan X, Karczmar GS, Abe H, Schmidt RA, Newstead GM. Differentiation between benign and malignant breast lesions detected by bilateral dynamic contrast-enhanced MRI: a sensitivity and specificity study. Magn Reson Med. 2008; 59(4):747–754

[18] Jansen SA, Fan X, Karczmar GS, et al. DCEMRI of breast lesions: is kinetic analysis equally effective for both mass and nonmass-like enhancement? Med Phys. 2008; 35(7):3102–3109

[19] Moate PJ, Dougherty L, Schnall MD, Landis RJ, Boston RC. A modified logistic model to describe gadolinium kinetics in breast tumors. Magn Reson Imaging. 2004; 22(4):467–473

[20] Platel B, Mus R, Welte T, et al. Automated Characterization of breast lesions imaged with an ultrafast DCE-MR protocol. IEEE T Med Imaging. 2014; 33(2):225–232

[21] Orth RC, Bankson J, Price R, Jackson EF. Comparison of single- and dual-tracer pharmacokinetic modeling of dynamic contrast-enhanced MRI data using low, medium, and high molecular weight contrast agents. Magn Reson Med. 2007; 58(4):705–716

[22] Gliozzi AS, Mazzetti S, Delsanto PP, Regge D, Stasi M. Phenomenological universalities: a novel tool for the analysis of dynamic contrast enhancement in magnetic resonance imaging. Phys Med Biol. 2011; 56(3):573–586

[23] Fram EK, Herfkens RJ, Johnson GA, et al. Rapid calculation of T1 using variable flip angle gradient refocused imaging. Magn Reson Imaging. 1987; 5(3):201–208

[24] Deoni SCL, Rutt BK, Peters TM. Rapid combined T1 and T2 mapping using gradient recalled acquisition in the steady state. Magn Reson Med. 2003; 49(3):515–526

[25] Schabel MC, Morrell GR. Uncertainty in T(1) mapping using the variable flip angle method with two flip angles. Phys Med Biol. 2009; 54(1):N1–N8

[26] Cheng H-LM, Wright GA. Rapid high-resolution T(1) mapping by variable flip angles: accurate and precise measurements in the presence of radiofrequency field inhomogeneity. Magn Reson Med. 2006; 55(3):566–574

[27] Brown RW, Cheng Y-CN, Haacke EM, Thompson MR, Venkatesan R. Magnetic Resonance Imaging: Physical Principles and Sequence Design. Hoboken, NJ: Wiley; 2014

[28] Barral JK, Gudmundson E, Stikov N, Etezadi-Amoli M, Stoica P, Nishimura DG. A robust methodology for in vivo T1 mapping. Magn Reson Med. 2010; 64(4):1057–1067

[29] Henderson E, McKinnon G, Lee TY, Rutt BK. A fast 3D look-locker method for volumetric T1 mapping. Magn Reson Imaging. 1999; 17(8):1163–1171

[30] Messroghli DR, Radjenovic A, Kozerke S, Higgins DM, Sivananthan MU, Ridgway JP. Modified Look-Locker inversion recovery (MOLLI) for high-resolution T1 mapping of the heart. Magn Reson Med. 2004; 52(1):141–146

[31] Medved M, Karczmar G, Yang C, et al. Semiquantitative analysis of dynamic contrast enhanced MRI in cancer patients: variability and changes in tumor tissue over time. J Magn Reson Imaging. 2004; 20(1):122–128

[32] Merchant TE, Thelissen GR, de Graaf PW, Nieuwenhuizen CW, Kievit HC, Den Otter W. Application of a mixed imaging sequence for MR imaging characterization of human breast disease. Acta Radiol. 1993; 34(4):356–361

[33] Graham SJ, Ness S, Hamilton BS, Bronskill MJ. Magnetic resonance properties of ex vivo breast tissue at 1.5 T. Magn Reson Med. 1997; 38(4):669–677

[34] Rakow-Penner R, Daniel B, Yu H, Sawyer-Glover A, Glover GH. Relaxation times of breast tissue at 1.5 T and 3 T measured using IDEAL. J Magn Reson Imaging. 2006; 23(1):87–91

[35] Pineda FD, Medved M, Fan X, Karczmar GSB. B1 and T1 mapping of the breast with a reference tissue method. Magn Reson Med. 2016; 75(4):1565–1573

[36] Kuhl CK, Kooijman H, Gieseke J, Schild HH. Effect of B1 inhomogeneity on breast MR imaging at 3.0 T. Radiology. 2007; 244(3):929–930

[37] Azlan CA, Di Giovanni P, Ahearn TS, Semple SI, Gilbert FJ, Redpath TW. B1 transmission-field inhomogeneity and enhancement ratio errors in dynamic contrast-enhanced MRI (DCE-MRI) of the breast at 3 T. J Magn Reson Imaging. 2010; 31(1):234–239

[38] Willinek WA, Gieseke J, Kukuk GM, et al. Dual-source parallel radiofrequency excitation body MR imaging compared with standard MR imaging at 3.0 T: initial clinical experience. Radiology. 2010; 256(3):966–975

[39] Rahbar H, Partridge SC, Demartini WB, Gutierrez RL, Parsian S, Lehman CD. Improved B1 homogeneity of 3 Tesla breast MRI using dual-source parallel radiofrequency excitation. J Magn Reson Imaging. 2012; 35(5):1222–1226

[40] Schabel MC, Parker DL. Uncertainty and bias in contrast concentration measurements using spoiled gradient echo pulse sequences. Phys Med Biol. 2008; 53(9):2345–2373

[41] Yarnykh VL. Actual flip-angle imaging in the pulsed steady state: a method for rapid three-dimensional mapping of the transmitted radiofrequency field. Magn Reson Med. 2007; 57(1):192–200

[42] Nehrke K. On the steady-state properties of actual flip angle imaging (AFI). Magn Reson Med. 2009; 61(1):84–92

[43] Sung K, Saranathan M, Daniel BL, Hargreaves BA. Simultaneous T(1) and B(1) (+) mapping using reference region variable flip angle imaging. Magn Reson Med. 2013; 70(4):954–961

[44] Deoni SCL. Correction of main and transmit magnetic field (B0 and B1) inhomogeneity effects in multicomponent-driven equilibrium single-pulse observation of T1 and T2. Magn Reson Med. 2011; 65(4):1021–1035

[45] Cunningham CH, Pauly JM, Nayak KS. Saturated double-angle method for rapid B1 + mapping. Magn Reson Med. 2006; 55(6):1326–1333

[46] Nehrke K, Börnert P. DREAM–a novel approach for robust, ultrafast, multislice B1 mapping. Magn Reson Med. 2012; 68(5):1517–1526

[47] Sacolick LI, Wiesinger F, Hancu I, Vogel MW. B1 mapping by Bloch-Siegert shift. Magn Reson Med. 2010; 63(5):1315–1322

[48] Nehrke K, Sprinkart AM, Börnert P. An in vivo comparison of the DREAM sequence with current RF shim technology. MAGMA. 2015; 28(2):185–194

[49] Rohrer M, Bauer H, Mintorovitch J, Requardt M, Weinmann H-J. Comparison of magnetic properties of MRI contrast media solutions at different magnetic field strengths. Invest Radiol. 2005; 40(11):715–724

[50] Pintaske J, Martirosian P, Graf H, et al. Relaxivity of Gadopentetate Dimeglumine (Magnevist), Gadobutrol (Gadovist), and Gadobenate Dimeglumine (MultiHance) in human blood plasma at 0.2, 1.5, and 3 Tesla. Invest Radiol. 2006; 41(3):213–221

[51] Treier R, Steingoetter A, Fried M, Schwizer W, Boesiger P. Optimized and combined T1 and B1 mapping technique for fast and accurate T1 quantification in contrast-enhanced abdominal MRI. Magn Reson Med. 2007; 57(3):568–576

[52] Zhang JL, Rusinek H, Bokacheva L, Chen Q, Storey P, Lee VS. Use of cardiac output to improve measurement of input function in quantitative dynamic contrast-enhanced MRI. J Magn Reson Imaging. 2009; 30(3):656–665

[53] Yang C, Karczmar GS, Medved M, Stadler WM. Multiple reference tissue method for contrast agent arterial input function estimation. Magn Reson Med. 2007; 58(6):1266–1275

[54] Lavini C, Verhoeff JJC. Reproducibility of the gadolinium concentration measurements and of the fitting parameters of the vascular input function in the superior sagittal sinus in a patient population. Magn Reson Imaging. 2010; 28 (10):1420–1430

[55] Parker GJM, Roberts C, Macdonald A, et al. Experimentally-derived functional form for a population-averaged high-temporal-resolution arterial input function for dynamic contrast-enhanced MRI. Magn Reson Med. 2006; 56(5): 993–1000

[56] Tofts PS, Kermode AG. Measurement of the blood-brain barrier permeability and leakage space using dynamic MR imaging. 1. Fundamental concepts. Magn Reson Med. 1991; 17(2):357–367

[57] Su M-Y, Jao J-C, Nalcioglu O. Measurement of vascular volume fraction and blood-tissue permeability constants with a pharmacokinetic model: studies in rat muscle tumors with dynamic Gd-DTPA enhanced MRI. Magn Reson Med. 1994; 32(6):714–724

[58] Simpson NE, He Z, Evelhoch JL, He Z, Evelhoch JL. Deuterium NMR tissue perfusion measurements using the tracer uptake approach: I. Optimization of methods. Magn Reson Med. 1999; 42(1):42–52

[59] Yankeelov TE, Luci JJ, Lepage M, et al. Quantitative pharmacokinetic analysis of DCE-MRI data without an arterial input function: a reference region model. Magn Reson Imaging. 2005; 23(4):519–529

[60] Wang S, Fan X, Medved M, et al. Arterial input functions (AIFs) measured directly from arteries with low and standard doses of contrast agent, and AIFs derived from reference tissues. Magn Reson Imaging. 2016; 34(2):197–203

[61] Lammertsma AA, Bench CJ, Hume SP, et al. Comparison of methods for analysis of clinical [11C]raclopride studies. J Cereb Blood Flow Metab. 1996; 16(1):42–52

[62] Kovar DA, Lewis M, Karczmar GS. A new method for imaging perfusion and contrast extraction fraction: input functions derived from reference tissues. J Magn Reson Imaging. 1998; 8(5):1126–1134

[63] Tofts PS, Berkowitz B, Schnall MD. Quantitative analysis of dynamic Gd-DTPA enhancement in breast tumors using a permeability model. Magn Reson Med. 1995; 33(4):564–568

[64] Tofts PS, Brix G, Buckley DL, et al. Estimating kinetic parameters from dynamic contrast-enhanced T(1)-weighted MRI of a diffusable tracer: standardized quantities and symbols. J Magn Reson Imaging. 1999; 10(3):223–232

[65] Kety SS. The theory and applications of the exchange of inert gas at the lungs and tissues. Pharmacol Rev. 1951; 3(1):1–41

[66] Yang C, Karczmar GS, Medved M, Stadler WM. Estimating the arterial input function using two reference tissues in dynamic contrast-enhanced MRI studies: fundamental concepts and simulations. Magn Reson Med. 2004; 52 (5):1110–1117

[67] Walker-Samuel S, Leach MO, Collins DJ. Evaluation of response to treatment using DCE-MRI: the relationship between initial area under the gadolinium curve (IAUGC) and quantitative pharmacokinetic analysis. Phys Med Biol. 2006; 51(14):3593–3602

[68] Tofts PS. Modeling tracer kinetics in dynamic Gd-DTPA MR imaging. J Magn Reson Imaging. 1997; 7(1):91–101

[69] Aime S, Caravan P. Biodistribution of gadolinium-based contrast agents, including gadolinium deposition. J Magn Reson Imaging. 2009; 30(6):1259–1267

[70] Jansen SA, Paunesku T, Fan X, et al. Ductal carcinoma in situ: X-ray fluorescence microscopy and dynamic contrast-enhanced MR imaging reveals gadolinium uptake within neoplastic mammary ducts in a murine model. Radiology. 2009; 253(2):399–406

[71] Yang C, Karczmar GS, Medved M, Oto A, Zamora M, Stadler WM. Reproducibility assessment of a multiple reference tissue method for quantitative dynamic contrast enhanced-MRI analysis. Magn Reson Med. 2009; 61(4): 851–859

[72] Brix G, Kiessling F, Lucht R, et al. Microcirculation and microvasculature in breast tumors: pharmacokinetic analysis of dynamic MR image series. Magn Reson Med. 2004; 52(2):420–429

[73] Morales MF, Smith RE. On the theory of blood-tissue exchange of inert gases; validity of approximate uptake expressions. Bull Math Biophys. 1948; 10(3): 191–200

[74] Patlak CS, Fenstermacher JD. Measurements of dog blood-brain transfer constants by ventriculocisternal perfusion. Am J Physiol. 1975; 229(4):877–884

[75] Patlak CS, Blasberg RG, Fenstermacher JD. Graphical evaluation of blood-to-brain transfer constants from multiple-time uptake data. J Cereb Blood Flow Metab. 1983; 3(1):1–7

[76] Huang W, Li X, Morris EA, et al. The magnetic resonance shutter speed discriminates vascular properties of malignant and benign breast tumors in vivo. Proc Natl Acad Sci U S A. 2008; 105(46):17943–17948

[77] Huang W, Li X, Chen Y, et al. Variations of dynamic contrast-enhanced magnetic resonance imaging in evaluation of breast cancer therapy response: a multicenter data analysis challenge. Transl Oncol. 2014; 7(1):153–166

[78] Huang W, Tudorica LA, Li X, et al. Discrimination of benign and malignant breast lesions by using shutter-speed dynamic contrast-enhanced MR imaging. Radiology. 2011; 261(2):394–403

[79] Li X, Huang W, Yankeelov TE, Tudorica A, Rooney WD, Springer CS, Jr. Shutter-speed analysis of contrast reagent bolus-tracking data: Preliminary observations in benign and malignant breast disease. Magn Reson Med. 2005; 53(3):724–729

[80] Li X, Huang W, Morris EA, et al. Dynamic NMR effects in breast cancer dynamic-contrast-enhanced MRI. Proc Natl Acad Sci U S A. 2008; 105(46): 17937–17942

[81] Tudorica A, Oh KY, Chui SYC, et al. Early prediction and evaluation of breast cancer response to neoadjuvant chemotherapy using quantitative DCE-MRI. Transl Oncol. 2016; 9(1):8–17

[82] Springer CS, Jr, Li X, Tudorica LA, et al. Intratumor mapping of intracellular water lifetime: metabolic images of breast cancer? NMR Biomed. 2014; 27 (7):760–773

[83] Fan X, Karczmar GS. A new approach to analysis of the impulse response function (IRF) in dynamic contrast-enhanced MRI (DCEMRI): a simulation study. Magn Reson Med. 2009; 62(1):229–239

[84] Schabel MC. A unified impulse response model for DCE-MRI. Magn Reson Med. 2012; 68(5):1632–1646

[85] St Lawrence KS, Lee T-Y. An adiabatic approximation to the tissue homogeneity model for water exchange in the brain: II. Experimental validation. J Cereb Blood Flow Metab. 1998; 18(12):1378–1385

[86] Kershaw LE, Cheng HLM. Temporal resolution and SNR requirements for accurate DCE-MRI data analysis using the AATH model. Magn Reson Med. 2010; 64(6):1772–1780

[87] Fusco R, Sansone M, Maffei S, Raiano N, Petrillo A. Dynamic contrast-enhanced MRI in breast cancer: A comparison between distributed and compartmental tracer kinetic models. J Biomed Graph Comput. 2012; 2 (2):23–36

[88] Knight SP, Browne JE, Meaney JFM, Fagan AJ. Quantitative effects of acquisition duration and temporal resolution on the measurement accuracy of prostate dynamic contrast-enhanced MRI data: a phantom study. MAGMA. 2017; 30(5):461–471

[89] Planey CR, Welch EB, Xu L, et al. Temporal sampling requirements for reference region modeling of DCE-MRI data in human breast cancer. J Magn Reson Imaging. 2009; 30(1):121–134

[90] Radjenovic A, Dall BJ, Ridgway JP, Smith MA. Measurement of pharmacokinetic parameters in histologically graded invasive breast tumours using dynamic contrast-enhanced MRI. Br J Radiol. 2008; 81(962):120–128

[91] Furman-Haran E, Schechtman E, Kelcz F, Kirshenbaum K, Degani H. Magnetic resonance imaging reveals functional diversity of the vasculature in benign and malignant breast lesions. Cancer. 2005; 104(4):708–718

[92] Padhani AR, Hayes C, Assersohn L, et al. Prediction of clinicopathologic response of breast cancer to primary chemotherapy at contrast-enhanced MR imaging: initial clinical results. Radiology. 2006; 239(2):361–374

[93] Vincensini D, Dedieu V, Eliat PA, et al. Magnetic resonance imaging measurements of vascular permeability and extracellular volume fraction of breast tumors by dynamic Gd-DTPA-enhanced relaxometry. Magn Reson Imaging. 2007; 25(3):293–302

[94] El Khouli RH, Macura KJ, Kamel IR, Jacobs MA, Bluemke DA. 3-T dynamic contrast-enhanced MRI of the breast: pharmacokinetic parameters versus conventional kinetic curve analysis. AJR Am J Roentgenol. 2011; 197(6):1498–1505

[95] Schabel MC, Morrell GR, Oh KY, Walczak CA, Barlow RB, Neumayer LA. Pharmacokinetic mapping for lesion classification in dynamic breast MRI. J Magn Reson Imaging. 2010; 31(6):1371–1378

[96] Ah-See M-LW, Makris A, Taylor NJ, et al. Early changes in functional dynamic magnetic resonance imaging predict for pathologic response to neoadjuvant chemotherapy in primary breast cancer. Clin Cancer Res. 2008; 14(20):6580–6589

[97] Li X, Arlinghaus LR, Ayers GD, et al. DCE-MRI analysis methods for predicting the response of breast cancer to neoadjuvant chemotherapy: pilot study findings. Magn Reson Med. 2014; 71(4):1592–1602

13 Future Applications: Radiomics and Deep Learning on Breast MRI

Maryellen L. Giger

Abstract

Effective cancer diagnosis and treatment rely on the integration of information from multiple patient tests involving clinical, molecular, imaging, and genomic data. Adapting the Precision Medicine Initiative into imaging includes studies in both discovery and translation in order to enable the conversion of current radiological interpretation from that of the average patient to the precise interpretation and patient-care management decisions specific to the individual patient. Over the past few decades, various investigators have been developing image analysis methods for computer-aided diagnosis (CAD) and the quantitative characterization of breast lesions on clinical images. Radiomics, an expansion of computer-aided diagnosis, is a growing effort that involves these computerized image analyses in attempt to further relate quantitative image data to other -omic data such as clinical, pathologic, and genomic data. Also, the integration of imaging data (radiomics) with genomic data, referred to as imaging-genomics or radiogenomics, allows for the study of associations between the radiomic tumor phenotypes and the genomic measurements of the same tumors. This chapter discusses the translation of radiomics to clinical practice, which requires, beyond the actual development of the quantitative radiomic features, a multi-stage process of discovery and translation.

Keywords: breast radiomics, computer-aided diagnosis, machine learning, radiogenomics, deep learning

13.1 Introduction

Effective cancer diagnosis and treatment rely on the integration of information from multiple patient tests involving clinical, molecular, imaging, and genomic data. Such integrations are expected to facilitate patient-specific research for precision medicine. Adapting the Precision Medicine Initiative into imaging research includes studies in both discovery and translation in order to enable the conversion of current radiological interpretation from that of the "average patient" to the precise interpretation and patient-care management decisions specific to the individual patient.

Over the past few decades, various investigators have been developing image analysis methods for computer-aided diagnosis (CAD) and the quantitative characterization of breast lesions on clinical images.[1] Radiomics, an expansion of CAD, is a growing effort that involves these computerized image analyses in attempt to further relate quantitative image data to other "-omic" data such as clinical, pathologic, and genomic data.[2] The integration of imaging data (radiomics) with genomic data, referred to as "imaging-genomics" or "radiogenomics," allows for the study of associations between the radiomic tumor phenotypes and the genomic measurements of the same tumors.[3,4,5] Radiomic phenotypes (i.e., features) that are highly correlated with important clinical, molecular, or genomic biomarkers can potentially serve as diagnostic or prognostic tools for patient monitoring and assessing therapeutic response, and thus augment the utility of medical imaging as a noninvasive technology for cancer care, like a "virtual digital biopsy."

It is useful to review the goals of CAD, which are to reduce search errors, reduce interpretation errors, reduce variation between and within observers, and/or improve the efficiency of the breast imaging interpretation process.[6] These goals can be achieved if the computer's output is presented in an effective and efficient manner and if the computer output is used appropriately by the radiologist. However, the potential of various developments in CAD goes beyond the radiologist's interpretation process to future roles in radiomics such as image-based biomarkers (phenotypes) for assessing prognosis and estimating response to therapy as well as in imaging genomics and cancer (disease) discovery. Note that CADe is computer-aided detection and CADx is computer-aided diagnosis; both of these approaches require radiologists to use the computer output as an aid in their interpretation.

It is important to note that with CAD as well as radiomics, the extraction of features from digital medical images without the association with disease characteristics is basically only *extracted information*. Through investigations into the applications of these computer vision techniques, within CAD and beyond, *knowledge* is gained in the management of the (cancer) patient and in the understanding of the disease. As will be discussed throughout this chapter, the translation of radiomics to clinical practice requires, beyond the actual development of the quantitative radiomic features, a multistage process of discovery and translation.

In the discovery stage, one attempts to find relationships between images (through quantitative radiomics) and clinical data, molecular data, genomic data, and outcome data. Discovery is a multidisciplinary data mining effort involving researchers such as radiologists, medical physicists, statisticians, oncologists, computer scientists, engineers, and computational geneticists. Similar to how the genomics community approached the big biology of the Cancer Genome project, the radiological community needs to continue to conduct robust collection, annotation, analysis, and evaluation of images of large populations.

In the application stage, one aims to develop predictive models for use in risk assessment, screening, detection, diagnosis, prognosis, therapeutic response, risk of recurrence, and other clinical tasks, as discussed later in this chapter. Here, radiomics serve as contributions to "virtual digital biopsies" for use when actual biopsies are not practical such as in screening and repeated assessments of treatment response (▶ Fig. 13.1).

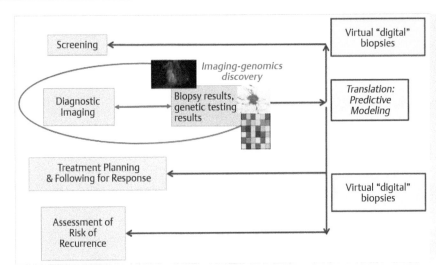

Fig. 13.1 Illustration of the multistage process of radiomics, discovery, and translation, including the development and validation of quantitative radiomic features, the discovery of their relationships to other "-omics," and the translation into clinical predictive models for use as "virtual digital biopsies," such as in screening and assessing response to therapy where actual biopsies are not practical.

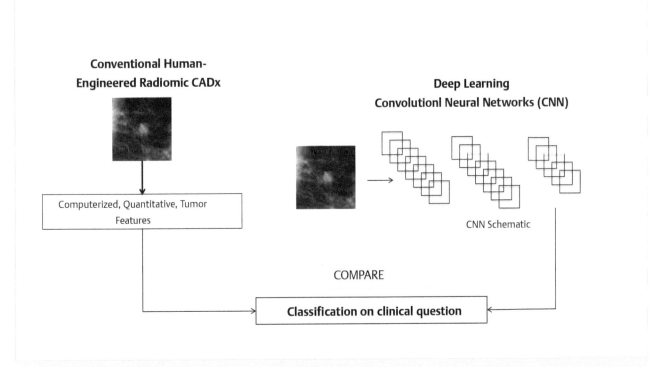

Fig. 13.2 Schematic pipeline comparing conventional CAD (*left*) and deep learning (*right*).

13.2 Quantitative Radiomics of Tumors and Their Microenvironment

In the general definition of "radiomics," that of converting images to minable data, one could potentially have radiologists interpret images and assign numerical ratings to different characteristics, such as degree of circularity for lesion shape or amount of uptake for kinetic enhancement. However, assessment of image-based tumor characteristics by radiologists is usually qualitative with interradiologist's variation as well as time consuming. Thus, it is beneficial to use computer analysis methods and machine learning methods to quantitatively, objectively, and automatically extract characteristics from images, i.e., quantitative radiomics. Such features could be descriptive of a tumor with or without its microenvironment or a normal region. The remainder of this chapter will mainly focus on quantitative radiomics.

Given the rise in the application of deep learning to the general task of image interpretation, it is beneficial to explore radiomics in terms of lesion segmentation–based methods as well as deep learning–based methods, and then look for opportunities to merge such techniques into advanced predictors (▶ Fig. 13.2).

Table 13.1 Representative examples of MRI phenotyping descriptors

Tumor phenotypes	Mathematical descriptors	MRI protocol	Selected references
Size	Volume		7,8
Shape	Sphericity or irregularity	DCE	7,9
Morphology	Margin sharpness	T2w	7,9
	Texture	T2w	9
	ADC	DWI	10
Enhancement heterogeneity	Fourier descriptors of texture postcontrast	DCE	13
Enhancement	Contrast	DCE	61
Kinetics	Uptake	DCE	7,61,63
Enhancement variance	Max enhancement-variance	DCE	11

Abbreviations: ADC, apparent diffusion coefficient; DCE, dynamic contrast-enhanced; DWI, diffusion-weighted imaging; T2w, T2-weighted.

13.2.1 Segmentation-Based CAD/Radiomics

In the computer characterization of a segmented tumor or region, multiple steps are available for automation along the radiomics pipeline (chain). These include tumor (or region) segmentation, feature extraction, and merging of features into a tumor signature (relevant to a specific clinical question).

Since with radiomics, we are interested in image-based phenotypes of the tumor or region, we can use examples from CADx, and not CADe, since detection is not the task. ▶ Table 13.1 lists various radiomic features along with their general phenotypic category and potential clinical application. References are given; however, many examples can be found in the literature over the past multiple decades.

For example, quantitative tumor radiomics, i.e., tumor phenotypes, can be automatically extracted from dynamic contrast-enhanced magnetic resonance (DCE-MR) images of the breast using methods and algorithms that automatically segment the tumor (▶ Fig. 13.3) from the surrounding parenchymal background within the DCE-MR images and extract lesion characteristics in six phenotypic categories (▶ Fig. 13.4): (1) size (measuring tumor dimensions), (2) shape (quantifying the 3D geometry), (3) morphology (margin characteristics), (4) enhancement texture (describing the heterogeneity within the texture of the contrast uptake in the tumor on the first postcontrast MRIs), (5) kinetic curve assessment (describing the shape of the kinetic curve and assessing the physiologic process of the uptake and washout of the contrast agent in the tumor during the dynamic imaging series, and (6) enhancement-variance kinetics (characterizing the time course of the spatial variance of the enhancement within the tumor).

Note that multiple mathematical descriptors can be used to calculate these phenotypes, with many being highly correlated within a specific phenotypic category. Uses of these features for specific clinical tasks will be discussed later in this chapter.

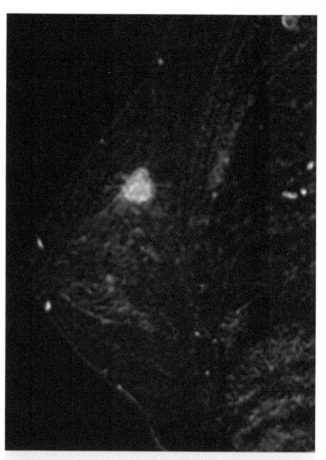

Fig. 13.3 Example case including the tumor outline obtained from the 4D automatic computer segmentation algorithm. This case is a Luminal A, ER-positive, PR-positive, HER2-negative, stage II, and with negative lymph nodes. From the computer analysis, the MRI radiomics size of effect diameter is 13.6 mm, the radiomics shape of irregularity is 0.49, and the radiomics enhancement texture (energy) is 0.00185.

Related features such as shape, margin, and texture can also be extracted using computer analysis from T2-weighted (T2w) and other common as well as exploratory MRI techniques, as listed in ▶ Table 13.1.[7,8,9,10,11,12]

For other tasks, radiomic features can be extracted from regions within images of normal tissue to characterize the density and texture of parenchyma for potential uses in breast cancer risk assessment. Texture-based phenotypes have been used extensively over the past decades, with the use rapidly increasing as a means to describe heterogeneity within tumors or regions.[13,14,15] While texture analysis on mammographic parenchyma has shown that women at high risk tend to have dense breast with coarse and low contrast patterns (▶ Fig. 13.5),[16,17,18] such analyses are also being conducted on breast MRI.[19,20]

13.2.2 Deep Learning in the Classification of Tumors and Normal Tissue

An alternative to having the computer extract specific lesion features (e.g., using mathematical descriptors to calculate margin sharpness) from the lesion image is to input the image data

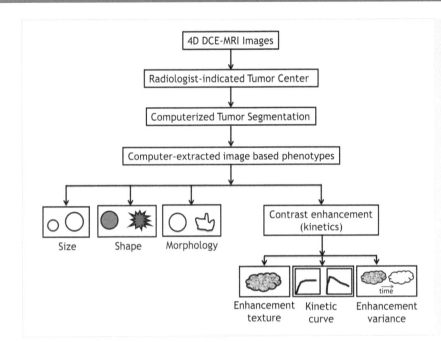

Fig. 13.4 Schematic diagrams illustrating the computer-extraction of the quantitative MRI-based tumor phenotypes. (Reproduced with permission from Li et al.[48])

to the computer and have the computer learn directly from the image data. Learning directly from the image data has led to deep learning methods for content-based retrieval, CAD, and data mining.[21] Note that the use of deep learning can contribute along the decision-making pipeline at multiple stages including filtering, segmentation, feature extraction, and/or classification.

In the early 1990s, convolutional neural networks (CNNs) were initially introduced to mammographic imaging for CAD using regions of interest (ROIs) from which to learn without explicit manual intervention.[22] Zhang et al used CNNs as a means to filter the image prior to subsequent feature extraction (▶ Fig. 13.6).[23] Others started using CNNs for classification of ROIs as either tumor or normal tissue.[24]

Although CNNs typically rely on massive datasets for training, it has been shown that transfer learning techniques such as fine-tuning or feature extraction based on ImageNet or other trained CNNs can be used to reduce the need for larger data-sets.[25,26] In this scenario, deep learning techniques are being implemented for feature extraction and are exhibiting strong predictive performances on CADx tasks without requiring data-intensive computing.[27,28]

Specifically, for radiomics using CNN features, the computer analysis involves the extraction of one or more network layers, which subsequently serve as "features," from a pretrained CNN. These CNN features are then further used to train classifiers. Examples are given for pretrained AlexNet and VGG19 net, each of which has been trained on the ImageNet dataset of "every-day" images. The architecture of VGG19 model includes five stacks—with each stack containing two or four convolutional layers and a max-pooling layer—followed by three fully connected layers. The VGG19 architecture and CNN feature-extraction pipeline is illustrated in ▶ Fig. 13.7. It should be noted that many of the elements in each layer that serve as the initial features may exhibit zero variance across the dataset, and thus can be eliminated as useful features.

In a study of CNNs in the classification of malignant and benign breast tumors, a VGG19 model was used across three imaging modalities—mammography, ultrasound, and DCE-MRI.[29] The VGG19 model has three "RGB color" channels for input, which is conducive to inputting, for example, three MR images across different contrast uptake points or three MR images across three neoadjuvant treatment points. Note that when using different images within the three channels, caution is needed in order to ensure proper registration of the input images. The output layers, i.e., the features, were then subsequently merged using a support vector machine (SVM) to develop classifiers for specific clinical questions.

As databases of breast MRIs increase, deep learning in which CNNs are trained from scratch will be possible; however, potentially millions of MRIs may be necessary.

13.2.3 Comparison of Conventional CADx to Deep Learning

Comparison of segmentation-based, hand-crafted radiomic features (as in conventional CADx) and CNN-based radiomic features (as in transfer learning) is expected to yield further understanding of the nonintuitive CNN-based features. ▶ Fig. 13.8 shows the comparison of diagnostic decision making from using segmentation-based features and CNN-based features on various modalities of breast imaging. While both conventional hand-crafted CADx features and CNN-based features perform relatively well in estimating the likelihood of malignancy, they each do not yield correct estimates for the same breast lesions, thus allowing for improved performance when combined, similar to consensus reads from two expert radiologists.

Thus, fusion methods can be employed in which the classifier outputs from segmentation-based methods and the CNN-based methods are combined, such as by averaging the separate

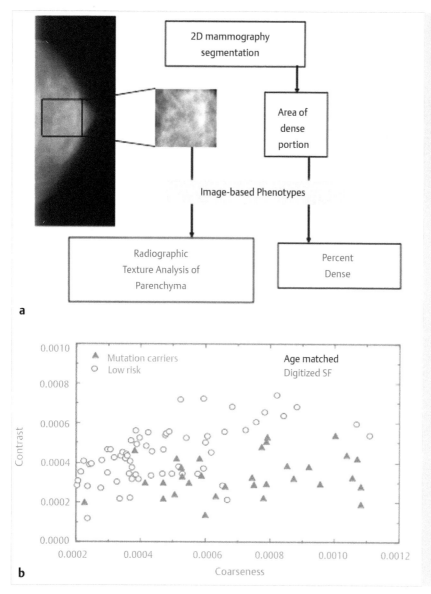

Fig. 13.5 Radiomic phenotypes of breast parenchyma as extracted from digital mammograms for use in estimating risk of future breast cancer. (Reproduced with permission from Huo et al.[16])

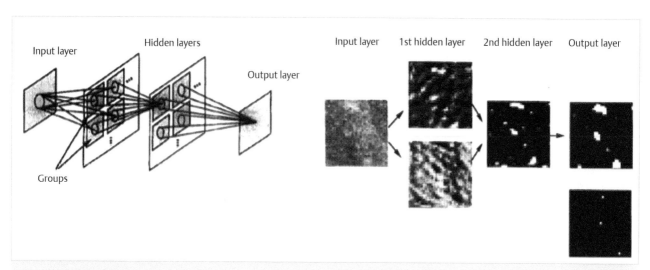

Fig. 13.6 Example of the first use of deep learning in medical imaging in which convolutional neural networks were employed in the detection of microcalcifications on mammograms. Here the CNN was used to yield an optimized image filter in which the output was sent for further processing. (Reproduced with permission from Zhang et al.[23])

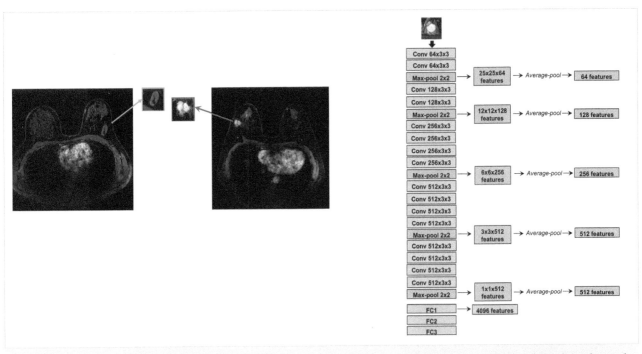

Fig. 13.7 Illustration of ROIs cut from a malignant breast cancer case and benign case for input to a pretrained VGGNet convolutional neural network. Architecture of the VGG19 model comprises five blocks, each of which contains two or four convolutional layers and a max-pooling layer. The five blocks are followed by three fully connected layers. Features are extracted from the five max-pooling layers, average-pooled across the channel (third) dimension, and normalized with L2 norm. The normalized features are concatenated to form our CNN feature vector.

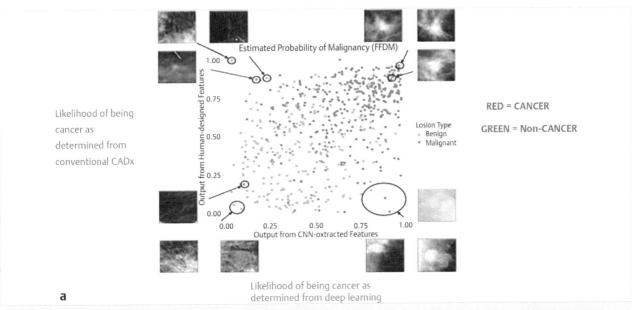

Fig. 13.8 (a) A diagonal classifier agreement plot between the CNN-based classifier and the conventional CADx classifier for full-field digital mammography cases. The x-axis denotes the output from the CNN-based classifier, and the y-axis denotes the output from the conventional CADx classifier. Each point represents an ROI for which predictions were made. Points near or along the diagonal from bottom left to top right indicate high classifier agreement; points far from the diagonal indicate low agreement. ROI pictures of extreme examples of agreement/disagreement are included. (*Continued*)

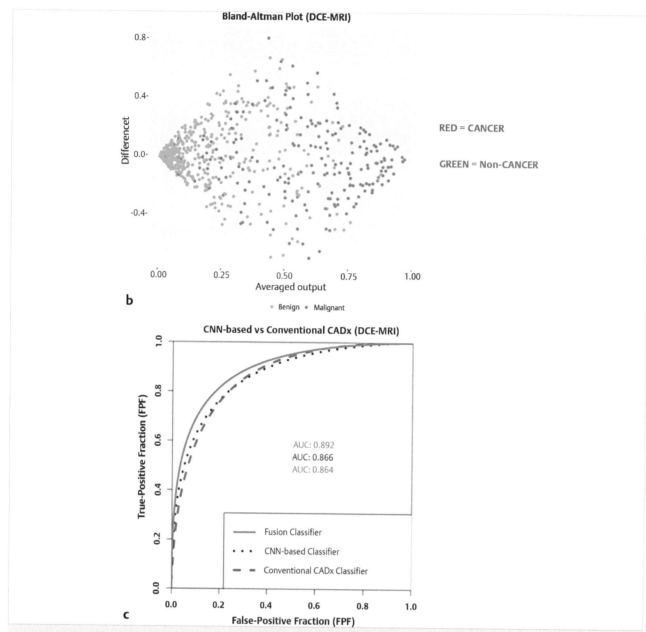

b

c

Fig. 13.8 (*continued*) (b) Bland–Altman plots for a DCE-MRI modality illustrating classifier agreement between the CNN-based classifier and the CADx-based classifier. The y-axis shows the difference between the SVM outputs of the two classifiers; the x-axis shows the averaged output of the two classifiers. Since the averaged output is also the output of the fusion classifier, these plots also help visualize potential decision boundaries between benign and malignant classifications. (c) Fitted binormal ROC curves comparing the performances of CNN-based classifiers, CADx-based classifiers, and fusion classifiers. The *solid green line* represents the fusion classifier. The *dotted black line* represents the CNN-based classifier using pooled features. The *dashed red line* represents the conventional CADx classifier using handcrafted features. (Reproduced with permission from Antropova et al.[29])

output to yield a combined output related to the likelihood of being cancerous.

13.2.4 Robustness of Radiomic Features

Despite computerized image interpretation having potential in aiding radiologists, it also faces many challenges. Variation in scanning protocols, MR system manufactures, and magnet strengths may lead to variability in the image data. With sufficient training and experience, human readers may adjust their interpretation, while computational radiomic analysis results may be dependent on the differences in acquisitions. Therefore, for computerized image analysis to be clinically useful, radiomic systems need to generate consistent results when they analyze images acquired at different conditions. The harmonization of feature values may be achieved by standardization of image data during acquisition and prior to feature extraction or through the harmonization of feature computing methods. Various investigators have studied different approaches to robustness with much of the literature in assessing the robustness of radiomic features of the lung.[30] Robustness of quantitative imaging is also a major focus of the National Cancer Institute's (NCI) Quantitative Imaging Network (QIN)[31] and the RSNA's Quantitative Imaging Biomarker Alliance (QIBA).[32] Recently, new metrics of robustness have been demonstrated to assess differences in radiomic features between different manufacturers' imaging systems.[33]

To ensure robustness of radiomic analysis, variation in current features must be investigated to allow further exploration of data harmonization. Limited literature is available on evaluation of feature variability across MR scanners and imaging protocols.[34] In one study in which breast DCE-MR images had been acquired with scanners from two different manufacturers, the equivalence of MRI radiomic features (phenotypes) and their performance in distinguishing breast cancers in terms of lymph node status and molecular classification were investigated.[34]

Each case was subject to computerized feature extraction with a breast MRI radiomics workstation. Superiority testing was used to evaluate the differences in feature performance in the prognostic tasks of distinguishing lymph node and hormone receptor statuses, with area under the receiver operating characteristic curve (AUC) serving as a figure of merit. The features that failed to show statistically significant differences in performance were further evaluated with noninferiority testing. Finally, classification models were built for assessment of clinical tasks. Leave-one-out cross-validation and independent testing were conducted to assess performance robustness. In prognostic tasks, features showed varying levels of robustness. The best agreement in performance was seen in a lymph node classification for two features—tumor morphology and tumor heterogeneity—with absolute value of the lower bound of the 90% confidence interval for ΔAUC < 0.05.

Quantitative breast radiomic features show varying robustness in their average values and in performance across MRI scanners. Noninferiority testing can reveal radiomic features with robust performance in the classification tasks. In practice, features showing different performance levels need to be tuned based on the MRI scanner used during imaging procedure.

13.3 Computerized Image–Based Cancer Risk

Association of mammographic density with breast cancer risk has led to DCE-MRI being recommended for screening of high-risk women. Radiomic features related to risk include breast density and parenchyma texture pattern, as discussed earlier in this chapter. However, most of such developments are conducted on digital mammograms.[22,35] More studies are needed to understand how breast background parenchymal enhancement (BPE) on DCE-MRI is associated with breast density and breast cancer risk.[36,37,38] The characterization of normal breast tissue on DCE-MRI has become more important in assessing the breast cancer risk.[39,40]

In one study on a high-risk population of 92 asymptomatic women, breast BPE on DCE-MRI was compared to parenchymal density and texture on full-field digital mammograms (FFDMs).[41] Breast volume on MRI was computed using a volume-growing algorithm and classified into fibroglandular and fatty regions. Kinetic curves within breast fibroglandular regions were extracted and categorized using fuzzy c-means (FCM) clustering yielding BPE. On corresponding FFDM images, mammographic density and textures were calculated. Correlation analysis between the two-modality density measures yielded a correlation coefficient of 0.80 (p < 0.0001). From kinetic analyses, 70% of the most enhancing curves showed persistent curve type and reached peak parenchymal intensity at the last postcontrast time point, with 89% of most enhancing curves reaching peak intensity at the fourth or fifth postcontrast time points. Dense breasts were found to have a higher peak enhancement with an average of 116.5%, while fatty breasts demonstrated an average peak enhancement of 66.0%. Dense breasts, with coarser, low-contrast mammographic patterns tended to have more BPE at peak time point. Thus, BPE may be potentially useful in assessing breast cancer risk.

13.4 High-Throughput MRI Phenotyping of Breast Tumors for Diagnosis and Prognosis Relative to Molecular Subtyping

Use of quantitative radiomics in big data analysis requires that there is an effective and efficient pipeline to convert acquired breast MR images into a set of quantitative phenotypic descriptors as described earlier in the chapter, as shown earlier in ▶ Fig. 13.4, which is a schematic of a breast MRI workstation that takes as input the 4D DCE-MR images and outputs radiomic features.

It is useful to emphasize that radiomic feature chosen for one clinical task may not be that useful for another clinical task. However, if one's "big data" dataset is sufficiently large, one can assess the features across different tasks. Examples of such are demonstrated in the next sections that highlight the MRI phenotyping research conducted on The Cancer Genome Atlas/The Cancer Imaging Archive (TCGA/TCIA) datasets.[42,43,44]

While imaging is used in the clinical staging of a breast cancer to initially manage the patient, it is the biopsy-determined "pathologic" stage that drives further decision making. In order to augment the TNM staging system, investigators are developing radiomic biomarkers, e.g., on breast MRI, to help predict pathologic stage and thus inform patient management and appropriate treatment, such as neoadjuvant chemotherapy, surgery, and/or radiation therapy.

Using the collected de-identified datasets of invasive breast carcinomas from TCGA and TCIA, cancer research resources supported by the NCI of the U.S. National Institutes of Health,[42, 43] the TCGA Breast Phenotype Group[44] investigated relationships between computer-extracted quantitative radiomic MRI lesion features and various clinical, molecular, and genomics markers of prognosis and risk of recurrence, including gene expression profiles. At the time of analysis, 91 biopsy-proven invasive breast cancers from the TCGA had DCE-MR images were available and underwent analysis, as schematically shown in ▶ Fig. 13.9. On these cases, the predictive ability of the quantitative radiomic MRI features was assessed relative to the tasks of pathologic stage and cancer subtypes.

Tumors were characterized according to: (1) radiologist-measured size and (2) computer-extracted quantitative radiomic features. Then, models were built to predict tumor pathologic stage and lymph node involvement. It was found that tumor size was the most powerful predictor of pathologic stage, but radiomic features that captured biologic behavior also emerged as predictive (e.g., stage I and II vs. stage III yielded an AUC of 0.83).[45] It was concluded that computer-extracted MRI phenotypes have promise for predicting breast cancer pathologic stage and lymph node status.

On the basis of receptor status (estrogen receptor [ER], progesterone receptor [PR], and human epidermal growth factor receptor 2 [HER2]), breast cancer can be classified into different subtypes. By considering gene expression profiles, breast cancer can be also categorized into molecular subtypes, such as normal-like, luminal A, luminal B, HER2-enriched, and basal-like.[46, 47] Cancers of different subtypes have different prognoses and respond differently to different therapies. Thus, the correlation between the quantitative MRI radiomic features and various cancer subtypes was studied.[14] MRI-based tumor phenotypes were able to distinguish between molecular prognostic indicators through tasks of distinguishing between ER + versus ER–, PR + versus PR–, HER2 + versus HER2–, and triple-negative cancers versus all others, respectively. Statistically significant associations between tumor phenotypes and receptor status were observed. More aggressive cancers were found to more likely be larger in size with more heterogeneity demonstrated quantitatively in their contrast enhancement texture. Even after controlling for tumor size, statistically significant trends were observed between enhancement texture (entropy) and molecular subtypes (normal-like, luminal A, luminal B, HER2-enriched, basal-like) (▶ Fig. 13.10). In conclusion, computer-extracted MRI phenotypes show promise for high-throughput discrimination of breast cancer subtypes and may yield a quantitative predictive signature for assessing prognosis.

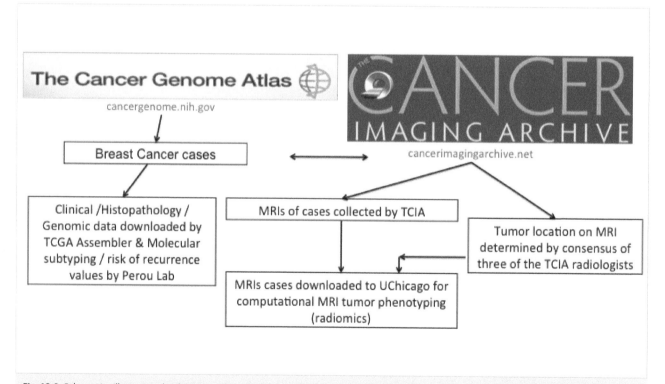

Fig. 13.9 Schematics illustrating the datasets and some of the analyses of invasive breast carcinomas from The Cancer Genome Atlas (TCGA) and The Cancer Imaging Archive (TCIA), cancer research resources supported by the National Cancer Institute (NCI) of the U.S. National Institutes of Health, which were conducted by TCGA Breast Phenotype Group to investigate relationships between computer-extracted quantitative radiomic MRI lesion features and various clinical, molecular, and genomics markers of prognosis and risk of recurrence, including gene expression.

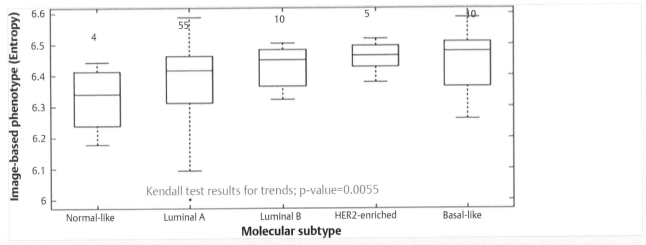

Fig. 13.10 Relationship between the MRI phenotypes of enhancement texture (entropy) and molecular subtypes. The enhancement texture is calculated from data of the first postcontrast MR image, thus quantitatively characterizing the heterogeneous uptake of contrast within the tumor. Shown is a statistically significant trend between entropy and molecular subtype (*p*-value of 0.006 from the Kendall test). (Reproduced with permission from Li et al.[14])

13.5 High-Throughput MRI Phenotyping of Breast Tumors for Assessing Risk of Recurrence

Use of computer vision and machine learning to further analyze breast tumors on MRI has led to predictive methods for assessing the risk of recurrence of breast cancer.[48,49]

Investigators have developed multigene assays with which to relate breast cancer expression profiles to risk of cancer recurrence, including the 21-gene Oncotype DC assay, the 50-gene PAM50 assay, and the 70-gene MammaPrint microarray assay.[47,50,51,52,53] To investigate the relationships between quantitative MRI radiomic features and risk of breast cancer recurrence, association studies were conducted within the TCGA Breast Phenotype group using research versions of these multigene assays.[47] ▶ Fig. 13.11 shows a color map illustrating relationships between the computer-extracted MRI features and the microarray recurrence models.[48] Multiple linear regression analyses demonstrated significant associations between the MRI radiomics signatures (incorporating tumor size and enhancement heterogeneity) and the multigene assay recurrence scores.[48] Such computer-extracted MRI radiomics shows potential for image-based phenotyping in assessing the risk of cancer recurrence.

13.6 High-Throughput MRI Phenotyping of Breast Tumors for Predicting Therapeutic Response

As repeatedly mentioned throughout this chapter, computer-extracted phenotypic features can be extracted but used in multiple clinical tasks. For the tasks of assessing response to treatment as well as predicting disease-free survival, investigators are evaluating various computer-extracted features from

breast MRI—some semiautomated and some automated.[54,55,56,57,58,59] Note here that one is reusing methods for quantitative radiomics analysis on breast cancer MR images at different treatment time points (such as pretreatment and early treatment) to investigate the use of these features and their change over time for response assessment. In addition, since the MR images are acquired over multiple treatment times, image registration methods may be necessary to track similar regions of the breast during neoadjuvant treatment.[60]

For example, using a dataset of DCE-MR images from the American College of Radiology Imaging Network (ACRIN) trial 6657,[55] investigators have used both semiautomated approaches[56,57,58] and automated methods[59,61] to study tumor response to neoadjuvant chemotherapy. The "functional tumor volume"[57] or similarly a "most-enhancing tumor volume"[59] showed association with recurrence-free survival. The automatic quantitative radiomics method yielding the most enhancing tumor volume serves as an image-based biomarker in the task of predicting recurrence and association with recurrence-free survival.

13.7 MRI Phenotypes and Genomics

As noted earlier, the integration of imaging data (radiomics) with genomic data (i.e., "imaging-genomics" or "radiogenomics"), as well as other "-omics," allows for investigations of associations between the radiomic tumor phenotypes and the genomic measurements of the same tumors.[3,4,5,62] Knowledge of significant correlations will advance the use of medical imaging as a noninvasive technology for cancer care, like a "virtual digital biopsy."

Using again the datasets of invasive breast carcinomas from TCGA and TCIA,[42,43] the TCGA Breast Phenotype Group[44] investigated associations between the computer-extracted quantitative radiomic MRI lesion features and genomic features

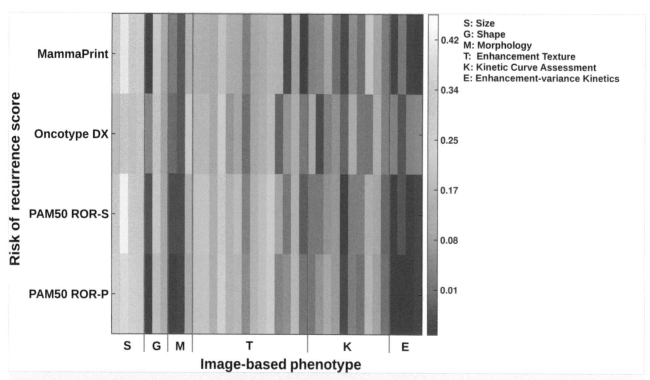

Fig. 13.11 Color map shows the correlation of the MRI-based phenotypes with the recurrence predictor models of MammoPrint, Oncotype DX, PAM50 ROR-S, and PAM50 ROR-P. For this color scale, *yellow* indicates higher correlation as compared with *blue*. The different gene assays (recurrence predictor models) serve as the "reference standard" in this study. (Reproduced with permission from Li et al.[48])

downloaded from the TCGA (including DNA mutation, miRNA expression, protein expression, pathway gene expression, and copy number variation).[5,62] Employing unsupervised clustering analyses, they found clusters based on radiomic features that overlapped those of molecular subtypes (▶ Fig. 13.12).

From the radiomics–genomics studies, associations of radiomics with two types of genomic features were found: transcriptional activities of pathways and miRNA expressions (▶ Fig. 13.13). Note, that these associations are being used in the "discovery stage" in which one tries to understand the radiomic phenotype of breast cancers.[5,62] For example, pathway transcriptional activities were found to be associated, at a statistically significant level, with all six types of MRI tumor radiomic phenotypes (size, shape, margin morphology, enhancement texture, kinetics, and enhancement-variance kinetics), indicating that they may be regulating various aspects of the tumor radiomics. Since larger tumors were associated with mostly higher pathway activities, one might infer that many pathways are upregulated during tumor growth. Also, since pathway transcriptional activities were mostly negatively associated with morphological phenotypes that characterize tumor margin sharpness, one might infer a positive correlation between the transcriptional activities of genetic pathways and a blurred tumor margin, which could be a sign of tumor invasion into the surrounding tissue. Other identified radiogenomic associations suggested that miRNAs may mediate the growth and the heterogeneity of angiogenesis in tumors.

Overall, the investigators discovered some highly specific imaging-genomic associations. Such discovery insights may yield a future understanding of cancer to contribute to the design of new treatments and patient managements, augmenting the medical practice of actual tumor biopsies with "virtual digital biopsies," which have the benefit of yielding an analysis of the entire tumor to assess heterogeneity, being basically non-invasive, and being repeatable over time, such as in the case of monitoring treatment.

13.8 Summary and Overview

This chapter has presented an overview of the potential of quantitative radiomics and deep learning in breast cancer imaging and patient management. The future of breast cancer diagnosis and treatment is expected to benefit from: (1) the objective information that is being extracted from breast MRIs through quantitative radiomics and (2) from the creation of new knowledge through discoveries between radiomics and other "-omics" (such as genomics). Novel predictive models of MR radiomics, serving as "virtual digital biopsies," will potentially enhance patient management at stages when actual biopsies are not practical or possible.

13.9 Acknowledgments

M.L.G. acknowledges the many current and past members of her Lab at the University of Chicago, including Hui Li, PhD, Karen Drukker, PhD, Natalia Antropova, Kayla Mendel, Ben Huynh, Li Lan, MS, Sasha Edwards, MS, John Papaioannou, MS, and Chun-Wai Chen, MS, who have contributed through engaging discussions and research.

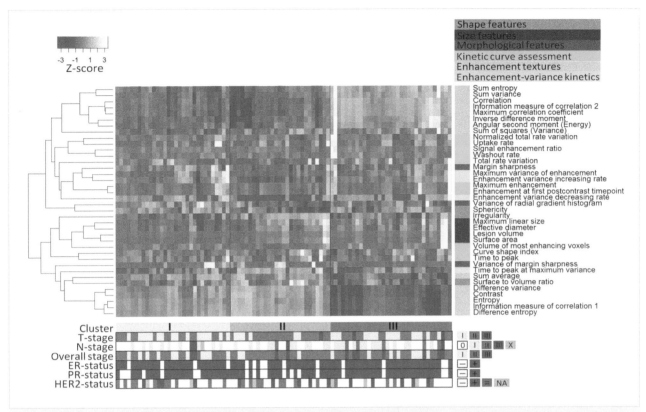

Fig. 13.12 Clustering analysis of tumor samples based on different data platforms. In the heatmaps, the tumor samples (columns in the heatmaps) are grouped by the Affinity Propagation Clustering (APC) into clusters divided by *red lines*. All features (rows in the heatmaps) are organized by the hierarchical clustering based on the euclidean distance and complete linkage function, for which a dendrogram is shown on the left. All features were transformed and standardized to obtain Z scores, based on which the clustering and heatmap drawing were done. The pathological stages and the molecular receptor status of tumors are shown under the heatmaps for the radiomics imaging data. (Reproduced with permission from Zhu et al.[5])

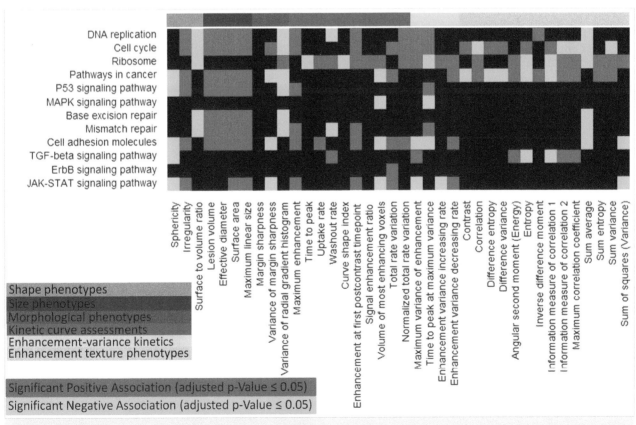

Fig. 13.13 Heatmap representation of statistically significant associations between radiomic phenotypes and transcriptional activities of some cancer-related genetic pathways. In the heatmap, genetic pathways are rows and radiomic phenotypes are columns. (Reproduced with permission from Zhu et al.[5])

M.L.G. also acknowledges her appreciation to the NCI and NIBIB of the NIH for their grant support of her research.

M.L.G. is a stockholder in R2 technology/Hologic, is a cofounder of and equity holder in Quantitative Insights, and receives royalties from Hologic, GE Medical Systems, MEDIAN Technologies, Riverain Medical, Mitsubishi, and Toshiba.

References

[1] Giger ML, Karssemeijer N, Schnabel JA. Breast image analysis for risk assessment, detection, diagnosis, and treatment of cancer. Annu Rev Biomed Eng. 2013; 15:327–357

[2] Lambin P, Rios-Velazquez E, Leijenaar R, et al. Radiomics: extracting more information from medical images using advanced feature analysis. Eur J Cancer. 2012; 48(4):441–446

[3] Aerts HJ, Velazquez ER, Leijenaar RT, et al. Decoding tumour phenotype by noninvasive imaging using a quantitative radiomics approach. Nat Commun. 2014; 5:4006

[4] Gillies RJ, Kinahan PE, Hricak H. Raodiomics: images are more than pictures, they are data. Radiology. 2016; 278(2):563–577

[5] Zhu Y, Li H, Guo W, et al. Deciphering genomic underpinnings of quantitative MRI-based radiomic phenotypes of invasive breast carcinoma. Sci Rep. 2015; 5:17787

[6] Giger ML, Chan H-P, Boone J. Anniversary paper: history and status of CAD and quantitative image analysis: the role of Medical Physics and AAPM. Med Phys. 2008; 35(12):5799–5820

[7] Gilhuijs KGA, Giger ML, Bick U. Computerized analysis of breast lesions in three dimensions using dynamic magnetic-resonance imaging. Med Phys. 1998; 25(9):1647–1654

[8] Chen W, Giger ML, Bick U. A fuzzy c-means (FCM)-based approach for computerized segmentation of breast lesions in dynamic contrast-enhanced MR images. Acad Radiol. 2006; 13(1):63–72

[9] Bhooshan N, Giger M, Lan L, et al. Combined use of T2-weighted MRI and T1-weighted dynamic contrast-enhanced MRI in the automated analysis of breast lesions. Magn Reson Med. 2011; 66(2):555–564

[10] Partridge SC, Mullins CD, Kurland BF, et al. Apparent diffusion coefficient values for discriminating benign and malignant breast MRI lesions: effects of lesion type and size. AJR Am J Roentgenol. 2010; 194(6):1664–1673

[11] Chen W, Giger ML, Lan L, Bick U. Computerized interpretation of breast MRI: investigation of enhancement-variance dynamics. Med Phys. 2004; 31(5):1076–1082

[12] Weiss WA, Medved M, Karczmar GS, Giger ML. Preliminary assessment of dispersion versus absorption analysis of high spectral and spatial resolution magnetic resonance images in the diagnosis of breast cancer. J Med Imaging (Bellingham). 2015; 2(2):024502

[13] Chen W, Giger ML, Li H, Bick U, Newstead GM. Volumetric texture analysis of breast lesions on contrast-enhanced magnetic resonance images. Magn Reson Med. 2007; 58(3):562–571

[14] Li H, Zhu Y, Burnside ES, et al. Quantitative MRI radiomics in the prediction of molecular classifications of breast cancer subtypes in the TCGA/TCIA data set. NPJ Breast Cancer. 2016; 2:16012

[15] Sutton EJ, Oh JH, Dashevsky BZ, et al. Breast cancer subtype intertumor heterogeneity: MRI-based features predict results of a genomic assay. J Magn Reson Imaging. 2015; 42(5):1398–1406

[16] Huo Z, Giger ML, Olopade OI, et al. Computerized analysis of digitized mammograms of BRCA1 and BRCA2 gene mutation carriers. Radiology. 2002; 225(2):519–526

[17] Li H, Giger ML, Lan L, et al. Computerized analysis of mammographic parenchymal patterns on a large clinical dataset of full-field digital mammograms: robustness study with two high-risk datasets. J Digit Imaging. 2012; 25(5):591–598

[18] Gierach GL, Li H, Loud JT, et al. Relationships between computer-extracted mammographic texture pattern features and BRCA1/2 mutation status: a cross-sectional study. Breast Cancer Res. 2014; 16(24):424

[19] Nie K, Chang D, Chen JH, Hsu CC, Nalcioglu O, Su MY. Quantitative analysis of breast parenchymal patterns using 3D fibroglandular tissues segmented based on MRI. Med Phys. 2010; 37(1):217–226

[20] Li H, Weiss WA, Medved M, et al. Breast density estimation from high spectral and spatial resolution MRI. J Med Imaging (Bellingham). 2016; 3(4):044507

[21] Zheng L, Zhao Y, Wang S, et al. Good practice in CNN feature transfer. 2016; arXiv:1604.00133

[22] Li H, Giger ML, Huynh BQ, Antropova NO. Deep learning in breast cancer risk assessment: evaluation of convolutional neural networks on a clinical dataset of full-field digital mammograms. J Med Imaging (Bellingham). 2017; 4(4):041304

[23] Zhang W, Doi K, Giger ML, Wu Y, Nishikawa RM, Schmidt RA. Computerized detection of clustered microcalcifications in digital mammograms using a shift-invariant artificial neural network. Med Phys. 1994; 21(4):517–524

[24] Sahiner B, Chan H-P, Petrick N, et al. Classification of mass and normal breast tissue: a convolution neural network classifier with spatial domain and texture images. IEEE Trans Med Imaging. 1996; 15(5):598–610

[25] Yosinski J, Clune J, Bengio Y, Lipson H. How transferable are features in deep neural networks? Paper presented at: NIPS'14 Proceedings of the 27th International Conference on Neural Information Processing Systems - Volume 2; December 8–13, 2014; Montreal, Canada

[26] Donahue J, Jia Y, Vinyals O, et al. DeCAF: a deep convolutional activation feature for generic visual recognition. Paper presented at: Proceedings of the 31st International Conference on Machine Learning; 2014; Beijing, China

[27] Bar Y, Diamant I, Wolf L, Greenspan H. Deep learning with non-medical training used for chest pathology identification. Paper presented at: SPIE Proceedings Vol 9414: Medical Imaging 2015: Computer-Aided Diagnosis; 2015

[28] Huynh BQ, Li H, Giger ML. Digital mammographic tumor classification using transfer learning from deep convolutional neural networks. J Med Imaging (Bellingham). 2016; 3(3):034501

[29] Antropova N, Huynh BQ, Giger ML. A deep feature fusion methodology for breast cancer diagnosis demonstrated on three imaging modality datasets. Med Phys. 2017; 44(10):5162–5171

[30] Kalpathy-Cramer J, Mamomov A, Zhao B, et al. Radiomics of lung nodules: a multi-institutional study of robustness and agreement of quantitative imaging features. Tomography. 2016; 2(4):430–437

[31] Clarke LP, Nordstrom RJ, Zhang H, et al. The Quantitative Imaging Network: NCI's historical perspective and planned goals. Transl Oncol. 2014; 7(1):1–4

[32] Sullivan DC, Obuchowski NA, Kessler LG, et al. RSNA-QIBA Metrology Working Group. Metrology standards for quantitative imaging biomarkers. Radiology. 2015; 277(3):813–825

[33] Mendel KR, Li H, Lan L, et al. Quantitative texture analysis: robustness of radiomics across two digital mammography manufacturers' systems. J Med Imaging (Bellingham). 2018; 5(1):011002

[34] Bhooshan N, Giger ML, Jansen SA, Li H, Lan L, Newstead GM. Cancerous breast lesions on dynamic contrast-enhanced MR images: computerized characterization for image-based prognostic markers. Radiology. 2010;254(3):680-690

[35] Kallenberg M, Petersen K, Nielsen M, et al. Unsupervised deep learning applied to breast density segmentation and mammographic risk scoring. IEEE Trans Med Imaging. 2016; 35(5):1322–1331

[36] Klifa C, Suzuki S, Aliu S, et al. Quantification of background enhancement in breast magnetic resonance imaging. J Magn Reson Imaging. 2011; 33(5):1229–1234

[37] Pike MC, Pearce CL. Mammographic density, MRI background parenchymal enhancement and breast cancer risk. Ann Oncol. 2013; 24(Suppl 8):viii37–viii41

[38] Wu S, Weinstein SP, DeLeo MJ, III, et al. Quantitative assessment of background parenchymal enhancement in breast MRI predicts response to risk-reducing salpingo-oophorectomy: preliminary evaluation in a cohort of BRCA1/2 mutation carriers. Breast Cancer Res. 2015; 17:67

[39] Jansen SA, Lin VC, Giger ML, Li H, Karczmar GS, Newstead GM. Normal parenchymal enhancement patterns in women undergoing MR screening of the breast. Eur Radiol. 2011; 21(7):1374–1382

[40] King V, Brooks JD, Bernstein JL, Reiner AS, Pike MC, Morris EA. Background parenchymal enhancement at breast MR imaging and breast cancer risk. Radiology. 2011; 260(1):50–60

[41] Li H, Giger ML, Yuan Y, et al. Computerized breast parenchymal analysis on DCE-MRI. Paper presented at: Proceedings of the SPIE, Vol 7260: Medical Imaging Conference; 2009

[42] Cancer Genome Atlas Network. Comprehensive molecular portraits of human breast tumours. Nature. 2012; 490(7418):61–70

[43] Clark K, Vendt B, Smith K, et al. The Cancer Imaging Archive (TCIA): maintaining and operating a public information repository. J Digit Imaging. 2013; 26(6):1045–1057

[44] TCGA Breast Phenotype Research Group. Available at: https://wiki.cancerimagingarchive.net/display/Public/TCGA+Breast+Phenotype+Research+Group

[45] Burnside ES, Drukker K, Li H, et al. Using computer-extracted image phenotypes from tumors on breast magnetic resonance imaging to predict breast cancer pathologic stage. Cancer. 2016; 122(5):748–757

[46] Perou CM, Sørlie T, Eisen MB, et al. Molecular portraits of human breast tumours. Nature. 2000; 406(6797):747–752

[47] Parker JS, Mullins M, Cheang MC, et al. Supervised risk predictor of breast cancer based on intrinsic subtypes. J Clin Oncol. 2009; 27(8):1160–1167

[48] Li H, Zhu Y, Burnside ES, et al. MR imaging radiomics signatures for predicting the risk of breast cancer recurrence as given by research versions of MammaPrint, Oncotype DX, and PAM50 gene assays. Radiology. 2016; 281(2):382–391

[49] Mahrooghy M, Ashraf AB, Daye D, et al. Pharmacokinetic tumor heterogeneity as a prognostic biomarker for classifying breast cancer recurrence risk. IEEE Trans Biomed Eng. 2015; 62(6):1585–1594

[50] van de Vijver MJ, He YD, van't Veer LJ, et al. A gene-expression signature as a predictor of survival in breast cancer. N Engl J Med. 2002; 347(25):1999–2009

[51] Paik S, Shak S, Tang G, et al. A multigene assay to predict recurrence of tamoxifen-treated, node-negative breast cancer. N Engl J Med. 2004; 351(27):2817–2826

[52] Cronin M, Sangli C, Liu M-L, et al. Analytical validation of the Oncotype DX genomic diagnostic test for recurrence prognosis and therapeutic response prediction in node-negative, estrogen receptor-positive breast cancer. Clin Chem. 2007; 53(6):1084–1091

[53] Prat A, Parker JS, Fan C, Perou CM. PAM50 assay and the three-gene model for identifying the major and clinically relevant molecular subtypes of breast cancer. Breast Cancer Res Treat. 2012; 135(1):301–306

[54] Santamaría G, Bargalló X, Fernández PL, Farrús B, Caparrós X, Velasco M. Neoadjuvant systemic therapy in breast cancer: association of contrast-enhanced MR imaging findings, diffusion-weighted imaging findings, and tumor subtype with tumor response. Radiology. 2017; 283(3):663–672

[55] Esserman LJ, Berry DA, Cheang MC, et al. I-SPY 1 TRIAL Investigators. Chemotherapy response and recurrence-free survival in neoadjuvant breast cancer depends on biomarker profiles: results from the I-SPY 1 TRIAL (CALGB 150007/150012; ACRIN 6657). Breast Cancer Res Treat. 2012; 132(3):1049–1062

[56] Hylton NM, Blume JD, Bernreuter WK, et al. ACRIN 6657 Trial Team and I-SPY 1 TRIAL Investigators. Locally advanced breast cancer: MR imaging for prediction of response to neoadjuvant chemotherapy–results from ACRIN 6657/I-SPY TRIAL. Radiology. 2012; 263(3):663–672

[57] Hylton NM, Gatsonis CA, Rosen MA, et al. ACRIN 6657 Trial Team and I-SPY 1 TRIAL Investigators. Neoadjuvant chemotherapy for breast cancer: functional tumor volume by mr imaging predicts recurrence-free survival-results from the ACRIN 6657/CALGB 150007 I-SPY 1 TRIAL. Radiology. 2016; 279(1):44–55

[58] Mazurowski MA, Grimm LJ, Zhang J, et al. Recurrence-free survival in breast cancer is associated with MRI tumor enhancement dynamics quantified using computer algorithms. Eur J Radiol. 2015; 84(11):2117–2122

[59] Drukker K, Li H, Antropova N, Edwards A, Papaioannou J, Giger ML. Most-enhancing tumor volume by MRI radiomics predicts recurrence-free survival "early on" in neoadjuvant treatment of breast cancer. 2018; 18(1):12

[60] Ou Y, Weinstein SP, Conant EF, et al. Deformable registration for quantifying longitudinal tumor changes during neoadjuvant chemotherapy. Magn Reson Med. 2015; 73(6):2343–2356

[61] Chen W, Giger ML, Bick U, Newstead GM. Automatic identification and classification of characteristic kinetic curves of breast lesions on DCE-MRI. Med Phys. 2006; 33(8):2878–2887

[62] Guo W, Li H, Zhu Y, et al. Tcga Breast Phenotype Research Group. Prediction of clinical phenotypes in invasive breast carcinomas from the integration of radiomics and genomics data. J Med Imaging (Bellingham). 2015; 2(4):041007

[63] Hylton N. Dynamic contrast-enhanced magnetic resonance imaging as an imaging biomarker. J Clin Oncol. 2006; 24(20):3293–3298

[64] Grimm LJ. Breast MRI radiogenomics: Current status and research implications. J Magn Reson Imaging. 2016; 43(6):1269–1278

Index